a LANGE medical book

CURRENT
Diagnosis & Treatment
Pediatric Neurology

Andrew D. Hershey, MD, PhD, FAAN, FAHS
Endowed Chair and Director of Neurology
Professor of Pediatrics and Neurology
University of Cincinnati, College of Medicine
Cincinnati Children's Hospital Medical Center
Cincinnati, Ohio

New York   Chicago   San Francisco   Athens   London   Madrid   Mexico City   Milan
New Delhi   Singapore   Sydney   Toronto

CURRENT Diagnosis & Treatment Pediatric Neurology

1 2 3 4 5 6 7 8 9 LCR 27 26 25 24 23 22

ISBN 978-1-260-45752-0
MHID 1-260-45752-4

This book was set in Minion Pro by KnowledgeWorks Global Ltd.
The editors were Leah Carton and Christina M. Thomas.
The production supervisor was Rick Ruzycka.
Project management was provided by Nitesh Sharma, KnowledgeWorks Global Ltd.

This book is printed on acid-free paper.

Library of Congress Cataloging-in-Publication Data

Names: Hershey, Andrew D., editor.
Title: Current diagnosis & treatment. Pediatric neurology / [edited by]
    Andrew D. Hershey.
Other titles: Current diagnosis and treatment. Pediatric neurology | Lange
    medical book 1549-5736
Description: New York : McGraw Hill, [2023] | Series: Lange medical book |
    Includes bibliographical references and index. | Summary: "An
    up-to-date, quick reference guide to the diagnosis and treatment of
    neurologic disorders in infants, children, and adolescents for residents
    in pediatrics, neurology, internal medicine/pediatrics, family medicine,
    and child/adolescent psychiatry, as well as pediatric nurse
    practitioners and physician assistants"—Provided by publisher.
Identifiers: LCCN 2022038303 | ISBN 9781260457520 (paperback) | ISBN
    9781260457537 (ebook)
Subjects: MESH: Nervous System Diseases—diagnosis | Nervous System
    Diseases—therapy | Infant | Child | Adolescent
Classification: LCC RJ486 | NLM WS 340.5 | DDC 618.92/8—dc23/eng/20220914
LC record available at https://lccn.loc.gov/2022038303

Contents

9. Autism Spectrum Disorder and Regressive Developmental Disorders   62

Heather M. Wied, MD, PhD
Shannon M. Standridge, DO, MPH

10. Neurocutaneous Disorders   69

David M. Ritter, MD, PhD
David N. Franz, MD
Darcy A. Krueger, MD, PhD

Section IV. Pain and Other Disorders of Somatic Sensation, HA, BA

11. A General Approach to Pediatric Pain   77

Kenneth R. Goldschneider, MD
Cheryl J. Hartzell, MD

12. Pediatric Migraine Presentation and Treatment Algorithm   82

Sharoon Qaiser, MBBS, MD
Antoinette Green, BS
Marielle Kabbouche, MD, FAAN, FAHS

13. Migraine Equivalent or Episodic Syndromes in Children 89

Sharoon Qaiser, MBBS, MD
Antoinette Green, BS
Marielle Kabbouche, MD, FAAN, FAHS

14. Primary Headache Disorders: Types and Management 92

Sharoon Qaiser, MD
Marielle Kabbouche, MD, FAAN, FAHS

15. Secondary Headaches in Children and Adolescents 106

Marielle Kabbouche, MD, FAAN, FAHS

Section VI. Major Categories of Neurologic Disease

Authors

Samuel Alperin, MD
Attending Neurologist
Division of Neurology at Children's Hospital of Philadelphia
Assistant Professor of Neurology
Perelman School of Medicine at the University of Pennsylvania
Philadelphia, Pennsylvania
Chapter 26

Todd Arthur, MD
Associate Professor of Pediatrics
Division of Neurology
Cincinnati Children's Hospital Medical Center
University of Cincinnati, College of Medicine
Cincinnati, Ohio
Chapter 37

Gewalin Aungaroon, MD
Associate Professor
Cincinnati Children's Hospital Medical Center
University of Cincinnati College of Medicine
Cincinnati, Ohio
Chapters 19 and 21

Peter de Blank, MD, MSCE
Associate Professor of Pediatrics
Division of Oncology
Cincinnati Children's Hospital Medical Center
University of Cincinnati, College of Medicine
Cincinnati, Ohio
Chapter 33

Eileen Broomall, MD
Assistant Professor of Pediatrics
Division of Neurology
Cincinnati Children's Hospital Medical Center
University of Cincinnati College of Medicine
Cincinnati, Ohio
Chapter 1

Colleen Buhrfiend, MD
Assistant Professor of Pediatrics
Department of Pediatrics
Division of Pediatric Neurology
Rush University Medical Center
Chicago, Illinois
Chapter 18

Anna Weber Byars, PhD
Professor of Pediatrics, Division of Neurology
Cincinnati Children's Hospital Medical Center
University of Cincinnati, College of Medicine
Cincinnati, Ohio
Chapter 3

Clifford S. Calley, MD
Assistant Professor of Neurology, Neurosurgery, and Pediatrics
University of Texas at Austin School of Medicine
Dell Children's Medical Center
Austin, Texas
Chapter 24

Marie Clements, MD
Resident in Neurology
Division of Neurology
Cincinnati Children's Hospital Medical Center
University of Cincinnati, College of Medicine
Cincinnati, Ohio
Chapter 19

Thomas J. Dye, MD, FAASM
Associate Professor of Pediatrics
Division of Neurology
Division of Pulmonary, Sleep Medicine
Cincinnati Children's Hospital Medical Center
University of Cincinnati, College of Medicine
Cincinnati, Ohio
Chapters 28,29

Kristen Fisher, DO
Assistant Professor
Baylor College of Medicine
Department of Pediatrics
Section of Neurology and Developmental Neuroscience
Texas Children's Hospital
Houston, Texas
Chapters 35, 36

David N. Franz, MD
Professor of Pediatrics and Neurology
Division of Neurology
Cincinnati Children's Hospital Medical Center
University of Cincinnati, College of Medicine
Cincinnati, Ohio
Chapter 10

Susan L. Fong, MD, PhD
Assistant Professor
Department of Pediatrics
Division of Neurology, Cincinnati Children's Hospital
    Medical Center
University of Cincinnati, College of Medicine
Cincinnati, Ohio
Chapter 20

Ankita Ghosh, MD
Assistant Professor of Neurology
Le Bonheur Children's Hospital
University of Tennessee Health Science Center
Memphis, Tennessee
Chapter 16

Donald L. Gilbert, MD, MS
Professor of Pediatrics, Division of Neurology
Cincinnati Children's Hospital Medical Center
University of Cincinnati, College of Medicine
Cincinnati, Ohio
Chapters 4, 5, 6

Kenneth R. Goldschneider, MD
Director, Pain Management Center
Professor, Clinical Anesthesia and Pediatrics
Cincinnati Children's Hospital Medical Center
University of Cincinnati, College of Medicine
Cincinnati, Ohio
Chapters 11, 17

Krista Grande, MD
Clinical Fellow in Epilepsy Fellowship
Division of Neurology
Cincinnati Children's Hospital Medical Center
University of Cincinnati, College of Medicine
Cincinnati, Ohio
Chapters 25, 31

Antoinette Green, BS
Department of Pediatrics
Division of Neurology
Cincinnati Children's Hospital Medical Center
University of Cincinnati, College of Medicine
Cincinnati, Ohio
Chapters 12, 13

Cheryl J. Hartzell, MD
Assistant Professor
Department of Pediatric Anesthesiology and Pain Management
Cincinnati Children's Hospital Medical Center
University of Cincinnati, College of Medicine
Cincinnati, Ohio
Chapters 11, 17

Andrew D. Hershey, MD, PhD, FAAN, FAHS
Endowed Chair and Director of Neurology
Professor of Pediatrics and Neurology
Cincinnati Children's Hospital Medical Center
University of Cincinnati, College of Medicine
Cincinnati, Ohio

Katherine Holland, MD, PhD
Professor of Pediatrics
Division of Neurology
Cincinnati Children's Hospital Medical Center
University of Cincinnati, College of Medicine
Cincinnati, Ohio
Chapters 22, 25

S. Katie Zeller Ihnen, MD, PhD
Assistant Professor of Pediatrics
Division of Neurology
Cincinnati Children's Hospital Medical Center
University of Cincinnati, College of Medicine
Cincinnati, Ohio
Chapters 1, 20, 39

Marielle Kabbouche, MD, FAAN, FAHS
Director Headache Center
Professor of Pediatrics and Neurology
Division of Neurology
Cincinnati Children's Hospital Medical Center
University of Cincinnati, College of Medicine
Cincinnati, Ohio
Chapters 12, 13, 14, 15

Joanne Kacperski, MD, FAHS
Assistant Professor of Pediatrics, Division of Neurology
Cincinnati Children's Hospital Medical Center
University of Cincinnati, College of Medicine
Cincinnati, Ohio
Chapters 16, 37

Beth Kline-Fath, MD
Professor of Radiology
Cincinnati Children's Hospital Medical Center
University of Cincinnati, College of Medicine
Cincinnati, Ohio
Chapter 30

Kelly Kremer, MD
Assistant Professor of Pediatrics and Neurology
Cincinnati Children's Hospital Medical Center
University of Cincinnati, College of Medicine
Cincinnati, Ohio
Chapter 23

Darcy A. Krueger, MD, PhD
Clack Endowed Professor in Tuberous Sclerosis
Professor of Clinical Pediatrics and Neurology
Cincinnati Children's Hospital Medical Center
University of Cincinnati, College of Medicine
Cincinnati, Ohio
Chapter 10

Wendy Lai, MD, FAAP
General Pediatrician
Pecan Tree Pediatrics
Wylie, Texas
Chapter 2

Travis R. Larsh, MD
Assistant Professor of Pediatrics
Division of Neurology
Cincinnati Children's Hospital Medical Center
University of Cincinnati, College of Medicine
Cincinnati, Ohio
Chapter 7

Karen Leonard, RN, BSN
Division of Neurology
Cincinnati Children's Hospital Medical Center
University of Cincinnati, College of Medicine
Cincinnati, Ohio
Chapter 27

Nan Lin, MD
Assistant Professor of Pediatrics, Division of Neurology
Cincinnati Children's Hospital Medical Center
University of Cincinnati, College of Medicine
Cincinnati, Ohio
Chapter 18

Ashley McGill, RN, BSN
Heart Institute
Cincinnati Children's Hospital Medical Center
University of Cincinnati, College of Medicine
Cincinnati, Ohio
Chapter 27

Paola Maria Mendoza-Sengco, MD
Assistant Professor of Clinical Pediatrics and Clinical
   Neurology and Rehabilitation Medicine
Cincinnati Children's Hospital Medical Center
University of Cincinnati, College of Medicine
Cincinnati, Ohio
Chapter 7

Usha D. Nagaraj, MD
Associate Professor of Radiology
Cincinnati Children's Hospital Medical Center
University of Cincinnati, College of Medicine
Cincinnati, Ohio
Chapter 30

Kelsey Poisson, MD
Clinical Neuroimmunology Fellow
Birmingham, Alabama
University of Alabama
Chapter 36

Sharoon Qaiser, MBBS, MD
Assistant Professor of Neurology
University of Kentucky, College of Medicine
Lexington, Kentucky
Chapters 12, 13, 14

David M. Ritter, MD, PhD
Assistant Professor of Pediatrics
Division of Neurology
Cincinnati Children's Hospital Medical Center
University of Cincinnati, College of Medicine
Cincinnati, Ohio
Chapter 10

Mark B. Schapiro, MD
Professor
Department of Pediatrics
Division of Neurology
Cincinnati Children's Hospital Medical Center
University of Cincinnati, College of Medicine
Cincinnati, Ohio
Chapter 8

Veeral Shailesh Shah, MD, PhD, FAAO, FAAP
Assistant Professor of Ophthalmology, Pediatric
   Neuro-Ophthalmology
Cincinnati Children's Hospital Medical Center
Abrahamson Pediatric Eye Institute
University of Cincinnati, College of Medicine
Cincinnati, Ohio
Chapters 41 and 42

Lori M. Singleton, MD
Associate Professor
Department of Pediatrics
Morehouse School of Medicine
Atlanta, Georgia
Chapter 2

Melissa Squires, MD, MPH
Assistant Professor of Pediatrics
Division of Neurology
Cincinnati Children's Hospital Medical Center
University of Cincinnati, College of Medicine
Cincinnati, Ohio
Chapter 26

Shannon M. Standridge, DO, MPH
Professor of Pediatrics
Division of Neurology
Cincinnati Children's Hospital Medical Center
University of Cincinnati, College of Medicine
Cincinnati, Ohio
Chapter 9

J. Michael Taylor, MD
Associate Professor of Pediatrics
Division of Neurology
Cincinnati Children's Hospital Medical Center
University of Cincinnati, College of Medicine
Cincinnati, Ohio
Chapter 32

Jeffrey R. Tenney, MD, PhD
Associate Professor of Pediatrics
Cincinnati Children's Hospital Medical Center
University of Cincinnati, College of Medicine
Cincinnati, Ohio
Chapter 24

Cameron Thomas, MD, MS
Associate Professor of Pediatrics, Division of Neurology
Cincinnati Children's Hospital Medical Center
University of Cincinnati, College of Medicine
Cincinnati, Ohio
Chapter 27

Cuixia Tian, MD
Associate Professor
Department of Pediatrics
Cincinnati Children's Hospital Medical Center
University of Cincinnati, College of Medicine
Cincinnati, Ohio
Chapters 43, 44, 45, 46, 47, 48, and 49

Marisa Vawter-Lee, MD
Associate Professor of Pediatrics
Division of Neurology
Cincinnati Children's Hospital Medical Center
University of Cincinnati, College of Medicine
Cincinnati, Ohio
Chapters 2 and 34

Charu Venkatesan, MD, PhD
Associate Professor of Pediatrics, Division of Neurology
Cincinnati Children's Hospital Medical Center
University of Cincinnati, College of Medicine
Cincinnati, Ohio
Chapters 30,31

Kris Wesselkamper, MD
Assistant Professor
Department of Pediatrics
Division of Neurology
Cincinnati Children's Hospital Medical Center
University of Cincinnati, College of Medicine
Cincinnati, Ohio
Chapters 38 and 40

Heather M. Wied, MD, PhD
Assistant Professor of Pediatrics, Division of Neurology
Cincinnati Children's Hospital Medical Center
University of Cincinnati, College of Medicine
Cincinnati, Ohio
Chapter 9, 33

Martha W. Willis, MS, RN, CPNP-AC/PC, CNS
Nurse Practitioner
Division of Cardiology
Heart Institute
Cincinnati Children's Hospital Medical Center
University of Cincinnati, College of Medicine
Cincinnati, Ohio
Chapter 27

Zachary I. Willis, MD, MPH
Assistant Professor of Pediatrics
Division of Pediatric Infectious Diseases
University of North Carolina School of Medicine
Chapel Hill, North Carolina
Chapter 34

Heather Wilson, RN, BSN
Division of Neurology
Cincinnati Children's Hospital Medical Center
University of Cincinnati, College of Medicine
Cincinnati, Ohio
Chapter 27

Amy L. Wiseman, RN, BSN
Heart Institute
Cincinnati Children's Hospital Medical Center
University of Cincinnati, College of Medicine
Cincinnati, Ohio
Chapter 27

Rochelle M. Witt, MD, PhD
Assistant Professor of Pediatrics, Division of Neurology
Cincinnati Children's Hospital Medical Center
University of Cincinnati, College of Medicine
Cincinnati, Ohio
Chapters 28, 29

Helen Wu, MD, PhD
Resident in Neurology, Division of Neurology
Cincinnati Children's Hospital Medical Center
University of Cincinnati, College of Medicine
Cincinnati, Ohio
Chapter 35

Steve W. Wu, MD
Associate Professor of Pediatrics
Division of Neurology
Cincinnati Children's Hospital Medical Center
University of Cincinnati, College of Medicine
Cincinnati, Ohio
Chapter 7

Kevin X. Zhang, MD, PhD
Resident in Ophthalmology
Department of Ophthalmology
Northwestern Medicine
Feinberg School of Medicine
Chicago, Illinois
Chapters 41, 42

Alexander M. Zygmunt, MD
Assistant Professor of Pediatrics
Division of Neurology
Cincinnati Children's Hospital Medical Center
University of Cincinnati, College of Medicine
Cincinnati, Ohio
Chapters 7, 46, 47

Preface

The first edition of *Current Diagnosis & Treatment: Pediatric Neurology* joins the LANGE SERIES to cover the field of child neurology with a practical, up-to-date approach across the wide spectrum of neurologic diseases that impact children, adolescents, and young adults and their families. Although the unique nature of neurologic illness in children and adolescents has been long recognized with many of the illnesses described centuries ago, the recognition of child neurology has come to its own more recently. This is highlighted by the Child Neurology Society celebrating its start of the next 50 years with its meeting in Cincinnati, Ohio. This book addresses many of the new advances in child neurology while remaining relevant to trainees and general practitioners to be used as a quick reference guide on treating patients who you may see every day. This easy-to-read format not only includes the basics needed to treat patients but also discusses many of the tools and some of the pathophysiology that underlies these diagnoses and tools. In doing so, this reference can fill a void and help us improve the lives of the patients and families we treat.

INTENDED AUDIENCE

Like all Lange medical books, this book provides a concise approach, while including comprehensive sources of up-to-date information. This balance between brevity and depth is expected to meet the needs of a wide variety of readers, from students with a beginning interest in neurologic disorders in this age range to subspecialists in child neurology who may want a refresher on advances in areas in which they have become less familiar. For residents in pediatrics, neurology, or child neurology, this book can serve as a frequent reference, while pointing the way to more in-depth study. For clinicians including pediatricians, family practitioners, nurses, nurse practitioners, physician assistants, and other healthcare providers, this book is designed to be used on a daily basis, addressing both frequent and rare diseases.

COVERAGE

This book includes 49 chapters and covers a wide range of topics, divided into 7 sections. This starts with a general approach that includes the neurologic evaluation, neuropsychological evaluation, and normal development. The text then dives into areas of movement disorders, developmental disorders, pain disorders with an expanded section on headaches, epilepsies, intracranial disorders of neonatal neurology, tumors and neuroimmunology diseases, traumatic injury, diseases of the senses, and a special discussion on neuro-ophthalmologic disease and neuromuscular disease. This is accomplished with brief overviews, highlighted areas of importance, and numerous figures and tables to improve the readability of the chapters.

AUTHORS

Each chapter is written by experts in their own subspecialty. All authors have an association with Cincinnati Children's Hospital Medical Center and University of Cincinnati College of Medicine. This includes faculty within both the Division of Neurology and other divisions to include their own special knowledge. Many of the residents and fellows have participated in this writing, thus assuring that the needs of all levels of readers are met. While some of these authors have moved to new careers at other institutions, the connectedness of working together on this book has helped its cohesiveness, and I am grateful to all the authors' work and diligence to help produce this very useful textbook.

Andrew D. Hershey, MD, PhD, FAAN, FAHS

Cincinnati, Ohio

Approach to the Child With a Neurologic Disease

S. Katie Zeller Ihnen, MD, PhD

Eileen Broomall, MD

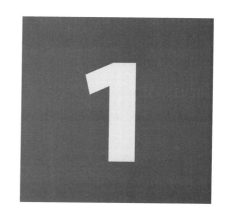

INTRODUCTION

Disorders of the central and peripheral nervous systems run the gamut from mild to severe, hyperacute to chronic, and extremely common to exceedingly rare. This large group of disorders reflects pathology that can be localized anywhere along the neuraxis, from the level of the molecule to the level of complex thalamic-subcortical-cortical circuits and at every level in between. Additionally, the nervous system can be involved in a multitude of systemic diseases across the life span. Because of this heterogeneity of pathologies and presentations, the management of neurologic problems occurs in a multitude of clinical settings, from the outpatient office to the intensive care unit. In caring for patients in these various settings, neurologists often collaborate closely with other medical specialists. Despite the increasing availability of sophisticated diagnostic tools such as genetic testing, magnetic resonance imaging (MRI), and electroencephalography (EEG), neurologists still rely substantially on a comprehensive examination to localize the lesion along the neuraxis, narrow the differential diagnosis, and guide subsequent evaluations. Child neurology is particularly unique in its use of play to obtain the best version of this examination, much to the delight of those lucky enough to practice in this field.

In the adult neurology clinic, the history and physical examination are typically conducted in a standardized manner so that nothing is missed. A similarly systematic approach is ideal but not always obtainable in pediatric patients. As the adage goes, children are not just little adults. Indeed, part of what makes child neurology both challenging and fun is that both diagnosis and treatment must account for the maturational stage of the patient, whether the relevant developmental issues are subtle or striking. Thus, the neurologic exam of a pediatric patient must often be focused or at least adapted and prioritized. Sometimes the history must be similarly abbreviated.

This book is intended to serve as a useful reference that is accessible to child neurology practitioners at multiple levels, including learners. This chapter in particular is intended to serve as a framework or foundation upon which one can build their own approach to a child with a neurologic problem. We encourage those who are new to the field to dive into an active role in the evaluation of patients as soon as possible, since the best learning comes by doing rather than observing. With the neurologic exam of an infant or child, frequent practice develops confidence, deepens our knowledge base, and (as anyone who works with children knows) keeps us humble and laughing. Although the authors of this book admit to bias, we consider child neurology to be the richest and most rewarding field of medicine, and we are thrilled to share with you some of what we have learned from our patients.

GENERAL APPROACH TO THE ENCOUNTER

The key to a successful patient encounter is rapport. Within the first minute or two of the encounter, it is crucial to establish a connection with both the patient *and* the parent(s)/caregiver(s) so that the rest of the visit can be productive. The behavior of small children and those with developmental disabilities is not necessarily governed by social norms, and their response to doctors' offices may be based on prior scary or painful interactions. Often your best clue to how to approach the patient is to listen to how they responded to the medical assistant who roomed them and/or obtained vital sign measurements. Some children require a warming-up period, and some children will be interested in interacting with you immediately. When encountering a toddler, ask the parents a question such as "How is the stranger danger in this one?"—this provides an insight into past experiences and a guide to how to move forward. This question reassures the parent that you want to make the clinic visit as pleasant as possible for their child. The presence of a sibling can be the key to a fantastic interaction—the most fun in clinic may be checking 3 siblings' patellar tendon reflexes, as everyone wants in on the fun. Guided by your own communication style and the age and disposition of the patient, make a habit of observing the patient and adjusting your visit as needed. Reassure the patient with statements such as "Most kids have fun, and nothing today will hurt."

After introductions and pleasantries, the most important question you ask should be simple: "How can I help you today?" Following this question, one should strive to provide adequate time (uninterrupted) for the patient and family to express their concern(s). Studies show that doctors tend not to give enough uninterrupted to patients to allow them to express their concerns[1], and that listening longer leads to improved patient satisfaction[2] and better compliance with treatment plans[3].

As the history taking and exam proceed from there, one must be continually considering and reconsidering multiple levels of categorization of the presenting problem, including anatomic localization, possible etiologies, and severity, all the while thinking about which additional data points will help refine the diagnostic formulation.

HISTORY

We describe key features of each section of the history.

▶ History of Present Illness

Specify from whom and which sources the history was obtained—for simplicity sake, we will say parent, but caregivers come in all forms.

While some complaints are self-evident (eg, "My child had a seizure last week"), others need more team work (eg, developmental delay or regression evaluations). Helpful questions may include "When were you first worried about your child?" and "Does your child keep up with siblings/friends when playing?" These questions allow the parent to share their knowledge and worries about the child.

Describe the chief complaint in detail and include the following key components: quality; onset (ie, chronic, recurrent, or new); if episodic in nature, frequency, duration, and most recent instance; trajectory (ie, better, worse, or same); triggers; mitigating factors; and associated symptoms.

Teenage patients should be approached with respect and included in the conversation, with sensitivity given to discrepancies in patient- and parent-provided information that often cause tension in the exam room. Teens may not be upfront with social or behavioral risk factors at the first visit, with parents present, or until subsequent visits when you have gained their trust.

▶ Videos

Easy availability of video recordings is perhaps the biggest advancement in neurologic history taking, allowing unbiased evidence of the event of concern. However, some parents may be taken aback when asked about a video, as they may view video recordings as a source of fun or entertainment and not as a source of key medical data. To ease that parental reaction, it can be helpful to frame the question as follows: "Once you were sure your child was safe, did anyone take a video to share in the future with medical providers? I know it was a scary moment, and most parents don't think to do so, but it could be helpful."

Ask if the parents have videos or if anyone else who cares for the child (eg, grandparent, teacher) might have a video. Some patients have arrived at a clinic with videos from school security cameras of events that occurred in the hallway or cafeteria. If they do not have videos, encourage caregivers to videotape events once the safety of the patient is established and parents feel control over the situation.

Patients and parents have usually been searching the Internet to find answers to their questions and concerns, and these unstated fears may overshadow the visit. We find it best to address this early—"Have you been researching this concern? What does Dr Google say?" is a lighthearted way to learn about these behaviors and presents an opportunity to offer reassurance or redirection and to congratulate patients who have diagnosed themselves correctly.

▶ Birth History

Birth history should include gestational age; maternal medications or medical issues during pregnancy; presence of any prenatal concerns such as growth restriction or anatomic abnormalities; complications during delivery, including the need for urgent delivery or resuscitation; and indication for and duration of neonatal intensive care unit/special care nursery stay, if applicable.

Particularly in infants, confirm whether newborn screening was conducted and whether there were any abnormal results. Note that what is included on the newborn screen varies by state.

▶ Developmental History

Developmental pace and attainment are adjusted to corrected gestational age for the first 3 years of life, similar to growth chart measurements for premature infants.

Comment on each major category, including gross motor, fine motor, language, and social. Various tools and charts exist to aid the clinician in this assessment, which may include parental checklists prior to visits or guided questions. This may be an intimidating area for clinicians without much experience caring for patients with developmental disabilities or physical handicaps—Where to start? How not to offend the parent? Often the simplest questions provide the best insight into understanding: "What does your child do for fun?", "How does your child tell you what they want?", and the one that is sure to provoke a smile from the parent or caregiver, "How would you describe your child's personality?"

Parental observations of muscle tone are valuable: Ask if their child is too loose or too tight, if they are strong when they are mad, or if they are difficult to carry due to being too loose. All of these are important clues.

Note whether there have been periods of stagnation or loss of previously acquired milestones and whether these occurred in the context of another illness or injury or with onset of other neurologic symptoms.

Medical History

Note prior hospitalizations, current or prior medical subspecialists, quality and duration of sleep, and presence of psychiatric comorbidities.

Surgical History

Note history of any reactions to anesthesia or bleeding problems.

Diet and Feeding History

Note dietary restrictions and food allergies.

Family History

This can be tailored to the history of present illness, but consider including epilepsy; febrile seizures; migraines; movement disorders; neuromuscular disorders; metabolic disorders; autism or neurodevelopmental disabilities; intellectual disability or problems with learning; stroke in childhood or young adulthood; early childhood deaths; and nonneurologic diseases with childhood onset, including psychiatric illnesses.

Depending on the medical literacy of the patient and family, you may have to ask a question using several different words. For example, you may ask about "epilepsy," "seizure disorders," and "convulsions."

Academic History

Note current grade level and whether this is age appropriate; current grades the child is receiving; and whether an Individualized Education Program, 504 Plan, or other learning services are in place.

Services Received

Note indication and frequency of any services such as physical therapy, occupational therapy, or speech therapy. Ask the parent or caregiver if these services seem to be beneficial to the patient.

Social History

Questions should be tailored to the patient's age and problem but typically include the following: With whom does the patient live? Who helps to care for the child? Are there cultural or religious factors that may impact care? Are there concerns about abuse or neglect?

Medications With Dosages and Frequencies

Note over-the-counter medications, supplements, and vitamins. Some caregivers need prodding to "admit" to administering certain supplements. History of previous tried medications may be informative.

Allergies

Note the presence and nature of any allergic reactions.

Immunization Status

If the patient is not up to date, ask why and demonstrate a willingness to address parental concerns and share medical knowledge in hopes of providing the best medical care to the patient.

Review of Previous Data

Ideally, obtain and review source data for relevant imaging, neurophysiology, labs, neuropsychological testing, genetic testing, and any other tests as indicated (eg, electrocardiogram if the chief complaint is paroxysmal spells).

PHYSICAL EXAMINATION

Vitals

Note heart rate, blood pressure, respiratory rate, and oxygen saturation (when relevant, typically for hospitalized patients receiving oxygen therapy).

Growth Parameters

These should include weight, height, and head circumference with age- and sex-specific percentiles as well as historical trends. You may need to obtain historical data from primary care provider.

General Exam

Ideally, the general exam should be comprehensive. However, if it must be prioritized, aspects that should not be omitted include the following: observation of facial or other dysmorphic features; skin exam to screen for clues to neurocutaneous disorders; abdominal exam to screen for organomegaly; and detailed cardiac, ophthalmologic, and other systemic exams as appropriate. See also the later section on the infant exam.

Neurologic Exam

The most important point to emphasize regarding the neurologic exam is that a significant amount of useful information can be gleaned from passive observation. This does not mean that intentional exam maneuvers are not also useful.

However, the exam begins as soon as the physician enters the room. The observation of the patient's level of activity, interaction with caregiver(s), reaction to the examiner, natural gait, and spontaneous use of objects in the room can all provide information applicable to the patient's neurologic status. One must be flexible regarding the order in which exam components are obtained to maintain the engagement of the child.

For a cooperative and ambulatory child, it is prudent to begin with a gait exam because it is high yield (requiring attention, strength, coordination, and vision), requires the patient to be awake and engaged, and is fun—most children love to show off their running and jumping skills, building comfort with the examiner from a safe distance (ie, as far away as they can run).

With younger and less cooperative patients, it may make more sense to begin with the patient in a parent's lap, where they feel safest. With the goal of minimizing stress to the patient, consider the least invasive way to obtain the needed information. For patients in the inpatient setting, it may be necessary (and, in fact, can be quite instructive) to split the exam up over a couple of sessions and/or to repeat particular exam maneuvers to assess their reliability. Never be afraid to repeat part of the exam about which you are not confident. Never be afraid to get down on your patient's level (sitting on the floor if possible), and never be afraid to have fun or be silly—parents often recount these moments as times when they knew the provider was interested in their child and when a patient-doctor relationship was established.

In the following sections, we describe key considerations for each part of the neurologic exam. Table 1–1 shows a template for a neurologic exam on a child. Table 1–2 shows a template for a neurologic exam on an infant. Table 1–3 shows a template for a neurologic exam on a comatose patient.

Mental Status

Mental status can and should always be described with some level of detail, regardless of patient age, intellectual level, or level of alertness. For patients for whom responsivity and level of engagement with exam are low, it is critical to document what specific maneuvers and stimuli were used to attempt to evoke a response. For example, in an infant with a severe brain injury and presumed hearing impairment, what stimuli were used to assess for sound localization? Loud clap? Rattle? Voice of examiner? Voice of parent?

Cranial Nerves

All cranial nerves except for cranial nerve I (olfactory nerve) are typically assessed. Even before children are able to follow commands (eg, "Puff out your cheeks"), they can demonstrate a wide range of facial expressions and mimic the facial expression of adults.

Motor

The 3 components of the motor exam are bulk, tone, and power.

Table 1–1. Neurologic exam in a noninfant child.

Mental status	Awake, responsive, attentive, and cooperative with exam
	Answered questions in an age-appropriate manner
	Makes appropriate eye contact
	Affect euthymic
Cranial nerves	
II	Visual fields full to finger counting
	Discs sharp bilaterally, with normal appearance of retinal vessels
III, IV, VI	Pupils equal, round, and reactive to light and near fixation
	Conjugate gaze in neutral position
	Extraocular movements full and symmetric in all directions
	No ptosis
V	Normal facial sensation bilaterally
	Strong mastication
VII	Full and symmetric facial movements
VIII	Hearing intact to finger rub and conversation
	No nystagmus
IX, X, XI	Midline cervical position without torticollis
	Normal phonation
	Palate elevates midline
XII	Tongue extrudes midline
Motor	Normal and symmetric muscle tone and bulk
	Strength at least 4+ in all 4 extremities, limited only by ability to cooperate with testing
	No pronator drift
	Normal finger tapping bilaterally
	No adventitial movements
Sensory	Vibratory sensation intact and symmetric in all 4 extremities
	Rough/smooth discrimination intact and symmetric in all 4 extremities
Coordination	No dysmetria or ataxia on spontaneous truncal or appendicular movements
	Age-appropriate performance on finger-nose-finger and heel-to-shin
	Negative Romberg
Deep tendon reflexes	2+ and symmetric in bilateral biceps, triceps, brachioradialis, patellas, and Achilles
	No ankle clonus
	Toes downgoing bilaterally
Gait	Stance and swing appropriate for age
	Heel-walks, toe-walks, and tandem walks at least 10 steps without difficulty
	Able to stand on 1 foot/hop

Table 1–2. Neurologic exam in an infant.

Mental status	Awake and responsive to exam
	Exhibited state change, without excessive irritability; consolable
	Cry normal, neither weak nor high-pitched
Cranial nerves	
II, III	Dazzle reflex present
II, III	Pupils equal, round, and reactive to light
III, IV, VI, VIII	Conjugate gaze in neutral position
	Extraocular movements full and conjugate in all directions
	No transient or persistent roving eye movements
	No ptosis
	Doll's eye maneuver elicits contralateral eye deviation
V	Reacts to light facial touch bilaterally
	Strong suck
VII	Full and symmetric facial movements
VIII	Startles to clap
	No transient or persistent nystagmus
IX, X	Gag reflex present
XI	Midline cervical position without torticollis
XII	Tongue extrudes midline
Motor	Normal and symmetric muscle tone: mainly flexion at rest; negative scarf sign; no slip through on vertical suspension; appropriate extension on ventral suspension; no pronounced head lag
	Normal and symmetric muscle bulk
	Moves all 4 extremities equally, asynchronously, at least antigravity, and with normal frequency
	No jitteriness
	Keeps hands mainly but not exclusively fisted
	No adventitial movements
Sensory	Reacts equally to light touch in all 4 extremities
Deep tendon reflexes	2+ and symmetric in bilateral biceps, patellas, and Achilles
	No ankle clonus
Primitive reflexes	Suck strong and sustained
	Rooting reflex present
	Moro full and symmetric
	Palmar grasp present bilaterally (expected starting at 27 weeks)
	Plantar grasp present bilaterally (expected starting at 26 weeks)
	Placing reflex present bilaterally

Table 1–3. Neurologic exam in a comatose pediatric patient.

Mental status	State in patient room (intubated/supine/eyes open or closed, spontaneous movement, or other activity)
	Response to greeting, verbal commands, tactile stimulation (eg, removing blankets)
	Reactivity to examination in terms of any discernible autonomic changes
Cranial nerves	
II, VII	Blink to threat
II, III	Pupils __ mm, equal, round, reactivity to light; pupillometry used
	Eyes conjugate/dysconjugate and in primary gaze
III, IV, VI, VIII	Fixing or following, even with eyes held open
	Doll's eye maneuver (oculocephalic) reflex present or absent (ie, eyes move in same direction as forced head deviation)
	Cold calorics (oculovestibular reflex) present or absent (irrigate external auditory meatus with 50 mL cold water; normally, eyes should deviate conjugately toward irrigated ear, with nystagmus with rapid phase away from irrigated ear)
V, VII	Corneal reflex to saline drop bilaterally
	Reaction to noxious stimulation of Q-tip to nares bilaterally
	Reaction to noxious pressure on supraorbital ridge bilaterally
VII	Facial symmetry, if possible assessed when supine and more upright
	Spontaneous or reactive facial movements
IX	Response to cotton swab stimulation of the posterior pharynx
X	Response to stimulation of the trachea using suction per endotracheal tube
Motor	Normal and symmetric muscle tone and bulk
	Spontaneous movements of any extremity
	Reactive movements to noxious stimuli, either central (sternal rub, axillary pinch, thigh pinch) or peripheral (deep nailbed pressure), as per the above
Sensory	Response to noxious stimuli, either central (sternal rub, axillary pinch, thigh pinch) or peripheral (deep nailbed pressure), as per the above
Coordination	Resting or provoked tremor
	Bilateral biceps, brachioradialis, triceps, patellas, and Achilles
	Abdominal reflex
Deep tendon reflexes	Assess for reflexes, ankle clonus, and plantar response
Gait/station	Gait obviously cannot be assessed, but for station, consider patient positioning in bed and need for restraints

Muscle tone is best assessed with the patient in a calm, quiet state, although it is extremely informative if the child is still hypotonic even when crying or angry.

Power can be assessed at the level of individual muscles; however, it is more practical and appropriate in most patients to test instead at the level of flexion and extension of various compartments (eg, flexion of the ankle).

For power, be sure to test each side separately (except for the trapezius, so as to avoid causing the patient to fall over). For direct comparison, alternate between left and right sides for each maneuver.

Some very slight asymmetry in power can be normal and accounted for by the patient's dominant side.

For power, the Medical Research Council scale includes scores of 0 through 5.[3] A rating of 4 can be further specified by a + or − to indicate a gradation of power within that category of movement against resistance without full strength. See Table 1–4.

Sensory

You can use a tongue blade or cotton swab (one end broken to create a rough edge and one end intact to provide a smooth edge), a tuning fork (cold or buzzy), or a patient's own toys (eg, soft, squishy).

Deep Tendon Reflexes

Scoring is conventionally 0, +, ++, +++, or ++++, although the notation of 0, 1+, 2+, 3+, and 4+ is commonly seen. Note that notation does not include numerals without a plus sign.

Distraction maneuvers can help elicit deep tendon reflexes (DTRs) when they are difficult to obtain. These include engaging the patient in conversation or asking the patient to clasp their hands together at the time the tendon is tapped.

Gait and Stance

Observation of gait along a hallway or larger space is recommended. Children are often happy to demonstrate running, skipping or galloping skills, which provides further information into balance, coordination and strength. Tandem gait should be assessed for a minimum of 10 steps. This can usually be done fairly well by age 6 to 7 years. Younger patients may instead be able to demonstrate standing or hopping on one foot.

▶ Exam Considerations for Infants

It is imperative to document occipitofrontal circumference with percentile and trend, if available.

The general exam should include observations regarding skull shape and patency of fontanelles; red reflex; organomegaly; and any tufts, pits, or hair along the midline of the back.

Several parts of the neurologic exam will be different, as noted in Table 2–1, including testing of primitive reflexes as appropriate.

If a Dubowitz neurological exam was done (applies to neonates), include the score for each of six categories (tone, tone pattern, reflexes, movement, abnormal signs, orientation, and behavior)[4].

▶ Exam Considerations for Comatose Patients

For the documentation of the exam of a comatose patient, one must comment on any sedating medications the patient has received and the dates and times of most recent doses. The examiner should pay particular attention to signs of contracture, atrophy, foot deformity, etc, which may provide additional clues to the patient's baseline neurologic functioning.

▶ Exam Considerations for Telemedicine

Since the start of the COVID-19 pandemic, child neurologists, like other physicians and care providers, have adapted creatively to the use of telemedicine for some patients in some scenarios. The use of telemedicine will likely continue in some capacity after the pandemic ends. Telemedicine offers both advantages and disadvantages as compared to in-person evaluations. In particular, for established patients in whom the general and neurologic exams have been stable, telemedicine appointments have provided an unexpected convenience. In contrast, for new patients, a telemedicine visit does not allow for a full examination. For both new visits and follow-up visits, it is of utmost importance that patients and their parents are in safe, quiet environments with sufficient space to demonstrate any necessary maneuver. Absolute contraindications to televisits include participants situated in moving vehicles or crowded public environments.

History taking can proceed as it does for in-person visits. Examination, both general and neurologic, obviously must be adapted. However, an astute neurologist can obtain a significant amount of information via a telemedicine encounter. Patients can demonstrate motor skills such as skipping, walking, or jumping jacks; lifting common household objects such as a jug of milk or juice can demonstrate strength; and most patients have sufficient toys to be able to demonstrate

Table 1–4. Medical Research Council rating scale for muscle power.

Observed Muscle Function	Rating
No movement, no twitch	0
Trace movement only	1
Movement in the plane of gravity, but not against	2
Movement against gravity, but not against resistance	3
Movement against some resistance, but not full	4 (or 4+ or 4−)
Full strength against full resistance	5

stacking, reaching, and pointing. One important point is that the examiner can observe the patient in their home setting, which can help contextualize the problem.

Suggested Tools

Suggested tools include the following: stethoscope, reflex hammer (heavier weight reflex hammers such as Queen Square or Troemner hammer are typical favorites), tuning forks (512 Hz is ideal for testing hearing, 128 Hz is ideal for assessing vibratory sensation), penlight, ophthalmoscope (either standard or panoptic), and bedside vision card (eg, Snellen or Rosenbaum).

Additional tools to make the exam more enjoyable and more productive include the following: finger puppets, small blocks, small toys in a small container whose lid can be unscrewed, matchbox car, miniature animals, rattles, or light-up toys. Toys that can be easily washed, are not easily swallowed or broken, and do no hurt when flung at the examiner are particularly advised. See Figure 1–1.

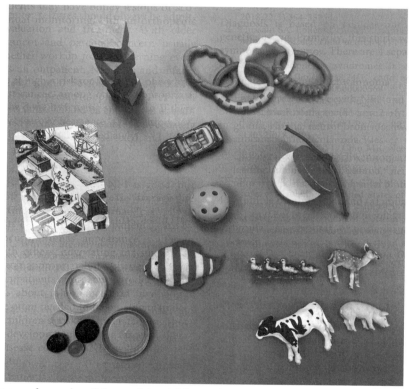

▲ **Figure 1–1.** Toys are a fun and useful part of the child neurologist's toolkit. Shown in this image are examples of toys that can help obtain an informative exam. The matchbox car and small orange ball allow for easy engagement in mutual play, which is helpful for assessing social skills and for building rapport. Several items are helpful for assessing coordination and fine motor dexterity at various developmental stages, including the teething rings (for infants) and plain stacking blocks (for toddlers on up). There is also a set of pebbles shown with a small container with a twist-on lid. In addition to helping assess coordination and fine motor skills, the pebble set can be used to test color knowledge and counting ability, when appropriate. All of these objects can be used to verify handedness, for example, by repeatedly placing at midline and observing for which hand reaches first and by directly comparing the dexterity with which each hand is used to manipulate the object. The red and yellow castanets are a fun and functional way to assess hearing and sound localization. The animal figurines (deer, pig, cow, and ducks) can be used to assess expressive and receptive language in a small child, with some children able to demonstrate animal sounds before they can produce the animal names. The picture card on the far left can be used to assess linguistic skills in a more sophisticated fashion in an older child. The red and white striped fish finger puppet is used by the examiner to assess extraocular movements. Note that the objects that the patient manipulates can be cleaned after each use.

SYNTHESIS AND DIAGNOSTIC FORMULATION

Differential diagnoses for various problems are discussed in detail in the content-based chapters. One general rubric for synthesizing information to formulate a differential diagnosis is to use some preferred mnemonic device to remember categories of etiologies. For example, some people use the mnemonic VITAMINS, where V stands for vascular, I stands for infectious (or inflammatory), T stands for traumatic (or toxic), A stands for autoimmune, M stands for metabolic, I stands for iatrogenic (or idiopathic), N stands for neoplastic, and S stands for social. Other mnemonics exist.

It is also helpful to keep in the differential both the most dangerous and the most common diagnoses, until they have been clearly ruled out. Parents are often fearful that they caused this medical problem in their child—reassurance should be provided unbidden and repeated as needed.

From among the differential diagnoses, one working diagnosis should be chosen. Even if this diagnosis is uncertain, it should be shared, provisionally, with the patient, family, and consulting physician (if applicable). The next step is to gather additional data that will either refute or support the working diagnosis.

ORDERING OBJECTIVE DATA: LABORATORY, RADIOLOGIC, NEUROPHYSIOLOGIC, AND OTHER TESTING

Commonly ordered diagnostic studies for child neurology patients include the following: laboratory studies (including serum and/or cerebrospinal fluid); brain and/or spinal cord imaging (most often MRI but sometimes ultrasound or other imaging modalities); EEG, either routine or prolonged; electromyogram; and nerve conduction study. Specific guidance for ordering tests can be found in the content-based chapters.

TREATMENT

It is important to confirm that the patient and parent(s)/caregiver(s) understand the treatment plan, including potential side effects of prescribed medications.

It is important to remember that evaluations and treatments of pediatric patients occur within a family, a larger social group, and school. Parents often have fears of worsening a medical condition. It is important to empower parents to continue parenting their child in a developmentally appropriate way. Common struggles for children with neurologic impairment include discipline, limit setting, bedtime rules, chores, school attendance, and homework. These issues need to be addressed at the initial visit and at each follow-up.

FOLLOW-UP PLAN AND REFERRALS

Medicine is a team sport. In addition to making use of auxiliary services within one's own division/department (including medical assistants, nurses, social workers, dieticians, and care coordinators), one should think, at the first encounter, about which other disciplines might be able to assist in the evaluation of the patient. In child neurology, these often include genetics, psychiatry, ophthalmology, physical medicine and rehabilitation, and developmental and behavioral pediatrics.

Include anticipatory guidance, with guidelines for what would warrant a phone call prior to the next visit. Choose a follow-up interval that is appropriate to the working diagnosis. Err on the side of setting a shorter follow-up interval for new diagnoses or when therapies are initiated or increased.

RESOURCES FOR FURTHER LEARNING

There is a series of helpful videos from the University of Utah that show how to conduct various parts of the child neurology exam at various ages; see https://neurologicexam.med.utah.edu/pediatric/html/home_exam.html.

The Internet is the most powerful tool for spreading information and disinformation; tread lightly and critically appraise the source of any information. The websites of children's hospitals, residency programs, national medical associations, and disease-specific support groups are usually verified sources of information; information on social media sites may be informative but should undergo additional scrutiny.

REFERENCES

1. Singh ON, Phillips KA, Rodriguez-Gutierrez R, et al. "Eliciting the patient's agenda-secondary analysis of recorded clinical encounters." *Journal of general internal medicine.* 2019;34(1):36–40.
2. Jagosh J, Boudreau JD, Steinert Y, et al. The importance of physician listening from the patients' perspective: Enhancing diagnosis, healing, and the doctor–patient relationship. *Patient education and counseling.* 2011;85(3):369–374.
3. Ogden J, Bavalia K, Bull M, et al. "I want more time with my doctor": a quantitative study of time and the consultation. *Family practice.* 2004;21(5):479–483.
4. Medical Research Council. Aids to examination of the peripheral nervous system. Memorandum no. 45. London: Her Majesty's Stationary Office; 1976.
5. Dubowitz LM, Dubowitz V, Palmer P, et al. A new approach to the neurological assessment of the preterm and full-term newborn infant. *Brain and Development.* 1980;2(1):3–14.
6. Dubowitz Lilly, Daniela Ricciw, and Eugenio Mercuri. The Dubowitz neurological examination of the full-term newborn. *Mental retardation and developmental disabilities research reviews.* 2005;11(1):52–60.

Development in the Normal Infant and Child

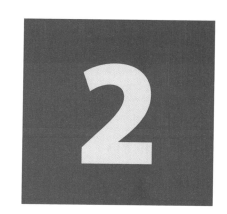

Marissa Vawter-Lee, MD

Wendy Lai, MD

Lori M. Singleton, MD

INTRODUCTION

Achieving developmental milestones on time is a cornerstone of healthy, normal development. As physicians, we expect children to achieve certain milestones by specific times. These milestones include gross motor and fine motor skills, expressive and receptive language, vision, hearing, and cognitive and social skills. Although it may seem clear-cut by which age a child should be able to perform each skill, there is some flexibility. It is important to keep in mind whether a skill should be achieved by 50% of kids by a certain age or by 90% of kids at a certain age. In this chapter, we discuss skills in terms of when 75% to 90% of typical children of that age should have achieved the skill.[1-8]

When tracking development, providers should correct the age to account for premature birth (birth prior to 37 weeks' gestational age) until a child is 2 years old.[9,10]

DEVELOPMENTAL MILESTONES

▶ Newborn

Gross Motor: The Moro startle, where a baby's head falls backward and they reflexively extend the arms and legs outward and then rapidly bring arms to midline, lasts until 2 to 3 months old. The plantar grasp reflex, where the infant's toes curl downward when you touch the sole of the foot behind the toes, is present from birth until 6 months old. The fencing reflex (also called asymmetrical tonic neck reflex) lasts until 5 to 7 months old; in this reflex, when a baby's head is turned to one side, the baby will reflexively straighten the arm on that side and flex their opposite arm. The Babinski reflex, where stroking the sole of the foot triggers the big toe to extend upward and other toes to fan outward, is present and can persist until 9 to 12 months old. In the stepping reflex, when a baby is held upright with soles touching the floor, they reflexively step one leg forward; this reflex is present from birth until 2 months old.

Fine Motor: The newborn grasp reflex (also called palmar grasp), where stroking the palm of the baby's hand triggers the baby to grip the finger, is present and lasts until 5 to 6 months old. Newborns preferentially hold hands fisted much of the time.

Language/Oral Skills: A newborn baby cries when there is discomfort. When an object touches the roof of their mouth, the sucking reflex triggers the baby to suck. Until 4 months old, when a baby's cheek or mouth is stroked on one side, they will turn their head to that side due to the rooting reflex.

Social: A newborn baby maintains brief periods of wakefulness.

Vision: A newborn can see 8 to 10 inches away from their face and is very sensitive to bright lights. Their vision is only in black, white, and gray.

▶ 1 Month Old

Gross Motor: Infants start to lift their heads up. Moro, fencing, Babinski, and stepping reflexes all persist.

Fine Motor: Grasping reflexes continue. Infants hold hands more open when at rest.

Language: Infants cry when uncomfortable but will respond to calming. They are alert to sounds.

Social: Infants have increased periods of wakefulness. Some infants have colic.

Vision: Infants start to visually fixate.

▶ 2 Months Old

Gross Motor: Infants lift their head with some control, usually to 45 degrees. Moro, fencing, Babinski, and stepping reflexes all persist.

Fine Motor: Grasping reflexes continue.

Language: Infants start to coo vowel sounds. They will turn toward noises.

Social: Infants look at their parents' faces and start to smile. They can indicate if they are happy or sad by their sounds.

Vision: Infants start to visually track objects and lights.

4 Months Old

Gross Motor: Infants hold their head with complete control, and in prone position, they push their chest off the ground. Some infants can roll over stomach to back.

Fine Motor: Infants can grasp a rattle. They will bring hands together to midline and will bring hands to their mouth. They begin to reach for toys with one hand with a palmar grasp.

Language: Cooing continues, and infants start to laugh and squeal.

Social: Infants continue to smile and enjoy looking around.

Vision: Infants can visually track objects. They are starting to develop color vision, and in the next month, they will have full color vision and develop depth perception.

6 Months Old

Gross Motor: Infants roll both stomach to back and back to stomach. Infants can briefly sit upright unsupported. When stood up and supported, they start to bounce and will support some weight.

Fine Motor: Infants transfer objects between their hands and start to pick up finger foods. They start to reach with a raking grasp (using fingers to hold the object).

Language: Infants begin to babble consonant sounds (eg, ga, ma, ba). They turn toward noises and voices. Many infants start to squeal and blow bubbles and raspberries.

Social: Infants recognize faces and can recognize strong emotions in others. They turn when their name is called.

Vision: Infants can see and recognize an object from across a room or through a window.

9 Months Old

Gross Motor: Infants can independently get into a sitting position. They should be able to stand holding onto something. They are starting to crawl. The infant will be able to pull to stand over the next month.

Fine Motor: By 9 months old, infants use their thumbs to grasp objects. They can handle finger foods well and can bang 2 cubes together.

Language: Infants' babbling should imitate speech and combine syllables. Infants should say "mamama" and "dadada" (or a similar term) nonspecifically. They consistently turn when their name is called.

Social and Cognitive Skills: Infants recognize family members versus strangers and may have stranger/separation anxiety. They lift their arms when they want to be picked up.

12 Months Old

Gross Motor: The child should be crawling and cruising and able to stand for at least 2 seconds.

Fine Motor: By 12 months, the child should have a mature pincer grasp (between finger and thumb) and they can drop a toy (such as a block) into a cup/container.

Language: A 1-year-old should say "mama," "dada," or similar terms specifically. They should be shaking their head no and waving bye. They understand "no."

Social and Cognitive Skills: The child should be able to play gesture games such as peek-a-boo or pat-a-cake. The child will look for hidden objects. When frustrated, aggressive behavior can emerge.

15 Months Old

Gross Motor: By 15 months old, children are able to stand alone and walk well without assistance. They can crawl up steps.

Fine Motor: The child should be able to stack blocks 2 high. The child may start to imitate parent's scribbling and can make marks with a crayon. They will indicate what they want nonverbally by pointing to things.

Language: Children at this age can say 1 to 3 words in addition to "mama" and "dada."

Social and Cognitive Skills: Children should be able to imitate things the family does and play with a ball. They should be able to follow a simple command. They will clap their hands when excited, and start to hug stuffed animals and toys.

18 Months Old

Gross Motor: By 18 months old, children are able to walk backward, and most children can run across a room with fair stability.

Fine Motor: By 18 months old, children are scribbling, can dump small items out of a bowl when demonstrated to them, and will turn book pages (though not always one page at a time).

Language: By 18 months old, most children will know 5 to 6 words. They should be able to follow 1-step commands.

Social and Cognitive Skills: By 18 months old, children can drink from an open cup, and most will use a spoon or fork. They are also interested in helping their parents (eg, they imitate sweeping). Temper tantrums emerge.

24 Months Old

Gross Motor: By 24 months old, children can walk up and down stairs with support. All children with normal development can run and kick a ball. Some are able to jump with both feet off the ground and are starting to climb playground ladders.

Fine Motor: By 24 months old, children can stack cubes 4 high and can turn book pages one at a time. They can copy or imitate a line drawn by others.

Language: By 24 months old, most children will know 25–50 words, and they should be able to put 2 or more words together. They should be able to point to 2 pictures in a book. They should be appropriately using "me" or "mine" and starting to use pronouns. They are starting to use words to ask for help.

Social and Cognitive Skills: By 24 months, most children will take off some of their clothes (eg, socks or shoes) and are starting to do imitation play (eg, feeding a doll) and parallel play. They should know 2 body parts. Some children are ready to start potty training; others will not be ready for several more months or years.

30 Months Old

Gross Motor: By 30 months old, a child can throw a ball overhand. All children with normal development can jump with both feet off the ground by 30 months old.

Fine Motor: By 30 months old, a child can stack cubes 6 high. They can scribble and draw a random line.

Language: Children with normal development will have at least 50 words by 30 months old. By 30 months old, a child's speech is 50% understandable. They can point at 4 pictures in a book and name 1 picture. They will say "Look at me" to get your attention and know their own first name. They should be able to follow 2-step commands.

Social and Cognitive Skills: By 30 months old, children are starting to wash and dry their hands, will help put their clothes on, and try to brush their own teeth. Most children know 6 body parts and one color.

3 Years Old

Gross Motor: Children can balance on 1 foot for 1 second and can jump forward. They can alternate feet when going upstairs and pedal a tricycle. They are proficient at climbing.

Fine Motor: Children can copy a circle and stack blocks 8 high. They are starting to button their clothing.

Most children have clear handedness. They can feed themselves independently.

Language: Children know more than 250 words, use plurals, and can say 3-word sentences. Children start to recognize single letters.[11] Speech is 75% understandable.

Social and Cognitive Skills: Children can independently wash and dry their hands. They start to ask "why" and "how" questions and can appropriately answer simple questions when prompted, such as "Where do you sleep at?" Most will be able to compare objects as bigger or smaller or taller or shorter. They can name a friend. They start to share toys, take turns, and play well with others. They can tell you their name, age, and gender. Most can put on a t-shirt. Nightmares and night terrors may occur.

Vision: Vision is nearing 20/20 acuity at 3 to 4 years old.

4 Years Old

Gross Motor: Children can balance on 1 foot for 2 seconds. They start to hop and alternate feet when going downstairs.

Fine Motor: By 4.5 years old, they can copy a plus sign and can draw a person with 3 body parts. They can catch a ball and use scissors.

Language: Four-year-olds start to use appropriate plural words and use sentences with more than 4 words. They will tell you stories based on shows or books. Speech is completely understandable. They can count 1 block.

Social and Cognitive Skills: Children can dress themselves on their own. They can sing a song from memory. By 4 years old, they can name 4 colors and correctly use "yesterday" and "tomorrow." They play well with a group of children. Fifty percent of children are potty trained overnight.

5 Years Old

Gross Motor: At age 5, children can balance on 1 foot for 3 to 4 seconds. Children start to skip and jump over small obstacles.

Fine Motor: Children can copy a square. By 5.5 years old, most can copy a triangle and can draw a person with 6 to 10 body parts. Most children can print their first name. The pictures they draw are recognizable, and most will stay in lines while coloring (especially by 5.5 years old).

Language: They can count 5 blocks. By 5.5 years old, they know 2 opposites. They can identify more than half of letters and can identify most numbers from 1 to 10. They use and recognize simple rhymes.

Social and Cognitive Skills: Children can correctly pick which line is the longest. They can play and follow rules in board games. They can make a bowl of cereal and brush their teeth independently. Seventy-five percent of children are potty trained overnight. They can tell you their first and last name.

▶ 6 Years Old

Gross Motor: They can balance on 1 foot for 6 seconds and walk with a heel-to-toe strike. Most children can ride a bicycle.

Fine Motor: Some children can copy a diamond (most not until 6.5 years old). Children can draw a person with 10 to 14 body parts.

Language: They can identify all letters of the alphabet.

Social and Cognitive Skills: Children can name the days of the week in the correct order. They can tell their right and left sides apart. They can explain how to use objects.

DEVELOPMENTAL SCREENING TESTS

Developmental surveillance should be done during each patient encounter, and screening is recommended by the American Academy of Pediatrics to be done by primary care doctors at the 9-, 18-, and 24- or 30-month-old well-child checks.[12] Unfortunately, there is not a standard approach to developmental assessment. The appropriate tool will depend on the child's age and the encounter type.

The Denver II Developmental Screening Test screens children 0 to 6 years old in the areas of gross motor, language, fine motor, and personal-social skills.[1] The Capute Scales consist of the Cognitive Adaptive Test (CAT) and Clinical Linguistic and Auditory Milestone Scale (CLAMS) and screen for delays in children 1 to 3 years old.[13,14] Both the Denver II and Capute Scales were developed from large studies with diverse populations. They require administration by a clinician and can take 10 to 20 minutes to complete, with Denver II being the shorter screening method.

The Ages and Stages Questionnaire (ASQ) and Parents' Evaluation of Development Status (PEDS) are developmental tools that have the benefit of being administered by the parents.[15,16] The ASQ takes approximately 10 to 15 minutes to complete and assesses the child's social-emotional development in addition to motor and language skills. The PEDS takes only 2 to 10 minutes to complete but does not assess social-emotional development. The ASQ is based on observations, while the PEDS tools is based on the assumption that parents know their child best and will naturally compare their child to others of similar age.

Although it has fallen out of favor, the Goodenough-Harris Draw-a-Person or Draw-a-Person Intellectual Ability tests can quickly be done in the clinic setting and provide a fun way for a child to demonstrate their fine motor and cognitive skills.[17,18] It should be noted that these drawing tests are no longer considered a valid way to precisely measure a child's intelligence quotient (IQ).

The Modified Checklist for Autism in Toddlers (mCHAT) is an excellent screening tool for families with concerns that a child may have autism.[19]

DEFINITION OF DEVELOPMENTAL DELAY

If children do not reach developmental milestones on time, physicians should closely monitor the development in the delayed areas and refer early for appropriate developmental therapies. A delay isolated to one area is defined as a specific delay, such as a gross motor delay or speech delay. The American Academy of Neurology and Child Neurology Society define global developmental delay as performing "more than 2 standard deviations below age-matched peers in 2 or more aspects of development."[20]

When children are older than age 6 years, it is preferred to start calling delays impairments, such as a gross motor impairment. Intellectual disability is defined as "significant limitations in both intellectual functioning and in adaptive behavior" as expressed in conceptual, social, and practical skills.[21] Intellectual disability is present before 18 years of age and is typically defined as an IQ score of less than 70.[21]

REFERENCES

1. Frankenburg WK, Dodds J, Archer P, Shapiro H, Bresnick B. The Denver II: a major revision and restandardization of the Denver Developmental Screening Test. *Pediatrics.* 1992; 89(1):91-97.
2. Sheldrick RC, Perrin EC. Evidence-based milestones for surveillance of cognitive, language, and motor development. *Acad Pediatr.* 2013;13(6):577-586. doi:10.1016/j.acap.2013 .07.001
3. Guddemi M, Sambrook A, Wells S, et al. Arnold Gesell's developmental assessment revalidation substantiates child-oriented curriculum. *SAGE OPEN.* 2014;April-June:1-18.
4. American Optometric Associaton. Infant vision: birth to 24 months of age. Accessed December 16, 2020. https://www .aoa.org/healthy-eyes/eye-health-for-life/infant-vision?sso=y
5. Boyd K, Lipsky S. Vision development: newborn to 12 months. American Academy of Ophthalmology. Accessed December 16, 2020. https://www.aao.org/eye-health/tips-prevention/baby-vision-development-first-year
6. Centers for Disease Control and Prevention. CDC milestone moments. Accessed January 27, 2021. https://www.cdc.gov/ ncbddd/actearly/pdf/parents_pdfs/milestonemomentseng508 .pdf
7. Hagan JF, Shaw JS, Duncan PM. *Bright Futures: Guidelines for Health Supervision of Infants, Children, and Adolescents* [pocket guide]. American Academy of Pediatrics. Accessed January 27, 2021. https://brightfutures.aap.org/Bright%20Futures%20 Documents/BF4_POCKETGUIDE.pdf
8. Zubler JM, Wiggins LD, Macias MM, et al. Evidence-informed milestones for developmental surveillance tools. *Pediatrics.* 2022;149(3).
9. Bernbaum JC, Campbell DE, Imaizumi SO. *American Academy of Pediatrics Textbook of Pediatric Care.* American Academy of Pediatrics; 2009.
10. D'Augostino JA. An evidentiary review regarding the use of chronological and adjusted age in the assessment of preterm infants. *J Spec Pediatr Nurs.* 2010;15(1):26-32.
11. Reach Out and Read. Milestones of early literacy. Accessed October 29, 2020. https://www.reachoutandread.org/what-we-do/resources-2/

12. Council on Children With Disabilities; Section on Developmental Behavioral Pediatrics; Bright Futures Steering Committee; Medical Home Initiatives for Children With Special Needs Project Advisory Committee. Identifying infants and young children with developmental disorders in the medical home: an algorithm for developmental surveillance and screening. *Pediatrics*. 2006;118(1):405-420. doi:10.1542/peds.2006-1231

13. Capute AJ, Palmer FB, Shapiro BK, Wachtel RC, Schmidt S, Ross A. Clinical linguistic and auditory milestone scale: prediction of cognition in infancy. *Dev Med Child Neurol*. 1986;28(6):762-771. doi:10.1111/j.1469-8749.1986.tb03930.x

14. Wachtel RC, Shapiro BK, Palmer FB, Allen MC, Capute AJ. CAT/CLAMS. A tool for the pediatric evaluation of infants and young children with developmental delay. Clinical Adaptive Test/Clinical Linguistic and Auditory Milestone Scale. *Clin Pediatr (Phila)*. 1994;33(7):410-415. doi:10.1177/000992289403300706

15. Squires J, Bricker D. *Ages & Stages Questionnaires®, Third Edition (ASQ®-3): A Parent-Completed Child Monitoring System*. Paul H. Brookes Publishing Co., Inc; 2009.

16. Glascoe F. *Collaborating With Parents: Using Parents' Evaluation of Developmental Status to Detect and Address Developmental and Behavioral Problems*. Ellsworth & Vandermeer Press; 1998.

17. Harris D. *Children's Drawings as Measures of Intellectual Maturity: A Revision and Extension of the Goodenough Draw-a-Man Test*. Harcourt, Brace & World; 1963.

18. Reynolds CR, Hickman JA. *Draw-a-Person Intellectual Ability Test for Children, Adolescents, and Adults Examiner's Manual*. Pro-Ed; 2004.

19. Robins DL, Fein D, Barton ML, Green JA. The Modified Checklist for Autism in Toddlers: an initial study investigating the early detection of autism and pervasive developmental disorders. *J Autism Dev Disord*. 2001;31(2):131-144. doi:10.1023/a:1010738829569

20. Michelson DJ, Shevell MI, Sherr EH, Moeschler JB, Gropman AL, Ashwal S. Evidence report: Genetic and metabolic testing on children with global developmental delay: report of the Quality Standards Subcommittee of the American Academy of Neurology and the Practice Committee of the Child Neurology Society. *Neurology*. 2011;77(17):1629-1635. doi:10.1212/WNL.0b013e3182345896

21. Schalock RL, Borthwick-Duffy SA, Bradley VJ, et al. *Intellectual Disability: Definition, Classification, and Systems of Supports*. 11th ed. American Association on Intellectual and Developmental Disabilities; 2010.

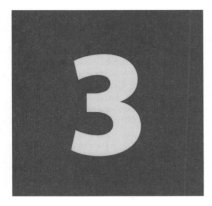

Neuropsychological Evaluation of Children and Adolescents

Anna W. Byars, PhD

Neuropsychological evaluation makes use of a set of clinical procedures that consists of standardized, evidence-based methods of assessment aimed at determining the integrity of brain-behavior relationships. It involves the individual administration of behavioral tests by a clinical neuropsychologist or by a trained technician (psychometrist) working with the neuropsychologist, with the goal of documenting the relationship between brain and behavior. It is useful in measuring many categories of cognitive functioning, including the following:

- Intellectual functioning
- Academic achievement
- Language processing
- Visuospatial processing
- Attention/concentration
- Verbal learning and memory
- Visual learning and memory
- Executive functions
- Speed of processing
- Sensory-perceptual functions
- Motor speed and strength
- Motivation/symptom validity
- Behavioral and emotional functioning

Examples of commonly used tests for each domain are listed in Table 3–1.

Neuropsychological evaluation can assist the child neurologist by providing quantifiable data to guide the evaluation of the cognitive effects of various medical disorders and associated treatments and interventions (eg, see Bosenbark et al[1]). It can aid in the assessment of central nervous system lesions before and after surgical interventions. In the epilepsy surgery setting, it is an integral part of the presurgical evaluation and postsurgical follow-up.[2,3] Neuropsychological data

can provide a basis for monitoring the effects of pharmacologic interventions. It is useful in documenting the cognitive effects of exposure to neurotoxins[4] and has been key in documenting the effects of radiation treatment on learning and cognition in children.[5] It is commonly used to confirm or clarify diagnoses that involve cognitive or intellectual symptoms, such as electrical status epilepticus in sleep (ESES).

Repeated or follow-up neuropsychological evaluation is often clinically useful in order to document changes in functioning since prior examinations, either a decline that may point to progressive or degenerative disease or an improvement that can help to quantify recovery and target remaining areas of deficit or concern. In this respect, repeated neuropsychological exams can help to guide rehabilitation programs and monitor patient progress.

As children approach adulthood, and in adults and the elderly, neuropsychological evaluation is sometimes used to inform decisions related to ongoing disease management, such as their ability to participate in decision-making about their medical conditions as well as larger competency issues related to legal and financial affairs. Neuropsychological data can inform caregivers about individuals' ability to live independently or with supervision as well as their readiness to return to work and school after significant injury or illness. Adults may undergo neuropsychological examination as part of the evaluation of their ability to consent to major interventions such as some complex surgeries or transplants.

Neuropsychological evaluation results are also quite useful to teachers as well as all types of therapists (speech, occupational, physical, and behavioral) who may work with the child or adolescent. Although the special education system in the United States tends to focus on children with intellectual disabilities and specific learning disabilities, each state also has mechanisms in place for students with health or neurologic impairments. However, these neurologic/neuropsychological problems are more uncommon, and the

Table 3–1. Examples of commonly used neuropsychological tests.

Domain	Neuropsychological Test
Intellectual functioning	Wechsler Scales Wechsler Adult Intelligence Scale–IV (WAIS–IV) Wechsler Intelligence Scale for Children–IV (WISC–IV) Wechsler Preschool and Primary Scale of Intelligence–IV (WPPSI– IV) Stanford-Binet Intelligence Scale–V
Academic achievement	Wechsler Individual Achievement Test (WIAT) Woodcock-Johnson Tests of Achievement, Fourth Edition
Language processing	Boston Naming Test Multilingual Aphasia Examination Peabody Picture Vocabulary Test Expressive One-Word Picture Vocabulary Test Verbal Fluency Token Test
Visuospatial processing	Rey-Osterrieth Complex Figure Block Design Judgment of Line Orientation Hooper Visual Organization Test
Attention/concentration	Digit Span Forward and Reversed Trail Making Test Cancellation Tasks (Letter and Symbol) Paced Auditory Serial Addition Test (PASAT)
Verbal learning and memory	Wechsler Memory Scale (WMS) Rey Auditory Verbal Learning Test California Verbal Learning Test Hopkins Verbal Learning Test Wide Range Assessment of Memory and Learning (WRAML)
Visual learning and memory	Wechsler Memory Scale Visual Reproduction I and II Rey-Osterrieth Complex Figure Continuous Recognition Memory Test Visual-Motor Integration Test
Executive functions	Wisconsin Card Sorting Test Category Test Stroop Test Trail Making Test–B WISC/WAIS subtests of Similarities and Block Design
Speed of processing	Simple and Choice Reaction Time Symbol Digit Modalities Test–Written and Oral
Sensory-perceptual functions	Halstead-Reitan Neuropsychological Battery (HRNB) Tactual Performance Test and Sensory Perceptual Examination
Motor speed and strength	Finger Tapping Test Grooved Pegboard Purdue Pegboard Grip Strength
Motivation	Test of Memory Malingering Forced-Choice Symptom Validity Testing
Personality assessment/behavior	Minnesota Multiphasic Personality Inventory (MMPI) Beck Depression Inventory (BDI) Child Behavior Checklist Behavior Assessment System for Children

Data from Lezak MD, Howieson DB, Bigler ED, et al. *Neuropsychological Assessment*, 5th ed. New York, NY: Oxford University Press; 2012.

guidance afforded by the neuropsychological evaluation, in concert with the recommendations provided by the medical team, is important for maximizing the applicability of the child's Individualized Education Plan (IEP). Approaches to therapy may be adjusted by an understanding of the child's memory or attention capacities or other neuropsychological limitations.

There are multiple neurologic conditions that might warrant neuropsychological evaluation, including:

- Epilepsy
- Brain tumor or other cancer
- Prematurity
- Failure to achieve developmental milestones
- Learning or attention deficits
- Traumatic brain injury
- Exposure to drugs, alcohol, or maternal illness in utero
- Exposure to chemicals, toxins, or heavy metals
- Stroke
- Parkinson disease
- Substance abuse
- Dementia
- Psychiatric disorders

The results of a neuropsychological evaluation must be considered in the context of the patient's age, education, sex, first language, and cultural background. These factors can affect test performance and limit the conclusions that can be drawn from the evaluation. In addition, test issues such as reliability, validity, sensitivity, and specificity need to be considered (see Baron[6] for a thorough discussion of all of these considerations). Large, population-based norms are available for relatively few measures. The main intellectual and academic achievement tests do have such norms and are very useful in the pediatric age groups but are sometimes of limited usefulness in an adult neuropsychological test battery. Ideally, patients should be compared with population-based norms, as well as with appropriate subgroups (ie, specific patient populations), to examine strengths and weaknesses. Significant gaps can be found in the normative data for all age, educational, and intellectual ranges; major deficiencies have also existed in the development of appropriate measures and norms for minority populations.

An important aspect of the neuropsychological evaluation is the review of the findings with the parent(s)/guardian(s)

and, if appropriate, the child or adolescent after the testing is completed. For some patients, providing an age- and developmentally appropriate understanding of their neuropsychological strengths and weaknesses, the pattern in which they present, and the underlying reason for them can be a therapeutic intervention in itself. For many individuals with neurologic illness, cognitive or neuropsychological symptoms are subtle in nature; they are not obvious and therefore are sometimes not easily understood by teachers, therapists, or friends in the community. Presenting a rationale for the inconsistencies in neuropsychological and behavioral functioning with which children and adolescents with neurologic illness must often cope can help teachers, friends, and others better appreciate their impact on functioning. For example, it is often the case that a child has an IQ score that is in the average range but significant difficulties in the classroom. It is only when a complete assessment of the range of neuropsychological skills is done that other potential explanations such as a memory deficit or language delay can be considered and addressed. The recommendations made based on neuropsychological findings can result in appropriate interventions and adjustments put in place to improve functioning.

REFERENCES

1. Bosenbark DD, Krivitzky L, Ichord R, Jastrzab L, Billinghurst L. Attention and executive functioning profiles in children following perinatal arterial ischemic stroke. *Child Neuropsychol.* 2018; 24:106-123.
2. Baxendale S, Wilson SJ, Baker GA, et al. Indications and expectations for neuropsychological assessment in epilepsy surgery in children and adults: report of the ILAE Neuropsychology Task Force Diagnostic Methods Commission: 2017–2021 neuropsychological assessment in epilepsy surgery. *Epileptic Disord.* 2019; 21:221-317.
3. Jones-Gotman M, Smith ML, Risse GL, et al. The contribution of neuropsychology to diagnostic assessment in epilepsy. *Epilepsy Behav.* 2010;18:3-12.
4. Ris M, Dietrich K, Succop P, Berger O, Bornschein R. Early exposure to lead and neuropsychological outcome in adolescence. *J Int Neuropsychol Soc.* 2004;10:261-270.
5. Jain N, Krull KR, Brouwers P, Chintagumpala MM, Woo SY. Neuropsychological outcome following intensity-modulated radiation therapy for pediatric medulloblastoma. *Pediatr Blood Cancer.* 2008;51:275-279.
6. Baron IS. *Neuropsychological Evaluation of the Child: Domains, Methods, and Case Studies.* 2nd ed. Oxford University Press; 2018.
7. Lezak MD, Howieson DB, Bigler ED, Tranel D. *Neuropsychological Assessment.* 5th ed. Oxford University Press; 2012.

Approach to Evaluation of Movement Problems in Children

Donald L. Gilbert, MD, MS

INTRODUCTION

This chapter addresses the key points of the clinical approach to evaluation of movement disorders in children. By convention, the term *movement disorders* designates conditions where one or both of the following occur: (1) impairment in initiation and/or execution of movement occurs that is not due to weakness; and/or (2) adventitious movements occur that are not automatic, purposeful, or goal directed. A common classification scheme divides phenomena into hyperkinetic and hypokinetic conditions, although this distinction can be imperfect when observing certain movement problems. Mastery of diagnosis involves a combination of visual pattern recognition and understanding principles of neuroanatomy and phenomenologic classification. This chapter and the following 2 chapters will emphasize practical approaches to more common conditions.

Parents, guardians, and general physicians have an expectation and understanding of the trajectory of typical development of motor control. Although there is variability, referrals to pediatric neurologists often involve recognition that motor control has fallen off the curve of expected gains, as in children who are ataxic or clumsy, or, more commonly, that an abnormally appearing movement is occurring, as in children with tics, stereotypies, or tremor. Comprehensive medical, developmental, family, and social history and general neurologic and physical examinations are vital for rarer presentations. Some typical straightforward presentations may be recognized quickly in the clinic room or based on a smartphone video brought to the visit.

The time-tested approach to diagnosis of movement disorders involves pattern recognition of phenomenology based on visual observation and findings on neurologic examination.[1] Understanding principles of normal function of cortical-striatal-pallidal-thalamo-cortical circuits as well as input and output pathways supporting cerebellar function is stimulating and can play a role in more complex presentations

but lies outside the scope of this text. Ultimately, the goals of initial clinical phenomenologic assessments are to make decisions about whether to obtain additional medical diagnostic testing and to determine approaches to treatment or management.

CLINIC WORKFLOW

Given the crucial role of observation, the clinician should observe the patient as much as possible, even while taking a history. Successful encounters with younger children may involve play, so age-appropriate toys may be offered during the history with the parent. With a verbal child, direct communication about the subjective experience of the movement and its impact on life at home, school, and with friends is very important. Taking time to establish a trusting relationship with parent and child is therefore important, and "small talk" about school, home life, and fun activities often helps accomplish this.

Some parents believe they are protecting their child by discussing the movement problem without the child present. This can create more, rather than less, emotional distress, while inhibiting the clinician's opportunity to obtain critical information directly from the child. Verbal, school-age children usually have sufficient awareness of their movement disorder phenomenology and may want to know more about it.

The first minutes of the clinic room encounter set the tone. After brief introductions among adults, the clinician should focus on the child as quickly as possible.

▶ Interviewing the Verbal Child

Opening the conversation with topics such as fun after-school activities, hobbies, sports, music participation, sibling, pets, and/or best friends serves 2 purposes. First, this can provide an opportunity for direct observation or other information gathering that aids in making the correct diagnosis. Second, this can be the basis for evaluation of movement disorder–related impairment (eg, "Does the shaking in your hands interfere with playing the violin?" "Does that head jerking movement slow down your reading?").

Conversing with and engaging emotionally with the child may bring out the abnormal movements in question; tics, stereotypies, and continuous abnormal movements like chorea may be observed if present. The description of key features of the movement as well as the impact on the child's life should be obtained from both the child and a parent. Important information includes the following: (1) awareness of the movement in real time; (2) sense of voluntariness of the movement; (3) for paroxysmal movements, preceding or premonitory sensations or urges and suppressibility; (4) effect of purposeful actions on the problem; (5) exacerbating or ameliorating factors; and (6) functional interference or effect on performance.

▶ Interviewing the Parents/Guardians

Input from adults in the child's life is critical as well. In addition to complementary information about the phenomenology, parents and guardians can provide the following information: (1) past diagnostic testing for the movement disorder; (2) prior treatments, if any; (3) current and past medications; (4) past perinatal, developmental, and medical history; (5) school performance data; (6) emotional/behavioral problems; (7) review of systems; and (8) 3-generation family history, emphasizing neurologic and psychiatric symptoms and diagnoses.

▶ The Physical and Neurologic Examinations

As previously noted, the examination begins at first sight of the patient. The goal of the general examination is to identify diagnostic clues and to aid in medical decision-making. A wide variety of findings across multiple nonneurologic body systems may be useful for diagnosis or treatment decisions.

An efficient neurologic examination (Table 4–1) for a child with a movement disorder is hypothesis-driven and sufficiently thorough but targeted. For example, tics and stereotypies seldom require a detailed examination, but discerning whether any chorea, dystonia, or parkinsonism is present is standard. The tremor examination should clearly document rest, posture, and approaching targets as well as other signs demonstrating function of the basal ganglia and cerebellum. Findings are interpreted in the context of the broad range of coordination and skills in typically developing young children. Occasionally, parents can be instructed on how to obtain neurologic examination findings at home and send a digital video file if cooperation in clinic is suboptimal or paroxysmal events cannot be induced to occur.

Table 4–1. Elements of movement disorder neurologic examination.

Exam Area	Selected Points Relevant to Movement Disorders
Mental status	Concerns for autism (communication, social skills, repetitive/restricted interests and behaviors); inattention; hyperactive/impulsive; obsessive-compulsive, anxious, depressed
Speech	Dysarthria, apraxia, dysprosody, abnormal cadence, mutism, dysphonia, stuttering
Cranial nerves	Presence of tics or involuntary movements in face, tongue
Eye movements	Nystagmus, impaired saccade initiation, hypo-/hypermetria
Motor examination	Tone, posture at complete rest, posture with limbs fully extended, persistence, presence of adventitious movements Finger to nose testing, fine rapid and alternating movements Gait at least walking and running Effect of various purposeful or cued movements on movement disorder Effect of complex (distraction) or rhythmic (entrainment) cued movements on movement disorder
Sensory	Targeted, hypothesis driven; Romberg

THE DIAGNOSIS

Diagnostic formulation initially involves phenomenology classification (Table 4–2).

Differential diagnosis follows from phenomenology plus time course. Likely acquired, acute and subacute movement disorders may have important historical clues such as other signs of a current or recent infection or inflammatory process, drug or toxin exposure, or psychological stressor.

Genetic diseases can increasingly be identified through whole-exome sequencing (WES) or large panels based on phenomenology. WES is often favored due to phenotypic heterogeneity. However, phenomenology can then be extremely useful in interpreting genetic results or driving further testing.

Multiple websites can aid in the complex process of diagnosis. Several particularly useful ones are as follows:

1. Online Mendelian Inheritance in Man (OMIM) (https://www.omim.org/ or https://www.ncbi.nlm.nih.gov/omim)

2. GeneReviews (https://www.ncbi.nlm.nih.gov/books/NBK1116/)

3. MDSGene (https://www.mdsgene.org)

4. Genetic Testing Registry (https://www.ncbi.nlm.nih.gov/gtr/)

5. VarSome (https://varsome.com)

Table 4–2. Movement disorder phenomenologic categories.

Broad Category	Phenomenologic Term
Hypokinetic	Parkinsonism
Hyperkinetic	
Paroxysmal/episodic	Tics
	Stereotypies
	Myoclonus
	Paroxysmal dyskinesias
	Other jerks
Continual	Tremor
	Dystonia
	Chorea
	Mixed
Uncoordinated	Clumsy
	Ataxic

SUMMARY

The diagnostic process should be systematic yet flexible. Given the explosion of relevant medical and neurologic knowledge, pediatric neurology divisions are increasingly creating movement disorder subspecialty clinics to manage these patients. The goal of the initial evaluation is to both classify the phenomenology and generate a reasonable differential diagnosis. Even experts may fail to reach consensus in some clinical situations about phenomenology or appropriate management strategies.

Although rational, disease-specific treatment is desirable, treatment is often based on phenomenology. In addition, the clinician has an important role as educator, providing information about diagnosis, prognosis, co-occurring disorders, and risk, as well as advocacy organizations and resources for obtaining appropriate services.

REFERENCE

1. O'Malley JA, Gilbert DL. Clinical approach to a child with movement disorders. *Semin Pediatr Neurol.* 2018;25:10-18.

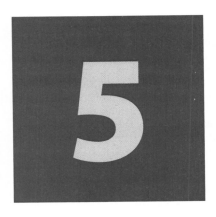

Hyperkinetic Disorders: Tics, Stereotypies, Tremor, and Less Common Abnormal Movements

Donald L. Gilbert, MD, MS

INTRODUCTION

As discussed in the previous chapter, a common schema in movement disorders is to classify movement problems broadly as hyperkinetic versus hypokinetic. The majority of movement disorder referrals from primary physicians to child neurologists are for hyperkinetic disorders, and of these, the most common are tics, stereotypies, and tremor.[1] Functional neurologic disorders are prevalent and may mimic tics or tremor. This chapter addresses the key points of the clinical approach to evaluation and management of these common presentations and then covers, briefly, less common movements of dystonia and chorea.

TICS

► Background

Tics are probably the most common pediatric movement disorder.[2] They occur at high rates in most community-based, school-age samples. A smaller proportion of patients and parents seek medical care, related to the severity (frequency, intensity, and/or impairment) of the tics, the presence of impairing co-occurring problems such as attention-deficit/hyperactivity disorder (ADHD) or obsessive-compulsive disorder (OCD), or parental anxiety.

► Phenomenology

Tics are patterned, repetitive, nonrhythmic movements, mostly within the repertoire of normal movements. They should look or, if vocal (phonic), sound pretty much the same each time they are performed. They can be readily performed or imitated. Simple tics are brief and involve a small cluster of muscles. Examples include blinking, eye darting, face scrunching, head jerking, throat clearing, sniffing, grunting, and humming. Complex tics last longer and involve more muscles in ways that sometimes overlap with the compulsions of OCD. Examples include looking to both sides sequentially, hand posturing followed by tapping, hopping, making animal sounds, and saying certain words or phrases. As is the case for many movements, these can be performed automatically throughout the day, with limited insight or awareness. However, particularly for older children or those with more complex tics, they can also be preceded by a premonitory sensation of some sort—an urge to do the movement. The urge is sometimes describable in sensory terms ("an itch") or as just a feeling ("I have to do it"), but in contrast to compulsions, it should not be related to a recurring, obsessive, intrusive, anxiety-producing thought ("to avoid germs"). The child will often say they feel like the tic is both voluntary ("I'm doing it") and involuntary ("I have to do it; I can't stop it"). Children who are aware of their tics should be able to suppress or postpone their tics at least briefly.[3] See Table 5–1 for comparative features with stereotypies and functional movements.

► Time Course

Tics can start at any time in life, but mostly they start after the age of 3 years and before the age of 10 years.[4] Onset may be gradual or fulminant. In children who manifest tics for more than 1 year, tics typically wax and wane in frequency and intensity and migrate in location over time. Initial tics are usually simple, involving muscles of the face or pharynx. Tics often peak in mid-childhood or adolescence and then begin to wane in late adolescence or adulthood.

► Diagnoses

The *Diagnostic and Statistical Manual of Mental Disorders, Fifth Edition*, classifies tic disorders as self-limited (provisional tic disorder, also known as transient tic disorder) or chronic, lasting greater than 1 year (Tourette disorder or syndrome [TS], chronic motor/vocal tic disorders).

Table 5–1. Phenomenology: signs and symptoms of tics, stereotypies, and functional tic/jerks.

	Tics	Stereotypies	Functional Tic-Like Behaviors
Appearance	Patterned, simple or complex	Patterned, complex	Patterned or pseudo-patterned (eg, head jerk direction varies); proximal muscle, large-amplitude jerks; may be predominantly complex (hitting self/others, prolonged and/or profane vocalizations)
Awareness	Younger children not always aware; older children are typically aware and feel an urge to perform some of them	Younger children not aware; older children are typically somewhat aware	Aware but dissociation may occur during and between bouts of movements
Clinical course	Onset age 3-10 years; may escalate in late childhood/adolescence and improve in late teens/adulthood	Onset usually before age 3 years; episodic, daily, remains relatively unchanged for years	After age 6 years, often after age 10 years
Suppressibility	Some ability to suppress, at least briefly, is common	Older children who are socially aware may limit occurrence to home/safe environments	Varies; adolescents may state movements are involuntary, random, nonsuppressible
Exacerbating factors	Stress, excitement, times of low activity demand, discussion of symptoms	Occur during times of happy excitement, boredom, anxiety, or when socially overwhelmed	Variable; may increase when observed or prior to nonpreferred or stressful activity (school, homework, chores)
Relationship to voluntary movement	Rarely occurs within purposeful, voluntary action (ask about sports, music)	Parents can always interrupt the behavior, but child may return to it	Variable; often occurs during purposeful movements of same body area on examination
Impact on activities of daily living	Usually none, but can interfere some with schoolwork and concentration	Usually none, but may delay onset of tasks	Usually none, which seems inconsistent in severe/dramatic presentations

TS criteria include childhood onset of tic disorder not explained by another cause, with 2 or more motor and 1 or more phonic/vocal tics, lasting greater than 12 months. Given the pervasive nature of throat clearing and sniffing in childhood, it is easy to "miss" the occurrence of these behaviors as phonic tics. In routine practice, if children have had 3 or more different motor tics, not necessarily concurrently, lasting over 1 year, a diagnosis of TS is reasonable, without quibbling about the lack of a known phonic/vocal tic. TS and chronic motor tic disorder are not meaningfully different in their genetic or biological bases.

Medical Diagnostic Testing

In the vast majority of cases, tic disorder diagnoses can be made with no lab testing, electroencephalography (EEG), or brain imaging,[5] although unfortunately, many clinicians continue to order such tests.[6] The common ongoing practice of searching for evidence of prior infection with group A β-hemolytic streptococci through obtaining throat swabs or blood tests for antibodies is not supported by clinical and epidemiologic studies.[7,8] Additional evaluations to clarify the presence or absence of ADHD, OCD, or other mood or anxiety disorders are often important as well.

Treatment

Education of the child and family is important. Most often in early childhood, it is best to ignore tics. In cases where tics do not cause injury or impairment, education about the tics and helping kids manage challenging social interactions and stigma may be sufficient. When tics cause excessive stress, social impairment, functional or school disruption, or physical injury, appropriate interventions can include behavioral therapies or medications.[5] Behavioral therapies are recommended when available.[9] Medications approved by the US Food and Drug Administration for tics include the D_2 receptor–blocking agents haloperidol, pimozide, and aripiprazole. Due to their side effect profiles, these are not preferred as initial medications. α_2-Adrenergic agonists given in single (long-acting) or divided doses are often tried first. These include guanfacine (1-4 mg daily) and clonidine (0.05-0.4 mg daily). A variety of other medicines have modest supportive published evidence as well.[5] If associated conditions such as

ADHD are present, optimizing their treatment is often important.

STEREOTYPIES

▶ Background

Stereotypies, sometimes called complex motor stereotypies, are less common than tics but are also very frequently observed.[10,11] These can be a feature of many conditions including autism spectrum disorder or Rett syndrome (classic midline stereotypies), but also can be present in isolation in children without another neurodevelopmental or genetic diagnosis.

▶ Phenomenology

Stereotypies are complex and usually bilateral, although not necessarily symmetric, movements. The movements may be rhythmic or tonic. Like tics, they are patterned and look the same or very similar each time; however, compared to tics, the duration of stereotypies is usually longer and much more variable, sometimes linked with some brief, interruptible dissociation from the environment. Examples include rocking, hand flapping, pacing, body clenching, and wiggling or fiddling with fingers in front of the center of face or body. These tend to occur much more automatically, without any premonitory awareness or urge. See Table 5–1 for comparative features with tics and functional movements.

▶ Time Course

Stereotypies generally start at a young age, before 3 years. Onset may be gradual or fulminant. In children who manifest stereotypies chronically, the appearance evolves slowly if at all. Pacing or grabbing a toy may be incorporated into the stereotypy, for example, but generally, the basic phenomenology will not vary. Children with typical development most often do stereotypies when they are engrossed mentally in something exciting or novel. This can also be a comforting mechanism for withdrawing from an environment that overloads the child's senses or is stressful. Although this movement disorder is involuntary and can begin automatically, older children may gain an improved ability to monitor their bodies and limit performing stereotypies during social times. Occasionally, stereotypies will increase markedly in older children and adolescents, occurring in long bouts, sometimes with pacing or vocalizations, generally in the home environment.

▶ Diagnoses

Stereotypies can be coded diagnostically as a stereotypic movement disorder.

▶ Medical Diagnostic Testing

In the vast majority of cases, no medical diagnostic testing is needed. Specifically, lab tests, magnetic resonance imaging (MRI), and EEG are not needed or useful. Parents may think their children are "unresponsive" and/or having a seizure while they are having these episodes and dissociating. Instructing parents to pick the child up or do noxious maneuvers during these events to clarify interruptibility helps to demonstrate that these events are not seizures and is more cost-effective than ordering a routine or continuous EEG "just to be sure it is not a seizure."

▶ Treatment

Education of the child and family is important. Most often in early childhood, it is best to ignore stereotypies. School diagnosis letters may also be useful. The indication for pharmacologic treatment is not strong because impairment is viewed as low. There are no approved pharmacologic treatments for stereotypies. Behavioral therapy may be reasonable once children are old enough to be motivated and to follow instructions.

FUNCTIONAL JERKS, TWITCHES, AND TIC-LIKE BEHAVIORS

▶ Background

In many research and clinical settings, the term *functional* has replaced *psychogenic* or *conversion* in referring to symptoms that mimic those found in neurologic diseases.[12] The role of volition in these clinical presentations is complex, as it is in tic disorders. The classical idea was that a proximate psychological stressor would overwhelm an individual such that, in their psychologically traumatized or dysfunctional state, they would voluntarily (malingering) or involuntarily (conversion disorder) manifest behaviors that resembled neurologic disease. Common forms included falling out, dissociating, having convulsive seizure-like events, and, relevant to this section, having jerks or tic-like movements. The classical diagnostic approach was to perform certain maneuvers designed to detect findings indicating a high likelihood of psychogenic etiologies, order multiple diagnostic tests to rule out other causes, and then refer the patient to psychology for identification of underlying stressors and/or mental illness, with no neurology follow-up. The new approach differs in several ways, including taking a more agnostic approach, at least initially, to the causal role of a single, severe, proximate, psychological stressor. The role of agency or secondary gain from the symptoms also has lower priority. The diagnosis is more often made clinically based on positive symptoms (eg, how the movement appears) as opposed to negative symptoms (eg, the absence of typical symptoms and neurologic signs).

Phenomenology

Functional tic-like behaviors are discrete, relatively rapid, and somewhat patterned movements that resemble tics or myoclonus. Prior to the coronavirus disease 2019 (COVID-19) pandemic, movements were generally more like simple tics or proximal muscle myoclonus. Commonly observed features included variable direction (eg, a head thrust might change direction), "attacks" of ongoing movements of varying intensity, and a tendency not to experience a premonitory urge. Whereas adolescents with tics described an ability, at least briefly, to suppress them, those with functional tics were more likely to state they could not suppress them. On examination, functional tics would persist to a much greater extent during the examination of muscles of the same body part (unlike tics). During the COVID-19 pandemic, several features of functional tic disorders changed. Adolescents were more likely to describe an urge, for example. Most prominently, the nature of the behaviors became much more complex, with long strings of words, profanity, hitting self and others, and high levels of disability with regard to school attendance but not with activities of daily living. The prevalence of this clinical presentation also skyrocketed, and many clinicians and investigators in North America, Europe, and Australia observed that the functional tic-like behaviors bore a very high resemblance to behaviors presented in TikTok videos.[13] Whether this represented a distinct mass social media–induced illness with a more volitional component than other functional disorders is controversial. See Table 5–1 for comparative features with tics and functional movements.

Time Course

Onset has tended to be quite abrupt as a new phenomenon or, in some cases, as a new severe phenomenon in youth with a prior history of mild and sometimes undiagnosed tics. Within minutes to hours, extreme fluctuations in these functional behaviors can occur. For example, at the beginning of the clinic visit, they may be relentless, and yet often they subside markedly as the diagnosis is being given to the adolescent and parents. In some cases, improvement is rapid, within 24 hours of the diagnosis. In other cases, the behaviors persist for weeks or months, and other functional symptoms such as nonepileptic, seizure-like events can occur.

Diagnoses

Multiple diagnostic codes exist for functional disorders, with specifications for type of neurologic presentation or "mixed" as subcategories.

Medical Diagnostic Testing

Typically no medical diagnostic testing is necessary or should be obtained for functional tic-like behaviors. Labs, imaging, and EEG are not useful.

Treatment

A biobehavioral and psychosocial approach is recommended, where neurologists make the diagnosis based on positive symptoms and signs and then, in collaboration and with continuity of care, the neurologist and psychologist teach strategies for mitigation of symptoms or rehabilitation. Education is extremely important. It is crucial for the family to be given a positive diagnosis. Saying what it is not (eg, "This is not Tourette") needs to be followed right away by saying what it is and giving a diagnostic label. *Functional neurologic disorder* is an agonistic term that can help avoid unproductive and sometimes confrontational discussions about psychological causes or mediators. This can be a biobehavioral explanation that, initially, may or may not include identification of stressors, especially if the family and patient are resistant to this formulation. The more important step is to develop a plan for how to manage symptoms. Staying home is not advisable. Returning to school and extracurricular activities full time is more adaptive and accelerates recovery in more cases. The neurologist may need to communicate this recommendation with the school in writing. For mitigating movement frequency and intensity, the clinician may recommend the patient practice physical "competing responses," which are movements in the same body area as the functional movement. These serve to occupy some of the patient's mental bandwidth and distract them from the abnormal functional behaviors. Regular exercise for mind-body engagement, stress relief, and further mind-body distractions from the abnormal movements may also be helpful.

In cases where there is a virtual disease model online (eg, TikTok tics in the pandemic era), there may be a tendency of the brain's motor circuits to involuntarily engage with and sometimes mimic behaviors observed on videos. Therefore, use of social media and watching any videos of tic-like behaviors should stop for at least 4 weeks or longer if symptoms are persisting. The neurosymptoms.org website and phone app are also recommended. Psychological referrals are strongly advised, along with treatment of co-occurring mental or physical health problems such as anxiety or depression and discernment about specific stressors or traumas that may trigger or perpetuate the condition.

TREMOR

Background

Tremor is a common referral.[14] The most common times for referrals are during the preschool years and adolescence.

Phenomenology

The term *tremor* indicates that the patient has an oscillation of a body part, causing displacement. The features of this movement include amplitude, frequency, and direction. A series of phenomenologic distinctions are important, elicited by history but also by careful examination and observation.

The first distinction is *at rest* versus *with action*. Rest tremor indicates that the oscillation is observable even when no work is being done with the body part, for example, when hands are resting in the patient's lap. Resting tremor is uncommon in children, and generally, a medical diagnostic workup is needed. Action tremor indicates that the oscillation is observable when a posture is maintained, so-called postural tremor, and/or when the body part approaches a target, so-called intention tremor. If isolated (ie, no other neurologic examination abnormalities are present), then the postural and/or intention tremor is most likely not a symptom of a serious disease.

The second distinction is *regular* versus *irregular*. A regular tremor (eg, postural tremor with hands outstretched) is often mild and relatively benign. A jerky irregular tremor, particularly with asymmetric hand posturing, may indicate a more severe disorder such as dystonia. Tremors with inconsistent muscle groups, tremor direction, tremor amplitude, and tremor frequency can be functional.

Time Course

Many children with tremor have an insidious onset with worsening that is gradual and episodic/situational (eg, when highly anxious). Tremor with acute or subacute onset should have, by history, some proximate cause identifiable or other findings on examination to help guide the clinician.

Medical Diagnostic Testing

Testing for tremor depends on age, time course, phenomenology of the tremor, and associated findings on neurologic examination. Jerky/irregular tremors, resting tremors, tremors with acute onset, and tremors with other neurologic findings or loss of any motor skills need a comprehensive diagnostic evaluation. The differential diagnosis for tremors is large. Broad or targeted laboratory assessment and neuroimaging are often appropriate in this setting. A toxicology screen may be appropriate.

Tremor or shakiness in a young child, classically noted first thing in the morning, with emotion or frustration, and while performing fine motor tasks, may be benign. If the examination is nonfocal and shows nothing more than mild clumsiness, a clinical observation approach with follow-up in 6 to 12 months is often adequate, without laboratory testing or neuroimaging. At this age, a common etiology is often a nonspecific static encephalopathy, and the tremor is accompanied by fine motor skill problems, clumsiness, and sometimes mild cognitive or behavioral difficulties.

Similarly, a clinical observation–only approach may be appropriate for an adolescent with relatively symmetric, regular postural or intention tremor. Other reassuring findings are a positive family history of bilateral hand tremor or the presence of significant anxiety and/or prescriptions for psychotropic or other tremorigenic medications. Laboratory testing may include general chemistries, a complete blood count to rule out anemia, thyroid-stimulating hormone, and other tests, but the yield is low. Imaging can often be deferred. At this age, a common etiology is essential/isolated tremor and enhanced physiologic or drug-induced tremor. The neurologic examination is critical. Findings supporting focal or diffuse neuropathology (eg, ataxia or dystonia) indicate the need for a comprehensive diagnostic evaluation.

Treatment

Decisions about treatment are based on tremor interference. Sometimes parents just want to make sure there is nothing more serious going on. If the tremor does not interfere with schoolwork, extracurricular activities, or performing activities of daily living, then it is likely not worth treating. Regular tremors can be treated as needed or daily with propranolol or daily with primidone. Irregular or dystonic tremors can be treated with carbidopa/levodopa or trihexyphenidyl. Drug-induced tremors may be treated by stopping or reducing dosages of the offending agent.

CHOREA, ATHETOSIS, AND BALLISM

Background

Some consider athetosis, chorea, and ballism to exist on a spectrum. Thus, athetosis can be considered to be a slow form of chorea. At the other end of the spectrum, ballism is fast chorea with severe, flinging, proximally generated muscle movements.[1] Most chorea in childhood is acquired as a result of pathology affecting the striatum or other areas in circuits involving the basal ganglia. Chorea, athetosis, and ballism can occur in many genetic diseases as well.

Phenomenology

The term *chorea* indicates that the patient has an ongoing, random-appearing sequence of discrete involuntary movements with variable timing, duration, rate, direction, and anatomic location. This gives the appearance of restlessness. Hypotonia and motor impersistence may also be present. Purposeful movements often exacerbate the chorea. *Athetosis* is slow, writhing, and continuous, more repetitive than chorea, and more likely to involve predominantly distal muscles of hands or feet. *Ballism*, or *ballismus*, designates high-amplitude, flinging movements, typically generated by proximal muscles. These may be brief or continual and may be unilateral, as in *hemiballismus*.

Time Course

Most neurologic conditions in childhood in which chorea is prominent present subacutely. In most cases, subacute-onset chorea occurs as part of a self-limited process and will resolve in days, weeks, or sometimes months, although recurrences are possible. Chorea can also be chronic and relatively static or chronic and progressive. Chorea can also emerge for brief periods of time in paroxysmal movement disorders such as paroxysmal or episodic kinesigenic dyskinesia, in which the movement disorder is a discrete choreic or mixed dyskinetic event triggered after the body goes from rest to an active state.

Medical Diagnostic Testing

Testing is critical for identifying treatable etiologies for chorea. A key factor is the time course of the clinical presentation.

Acute/subacute chorea generally involves a process in which basal ganglia function or structure is disrupted. The most common of these is rheumatic—poststreptococcal Sydenham chorea (SC). In a child or adolescent presenting with chorea, especially with motor impersistence of the hands and tongue, SC is the most likely cause. This diagnosis is established when there is a recent history of documented infection with group A β-hemolytic streptococcal infection, most often demonstrated by finding elevated blood anti-streptolysin O (ASO) or anti–DNAse B (ADB) antibodies. Concurrent skin rash and cardiac (systolic murmur) and joint (arthralgia, arthritis) conditions may be present. Due to the risk of recurrence and permanent damage to cardiac valves, it is important to be vigilant for cardiac status and to carefully follow evidence-based recommendations relating to rheumatic fever.[15]

Other inflammatory conditions and mitochondrial diseases should be considered in appropriate circumstances. These are much rarer. Neuroimaging should be performed if these are suspected, as well as appropriate inflammatory testing, including antiphospholipid antibody panels and/or metabolic laboratory testing, including lactate, pyruvate, and sequencing of mitochondrial DNA and *POLG1*. Anti–*N*-methyl-D-aspartate (NMDA) receptor encephalitis can also present with a dyskinetic movement disorder, but generally more diffuse symptoms are also present. Serum and cerebrospinal fluid studies and body imaging should be obtained if this is suspected, and treatment initiated promptly.

Chronic chorea may be acquired due to strokes, trauma, or injury to the basal ganglia in the perinatal or other periods. Neuroimaging with brain MRI is warranted in this setting, but this may be normal in genetic conditions, at least

initially. An α-fetoprotein level should be obtained to test for ataxia-telangiectasia. Genetic testing may be necessary. In the presence of characteristic features, certain genes, such as *SGCE*, *GNAO1*, or *ADCY5*, may be prioritized in smaller gene panels. Otherwise, whole-exome sequencing or a very large panel is appropriate to shorten the diagnostic odyssey. This testing has major implications for diagnosis, prognosis, and treatment.

Treatment

For SC, treatment has 3 parts: (1) secondary prevention of group A β-hemolytic streptococcal infections with penicillin (or other antibiotics), following published guidelines, until age 21; (2) immune suppression/modulation with steroids or intravenous immune globulin for more severe cases; and (3) symptom suppression when chorea is interfering with activities of daily living. The chorea of SC has been reported to respond well to valproic acid and levetiracetam, although, given the monophasic time course, interpreting clinical benefit versus effects of time can be unclear. Otherwise, the most effective treatments for SC and for other choreas are vesicular monoamine transporter 2 (VMAT2) inhibitors, which decrease dopamine production, or potent D_2 receptor–blocking agents such as risperidone or fluphenazine. Anticholinergic agents should not be used because they may worsen chorea. Withdrawal emergent dyskinesia benefits initially from restarting the previously prescribed D_2 receptor–blocking agent. Some genetic diseases have been demonstrated to have particularly beneficial treatments. For example, severe chorea in children with the dyskinetic neurodevelopmental disorder due to *GNAO1* mutations responds to pallidal deep brain stimulation. *ADCY5*-related dyskinesia–associated movements may improve with levodopa of caffeine. Current medical literature should be consulted and/or subspecialty consultation pursued.

DYSTONIA

Background

Dystonia is common as a symptom.[1] Many forms of brain injury affecting the basal ganglia or other interconnected structures can result in dystonia. Dystonia is often accompanied by tremor. Dystonia often occurs in children with cerebral palsy or with congenital brain malformation syndromes or after significant traumatic brain injuries. In these children, the dystonia may co-occur with spasticity, a mixed picture in which it is important to clarify the relative contributions of spasticity and dystonia to the child's impairment. Dystonia also occurs in neurodegenerative disorders. In these children, the dystonia may co-occur with other motor problems such as chorea, myoclonus, ataxia, or spasticity. Dystonia can also occur as a complication of psychiatric medications, and patients with functional disorders may have dystonic posturing. Thus, it is important to recognize dystonia and have an approach for diagnostic evaluation and management.

Phenomenology

The term *dystonia* applies to sustained or intermittent muscle contractions causing abnormal, often repetitive movements or postures. Dystonic movements may occur due to maladaptive co-contraction of flexors and extensors across a joint, generating patterned or twisting movements or jerky tremor. Dystonia is dynamic, meaning that the involuntary movements vary depending on the position, trajectory, or task occurring in the involved muscles. Some maneuvers such as sensory tricks or various antagonistic gestures may be employed by the patient to alleviate the tremor.

Time Course

Dystonia can emerge suddenly, when acquired due to a variety of reasons, or gradually. In children with prenatal or perinatal hypoxic-ischemic encephalopathy or brain malformations, dystonia may not become apparent for months or years as brain maturation or maladaptive plasticity occurring during injury recovery develops over the static injury. In genetic neurologic diseases in which dystonia is prominent, the timing and body distribution of dystonia emergence can vary depending on the underlying pathophysiology and unknown factors. For example, patients with dystonia due to a heterozygous variant in *TOR1A* tend to develop limb dystonia and, over months to years, generalized dystonia. The same variant in adults may result in only focal or task-specific dystonia, or no symptoms at all, as penetrance is incomplete. In dystonia due to variants in *GCH1*, which encodes the GTP cyclohydrolase 1 gene, various phenomenologies including parkinsonism, dystonia, and spasticity mimicking cerebral palsy or spastic paraplegia may occur. This disease is also known as dopa-responsive dystonia due to its underlying pathophysiology and dramatic beneficial response to levodopa. Dystonia can also emerge for brief periods of time in paroxysmal movement disorders such as paroxysmal or episodic kinesigenic dyskinesia due to *PRRT2* mutations, in which the movement disorder is a discrete dystonic event triggered after the body goes from rest to an active state.

Medical Diagnostic Testing

Testing is critical for identifying treatable etiologies for dystonia. In the majority of cases, brain imaging is appropriate as part of the diagnostic workup. This can yield vital information for medical decision-making in both acquired and genetic dystonias. In the proper clinical setting, genetic testing with focused or large panels or whole-exome sequencing is also indicated. A broad range of other laboratory tests including α-fetoprotein, ceruloplasmin, metabolic and

mitochondrial studies, inflammatory markers, autoimmune testing, and endocrine testing may be appropriate. Dystonia can be very challenging, and subspecialty referral is often advisable.

Treatment

Symptomatic pharmacologic treatment for dystonia typically involves trials of carbidopa/levodopa (1:4 ratio; 3-5 mg/kg/d initially) and trihexyphenidyl (gradual uptitration due to anticholinergic side effects), alone or in combination. Medications used for spasticity such as benzodiazepines and baclofen may provide some benefit. Pallidal deep brain stimulation yields phenomenal benefit in some childhood-onset, generalized dystonias.

SUMMARY

The diagnostic process for pediatric movement disorders should be systematic yet flexible. Referral to pediatric neurology movement disorder clinics is reasonable in more complex cases. Treatment is often based on phenomenology more than pathophysiology. Because many of these disorders and diseases are chronic, the clinician has an important role as educator as well.

REFERENCES

1. Singer HS, Mink JW, Gilbert DL, Jankovic J. *Movement Disorders in Childhood*. 2nd ed. Elsevier, Inc.; 2016.
2. Robertson MM, Eapen V, Singer HS, et al. Gilles de la Tourette syndrome. *Nat Rev Dis Primers*. 2017;3:16097.
3. Kim S, Greene DJ, Robichaux-Viehoever A, et al. Tic suppression in children with recent-onset tics predicts 1-year tic outcome. *J Child Neurol*. 2019;34:757-764.
4. Black KJ, Kim S, Yang NY, Greene DJ. Course of tic disorders over the lifespan. *Curr Dev Disord Rep*. 2021;8:121-132.
5. Pringsheim T, Okun MS, Muller-Vahl K, et al. Practice guideline recommendations summary: treatment of tics in people with Tourette syndrome and chronic tic disorders. *Neurology*. 2019;92:896-906.
6. Ganos C, Sarva H, Kurvits L, et al. Clinical practice patterns in tic disorders among Movement Disorder Society members. *Tremor Other Hyperkinet Mov (N Y)*. 2021;11:43.
7. Gilbert DL. Inflammation in tic disorders and obsessive-compulsive disorder: are PANS and PANDAS a path forward? *J Child Neurol*. 2019;34:598-611.
8. Martino D, Schrag A, Anastasiou Z, et al. Association of group A *Streptococcus* exposure and exacerbations of chronic tic disorders: a multinational prospective cohort study. *Neurology*. 2021;96:e1680-e1693.
9. Piacentini J, Woods DW, Scahill L, et al. Behavior therapy for children with Tourette disorder: a randomized controlled trial. *JAMA*. 2010;303:1929-1937.
10. Martino D, Hedderly T. Tics and stereotypies: a comparative clinical review. *Parkinsonism Relat Disord*. 2019;59:117-124.
11. Oakley C, Mahone EM, Morris-Berry C, Kline T, Singer HS. Primary complex motor stereotypies in older children and

adolescents: clinical features and longitudinal follow-up. *Pediatr Neurol.* 2015;52:398-403 e391.

12. Espay AJ, Aybek S, Carson A, et al. Current concepts in diagnosis and treatment of functional neurological disorders. *JAMA Neurol.* 2018;75:1132-1141.

13. Pringsheim T, Ganos C, McGuire JF, et al. Rapid onset functional tic-like behaviors in young females during the COVID-19 pandemic. *Mov Disord.* 2021;36:2707-2713.

14. Miskin C, Carvalho KS. Tremors: essential tremor and beyond. *Semin Pediatr Neurol.* 2018;25:34-41.

15. Gewitz MH, Baltimore RS, Tani LY, et al. Revision of the Jones criteria for the diagnosis of acute rheumatic fever in the era of Doppler echocardiography: a scientific statement from the American Heart Association. *Circulation.* 2015;131:1806-1818.

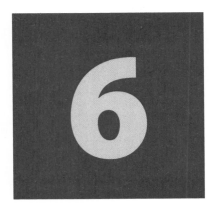

Coordination Disorders: Clumsiness and Ataxia

Donald L. Gilbert, MD, MS

INTRODUCTION

Typically developing children acquire motor skills at varying ages, and abnormal movements and motor control can occur in healthy children.[1] Understanding the course of motor development is a core skill in pediatric medicine. Divergence from the expected developmental course and subacute loss of motor control are common reasons for referral to child neurologists. This chapter addresses the key points of the clinical approach to evaluation and management of children with problems with coordination, gait and balance, and eye movement control. These occur in 3 broad categories: clumsiness, acute ataxia, and chronic progressive ataxia. Neuroanatomically, the conditions discussed in this chapter involve the cerebellum and/or its afferent or efferent connections, in most cases. *Ataxia* is defined as an inability to generate a normal or expected voluntary movement trajectory that cannot be attributed to weakness or involuntary movements (eg, chorea, dystonia, myoclonus, tremor).[2] In ataxia, the spatial pattern and/or timing of movements are affected. *Clumsiness* in this chapter refers to benign, nonprogressive difficulties with fine and gross motor function that are not due to a progressive neurologic disease. Key manifestations of cerebellar function/dysfunction are presented in Table 6–1.

THE CLUMSY CHILD

Background

A clumsy child is an otherwise healthy child who develops gait, balance, fine finger movements, and sometimes speech articulation along a developmental trajectory that is below the typical range. Determining what is benign clumsiness versus clumsiness due to an underlying neurologic disease can be challenging.[3] The most important historical feature indicative of a serious neurologic problem is loss of well-established motor skills. However, degenerative diseases can also initially present with slower-than-expected skill acquisition. Therefore, vigilance and longitudinal clinical follow-up with serial examinations is important.

Phenomenology

Parents may report tremor, particularly on awakening and during performance of fine motor tasks, and difficulty with tasks such as utensil use, drawing, or writing. Difficulties with cognition or emotional regulation are somewhat more common. Neurologic examination is critical. Benign clumsiness is often manifest primarily by slow, variable, inaccurate sequential finger tapping, with overflow during unimanual tasks. Walking, running, or tandem gait may also be clumsy. Red flags include any eye movement control difficulties including abnormal saccades or nystagmus, cranial nerve deficits, focal weakness, inability to stand with feet together as well as on either foot, a positive Romberg sign, or a lurching gait. Mild, symmetric postural or subtle intention tremor may accompany benign clumsiness. However, the presence of dystonic posturing, asymmetric jerky or resting tremor, chorea, or myoclonus indicates the need for a comprehensive evaluation.

Time Course

Improvement in motor function should occur over time. Benign clumsiness may be chronic, but it should not worsen.

Diagnoses

Descriptive terms may be used in the electronic health record. Some children may meet criteria for developmental coordination disorder,[4] in which case, the use of the term *ataxia* is generally not appropriate.

Medical Diagnostic Testing

In the absence of red flags discussed above on history or examination, clumsy children can be followed clinically

Table 6–1. Selected symptoms and signs of cerebellar disorders.

Eye movements	*Nystagmus* – oscillatory, rhythmical movements of the eyes
	Saccades – difficulties initiating or targeting rapid eye movement
	Pursuit – difficulties with smooth visual tracking
Speech	*Dysarthria* – imprecise production of consonant sounds
	Dysrhythmia – slow, irregularly timed sounds
Trunk movements	*Balance/position* – unsteadiness while standing or sitting
	Titubation – characteristic bobbing of the head and trunk
Limb movements	*Hypotonia* – diminished resistance to passive limb displacement
	Reflexes – pendular reflexes
	Dysmetria – overshoot/undershoot limb movements
	Intention tremor – on finger-to-nose and heel-to-shin testing
	Initiation – delayed initiation of movement
	Dysdiadochokinesia – errors in rate and regularity of movements
Gait	*Gait ataxia* – broad-based, staggering/lurching gait; inability to tandem walk

without any further medical diagnostic testing. Specifically, laboratory testing, electroencephalogram (EEG), and brain magnetic resonance imaging (MRI) are not needed in many cases. In the presence of red flags or a sufficiently concerning constellation of findings, brain MRI is the test of choice. Some children with static clumsy presentations may have mild versions of congenital cerebellar malformation syndromes such as rhombencephalosynapsis.

Treatment

Occupational (and, if needed, physical/speech) therapy referral through school-based services or, in more severe cases, through the medical system is advisable. At home, extracurricular activities that enhance motor skills, eye coordination, and so on can be recommended. Highly competitive team sports may not be a good fit, but generally, a helpful, coordination- and self-esteem–building activity can be found. The neural substrate for motor control is often not affected in isolation. Problems may emerge over time with attention, learning, impulse control, anxiety, or anger management. Advising parents of this possibility can promote vigilance

and early intervention. There are no pharmacologic interventions that reduce clumsiness.

ACUTE AND EPISODIC ATAXIA

▶ Background

Acute cerebellar ataxia is an iconic presentation in children with a broad differential diagnosis.[5,6] A large number of processes can affect cerebellar function. These include acute intoxications/ingestions, seizures, trauma, infections and inflammatory conditions, neoplasms, and rare metabolic diseases. A systematic approach is important to document domains of dysfunction and direct the clinical diagnostic evaluation. A thorough history and skilled medical and neurologic examination are vital.

▶ Phenomenology

Possible neurologic manifestations are listed in Table 6–2. Acute ataxia results from cerebellar dysfunction and usually presents with gait and balance problems. Symptoms and signs that may also occur include disordered eye movement control (oculomotor apraxia, hypo-/hypermetric saccades) or abnormal eye movements (nystagmus, opsoclonus), tremor, irregular amplitude and timing of movements, and dysarthria. The presence of seizures, confusion, focal weakness, and bowel or bladder dysfunction indicates more widespread neuropathology.

▶ Time Course

Emergence of symptoms occurs over minutes to hours or sometimes days. Careful documentation of neurologic examination findings, including using videos, is critical to understand if the underlying process is worsening. Duration varies with etiology and treatment.

▶ Diagnoses

Ataxia can be coded diagnostically as a stereotypic movement disorder.

▶ Medical Diagnostic Testing

In children with acute ataxia not preceded by trauma, brain MRI or head computed tomography without intravenous (IV) contrast is usually appropriate as part of the initial diagnostic evaluation. MRI has higher resolution and accuracy for a wider variety of pathologic processes, particularly in the posterior fossa. Screening blood testing, toxicology screening, and cerebrospinal fluid testing may be indicated depending on the history and suspected etiologies. Genetic testing and metabolic testing may be needed for recurring or episodic cases.

Table 6–2. Differential diagnosis, clinical presentation, and diagnostic testing for acute and recurrent ataxia.

Etiology	Common Examples	Features	Diagnostic Testing
Acute/subacute onset			
Inflammatory	Acute cerebellar ataxia	Gait impairment, truncal ataxia, titubation, nystagmus. Mental status normal or irritable.	Brain MRI (should be normal). Consider lumbar puncture for CSF studies.
	Acute disseminated encephalomyelitis (ADEM)	Delirium and multifocal neurologic deficits.	Brain MRI (should show multiple discrete lesions involving both gray and white matter). Lumbar puncture for CSF inflammatory markers.
	Guillain-Barré syndrome, including Miller Fisher variant	Oculomotor paresis, bulbar weakness, hyporeflexia, radicular pain.	Brain MRI (should be normal). CSF for cells, protein, infectious/inflammatory markers.
	Opsoclonus myoclonus ataxia syndrome (OMS, OMAS)	Truncal ataxia, multifocal myoclonus, opsoclonus (may be transient), behavioral irritability.	Image abdomen, pelvis, and chest for occult neuroblastoma. Urine catecholamines.
Infectious/inflammatory	Acute cerebellitis	Headaches, vomiting, papilledema, cranial nerve palsies.	Brain MRI with contrast.
Mass lesions	Posterior fossa neoplasms	Headaches, vomiting, papilledema, cranial nerve palsies.	Brain MRI with contrast.
Toxic acute ingestion	Alcohol, anticonvulsants, antihistamines, benzodiazepines, toluene	Delirium.	Brain MRI/head CT; urine/serum toxicology screen.
Trauma/vascular	Stroke, vertebrobasilar dissection	Consider after neck trauma or if hypercoagulable.	MRI brain/head CT, stroke protocol; vascular imaging of head and neck.
Recurring/episodic			
Metabolic	Inborn errors of metabolism	Illness trigger; preexisting intellectual disabilities, positive family history, encephalopathy and vomiting.	Biochemical, genetic testing.
Migrainous	Basilar, complex migraine		Brain MRI.
Episodic ataxias	Genetic episodic ataxias	Bouts of dysarthria, gait ataxia, sometimes with characteristic provoking factors.	Genetic testing.
Functional		Uneconomical gait, excessive sway without falling.	Often none.

CSF, cerebrospinal fluid; CT, computed tomography; MRI, magnetic resonance imaging.

Treatment

Treatment depends on etiology. Intoxications are usually self-limited. Inflammatory etiologies have established protocols to reduce disability and shorten disease courses with steroids, intravenous immune globulin, plasmapheresis, and more targeted immunomodulatory agents. Paroxysmal disorders such as migraines and episodic ataxias have an increasing variety of treatment options. A mainstay for episodic ataxias initially is acetazolamide. Functional disorders benefit from a biobehavioral approach. When ataxia is a major component of a functional disorder, physical therapy can play an important role in rehabilitating gait.

CHRONIC PROGRESSIVE ATAXIA

Background

Genetic degenerative disorders affecting the cerebellum usually affect other neurologic systems as well. Thus, ataxia may be preceded or accompanied by other movement disorders, spasticity, cognitive impairment, and other findings, sometimes involving other organs as well. The presence of chronic ataxia accompanied by any of these other findings raises concerns for a progressive neurologic diagnosis, as does loss of motor skills. The pattern of inheritance is more commonly autosomal recessive than autosomal dominant. The 2 most common progressive genetic ataxias presenting in children are ataxia-telangiectasia and Friedreich ataxia, both autosomal recessive.

Phenomenology

Phenomenologic findings are listed earlier in Table 6–1. Two broad categories of phenomenology for cerebellar disease are primary cerebellar ataxia and sensory/afferent pathway ataxia.[7] Primary cerebellar ataxia localizes to the cerebellum. Sensory ataxia localizes to afferent pathways providing proprioceptive feedback critical for motor control. A classic finding is the Romberg sign, where the patient stands successfully with feet together by using visual input but loses balance control with eyes closed when proprioceptive information is needed but not available due to disease.

Ataxia-telangiectasia typically presents in early childhood and results in eventual near-total disability due to ataxia and involuntary movements. Early movement problems may include chorea, dystonia, myoclonus, and pancerebellar ataxia. Difficulty with eye movements, especially initiating saccades, is characteristic. Dysarthria also occurs. Telangiectasias, dilated small blood vessels visible in the skin and conjunctiva, follow the emergence of the movement disorder. Immunologic deficiencies and lymphoreticular neoplasms can also be features of this diagnosis.[8]

Friedreich ataxia presents as a sensory ataxia in later childhood and adolescence. Gait, limb control, and speech are affected. Distal weakness with spasticity, loss of reflexes, and abnormal extensor plantar reflexes in the legs develop, contributing to loss of ambulation. Cardiomyopathy, diabetes, scoliosis, and foot deformities are associated as well.[9]

Time Course

Commonly, progression is gradual, with rates varying in part based on age of presentation and severity. Some diseases involve stepwise, more severe periods of functional regression.

Medical Diagnostic Testing

Brain MRI without contrast is usually appropriate for children presenting with progressive ataxia. The use of IV contrast, spectroscopy, or spinal imaging may be appropriate in selective instances. A blood test for α-fetoprotein, which is elevated in ataxia-telangiectasia, should always be obtained. Other labs depend on the circumstances, but generally, if the

clinical presentation is not classic for ataxia-telangiectasia or Friedreich ataxia, then a broad genetic panel for ataxias or whole-exome sequencing is preferred. This has vastly increased the ability to make specific, molecular diagnoses; however, a substantial fraction of children remain undiagnosed. EEG is not usually useful. Nerve conduction/electromyography studies may have value in selected instances in which neuropathy is suspected clinically and its establishment as demyelinating versus axonal would be important for diagnostic clarification.

Treatment

Treatment of ataxia remains unsatisfying. Physical therapy and use of adaptive devices are mainstays. Symptomatic pharmacologic therapy can be more effective for associated movement disorders such as dystonia, when present. Ataxias are the focus of intensive research efforts, with a number of rational, disease-modifying therapies under investigation.

SUMMARY

In acute ataxias, history, examination, and a broad differential diagnosis with comprehensive evaluation are important. Brain imaging is usually appropriate. For chronic ataxias, it can be initially difficult to determine if the symptoms are static or progressive. Brain imaging is usually appropriate but may be deferred in mild, nonprogressive cases with good clinical follow-up. The diagnostic process depends on understanding of the trajectory of developmental motor control in typical children and longitudinal follow-up with serial neurologic examinations. Multiple brain malformation syndromes affect cerebellar function. A vast number of degenerative disorders also affect cerebellar function.

REFERENCES

1. Kuiper MJ, Brandsma R, Vrijenhoek L, et al. Physiological movement disorder-like features during typical motor development. *Eur J Paediatr Neurol.* 2018;22:595-601.
2. Singer HS, Mink JW, Gilbert DL, Jankovic J. *Movement Disorders in Childhood.* 2nd ed. Elsevier, Inc.; 2016.
3. Brandsma R, Lawerman TF, Kuiper MJ, Lunsing RJ, Burger H, Sival DA. Reliability and discriminant validity of ataxia rating scales in early onset ataxia. *Dev Med Child Neurol.* 2017;59: 427-432.
4. Lawerman TF, Brandsma R, Maurits NM, et al. Paediatric motor phenotypes in early-onset ataxia, developmental coordination disorder, and central hypotonia. *Dev Med Child Neurol.* 2020;62:75-82.
5. Segal E, Schif A, Kasis I, Ravid S. Acute ataxia in children: common causes and yield of diagnostic work-up in the era of varicella vaccination. *J Clin Neurosci.* 2019;68:146-150.
6. Kirik S, Aslan M, Ozgor B, Gungor S, Aslan N. Acute ataxia in childhood: clinical presentation, etiology, and prognosis of single-center experience. *Pediatr Emerg Care.* 2021;37:e97-e99.

7. Lynch DR, McCormick A, Schadt K, Kichula E. Pediatric ataxia: focus on chronic disorders. *Semin Pediatr Neurol.* 2018;25:54-64.

8. McGrath-Morrow SA, Rothblum-Oviatt CC, Wright J, et al. Multidisciplinary management of ataxia telangiectasia: current perspectives. *J Multidiscip Healthc.* 2021;14:1637-1644.

9. Lynch DR, Schadt K, Kichula E, McCormack S, Lin KY. Friedreich ataxia: multidisciplinary clinical care. *J Multidiscip Healthc.* 2021;14:1645-1658.

Gait Disorder

Travis R. Larsh, MD

Paola Maria L. Mendoza-Sengco, MD

Alexander M. Zygmunt, MD

Steve W. Wu, MD

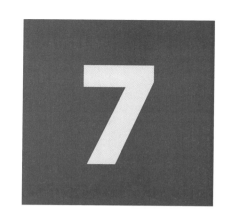

INTRODUCTION

Independent ambulation is a critical gross motor skill achieved early in childhood. Various neurologic disorders can manifest in infancy such that normal gait development is limited or delayed. In progressive neurologic conditions, children may never acquire independent walking or may regress, leading to loss of ambulation. Before discussing different abnormal gait phenomenologies, a brief review of normal gait development is provided. Included in this chapter is also a summary of nonneurologic causes for gait problems. Finally, as we discuss neurologic differential diagnoses for gait disorder, it is important to recognize that gait dysfunction often coexists with other abnormal neurologic symptoms in the context of global assessment of neurologic disorders in children and adolescents.

NORMAL GAIT DEVELOPMENT

Most gestationally full-term toddlers will walk unassisted by about 15 months of age. By age 3 years, children's gait pattern is mature. The gait cycle starts and ends with the ipsilateral heel striking the ground successively. Throughout the cycle, each leg alternates between the stance phase (~60%) when the foot is in contact with the ground and the swing phase (~40%). After heel strike, the foot rolls and lifts off at the toes to initiate the swing phase. Truncal posture is upright with head midline and arms reciprocally swinging at the side along with the contralateral leg. The distance between lateral aspects of both feet should approximate the width of the trunk.

As young infants learn to walk, they initiate the gait cycle by striking the ground with the entire plantar surface. Abducted arms along with a wide base help infants to maintain balance. There is pronounced flexion at the hip and knees. Legs are externally rotated. During stance phase, legs are fully extended at the knee. This gait pattern gradually matures with narrowing of the base. Heel strike develops around 18 months of age. Legs gradually start to rotate internally at the end of the swing phase. Full knee extension at midstance transitions to slight knee flexion to allow for smoother gait. Arms eventually are adducted and exhibit reciprocal swing. Gradually as children age, cadence (steps per minute) decreases while stride length and velocity increase.

APPROACH TO GAIT DISORDERS

Normal gait requires proper function of musculoskeletal and multiple neurologic systems (eg, visual, sensory, coordination, motor). Therefore, the assessment of a child with gait problems requires a detailed physical examination including a full neurologic exam.

Valuable insight into the cause of gait deviation without use of formal and expensive gait analysis equipment can be accomplished by observing the child walk in anterior, posterior, and lateral views, and describing movement and position of the swinging and stance limb across the foot, knee, and hip joints (Table 7–1). It is also important to note symmetry in step length and efficiency of walking pattern with either presence or absence of excessive body motion or other indicators of excessive energy consumption.

Prior to a more detailed discussion on gait dysfunction due to a neurologic disorder, a brief discussion on nonneurologic causes is important.

NONNEUROLOGIC CAUSES OF ABNORMAL GAIT

Antalgic gait is characterized by a shortened stance phase to minimize pain on the weight-bearing leg. Cause of pain could be due to traumatic (eg, fracture, soft tissue injury), infectious (eg, septic joint, osteomyelitis), rheumatologic (eg, juvenile idiopathic arthritis, rheumatic fever), hematologic (eg, hemophilia), or oncologic conditions.

Table 7–1. Practical questions to observe gait in a systematic approach.

	Stance	Swing
Foot	• Is ankle position in neutral or equinus? • Which portion of the foot contacts the floor first? • What is the foot progression angle during stance (and swing) relative to the knee? • Is the foot plantigrade in stance? • Does the foot maintain its appropriate arch contour during stance?	• What is the position of foot at end of swing—neutral, varus, valgus?
Knee	• Does the knee come into full extension? • Does the knee hyperextend, or is the extension controlled? • Is the knee aligned with the foot? • Is there a varus or valgus motion during loading?	• What is the knee position at the end of swing? • Is knee flexion in swing adequate for foot clearance?
Hip	• Are thigh and knee aligned? If not, is there internal or external malrotation? • Is there full hip extension at the end of stance? • Is the pelvis tilted anteriorly or posteriorly? • What are the trunk movements in each plane (bending forward/backward, side-to-side sway)?	• Is there excessive hip abduction in swing?
General	• Is the stride length adequate? • Is step length symmetric? • Is walking pattern efficient?	

Data from Gage JR, Schwartz MH, Koop SE, et al: *The Identification and Treatment of Gait Problems in Cerebral Palsy*, 2nd ed. London: Mac Keith Press; 2009.

Common orthopedic variations are also worth mentioning given the potential to affect gait. Leg length discrepancy and developmental dysplasia of the hip can cause a painless limping gait. Flat feet are very common in children. The medial arch typically develops around 2 to 3 years of age. The prevalence of flat feet in children around 3 to 4 years of age has been reported to be as high as 70%. Although this percentage drops with age, up to 40% of 5- to 8-year-old children can still have flat feet. Genu varum (bow legs) and valgum (knock knees) can also affect development of normal gait pattern. Vitamin D deficiency is a treatable condition that can cause genu varum. In-toeing is common in children and typically is a normal developmental variation. Out-toeing is common in young infants. As gait pattern matures, out-toeing should decrease. Progressive in-toeing or out-toeing may suggest either an orthopedic (tibial torsion or excessive hip rotation) or neurologic disorder (dystonia).

ABNORMAL GAIT RELATED TO NEUROLOGIC DISORDERS

▶ Idiopathic Toe-Walking

Toe-walking is very common in young infant during gait development. However, the persistence of toe-walking beyond toddler years remains common with a reported prevalence of 2.1% of children still actively toe-walking at 5.5 years of age. In the developmentally delayed population, this prevalence is significantly higher.

▶ Gait Deviations Due to Hypertonia

In most children with cerebral palsy or other upper motor neuron disorders including hereditary spastic diplegia, it is too simplistic to attribute the primary pathology to hypertonia (spasticity and dystonia) alone. Other primary impairments contribute to their gait and posture including weakness, poor balance, lack of selective control of muscles, delayed gross motor skills, bony malalignment, and joint deformities.

Spastic diplegic gait is characterized by a narrow base of support with tendency to scissor at the hips, excessive knee flexion in a crouched posture, and lack of heel contact or tendency to drag feet during swing due to a tiptoe pattern. These children may also elevate their arms with elbows flexed at shoulder level in a midguard posture to assist with balance. The scissoring pattern is most commonly due to hip adductor spasticity, but excessive hip and knee flexion combined with excessive internal hip rotation also play a significant role. Tight hamstrings can cause a flat back, posterior pelvic tilt, and lack of knee extension in swing and stance. Gastrocnemius spasticity can contribute to lack of heel contact in stance and a footdrop during swing known as equinus gait. It is important to distinguish between apparent versus true equinus. Apparent equinus is a compensatory tiptoe pattern due to knee extensor weakness and has been the cause of many cases of inappropriate heel cord lengthening. Stiff knee gait is another common pattern in children with spastic diplegia with an overactive rectus femoris muscle causing delayed or absent knee flexion in swing.

Children with spastic hemiplegia may circumduct at the hip during swing phase to clear their involved limb due to weakness over hip flexors and/or tightness at the ankle. Tiptoe pattern with lack of heel contact may signify spasticity over the gastrocnemius muscle, which is often accompanied by knee hyperextension in stance. There is often reduced or absent arm swing over the involved side.

Dystonia refers to a hyperkinetic movement disorder characterized by intermittent or sustained involuntary muscle contractions resulting in twisting, abnormal postures, or repetitive movements. Children with dystonia may manifest with similar gait deviations as those with spasticity. However, it is important to note that individuals with dystonia will have preserved or accentuated muscle bulk compared to patients with spasticity. In patients with mild dystonia, joint range of motion may be preserved, but for those with progressive dystonic syndrome, eventual joint contracture is likely to develop. Another unique feature of dystonia is the dynamic nature of the hypertonic pattern as dystonia is affected by movement intention/execution, other affected muscle groups (ie, overflow, mirror dystonia), type of activity (ie, task specificity), and various emotional states.

Ataxic Gait

Ataxic gait is characterized by variability in step length, direction, and duration. Children with ataxia appear "clumsy" when walking. Ataxic children also have poor upright balance and adapt a broad base of support to compensate. This broad base is seen during walking as well as upright standing. There is increased variability in step width, length, and duration. Steps are typically shorter. Veering side to side may be present as well. Ataxic patients have great difficulty in performing tandem walking. There may be increased truncal swaying. Titubation, a slow tremor of the trunk and head, may also be present. Patients with ataxia also frequently have axial hypotonia. Due to difficulty with coordinating movements and impaired postural balance, children with ataxia prefer to walk at higher speeds to mask some of the difficulty in coordinating complex joint movements necessary for ambulation.

Choreiform Gait

Choreiform gait involves the superimposed presence of chorea on the gait cycle. Irregular flowing movements can be observed at rest or when standing. Similar to ataxic gait, stepping appears uncoordinated with variability in step width, length, and duration. In fact, choreiform gait can resemble both ataxic and myoclonic gait. Some clues can be obtained from full neurologic examination. For instance, chorea and myoclonus can be seen when awake patients are fully at rest, whereas ataxic patients may have abnormal oculomotor findings.

Myoclonic Gait

Myoclonus can impair both quiet stance and swing phases. It can cause a "bouncing" appearance. This appearance is observed more frequently in negative myoclonus (sudden, brief interruption of muscle activity) compared to positive myoclonus (sudden muscle contraction). Myoclonus is the fastest movement disorder, and the velocity of myoclonus cannot be voluntarily produced, which helps to distinguish it from slower, bouncy movements that can be seen in the context of functional gait. Electrophysiology studies may be indicated to distinguish between myoclonic and choreiform gait since subtle chorea may be visually challenging to identify.

Parkinsonian Gait

Parkinsonism is characterized by bradykinesia (slowness of movement), rigidity, rest tremor, and postural instability. Particularly in children with parkinsonism, there is often co-occurring dystonia. Parkinsonism is uncommon in children. It is crucial to rule out iatrogenic parkinsonism before considering other differential diagnoses. Juvenile parkinsonism syndromes can have early onset, so some children never achieve independent ambulation. Parkinsonian gait is characterized by adopting a stooped posture with a narrow base. Gait is slow and arm swing is severely reduced. There is often a difficulty with initiating gait. Children may walk with short, shuffling steps, and festination (characterized by progressively increasing cadence with a co-occurring progressive decrease in step length) can occur. Postural instability is assessed by using the pull test.

Stiffness Gait

Stiff person syndrome in childhood is rare and can be due to underlying genetic or autoimmune causes. Stiffness syndrome is characterized by continuous motor unit activity at rest. When these abnormal motor activities affect truncal muscles (eg, abdominal, paraspinal), patients present with classic description of axial rigidity and lumbar hyperlordosis. They can also present with stiffness and reduced range of motion in joints of the lower extremity.

Functional Gait

Functional gait is a common manifestation of a functional neurologic disorder (FND). While it can be observed in isolation, approximately 90% of patients will have other co-occurring manifestations of FND. Clinical features suggestive of functional gait include exaggerated verbal and physical behaviors of effort disproportionate to the disability, extreme slowness, variability throughout the day, uneconomic or unusual postures, knee buckling, collapses, convulsive tremors, astasia-abasia, bouncing, and distractibility. Despite the seemingly severe and disabling appearance of the gait and reported disability, patients often will not report falling. If there is reported falling, often there is no significant associated injuries. Appearance of "controlled falls" may be observed. The clinical course can range from static/nonprogressive to extreme variability in phenomenology and severity over time. There may also be spontaneous remissions as well as sudden relapses. It is important to note that the presence of FND does not preclude the co-occurrence of organic neurologic disease.

Abnormal Gait Due to Peripheral Nervous System Disorders

Abnormal gait due to peripheral nervous system disturbances is characterized by the presence of weakness or sensory deficits. There may be footdrop resulting in a steppage gait. This gait pattern consists of excessively flexing at the hip and knee during the swing phase to avoid dragging the toes during stepping. Trendelenburg gait refers to compensation for weakness of the hip abductors during stance leading to dropping of the pelvis on the contralateral side during the swing phase. Children with Trendelenburg gait lean toward the stance leg to avoid dropping of the pelvis on the contralateral side.

Myopathic gait is characterized by usually progressive muscle weakness. On examination, muscular weakness will be evident and is more often pronounced in proximal muscle groups, which can be demonstrated with the Gower sign. Typical findings in the gait of myopathic children include reduced speed and range of motion, short stride length, reduced foot-floor clearance, increased energy expenditures, and increased lateral displacement of the center of gravity while walking. Due to hip extensor weakness, patients often exhibit lumbar lordosis. Toe-walking may also be observed as a compensatory mechanism for proximal weakness. Walking typically has a waddling appearance.

Patients with sensory deficits, particularly deficits in proprioception, develop a gait pattern similar to that of patients with cerebellar ataxia. Their steps are typically short, and the base of support can be broad. The entire foot seems to contact the ground at the same time to maximize afferent sensory inputs for gait stability. These patients will have marked increase in sway with the Romberg test and often fall. Deep tendon reflexes can be a helpful clue as to the location of the deficit, as patients with peripheral nerve deficits will typically have depressed or absent reflexes, whereas those with spinal cord lesions may have exaggerated reflexes. It is also worth noting that patients who have lesion localization at the nerve root level (eg, Guillain-Barré syndrome) may present with sensory changes as well as proximal muscle weakness.

CONCLUSION

In summary, independent ambulation is a complex motor function that develops early in childhood. Normal gait requires normal function of musculoskeletal and multiple neurologic systems. Careful observation and assessment of neurologic findings provide clues to accurately diagnose abnormal gait phenomenology.

Brain Malformations

Mark B. Schapiro, MD

CLASSIFICATION OF DISORDERS OF BRAIN DEVELOPMENT

Development of the central nervous system occurs in several stages: dorsal induction (3-4 weeks' gestation), ventral induction (3-4 weeks' gestation), cell proliferation (10-18 weeks' gestation), cell migration (3-5 months' gestation), synaptic development (5 months' gestation to postnatal), and myelination (postnatal). Depending on time of insult or error in programming, different disorders result (Table 8–1).

APPROACH

With development of computed tomography scanning and, later, magnetic resonance imaging (MRI) scanning, brain imaging has become the mainstay for the diagnosis of brain malformations. Historically, brain malformations have presented in children with developmental delay, motor disorder, seizures, and abnormalities in head size. However, with improved resolution of prenatal ultrasound complemented by fetal MRI scan, brain malformations are increasingly being recognized in utero.

As one approaches *brain images* of children suspected of having a brain malformation, the following should be examined: **midline structures** (interhemispheric fissure, septum pellucidum, corpus callosum, hypothalamus, pituitary gland, and optic nerves; presence of any interhemispheric lipomas or cysts), **cerebral cortex** (cortical thickness, gyral pattern, and cortical gray-white matter junction), **cerebral white matter** (myelination, presence of any heterotopia or clefts), **subcortical nuclei** (any dysmorphism, midline fusion), **ventricular system** (segmentation of lateral ventricles, size and shape of ventricles, patency of cerebral aqueduct), and **posterior fossa** (brainstem, cerebellum, and craniocervical junction; presence of any cysts).[1] Similarly, in approaching *spinal cord images* in a child with a suspected spinal cord malformation, one should examine the following: **spinal cord** (closure of

neural tube, intramedullary structure, central canal), **conus medullaris and cauda equina** (filum terminalis, level of termination), **vertebral arches**, and **overlying skin**.

If a developmental brain abnormality is discovered, then further *assessment of the underlying cause* should be considered to determine the need for assessment of other organ systems, prognosis, and recurrence risk assessment. A 3-generation family pedigree should be obtained, and family members should be examined if indicated, particularly if there is concern for subtle expression of a disorder. The child should be examined for dysmorphic features and abnormalities in other organ systems. Laboratory testing may include metabolic and/or genetic testing. The latter may involve a chromosomal karyotype to assess for aneuploidy, chromosomal microarray to assess for deletions/duplications, fluorescent in situ hybridization studies to detect microdeletion syndromes, and mutational analysis of individual or groups of genes. If no diagnosis is established, then consideration should be given to DNA extraction and storage or establishment of a lymphoblastoid cell line.

In the following sections, selected aspects of brain malformations will be discussed: imaging, embryology, etiology, assessment, and outcome.

VENTRAL INDUCTION

Ventral induction occurs at 3 to 4 weeks of gestation. Stimulus from prechordal mesoderm results in ventral induction and patterning of the anterior portion of the neural tube (prosencephalon), which is involved in the development of forebrain and facial structures. As a result, cleavage occurs in the sagittal plane to produce paired cerebral hemispheres, lateral ventricles, and basal ganglia; transversely to separate the telencephalon from the diencephalon; and horizontally to produce optic vesicles and olfactory bulbs and tracts. Brain disorders due to ventral induction abnormalities are listed in Table 8–1 (including holoprosencephaly, agenesis of

Table 8–1. Representative brain malformations.

Ventral induction
    Holoprosencephaly: alobar, semilobar, lobar, interhemispheric, septo-optic, holodiencephaly, microform
    Agenesis of the corpus callosum, interhemispheric cysts, pericallosal lipoma
    Septo-optic dysplasia, absent septum pellucidum
Dorsal induction
    Primary neurulation
        Craniorachischisis
        Meningomyelocele, myelocele, meningocele
        Anencephaly
    Secondary neurulation
        Meningocele
        Lumbosacral lipoma (lipoma, lipomeningocele)
        Tight filum terminalus
        Ventral dysraphism (sacral meningocele, neuroenterocyst, sacral agenesis)
        Dermoid tumor, dermoid sinus
        Myelocystocele
    Postneurulation defect
        Cephalocele: meningocele, encephalocele
Malformations of cortical development
    Malformations secondary to abnormal neuronal and glial proliferation or apoptosis (congenital microcephaly, megalencephaly, cortical dysgeneses with abnormal cell proliferation)
    Malformations due to abnormal neuronal migration (periventricular nodular heterotopia, lissencephaly, subcortical heterotopia, cobblestone malformations)
    Malformations secondary to abnormal postmigrational development (polymicrogyria, schizencephaly; focal cortical dysplasias type without dysmorphic neurons; postmigrational developmental microcephaly)
Posterior fossa
    Molar tooth–associated malformations (Joubert syndrome)
    Dandy-Walker malformation
    Pontocerebellar hypoplasia

Data from Barkovich AJ, Guerrini R, Kuzniecky RI, et al. A developmental and genetic classification for malformations of cortical development: update 2012. *Brain*. 2012;135(Pt 5):1348–1369.

the corpus callosum, absent septum pellucidum, and septo-optic dysplasia).

Clues to these disorders are found with examination of midline structures and the ventricular system on imaging. For example, if the **interhemispheric fissure** is absent with the cerebral cortex continuous across the midline and the **ventricle** is incompletely segmented, then holoprosencephaly is present. Other abnormalities in the ventricular system should be looked for, such as colpocephaly (disproportionate prominence of the occipital horns of the lateral ventricles), which often accompanies agenesis of the corpus callosum. The presence or absence of the **corpus callosum** with or without an interhemispheric cyst or pericallosal lipoma should be noted, as well as whether the **pituitary gland** is abnormal or ectopic. If the **septum pellucidum** is absent, then this may be isolated or may be associated with other midline abnormalities, such as optic nerve hypoplasia, abnormal or ectopic pituitary, or agenesis of the corpus callosum. Other clues to these brain malformations of ventral induction can be found on facial (cleft lip and palate, abnormalities in nose and teeth) and ophthalmologic (hypotelorism) appearance.

Neurodevelopmental abnormalities are typically present in disorders of ventral induction, most prominent in the more severe disorders. Hypothalamic-pituitary dysfunction is a concern in all of these disorders and can be life-threatening. Optic nerve hypoplasia is also a common association that may present with visual impairment or abnormal eye movements.

HOLOPROSENCEPHALY

▶ Imaging

In holoprosencephaly, in which there is incomplete cleavage of the prosencephalon into right and left hemispheres, into telencephalon and diencephalon, and into olfactory and optic bulbs and tracts, various degrees of abnormal hemispheric segmentation can occur and are evident on brain imaging (Figure 8–1).[2] Examination of the lateral ventricles, cerebral cortex, interhemispheric fissure, septum pellucidum, deep gray matter structures, and corpus callosum on brain imaging allows classification of the different variants in the holoprosencephaly spectrum based on the degree of separation of structures (see Table 8–2 for clinical subtypes).[3-8] A posterior dorsal cyst may be present in all variants, except the septo-optic variant and microform holoprosencephaly.

The disturbance in ventral induction additionally may cause abnormalities of the face and eyes, the severity of which often parallels those abnormalities in the brain. The range of abnormalities may include oral structures (cleft lip/palate to single maxillary central incisor), the nose (proboscis to closely spaced nares), and eyes (cyclopia to hypotelorism). Microcephaly will be present.

Additional clinical subtypes have been defined in recent years. In microform holoprosencephaly, there are holoprosencephaly-related craniofacial anomalies (milder anomalies, such as single incisor or hypotelorism) without major structural brain defects on imaging (cleavage of hemispheres occurs; may have subtle midline brain malformations, such as agenesis of corpus callosum), whereas in holodiencephaly, there is thalamic noncleavage without hemispheric noncleavage.

▶ Embryology

In the rostral neural tube, dorsal-ventral patterning occurs during the first 4 weeks of gestation through the interaction

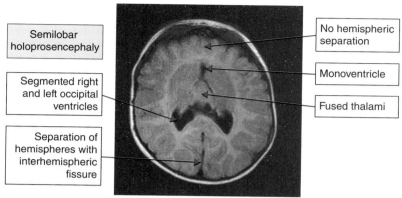

Semilobar holoprosencephaly

No hemispheric separation

Segmented right and left occipital ventricles

Monoventricle

Fused thalami

Separation of hemispheres with interhemispheric fissure

▲ **Figure 8–1.** Semilobar holoprosencephaly.

of ventral patterning signals (sonic hedgehog from the prechordal plate and, later, the floor plate) and dorsal patterning signals (eg, bone morphogenetic proteins and ZIC2 protein arising from the roof plate). It is hypothesized that holoprosencephaly results from a lack of production of ventralizing factors or an overproduction of dorsalizing factors resulting in noncleavage of the midline structures.[5,9]

▶ Etiology

The etiology is heterogeneous, including environmental (maternal diabetes in humans; statins, alcohol, retinoic acid in animal models) or heritable (chromosomal [numeric or structural abnormalities] or syndromic or nonsyndromic single-gene disorders) conditions. Common nonsyndromic single genes include *SHH*, *ZIC2*, *SIX3*, and *TGIF*. Facial malformations are frequent in *SHH* (ventral signal) mutations

and infrequent in *ZIC2* (dorsal signal) mutations. Overall, chromosomal abnormalities and syndromic disorders are the most common causes.

▶ Assessment

The assessment of holoprosencephaly begins with defining the severity of the brain malformation, identifying any associated interhemispheric cyst or other brain malformations, and noting any abnormalities of the face and eyes. Dysmorphic features or other organ system involvement should be searched for, which may suggest a chromosomal or syndromic cause. Hypothalamic-pituitary dysfunction should be tested for due to the high frequency of abnormalities. A maternal history for diabetes and toxic exposure should be queried. The parents should be examined for microforms of holoprosencephaly. Genetic studies may include

Table 8–2. Imaging features of different subtypes of holoprosencephaly.

	Ventricle	Cortex	IHF	Deep Nuclei	CC
Alobar	Monoventricle	No cerebral hemispheric separation	Absent	Lack of cleavage	Absent
Semilobar	Rudimentary occipital and temporal horns	Lack of cleavage anterior	Present posterior	Varying lack of cleavage	Absent, except splenium
Lobar	Small frontal horns	Partial lack of cleavage frontal lobes (basal)	Anterior incompletely developed	Separation	Rostrum, genu absent
MFV	Normal or hypoplastic frontal horns	Lack of cleavage posterior frontal/parietal lobes	Incomplete posterior frontal/parietal lobes	Separation (except fusion thalamus)	Absent body
SOV	Normal or small frontal horns; hypoplastic anterior III ventricle	Lack of cleavage septal/preoptic regions	Present		Rostrum absent or hypoplastic; genu hypoplastic

CC, corpus callosum; IHF, interhemispheric fissure; MFV, middle interhemispheric fusion variant; SOV, septo-optic variant.
Notes: Deep nuclei: basal ganglia, thalamus, and hypothalamus. Septum pellucidum absent in alobar, semilobar, and lobar variants.

high-resolution karyotype, chromosomal microarray, and specific gene testing.

Outcome

Frequent problems in children with holoprosencephaly include hydrocephalus, seizures, motor impairment, oromotor dysfunction, aspiration, gastrointestinal problems (poor gastric emptying, gastroesophageal reflux, and constipation), hypothalamic dysfunction (abnormal sleep-wake cycles, temperature instability, and impaired thirst mechanisms), and endocrine dysfunction.[10] Survival and developmental outcome are related to severity of brain malformation, severity of facial malformation, presence of chromosomal abnormality or syndromic cause, and presence of a multiple congenital anomaly syndrome or other organ involvement. However, virtually all children with classic holoprosencephaly (alobar, semilobar, and lobar) have developmental disabilities. Children with chromosomal abnormalities or syndrome causes have a higher perinatal mortality, whereas children with isolated holoprosencephaly (no associated chromosomal abnormality or syndrome) have the best survival.

AGENESIS OF THE CORPUS CALLOSUM

Imaging

Examination of the corpus callosum, the largest interhemispheric commissure, on brain imaging is an important step in assessing for a brain malformation of ventral induction (Figure 8–2). Imaging may show complete or partial agenesis of the corpus callosum, with or without an associated interhemispheric cyst or pericallosal lipoma. If agenesis of the corpus callosum is present, the gyri extend to the third ventricle ("radial spokes"), as seen on a midline sagittal image (Figure 8–3). The ventricles have a parallel appearance (like "railroad tracks") on axial slices (Figure 8–4), while they appear like "moose horns" or "Viking helmets" on coronal sections (Figure 8–5). Colpocephaly, a disproportionate prominence of the occipital horns of the lateral ventricles, may be present.

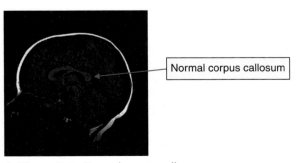

Normal corpus callosum

▲ **Figure 8–2.** Normal corpus callosum.

Embryology

The corpus callosum forms between the 8th and 20th weeks of gestation when commissural axons from the cortex are attracted to the midline massa commissuralis cells by chemoattractant proteins. These commissural axons then cross the midline without recrossing due to subsequent production of repellent proteins by the midline cells and continue on to their final targets in the contralateral hemispheres. The posterior genu and anterior body appear first, followed by the posterior body, inferior genu, splenium, and rostrum.

Agenesis of the corpus callosum may be primary, in which there is a failure of callosal fibers to develop or a failure to cross the midline (with resultant Probst bundles), or secondary, with association with other brain malformations, or degeneration or atrophy of the callosal fibers.

Etiology

The etiology is heterogeneous, including cytogenetic abnormalities, metabolic disorders (eg, maternal phenylketonuria, nonketotic hyperglycinemia, methylenetetrahydrofolate reductase deficiency), toxins (maternal alcohol use), infections (maternal rubella and cytomegalovirus), and genetic (eg, Aicardi syndrome [X-linked; characterized by the triad of chorioretinal lacunae, MRI brain abnormalities, and infantile spasms], *L1CAM*, and Mowat-Wilson syndrome).

Assessment

In the evaluation of agenesis of the corpus callosum, a maternal history for toxic exposure or infection should be obtained. An ophthalmologic exam is particularly important in girls to look for chorioretinal lacunae, a marker for Aicardi syndrome. The identification of dysmorphic features or other organ system involvement may suggest a syndromic disorder. Hypothalamic-pituitary dysfunction is most likely to occur if there is associated optic nerve hypoplasia (suggesting septo-optic dysplasia spectrum).

Outcome

The neurodevelopmental outcome is impacted by presence of other brain anomalies. The developmental outcome is normal in 60% to 80% if there is no other brain anomaly (or underlying etiology), as opposed to 25% if the agenesis of the corpus callosum is not isolated.[11,12] In addition, the underlying cause, if identified, also will influence developmental outcome. Prognosis is much less favorable if there is an associated brain malformation, genetic syndrome, cytogenetic abnormality, or infectious, metabolic, or toxic cause. Pericallosal lipomas typically remain asymptomatic and do not impact outcome.[13]

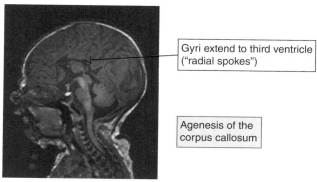

Gyri extend to third ventricle
("radial spokes")

Agenesis of the
corpus callosum

▲ **Figure 8–3.** Agenesis of the corpus callosum.

ABSENT SEPTUM PELLUCIDUM/ SEPTO-OPTIC DYSPLASIA

▶ Imaging

Examination of the septum pellucidum may provide clues to disorders in the septo-optic dysplasia spectrum. Brain imaging may show complete or partial agenesis of the septum pellucidum (Figure 8–6), either in isolation or in association with abnormalities in optic nerves (hypoplasia) and in the hypothalamic-pituitary axis (absence or ectopic location of the pituitary gland and changes in the infundibulum).

▶ Embryology

The septum pellucidum is a thin double membrane in the midline extending from the body of the corpus callosum superiorly to the fornix and rostrum of the corpus callosum inferiorly, separating the 2 sides of the anterior horns and body of the lateral ventricles. Although the septum pellucidum is not necessary for normal brain function, its absence can indicate the presence of other central nervous system abnormalities, including septo-optic dysplasia, absent corpus callosum, holoprosencephaly, and hydrocephalus.

The diagnosis of septo-optic dysplasia is established when 2 or more of the following features are present: (1) unilateral or bilateral optic nerve hypoplasia; (2) pituitary hormone abnormalities/abnormal function of the hypothalamic-pituitary axis; or (3) midline brain defects, including agenesis of the septum pellucidum and/or corpus callosum. All 3 features are present in 40% to 50% of cases, optic nerve hypoplasia and endocrine abnormalities (with normal septum pellucidum/corpus callosum; septo-optic dysplasia–like) in about 20% of cases, and optic nerve hypoplasia with absent septum pellucidum or agenesis of the corpus callosum (with normal endocrine function) in about 35% of cases; endocrine dysfunction with absent septum pellucidum or agenesis of the corpus callosum (with normal optic nerves) is rare. Septo-optic dysplasia plus (presence of associated malformations of cortical development, such as schizencephaly, polymicrogyria, and hippocampal malrotation) is more common with midline brain abnormalities (absent septum pellucidum or agenesis of the corpus callosum).

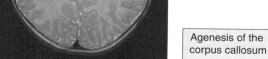

Ventricles parallel
("train track")

Agenesis of the
corpus callosum

▲ **Figure 8–4.** Agenesis of the corpus callosum.

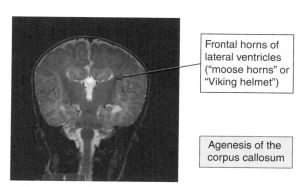

Frontal horns of
lateral ventricles
("moose horns" or
"Viking helmet")

Agenesis of the
corpus callosum

▲ **Figure 8–5.** Agenesis of the corpus callosum.

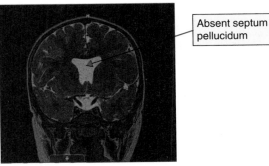

Absent septum pellucidum

▲ **Figure 8–6.** Absent septum pellucidum.

Etiology

In most cases of septo-optic dysplasia, no cause is identified. Mutations in developmental genes involved in the formation of eyes, pituitary, and forebrain structures (*HESX1*, *SOX2*, *SOX3*, and *OTX2*) have been identified, but only rarely. An increased prevalence in association with antenatal drug and alcohol abuse and younger maternal age, and the observation that the different components of the syndrome are embryonically unrelated in origin and timing of formation have led to the hypothesis that it is due to a vascular disruption syndrome.[14]

Assessment

In neonates with an absent septum pellucidum identified on fetal imaging, a careful assessment is needed after birth.[15] Nystagmus or strabismus raises the concern of optic nerve hypoplasia; this is best assessed with clinical exam by ophthalmology. Hypothalamic-pituitary dysfunction, which can be life threatening, is suspected with the presence of hypoglycemia, excessive or prolonged jaundice, microphallus with or without undescended testes, diabetes insipidus, hypothermia, hypotension, persistent bradycardia, and failure to thrive; this should be assessed with endocrinology testing. Pituitary hormone insufficiencies may evolve over time, so endocrinology follow-up will be needed, particularly in the presence of optic nerve hypoplasia. In babies with prior fetal MRI scan showing isolated absent septum pellucidum, a postnatal MRI of the brain is usually not immediately needed unless there are abnormalities found on postnatal endocrine or ophthalmologic assessments or concerns for additional findings (eg, hydrocephalus or seizures).

Outcome

The neurodevelopmental outcome is generally favorable in isolated absent septum pellucidum,[16] whereas it is more variable in septo-optic dysplasia, with developmental delay occurring in 50% to 75% of patients (more likely if there is bilateral vs unilateral optic nerve hypoplasia).[17,18] Outcome is not noted to be more severe in those with septo-optic dysplasia plus. Hypothalamic-pituitary dysfunction is noted in 55% or more of patients, likely influenced by referral pattern.[19]

DORSAL INDUCTION

Dorsal induction occurs in 2 stages: primary neurulation and secondary neurulation (caudal neural tube formation). Development of the neural plate from the ectodermal germ layer is induced by peptide growth factors and their inhibitors. **Primary neurulation**, the process of neural tube closure, occurs soon after, starting in the middle of the neural tube (hindbrain/cervical region) at approximately day 21 after fertilization and proceeding toward the anterior and posterior neuropores (open regions of the neural folds); closure of the neural tube is completed by 26 to 28 days. Different regions of the neural axis have different morphologic and molecular requirements for closure, so a neural tube defect typically affects only a portion of the neural tube.[20]

The rostral region of the neural tube becomes the brain, and the caudal region gives rise to the spinal cord. Patterning of the neural tube along the rostrocaudal axis (with subdivision of the neural plate into its major functional domains—telencephalon, diencephalon, mesencephalon, metencephalon, myelencephalon, and spinal cord) and dorsoventral axis (with differentiation into various neuronal and glial cell types) involves differential cell proliferation and signaling gradients from induction factors secreted from flanking endodermal and mesodermal cells and, later, secondary organizing centers within the neural tube interacting with genes whose expression defines individual territories or cell types.[21]

Disorders of primary neurulation, which are not skin covered, include failure of initiation of neural tube closure (resulting in craniorachischisis) or failure of neuropore closure (disturbances of anterior neuropore closure include anencephaly and dermal sinus, while defects of posterior neuropore closure include meningomyelocele, myelocele, and meningocele).

Secondary neurulation (caudal neural tube formation), the process by which the neural tube caudal to the mid-sacral region is formed, occurs by a distinct mechanism. There is coalescence of a caudal cell mass that then undergoes canalization to form the lumen of the neural tube for the lower sacral and coccygeal regions.[20] Disorders of secondary neurulation, in which the neural tube is skin covered, include meningocele, tight filum terminalus, myelocystocele, dermoid tumor, dermoid sinus, lumbosacral lipoma, and ventral dysraphism (sacral meningocele and sacral agenesis).

Clues to disorders of primary and secondary neurulation at the **spinal** level are found with clinical examination of the skin over the back and imaging of the spinal cord. For example, if examination of the **overlying skin** shows a sacral dimple (especially if a large cleft or >2.5 cm from the anus), hair tuff, lipoma, hemangioma, sinus tract, or nevus flammeus simplex, or if there is failure of closure of **vertebral arches**, then occult spinal dysraphism should be suspected.[22,23] The **spinal cord** should be examined to determine if there has been failure of closure of the neural tube, duplication, splitting, or central canal enlargement. The **conus medullaris** should be examined for level of termination and the **filum terminalis** for thickening or other abnormalities.

Clues to these disorders at the **rostral** level are found with imaging of the posterior fossa and other cerebral structures. The **posterior fossa** should be assessed to determine if it is small with associated crowding of structures and if there are any defects in the tentorium. Any herniation of the **cerebellar tonsils and vermis** through the foramen magnum, as well as any abnormal shape of the cerebellar tonsils, should be noted. The **ventricles** should be assessed for enlargement to suggest hydrocephalus. Associated **brain malformations**, such as agenesis of the corpus callosum and gray matter heterotopia, or **protrusion** of meninges and brain through a bony defect in the skull should be searched for.

FAILURE OF PRIMARY NEURULATION

Abnormal development during primary or secondary neurulation is known as dysraphia. Open neural tube (primary neurulation) defects result from failure of initiation or completion of neural tube closure. With incomplete neural tube closure, the neuroepithelium is exposed to amniotic fluid with resultant destruction.

▶ Craniorachischisis

Failure of the neural tube to initiate closure causes craniorachischisis with most of the brain and the entire spinal cord open. This is not compatible with survival.

▶ Meningomyelocele/Myelocele

Defects of posterior neuropore closure result in meningomyelocele (neural tissues are enclosed in a meninges-covered sac),

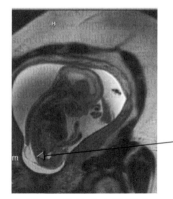

Fetal MRI demonstrating meningomyelocele

▲ **Figure 8–7.** Fetal MRI demonstrating meningomyelocele.

myelocele (neural tissues are exposed directly to amniotic fluid), or meningocele (meninges-covered sac without neural tissues). Secondarily, the vertebral arches fail to properly develop at the level of incomplete neural tube closure with resultant open vertebral column (spina bifida), allowing herniation of neural tissue and/or meninges-covered sac. Children with these defects have abnormalities of the spinal cord and brain with resultant neurologic impairment and secondary complications of other organ systems.[20,24]

Imaging

Spinal cord imaging, in addition to demonstrating meningomyelocele/myelocele (Figure 8–7), may show hydromyelia (abnormal widening of the central canal of the spinal cord), syringomyelia (fluid-filled cyst in spinal cord), diplomyelia (cord duplication), or diastematomyelia (longitudinal split in spinal cord). Typically, the conus medullaris is positioned lower in the spinal column due to attachment to the placode, with resultant tethering of the spinal cord (Figure 8–8).

Among the brain abnormalities noted on imaging in children with meningomyelocele, **hydrocephalus** occurs in the

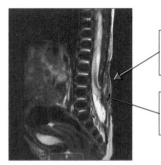

Meningomyelocele: Post-surgical and dysraphic changes at L3 through sacrum

Elongated spinal cord extending into an ill-defined placode in the dorsal thecal sac at L4

▲ **Figure 8–8.** Meningomyelocele.

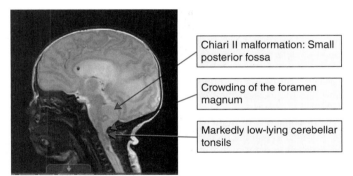

Chiari II malformation: Small posterior fossa

Crowding of the foramen magnum

Markedly low-lying cerebellar tonsils

▲ **Figure 8–9.** Chiari II malformation.

majority of children, being more common with higher-level lesions; it usually is treated with a ventricular shunt, which is subject to failure and infection. A **Chiari II malformation**, with a small posterior fossa, herniation of cerebellar vermis/tonsils, brainstem, and fourth ventricle through the foramen magnum into the cervical spinal canal, and elongation of the pons and fourth ventricle, occurs in almost all children whose meningomyelocele is above the sacral level (Figure 8–9).[24] **Other malformations** (eg, agenesis of the corpus callosum, absent septum pellucidum, gray matter heterotopia) and diffuse microstructural anomalies may also occur.[25]

Etiology

The causes of neural tube defects are multifactorial, with contributions from both genetic and environmental factors. Although most neural tube defects occur sporadically, there nonetheless is evidence for a genetic component contributing to the etiology of these defects. Genes that have been identified include human orthologs of genes whose mutation causes neural tube defects in mice and genes related to environmental risk factors.[20] Environmental factors that have been identified include maternal medications (valproic acid, carbamazepine, nonsteroidal anti-inflammatory drugs, opioid pain medications, and sulfonamides), fever, excessive use of hot tubs, obesity, diabetes, and low blood levels of folate.[26] It has been estimated that 50% to 60% of neural tube defects are preventable through preconceptional and periconceptional folic acid intake.[27] The Centers for Disease Control and Prevention recommended in 2 separate statements in 1991 and 1992 that (1) all reproductive-age women should consume 0.4 mg of folic acid in addition to a folate-rich diet; (2) women who have had an neural tube–affected pregnancy should consume 0.4 mg of folic acid per day, unless they are planning a pregnancy; and (3) women who have had a prior pregnancy affected by neural tube defects and are planning to start a new pregnancy, after consulting with their physician, should consume a 4.0-mg daily dose of folic acid, from at least 1 month before conception through the first 3 months

of pregnancy. The US Food and Drug Administration later mandated fortification of enriched cereal grain products such as flour, bread, and corn meal (January 1, 1998). These measures have resulted in a significant decrease in the prevalence of neural tube defects around the world.

Assessment

In the evaluation of myelomeningocele, a maternal history of prior neural tube defect, medication use (eg, valproate or folate acid antagonists), maternal fevers, excessive use of hot tubs, diabetes, obesity, and folate supplementation should be obtained.

The location of the neural tube defect should be noted, along with whether or not the placode is enclosed within a meninges-covered sac and whether exposed neural tissue was subjected to amniotic fluid, which may have resulted in neurologic damage in addition to that caused by the malformation itself. A neurologic exam should be performed looking for loss of motor and sensory function due to the spinal lesion; a mixture of upper and lower motor signs is typically present depending on the level of the lesion.[28]

Ventricular size should be determined on imaging; a ventricular drainage procedure is usually needed due to hydrocephalus, although not always in the neonatal period. In addition to searching for imaging evidence of a Chiari II malformation, clinical symptoms and signs should be assessed, including dysphagia, aspiration, hoarseness/stridor, apnea, and extremity motor dysfunction; posterior fossa decompression may be needed.[24] Other brain malformations should be noted.

Neurogenic bladder and bowel function will occur with lesions at all levels. Potential orthopedic complications should be assessed, such as contractures (including club feet), hip dislocation, scoliosis, kyphosis, and vertebral anomalies.

Standard of care for babies born with meningomyelocele/myelocele is postnatal repair within 3 postnatal days in order to prevent further injury and infection; this involves detethering the cord, restoring the tissue to the spinal canal, closing the dura, and providing skin coverage over the defect. Multiple subsequent surgeries are commonly required to alleviate re-tethering of the spinal cord, treat hydrocephalus, and/or address orthopedic, urologic, and/or bowel problems. Latex precautions are taken.

Fetal repair, either by open repair or fetoscopic repair, is being increasingly used since a clinical trial showed a significantly reduced need for ventriculoperitoneal shunt and improved composite score of mental development and motor function.[29] However, there is a risk of premature birth with associated complications.

Outcome (Spinal Cord)

With the spinal cord abnormality, there is typically both motor paralysis and sensory loss below the level of the lesion. Classification of the degree of impairment can be anatomic (level of neurologic impairment) or functional based on predictions for mobility (sacral level, low lumbar level, thoracic or high lumbar level).[30] Although lesion level is the primary determinant of motor outcome, motor function is also impacted by any associated hydromyelia/syrinx, diastematomyelia, diplomyelia, Chiari II malformation, hydrocephalus, complications of shunt treatment, and other brain malformations.

Loss of **motor** function in the lower extremities results in problems with limb movement (with the risk for joint contractures), posture (with development of scoliosis and kyphosis, impacted by associated vertebral anomalies), and mobility. Loss of **sensation** leads to decubitus ulcers, particularly at pressure points, and tissue damage from unrecognized hazards. Loss of efferent **autonomic** nerve function results in neurogenic bowel and bladder, which occurs in almost all patients with meningomyelocele.[24]

Due to the spinal cord lesion, which may be associated with diastematomyelia or diplomyelia, the spinal cord is typically positioned lower in the spinal column than in other individuals. With the surgical repair, the spinal cord is typically untethered. However, **re-tethering** can occur with development of new symptoms, such as leg weakness, atrophy, loss of deep tendon reflexes, sensory loss, pain, change in bladder or bowel function, new orthopedic contracture, or scoliosis.[24]

Outcome (Brain)

As a result of brain abnormalities, children with meningomyelocele have learning problems (particularly nonverbal disability and executive and attentional dysfunction), or intellectual disability, and behavioral problems (eg, attention-deficit/hyperactivity disorder). These deficits can be impacted by additional factors, such as shunt complications and seizures. Approximately 15% to 20% of individuals with myelomeningocele develop seizures, with a higher incidence in shunted (particularly in those with shunt revisions or infection) compared to nonshunted patients and in those with brain abnormalities (congenital or acquired). Intellectual disability is the strongest predictor for continued seizures.[31,32]

Children and adults with neural tube defects require ongoing surveillance and care that is best accomplished in a multidisciplinary clinic that specializes in care of such individuals.

Children with a meningocele do not have associated hydrocephalus or abnormal neurologic exam.[28]

▶ Anencephaly

Defects of anterior neuropore closure result in acrania-exencephaly-anencephaly sequence. The open neural folds undergo growth and differentiation, bulging from the cranium (exencephaly) due to absent calvarium (acrania). Exposure to amniotic fluid subsequently causes destruction of the exposed tissue with resultant anencephaly (absence of scalp, skull, cerebral hemispheres, and diencephalic structures and varying amounts of other parts of the brain with characteristic "frog eye" appearance) (Figure 8–10).[20,33] The diagnosis

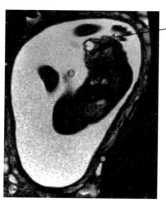

Anencephaly: Absence of cerebral hemispheres and abnormal craniofacial appearance

▲ **Figure 8–10.** Fetal MRI demonstrating Anencephaly.

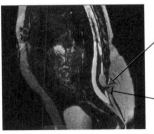

Lumbosacral lipoma: Terminal lipoma extends through a dorsal dysraphic defect at L5 to be contiguous with the subcutaneous fat

Beaking of neural tissue from dorsal aspect of the conus into the dysraphic defect

▲ **Figure 8–11.** L4-5 lipomyelomeningocele.

is usually made in utero with imaging supplemented by maternal serum α-fetoprotein level and/or amniotic fluid α-fetoprotein and acetylcholinesterase levels.

Postnatal criteria include the following: a large portion of the skull is absent; absent scalp over the skull defect; exposed hemorrhagic, fibrotic tissue; and absent recognizable cerebral hemispheres.[34] Infants who are alive at birth usually die within hours or days to weeks after birth, although there have been case reports of prolonged survival.[35]

FAILURE OF SECONDARY NEURULATION (CAUDAL NEURAL TUBE FORMATION)

Disorders of secondary caudal neural tube formation result in malformations with a skin-covered, closed neural tube[20] and include meningocele, tight filum terminalis, myelocystocele, dermoid tumor, dermoid sinus, lumbosacral lipoma (Figure 8–11), and ventral dysraphism (sacral meningocele and sacral agenesis). Clues to these disorders may be found in changes in the overlying skin: sacral dimple, hair tuff, lipoma, hemangioma, sinus tract, or nevus flammeus simplex. Frequently, there is associated tethering of the spinal cord with findings that may include scoliosis; lordosis; back pain (worse with activity); foot deformities; leg weakness, numbness, and pain; decreased deep tendon reflexes; difficulty walking; and incontinence.

POSTNEURULATION DEFECT

▶ Cephalocele

Imaging

In a congenital cephalocele, there is a protrusion of cranial contents in a sac (skin-covered unless rupture has occurred) through a defect in the skull either along the midline or at the skull base: meningocele with protrusion of meninges and cerebrospinal fluid, encephalocele with additional protrusion of brain tissue (usually through the narrow neck of the sac), and meningoencephalocystocele when ventricle is included. The sac may also include venous structures, which may complicate the surgical repair of the lesion.

Brain imaging will show the contents of the sac (whether brain, cerebral vessels, and/or ventricle are present) and the location of the cephalocele (occipital, parietal, basal, or sincipital/frontoethmoidal [nasofrontal, nasoethmoidal, or naso-orbital]) (Figures 8–12 and 8–13). Off-midline lesions (temporal lobe), on occasion, also may occur. Overall, the most common location is occipital, but there is geographic variation: Occipital cephaloceles are the most common type of cephalocele in North America, whereas sincipital/frontoethmoidal cephaloceles are more common in Southeast Asia.

Hydrocephalus frequently occurs and is not associated with location.[36] Other brain malformations may also

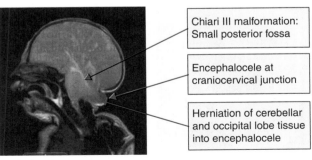

Chiari III malformation: Small posterior fossa

Encephalocele at craniocervical junction

Herniation of cerebellar and occipital lobe tissue into encephalocele

▲ **Figure 8–12.** Occipital encephalocele.

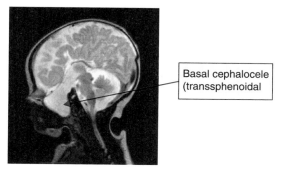

Basal cephalocele (transsphenoidal

▲ **Figure 8–13.** Basal cephalocele (transsphenoidal).

be present: Occipital cephaloceles may be associated with a Chiari III malformation (prolapse of the lower brainstem into the cervical spinal canal, herniation of the cerebellum into an occipito-cervical encephalocele, and small posterior fossa) (see Figure 8–12), Dandy-Walker syndrome, and abnormalities of the corpus callosum; sincipital cephaloceles may be associated with agenesis of the corpus callosum and arachnoid cysts.[37] For a basal cephalocele (see Figure 8–13), any impact on the airway should be noted.

Atretic encephaloceles, which are usually located in the parietal region and contain glial, meningeal (arachnoid), fibrous, and dermal elements, are noted by the vertical embryonic positioning of the straight sinus and prominent superior cerebellar cistern.[38]

Embryology

Different theories have been postulated for the etiology of cephaloceles, but most favor that the error occurs after closure of the neural tube given that the cephalocele is skin-covered. A prominent theory postulates that cephaloceles occur due to the failure of surface ectoderm to separate from the neural ectoderm in the fourth week of gestation, secondarily causing a midline mesodermal insufficiency that results in a bony defect in the skull and/or facial bones.[39] Another theory postulates a failure of neural crest migration, which prevents formation of centers of mesenchymal cells needed for development of bone, cartilage, and muscles of the skull and face.[40]

Other theories propose that neuroschisis occurs after neural tube closure, with resulting adhesions between the surface ectoderm and neural ectoderm preventing mesoderm from interposing between them to form bony structures; abnormal gene signaling from the neural tube; or amniotic bands (particularly for off-midline lesions, such as temporal bone defects).

In the case of sincipital/frontoethmoidal cephaloceles, such changes result in a failure of closure of normal bony foramina: fonticulus frontalis with resultant nasofrontal

cephalocele and foramen cecum with resultant nasoethmoidal and naso-orbital cephaloceles. Basal encephaloceles occur through the cribriform plate, ethmoid and sphenoid bones, craniopharyngeal canal, and superior and inferior orbital fissures.

Etiology

Cephaloceles are usually congenital, although there can be later acquired causes, such as from tumors or injury.[41] Most congenital cases occur sporadically. Genetic factors are thought to contribute to their occurrence, supported by the higher presence in families with neural tube defects and their presence in a number of genetic syndromes, including Meckel-Gruber syndrome and Walker-Warburg syndrome. Environmental factors, such as toxins or infections, are speculated to contribute, although none have been confirmed.

Assessment

Cephaloceles are often diagnosed in utero on prenatal imaging; this allows for prenatal counseling about the nature of the lesion and prognosis, appropriate antenatal monitoring, and planning for the delivery process and postnatal care. A cesarean section may be needed to avoid birth trauma to the sac. For basal cephaloceles, if there is evidence of high airway obstruction on prenatal imaging, then a decision will need to be made prior to delivery on how to manage the airway at birth; an airway to EXIT (ex utero intrapartum treatment) procedure for establishment of airway may be needed.

The postnatal assessment of a cephalocele will begin by determining whether or not the sac is skin-covered, the location, and the contents. Leaking cerebrospinal fluid may lead to infection. Transillumination of the sac may help determine if the sac contains cerebrospinal fluid, blood, or brain tissue. For large posterior cephaloceles, proper head positioning is needed to prevent forward flexion of neck with resultant airway compression; a neurologic exam should be performed, with attention to findings that might be seen with a Chiari malformation. For anterior cephaloceles, any craniofacial abnormalities, such as hypertelorism, broad nasal bridge, cleft palate, or evidence of nasal obstruction or cerebrospinal leak, should be noted. If ventriculomegaly is present, serial head circumferences and imaging may be needed to determine if a cerebrospinal fluid diversion procedure is indicated. A maternal history of prior neural tube defect should be queried. Extracranial manifestations should be looked for that might suggest a syndrome.

For cases without fetal imaging, most cephaloceles are noticeable after birth as a skin-covered mass near the midline of the skull. Exceptions are basal and small sincipital/frontoethmoidal cephaloceles, which may not be noticed and discovered until later when they present with a bulge in the pharynx, nasal mass/obstruction, cerebrospinal leak with recurrent meningitis, hypertelorism, broad nasal bridge, proptosis, frontal mass, or seizures due to associated brain abnormalities.

Outcome

Cephaloceles are treated with surgical excision of the sac and closure of the overlying cutaneous defects; for those with sincipital/frontoethmoidal cephaloceles, orbital translocation may also be needed if hypertelorism is present. Repair is performed electively, usually between birth and a few months of age, unless an urgent indication exists, such as thin or ulcerated skin covering, cerebrospinal fluid leakage with risk of meningitis, hemorrhage, obstructed airway with interference in breathing and feeding, or impairment of vision. The goals of surgery are removal of the sac with dural and skull closure to prevent rupture and infection and facilitate nursing care; preservation of functional neural tissue; wound closure with normal skin; and correction of any craniofacial abnormalities.[42,43] Poorer outcome is associated with hydrocephalus, seizure disorder, microcephaly, presence of associated intracranial abnormalities, and presence of brain tissue in the sac.[43] The location of the encephalocele does not have a statistically significant association with incidence of hydrocephalus or neurologic deficit.[36]

MALFORMATIONS OF CORTICAL DEVELOPMENT

The development of the cerebral cortex involves proliferation of progenitor cells, precursors of neurons and glial cells (oligodendrocytes and astrocytes), in the dorsal ventricular zone of the neural tube and in the ganglionic eminences, migration from dorsal ventricular zone along the processes of radial glial cells for excitatory neurons and by tangential migration from the ganglionic eminences for interneurons to their destination layers of the cortex, and postmigrational organization (dendritic extension and synaptogenesis).

Two classes of neurons populate the cerebral cortex, excitatory glutamatergic cortical neurons and inhibitory GABAergic cortical interneurons, which have different sites of origin. **Excitatory** neurons derive from 2 populations of progenitor cells: radial glial cells in the ventricular zone and intermediate progenitor cells in the subventricular zone. These neural progenitor cells proliferate rapidly in their proliferative zones between 8 and 16 weeks of gestation; the final number of neurons in mature cortex is determined by the number of neocortical founder cells, the proliferation of progenitor population during neurogenesis, and cell death. The radial glial cells, in addition to serving as progenitor cells, extend long processes from their bodies in the ventricular zone to the pial surface to serve as a structural scaffold for migration of generated neurons. Multiple generations of neuronal cells use the same glial fiber for migration. These neurons migrate along the radial glial fibers with the help of microtubules and the microtubule-associated dynein motor complex in the neuron, which provide the push/pull forces required for neuronal migration. Cues for migration regulate the microtubule-associated proteins Ndel1 and Lis1 (components of the dynein motor complex) to sustain function of the dynein and, along with DCX (a microtubule-associated protein), to stabilize the microtubule cytoskeleton. Tub1a is one component of the microtubule. During the migratory process, the cerebral cortex develops in 3 stages: a preplate, a cortical plate, and finally, the mature layered cortex. The preplate serves as a scaffolding for subsequently migrating neuronal cells. Migrating cells then split the preplate to form a superficial part (molecular layer—layer I) and a deep layer (subplate—layer VII; later disappears). The subsequent migrating cells (forming layers II-VI of the definitive cortex) migrate in an "inside out" manner ("birthday" determines position), with earlier migrating cells settling in the deepest cortical layers (large pyramidal cells of layers V and VI) and later generated cells settling in the most superficial layer (layer II) of the cortical plate.[44]

Inhibitory GABAergic cortical interneurons are generated in the medial and lateral ganglionic eminences in the ventral telencephalon and migrate tangentially into the cerebral cortex. This migration appears to follow preexisting axonal tracts. **Glial cells** derive from progenitor cells after neurogenesis is complete. For example, an astrocyte is generated from a glial cell once the cycles of neuronal generation and migration are completed on that glial cell.[44]

Brain disorders due to malformations of cortical development are listed in Table 8-1; the classification scheme,[45] based on the developmental and genetic processes that are disrupted, includes malformations secondary to **abnormal neuronal and glial proliferation or apoptosis** (congenital microcephaly, megalencephaly, cortical dysgeneses with abnormal cell proliferation), malformations due to **abnormal neuronal migration** (periventricular nodular heterotopia, lissencephaly, subcortical heterotopia and sublobar dysplasia, cobblestone malformations), and malformations secondary to **abnormal postmigrational** development (polymicrogyria, schizencephaly).

Clues to these disorders are found with examination of the cerebral cortex and white matter on imaging.[1,46] A change in the **craniofacial ratio** may indicate if the brain is too small or large. Any **asymmetry** in the size of the 2 hemispheres should be noted. The **thickness of the cortex** and the **degree of sulcation** should be determined, as well as any differences in the anterior-posterior pattern. The **cortical surfaces**, inner and outer, should be observed for irregularities. The **location of any polymicrogyria** and whether **unilateral/bilateral** should be assessed. **Heterotopia** should be searched for in periventricular or deep white matter regions; if present, it should be determined if they are nodular or laminar. The presence of **blurring of the gray-white junction** should be noted. In the cerebral white matter, the

myelination pattern should be assessed to determine if there is any delay for age or if diffuse hypomyelination is present (which may be due secondarily to a cortical malformation). Focal areas of abnormal myelination should be ascertained, as may be seen in hemimegalencephaly or focal cortical dysplasia.

As in disorders of induction, significant neurodevelopmental abnormalities are typically present in malformations of cortical development, although some exceptions exist (such as in periventricular nodular heterotopia from *FLNA* mutations). Additionally, seizures frequently are present and often intractable in these disorders.

▷ Malformations Secondary to Abnormal Neuronal and Glial Proliferation or Apoptosis

Imaging

Examination of brain size is the first step in assessing for a brain malformation of abnormal neuronal and glial proliferation or apoptosis. Imaging of the nonsyndromic congenital **microcephalic** brain (which may be 3 standard deviations or more below the mean for age and gender for severe microcephaly) may show normal gyri (suggesting premature exhaustion of neuronal progenitors) or simplified gyri (suggesting both decreased neurons and migration abnormality). The **megalencephalic** brain may be very large, 3 to 10 standard deviations above the mean for age and gender. Imaging will determine if there is bilateral or unilateral brain enlargement (hemimegalencephaly), either with complete or partial hemispheric involvement. If hemimegalencephaly is present, the underlying white matter also may be abnormal with indistinct gray-white matter junction, and heterotopia may be present (Figure 8–14). Additionally, specific regions in megalencephaly may show specific abnormalities more characteristic of specific disorders,

such as a thickened corpus callosum (megalencephaly capillary malformation [MCAP]), perisylvian polymicrogyria (MCAP and megalencephaly-polymicrogyria-polydactyly-hydrocephalus [MPPH]), and cerebellar tonsillar ectopia (MCAP and MPPH). Ventricular enlargement, including hydrocephalus, may be present. **Focal cortical dysplasia** may be suspected on brain MRI with findings of increased cortical thickness, blurring of the cortical gray-white matter junction with disappearance of subcortical white matter digitations, white matter signal abnormalities (increased signal on T2-weighted images) with or without a radially oriented linear or conical transmantle stripe of T2 hyperintensity, gray matter signal changes, abnormal gyral/sulcal patterns, and focal and/or lobar hypoplasia/atrophy.[47]

Embryology/Etiology

Congenital microcephaly results from impairment in neurogenesis due to disruption in pathways primarily involved in DNA replication, mitosis (including cell cycle length, spindle positioning, and centrosome maturation), and DNA repair.

Megalencephaly and cortical dysgeneses with abnormal cell proliferation appear to be due to abnormalities in the regulation of brain cellular proliferation, differentiation, cell cycle regulation, metabolism, survival, and apoptosis, and represent a spectrum of disorders.[48] Dysfunction of tumor suppressor pathways involved in these processes is the pathogenic basis for several representative disorders of megalencephaly and cortical dysgeneses with abnormal cell proliferation, the **phosphatidylinositol-3-kinase/Akt/mTOR pathway** in MPPH, MCAP, PTEN hamartoma tumor syndrome, dysplastic megalencephaly, hemimegalencephaly, and tuberous sclerosis, and the **patched-1/sonic hedgehog signaling pathway** in Gorlin syndrome. Mosaic mutations in the phosphatidylinositol-3-kinase/Akt/mTOR pathway are associated with segmental brain malformations, whereas

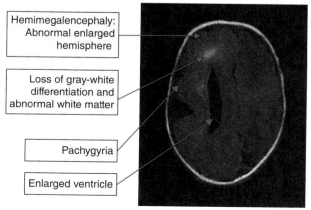

Hemimegalencephaly: Abnormal enlarged hemisphere

Loss of gray-white differentiation and abnormal white matter

Pachygyria

Enlarged ventricle

▲ **Figure 8–14.** Hemimegalencephaly.

germline mutations are associated with diffuse bilateral cortical malformations with megalencephaly.

Assessment/Outcome

Congenital microcephaly—Small brains can be due to acquired causes, inborn errors of metabolism, and genetic disorders (nonsyndromic or syndromic). In the evaluation of congenital microcephaly, a maternal history for exposure to drugs, toxins, or radiation, infection, hypoperfusion events, or trauma should be obtained. In the examination, height should be compared to head circumference: Proportional microcephaly (as part of small stature) may have a different outcome than microcephaly that is disproportionally small compared to height. The sutures should be assessed for evidence of craniosynostosis; if present, a primary versus secondary cause will need to be determined. Children with congenital microcephaly with head size smaller than 3 standard deviations below the mean usually have cognitive impairment to some degree.

Megalencephaly—Large brains can be due to metabolic/storage disease, such as Canavan disease or Alexander disease, or anatomic causes. The latter includes benign familial megalencephaly, overgrowth syndromes (eg, Sotos syndrome), neurocutaneous disorders (eg, neurofibromatosis), fragile X syndrome, and brain overgrowth disorders secondary to abnormal neuronal and glial proliferation or apoptosis (including disorders of tumor suppressor pathways [MPPH, MCAP, PTEN hamartoma tumor syndrome, Gorlin syndrome]).

In addition to imaging clues to brain overgrowth disorders, extracranial manifestations should also be noted, including whether there is polydactyly (MPPH and MCAP), segmental body overgrowth (MCAP), cutaneous vascular malformations (MCAP), dental cysts (Gorlin syndrome), dermatologic features (including lipomas, trichilemmomas, oral papillomas, and penile freckling; PTEN hamartoma syndrome), vascular features (eg, arteriovenous malformations or hemangiomas; PTEN hamartoma syndrome), and gastrointestinal polyps (PTEN hamartoma syndrome). Representative disorders are discussed.

In **MPPH**, the clinical diagnosis is established with the presence of megalencephaly (congenital or early postnatal onset), which is symmetric or mildly asymmetric, and bilateral perisylvian polymicrogyria. Ventricular enlargement is present that may progress to hydrocephalus. Progressive cerebellar ectopia may occur. Extracranial manifestations include postaxial polydactyly and distinct facies (frontal bossing, low nasal bridge, large eyes). Most individuals have a variable level of intellectual disability and seizures. Treatment is symptomatic, including addressing hydrocephalus, progressive and/or symptomatic cerebellar tonsillar ectopia, and epilepsy. Monitoring for hydrocephalus and cerebellar tonsillar herniation has been recommended. It is inherited in

an autosomal dominant manner. Mutations (mostly de novo germline) in 3 genes have been identified: *PIK3R2* and *AKT3* (2 genes in the phosphatidylinositol-3-kinase/Akt/mTOR pathway) and *CCND2* (encodes cyclin D2 protein, which regulates cell division and itself is regulated by the phosphatidylinositol-3-kinase/Akt/mTOR pathway).

The umbrella term **PIK3CA-related overgrowth spectrum (PROS)** is used to encompass a variety of segmental overgrowth phenotypes with somatic (rarely germline) activating *PIK3CA* mutations in the phosphatidylinositol-3-kinase/Akt/mTOR pathway. Within this umbrella, brain disorder phenotypes include MCAP, hemimegalencephaly, and dysplastic megalencephaly.[49] In MCAP, there is megalencephaly that can be significantly asymmetric. In addition to this brain overgrowth, there may be secondary overgrowth of specific brain structures, such as a markedly thick corpus callosum and progressive cerebellar enlargement (which can result in sudden death).[50] MCAP shares phenotypic similarities to MPPH, including congenital or early postnatal megalencephaly, perisylvian polymicrogyria (in a large subset of children), progressive ventriculomegaly that may lead to hydrocephalus, progressive cerebellar tonsillar ectopia, intellectual disability, and seizures. Unlike MPPH, MCAP may be associated with significantly asymmetric brain enlargement and with recognizable somatic features, such as segmental somatic overgrowth and cutaneous vascular malformations. Phenotypic variability is significant, related to the mosaic nature of MCAP syndrome. Treatment is symptomatic, as in MPPH, although research studies are being done on drugs that target the phosphatidylinositol-3-kinase/Akt/mTOR pathway.

For **Gorlin syndrome** (nevoid basal cell carcinoma syndrome), a cancer predisposition syndrome with congenital or postnatal megalencephaly, major and minor criteria for the diagnosis have been established: **Major** criteria include lamellar or early (prior to age 20 years) calcification of the falx, jaw keratocyst, palmar/plantar pits (≥2), multiple basal cell carcinomas (>5 in a lifetime or 1 prior to age 30 years), and first-degree relative with Gorlin syndrome; **minor** anomalies include childhood medulloblastoma, lymphomesenteric or pleural cysts, macrocephaly, cleft lip/palate, vertebral/rib anomalies, preaxial or postaxial polydactyly, ovarian/cardiac fibromas, and ocular anomalies. A diagnosis is made with 2 major or 1 major and 2 minor criteria fulfilled.[51,52] Many individuals also have frontal bossing and hypertelorism. Some motor delay may occur, but cognitive delay is not reported. It is inherited in an autosomal dominant manner. Causative germline mutations in *PTCH1* and *SUFU* (2 genes in the patched-1/sonic hedgehog signaling pathway) and microdeletion of chromosome 9q22.3 have been identified.[53-56] There is differential risk of development of medulloblastoma: 33% risk with *SUFU* pathogenic variant compared to 2% with *PTCH1* pathogenic variant.[57] Preventative measures for primary manifestation include limiting direct sun exposure, and avoiding unnecessary diagnostic radiation and radiotherapy if alternative measures are available. Specific treatments include surgical removal of keratocysts, early treatment of basal cell carcinomas, and sonic hedgehog inhibitors to treat severe basal cell carcinomas. Surveillance is necessary to monitor for tumor and jaw keratocyst development.[52]

PTEN hamartoma tumor syndrome is also a cancer predisposition syndrome that causes overgrowth with tall stature, megalencephaly, cognitive delay, and autism. Pediatric criteria for genetic testing based on clinical features have been established[58] and include macrocephaly and at least one of the following: autism or developmental delay; dermatologic features, including lipomas, trichilemmomas, oral papillomas, or penile freckling; vascular features, such as arteriovenous malformations or hemangiomas; and gastrointestinal polyps. Testing should also be considered with the occurrence of pediatric-onset thyroid cancer and germ cell tumors (testicular cancer and dysgerminoma). The syndrome is due to heterozygous germline mutations in the *PTEN* gene, a tumor suppressor gene in the phosphatidylinositol-3-kinase/Akt/mTOR pathway. Tumor surveillance in pediatrics includes an annual thyroid ultrasound and skin evaluation.

Cortical dysgenesis with abnormal cell proliferation— Included in this group are focal cortical dysplasia type II; hemimegalencephaly; dysplastic megalencephaly (bilateral hemimegalencephaly), now thought to form a spectrum of disorders due to somatic (rarely germline) activating *PIK3CA* and *AKT3* mutations[59]; and tuberous sclerosis complex, due to germline mutations in the *TSC1* or *TSC2* genes.

Focal cortical dysplasias are localized regions of malformed cerebral cortex characterized by cortical dyslamination with or without disordered cell types.[60] Focal cortical dysplasia type II, a malformation due to abnormal proliferation of glioneuronal progenitor cells, is characterized by disruption of cortical lamination associated with dysmorphic neurons without (type IIa) or with (type IIb) balloon cells. Focal cortical dysplasias are a frequent cause of intractable focal epilepsy.

Hemimegalencephaly, which involves overgrowth of one or more lobes of a hemisphere, and the rare dysplastic megalencephaly, which involves both hemispheres, are characterized by cortical dysplasia, white matter abnormalities, and polymicrogyria. They are associated with early onset-intractable epilepsy, contralateral hemiparesis, and intellectual disability. Treatment of epilepsy usually requires hemispherectomy.

▶ Malformations Due to Abnormal Neuronal Migration

Heterotopia (Malformations With Neuroependymal Abnormalities: Periventricular Heterotopia)

Imaging—In assessing for disorders of migration, clusters of heterotopic gray matter, which are isointense to normal gray matter on all MRI sequences and do not enhance with contrast, should be looked for in the periventricular region or deep white matter and categorized by location and morphology. These are an indication of arrested migration. In **periventricular nodular heterotopia**, there will be nodules of heterotopic gray matter of varying size that are localized to the immediate subependymal/periventricular region (Figure 8–15). There may be distortion of the outline of the ventricles. These nodules can be single or multiple (rarely laminar) or bilateral or unilateral, and different brain regions may be involved; for example, with *FLNA* gene mutations, there is diffuse heterotopia that typically spares the temporal regions.[61] The nodules are differentiated from the subependymal nodules of tuberous sclerosis, which are not isointense with gray matter, have variable contrast enhancement, and are calcified in 90% of cases.[62] Periventricular nodular heterotopia may be isolated or may develop in conjunction with central nervous system malformations or metabolic (peroxisomal) disorders.[63] **Subcortical heterotopias** may also occur, which may be transmantle gray (continuous from the ependyma to the cortex) or multiple nodules localized to the deep cerebral white matter; these are classified separately from periventricular nodular heterotopia due to presumed

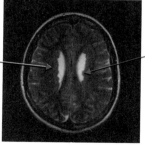

Periventricular nodular heterotopia: Nodular heterotopia lining the periventricular regions bilaterally

Distortion of the ventricles by the heterotopia

▲ **Figure 8–15.** Periventricular nodular heterotopia due to a *FLNA* mutation.

different embryogenesis. When subcortical heterotopia is present, the basal ganglia may be dysmorphic in appearance, as this region's formation is dependent on migration of neurons derived in the medial and lateral ganglionic eminences, areas that generate GABAergic inhibitory neurons that migrate tangentially to the cerebral cortex (see section on subcortical heterotopia and sublobar dysplasia). Finally, **subcortical band heterotopia** should be looked for; this too has a different embryogenesis from the other heterotopia groups (see section on lissencephaly).

Embryology/etiology—In periventricular nodular heterotopia, there are abnormal collections of late-born neurons in the subependymal/periventricular region; the overlying cortex is typically normal. Periventricular nodular heterotopia appears to have a different embryogenesis than other heterotopia and is categorized differently.[45] In periventricular nodular heterotopia due to *FLNA* mutations, it has been suggested that the gene product is important for the development and maintenance of the radial glial scaffold during corticogenesis and that disruption of the polarized radial glial scaffold in the ventricular zone impairs radial glia functions as neural progenitors and guides of neuronal migration with resultant ectopic neuronal nodules.[64]

Periventricular nodular heterotopia is a genetically heterogeneous condition.[65] Mutations in the filamin A (*FLNA*) gene located on chromosome Xq28 (X-linked dominant) and the ADP-ribosylation factor guanine exchange factor 2 (*ARFGEF2*) gene (autosomal recessive) on chromosome 20q13.13 are the most common causes; there are several other less common genetic causes.

Assessment/outcome—Periventricular nodular heterotopia can occur sporadically or be associated with identified genetic mutations or other brain malformations. Those due to *FNLA* mutations, which is X-linked dominant, occur predominantly in woman; there is a high rate of in utero lethality in hemizygous males, and surviving males have greater neurodevelopmental impairment. Affected females usually have epilepsy with intelligence in the normal or mildly impaired range. Other manifestations include cardiovascular defects (valvular heart disease and aortic root dilation) and connective tissue abnormalities (joint hypermobility, skin hyperextensibility, striae, and fragile blood vessels) that may meet criteria for hypermobile Ehlers-Danlos syndrome. In periventricular nodular heterotopia due to *ARFGEF2* mutations, microcephaly is prominent; other phenotypic features include a severe developmental delay, movement disorder, and putaminal hyperintensities.[66]

Lissencephaly (Malformation due to Generalized Abnormal Transmantle Migration)

Imaging—In lissencephaly/pachygyria, there is a **thick cerebral cortex** (more than the normal 2-3 mm; typically 12-20 mm) with few sulci (pachygyria) or absent sulcation (lissencephaly) (Figure 8–16). There may be a **spectrum** of changes, from agyria to pachygyria to subcortical band heterotopia (grading system by Dobyns and Truwit[67]). If there is diffuse agyria, then the brain has an "hourglass" or "figure 8" appearance on imaging (see Figure 8–16). The **anterior-posterior pattern** of any pachygyria/lissencephaly should be noted; a more severe anterior pattern is noted with *DCX* mutations, whereas a more posterior pattern is noted in *PAFAH1B1* and *TUBA1A* mutations. The inner margin of the cortex is smooth. The white matter appears as a narrow ribbon along the ventricles. Other brain malformations, such as cerebellar hypoplasia, may be present. In **subcortical band heterotopia**, there is a laminar layer of gray matter between the cortex and ventricle (often follows the curvature of the overlying cortex), giving a 3-layer appearance (double cortex): cortex and subcortical layer of band heterotopia separated by a thin white matter band.[68]

Embryology/etiology—In the lissencephaly spectrum, there is arrested neuronal migration leading to reduced

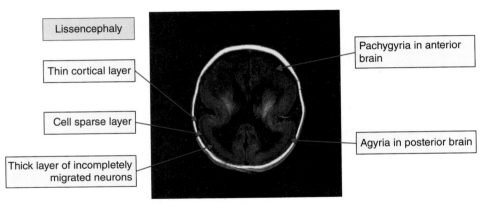

▲ **Figure 8–16.** Lissencephaly due to *PAFAH1B1* gene mutation.

folding (pachygyria or agyria) or subcortical band heterotopia. With agyria in classical lissencephaly, the cerebral cortex is significantly thicker (12-20 mm) than normal and contains 4 layers (molecular layer, cellular layer, cell sparse layer, and thick layer of incompletely migrated neurons extending to the ependyma), rather than the normal 6 layers. The white matter appears as a narrow ribbon along ventricles. With subcortical band heterotopia, there is a distinct band of neurons that is abnormally placed between the ventricle and the superficial cortical layers.

Mutations in genes that regulate components of the microtubule-associated dynein motor complex (*PAFAH1B1*) and microtubules (*DCX* and *TUBA1A*) are found in classical lissencephaly, whereas other genes have been identified in other forms of lissencephaly, including *RELN*, *ARX*, *VLDLR*, and *NDE1*.

Assessment/outcome—The severity of clinical manifestations in lissencephaly spectrum depends on the degree of cortical malformation; however, seizures, intellectual disability, microcephaly, and spasticity to some degree are present.

Several genes have been identified in classical lissencephaly and variant lissencephaly. Classical lissencephaly may be due to a heterozygous deletion or autosomal dominant mutation in the *PAFAH1B1* gene located on chromosome 17p13.3. The former results in Miller-Dieker syndrome, which is characterized by a more severe lissencephaly and dysmorphic facial features (bitemporal narrowing, a high forehead, small nose with anteverted nostrils, upslanted palpebral fissures, protuberant upper lip, and micrognathia). The deletion in these patients includes the *PAFAH1B1* gene, along with several nearby genes including the *YWHAE* (14-3-3e) gene, thus representing a contiguous gene syndrome. In isolated lissencephaly due to *PAFAH1B1* mutation or intragenic deletion of *PAFAH1B1*, the lissencephaly is less severe and dysmorphic features are not significant. The posterior brain region is more affected than the anterior region in classical lissencephaly due to germline mutations of the *PAFAH1B1* gene,[69] as well in rare cases of subcortical band heterotopia due to mosaic mutations in the *PAFAH1B1* gene.[70]

The lissencephaly spectrum disorders due to an X-linked recessive mutation in the doublecortin (*DCX*) gene located on chromosome Xq22.3-q24 often cause a different presentation in males and females, with males having the full spectrum of classical lissencephaly changes, while heterozygous females tend to have subcortical band heterotopia (due to 2 populations of neurons resulting from X chromosome inactivation—one with and one without the mutated gene). Somatic mosaicism for *DCX* may cause sporadic subcortical band heterotopia in both males and females.[71] The anterior brain is more affected than the posterior region in lissencephaly due to a *DCX* mutation.

Autosomal dominant mutations in the *TUBA1A* gene are a rare cause of classical lissencephaly (4-layered with posterior more affected than anterior brain) and a more common cause of variant lissencephaly with cerebellar hypoplasia. The former can have a dysmorphic corpus callosum, whereas the latter can have a cortex that is not as thick as classical lissencephaly, severe cerebellar hypoplasia, dysgenesis/agenesis of the corpus callosum, and a thin brainstem.[72]

Malformations have been found in other genes coding tubulin subunits besides *TUBA1A*, including *TUBA8*, *TUBB2B*, *TUBB3*, *TUBB5*, and *TUBG1*. The resulting disorders, known as tubulinopathies, are characterized by 5 cortical malformation patterns: (1) microlissencephaly; (2) lissencephaly; (3) central pachygyria and polymicrogyria-like cortical dysplasia; (4) generalized polymicrogyria-like cortical dysplasia; and (5) a simplified gyral pattern with area of focal polymicrogyria. Dysmorphic basal ganglia are a characteristic feature of tubulinopathies; agenesis of the corpus callosum and cerebellar hypoplasia are also prevalent.

Mutations in other genes cause lissencephaly, including *ARX*, an X-linked recessive disorder with a 3-layered (no cell sparse zone) moderately thick cortex, posterior brain more affected than anterior, other brain abnormalities (agenesis of the corpus callosum and abnormal basal ganglia), and clinical features of ambiguous genitalia in affected males; *RELN*, an autosomal recessive disorder with inverted cortical lamination (no cell sparse zone), anterior brain more affected than posterior, and severe abnormalities of cerebellum, brainstem, and hippocampus; and *NDE1* (nuclear distribution factor E-homolog 1) gene, an autosomal recessive cause of microlissencephaly.

Subcortical Heterotopia and Sublobar Dysplasia (Malformations Presumably due to Localized Abnormal Late Radial or Tangential Transmantle Migrations)

Subcortical heterotopias may be transmantle gray (continuous from the ependyma to the cortex; columnar or curvilinear) or multiple nodules localized to the deep cerebral white matter. The overlying cortex appears thin with shallow sulci, and the affected hemisphere is abnormally small. They may occur with other migration disorders. The embryogenesis is unknown.[45]

Cobblestone Malformations (Malformations due to Abnormal Terminal Migration and Defects in Pial Limiting Membrane)

Imaging—In cobblestone malformations, with high-resolution imaging, there will be an irregular nodular cortical surface with a thick cortex (~10 mm), although the thickness will not be to the degree seen in classical 4-layered lissencephaly (Figure 8–17). The malformation is usually bilateral and symmetric, typically involving most if not all of the cerebral cortex. The cortical white matter junction will be irregular and the underlying white matter will be hypomyelinated.

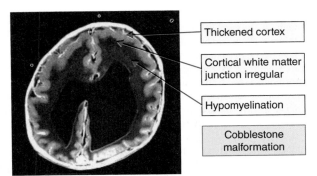

Thickened cortex

Cortical white matter junction irregular

Hypomyelination

Cobblestone malformation

▲ **Figure 8–17.** Cobblestone malformation.

Other abnormalities may include ventricular dilation, brainstem (hypoplasia, clefts) and cerebellar (hypoplasia, cysts) abnormalities, and encephalocele.[68,69]

Embryology/etiology—In cobblestone malformation, there is defective basement membrane formation in the cerebrum/cerebellum, skeletal muscle, and retina due to defective O-glycosylation of α-dystroglycan, a cell surface glycoprotein. In the brain, there is defective attachment of radial glial cells to the defective cortical pial basement membrane, resulting in undermigration of some neurons with resultant abnormal cortical lamination and overmigration of other neurons and glia through gaps in the pial basement membrane into the pial layer and subarachnoid space with resultant irregular nodular cortical surface. In muscle, there is defective binding of α-dystroglycan to extramatrix proteins, such as laminin-2, at the muscle membrane, disrupting the link between the intracellular cytoskeleton and extracellular matrix in skeletal muscle.

The etiology is most often due to autosomal recessive defects in O-glycosylation of α-dystroglycan. Multiple genes have been identified in patients with dystroglycanopathies, most commonly *POMT1*, *POMT2*, *POMGNT1*, *LARGE*, and *B3GALNT2* (coding for glycosyltransferases) and *FKTN* and *FKRP* (coding for proteins of unknown function). An individual gene may be associated with multiple phenotypes. Classic phenotypes, ranging from mild to severe disease respectively, include Fukuyama congenital muscular dystrophy, muscle-eye-brain disease, and Walker-Warburg syndrome.

Assessment/outcome—In the evaluation of cobblestone malformation, head size should be monitored due to the risk of hydrocephalus. A formal exam by an ophthalmologist should occur to assess for such problems as severe myopia, microphthalmia, glaucoma, cataracts, optic nerve hypoplasia, and retinal dysplasias. An evaluation of muscle strength and measurement of creatine phosphokinase is needed to assess for muscular dystrophy, and secondary complications should be looked for, such as respiratory insufficiency,

obstructive sleep apnea, feeding and swallowing problems, contractures, and episodes of rhabdomyolysis. Children with cobblestone malformation have severe intellectual disability, motor impairment (walking rarely achieved), and seizures. Those with Walker-Warburg syndrome, the most severe phenotype, do not survive past age 3 years.

▶ Malformations Secondary to Abnormal Postmigrational Development

Polymicrogyria and Schizencephaly

Imaging—In **polymicrogyria**, which pathologically is characterized by abnormal cortical lamination with resultant abnormal folding manifested as numerous small gyri and shallow sulci, the MRI morphology of the cortical surface can be varied: a thick cortex that often has palisades of sulcation (thick polymicrogyria); multiple small, delicate gyri with small branches of myelinated white matter intercalating into a finely microgyric cortex (delicate polymicrogyria); and thin gyri (composed of microgyri) separated by deep sulci (sawtooth pattern).[73] The variation in pattern may be due to topographical location, etiology, stage of myelination, fusion of the molecular layer between sulci, and MRI resolution and gray-white contrast. At the gray-white junction, there may be an irregular or bumpy contour or blurring, depending on the polymicrogyria pattern and imaging resolution. The underlying white matter is often hyperintense on T2-weighted sequences. Calcifications, often periventricular, may be seen in acquired causes, such as congenital infection. Superficial venous anomalies are frequently associated. The distribution of the areas of polymicrogyria can be unilateral or bilateral (most common) and focal or diffuse. Several bilateral topographical patterns have been described with MRI scan and are suspected to be genetic: frontal, frontoparietal, perisylvian (most common pattern), parieto-occipital, and generalized.[74] The perisylvian polymicrogyria is best seen on sagittal imaging; on axial and coronal images, the Sylvian fissures may appear flattened and elongated (Figure 8–18). Polymicrogyria can be an isolated finding or can occur in association with

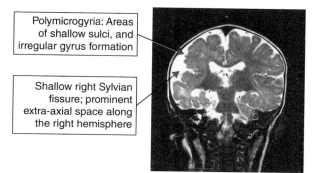

Polymicrogyria: Areas of shallow sulci, and irregular gyrus formation

Shallow right Sylvian fissure; prominent extra-axial space along the right hemisphere

▲ **Figure 8–18.** Polymicrogyria.

other brain malformations, including heterotopia, and abnormalities of the white matter, corpus callosum, brainstem, and cerebellum.

In **schizencephaly**, there is a cleft that extends from the ependyma of the ventricular surface to subarachnoid space at the pial surface. The cleft is typically lined by polymicrogyria or heterotopic neurons. The margins of the clefts may be opposed (closed lip) or separated by cerebrospinal fluid (open lip) (Figure 8–19). A dimple extending out from a ventricular margin is a subtle indicator of the closed lip form. An initially closed lip schizencephaly may later transform into open lip. The clefts can be unilateral or bilateral; when unilateral, there may be cortical dysplasia of the opposite hemisphere. Schizencephaly can be a part of the septo-optic dysplasia plus spectrum.[75]

Embryology—Polymicrogyria and schizencephaly are **classified together** due to coexistence in an individual patient and to their occurrence with common etiologies: polymicrogyria with schizencephalic clefts or calcifications

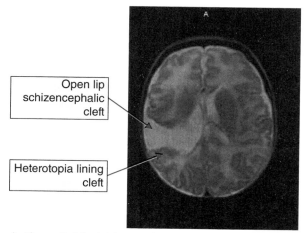

Open lip schizencephalic cleft

Heterotopia lining cleft

▲ **Figure 8–19.** Schizencephaly (open lip).

(presumably due to infection or vascular causes); polymicrogyria without clefts or calcifications (which may be genetic or disruptive); polymicrogyria as part of genetically defined multiple congenital anomaly syndromes; and polymicrogyria in conjunction with inborn errors of metabolism.[45]

Two histologic types of polymicrogyria have been identified, each with a different timing of the insult and alteration in the normal 6-layered lamination of the cerebral cortex. In the **unlayered** pattern, the molecular and upper cellular layers of the affected cortex are disorganized, while the remainder of the cortex is poorly laminated or nonlaminated, often with associated heterotopia in the subcortical white matter or cerebellum. This pattern results from disordered migration of neurons to the superficial cortical layers, thought to occur during the final phase of neuronal migration between 13 and 17 weeks of gestation as a result of clastic, genetic, or metabolic causes. In the **layered** pattern, cortical layers IV and V are gliotic with few neurons resulting from laminar necrosis of these layers from a perfusion or oxygenation deficit in previously normally developing cerebral cortex, during late migration between 16 and 20 weeks[76] or, on occasion, after termination of neuronal migration.[77] A mechanical model proposes that the injury affects the differential growth between the outer and inner portions of the cortex, causing excessive cortical folding.[78] Schizencephaly embryogenesis is not definitively defined.

Etiology—The causes for polymicrogyria are heterogeneous and include genetic, metabolic, and clastic (ischemic/hypoperfusion insults) causes. **Genetic causes** of polymicrogyria include both contiguous-gene and single-gene disorders: the former include, most commonly, 22q11.2 deletion (perisylvian polymicrogyria of variable severity; frequently asymmetric with predisposition for right hemisphere) and 1p36 deletion (bilateral perisylvian polymicrogyria), while other copy variant numbers that cause polymicrogyria are less frequent; the latter include genes implicated in other brain malformations, including phosphatidylinositol-3-kinase/Akt/mTOR pathway, tubulinopathies, α-dystroglycanopathies, laminopathies, and congenital disorders of glycosylation, as well as other genes.[79,80] Additionally, named syndromes, such as Aicardi syndrome and Mowat-Wilson syndrome, have polymicrogyria as a feature. **Metabolic** disorders include peroxisomal disorders, nonketotic hyperglycinemia, fumarase deficiency, glutaric aciduria type II, histidinemia, maple syrup urine disease, and mitochondrial disorders. **Clastic lesions** include disorders that result in ischemia to the brain; these may be due to fetal infection or hypoperfusion (eg, from maternal hypotension, carbon monoxide, or twin-twin transfusion).

Schizencephaly causes are clastic, including infection or vascular causes, supported by association with young parental age, monozygotic twins, septo-optic dysplasia, and non–central nervous system abnormalities due to vascular disruption.[81] Rarely, other causes are reported, although it is unclear if they are pathogenic.

Assessment—In the evaluation of polymicrogyria and schizencephaly, maternal age should be noted, along with whether there was a multiple gestation or any maternal infections, hypotensive events, trauma, or toxic exposures. Head size should be noted, as macrocephaly may suggest a disorder of the phosphatidylinositol-3-kinase/Akt/mTOR pathway, such as MPPH or PROS, whereas microcephaly may suggest clastic causes, such as a congenital infection or hypoperfusion insult. If there is concern for a congenital infection, then appropriate organ systems should be investigated. With schizencephaly, the optic nerves should be assessed for optic atrophy to suggest septo-optic dysplasia plus. A speech and oromotor apraxia should be looked for in the presence of perisylvian polymicrogyria. The presence of unilateral polymicrogyria, particularly of the right hemisphere, should initiate a search for other manifestations of 22q11.2 deletion syndrome. A hemiparesis or quadriparesis associated with unilateral or bilateral lesions, respectively, is often present. Seizures are frequent in these disorders. Serial head circumferences and imaging may be needed with open schizencephaly due to the risk of hydrocephalus. Testing for metabolic disorders should be guided by supportive features.

Outcome—With polymicrogyria, the severity of the clinical presentation depends on the extent of cortical involvement: Bilateral diffuse involvement has the poorest prognosis for language, cognition, and motor function, whereas those with unilateral focal involvement are least affected. Other factors that influence outcome include location of the polymicrogyria, underlying cause, presence of other brain malformations, and complicating features such as epilepsy.[79,82] The location will impact presentation: Frontal involvement is accompanied by a hemiparesis, whereas bilateral perisylvian polymicrogyria will present with oromotor and speech apraxia.

With schizencephaly, the severity of the clinical presentation and pattern of neurologic deficits also depend on the extent and location of cortical involvement. Overall, 60% to 80% of affected individuals have cognitive delay, although much less with unilateral closed lip schizencephaly. The cognitive prognosis is better for unilateral compared to bilateral schizencephaly and closed lip compared to open lip schizencephaly. Motor impairment is more likely to occur if there is frontal lobe involvement.[83,84] Seizures are present in over 50% of cases.

POSTERIOR FOSSA

The formation of the cerebellum begins at the brain 3-vesicle stage with bending at the cephalic (at the boundary between the mesencephalon and rhombencephalon) and cervical (between the rhombencephalon and spinal cord) flexures between 3 and 5 weeks and subdivision of the rhombencephalon into rhombomeres. This is followed by bending at the pontine flexure between the metencephalon and myelencephalon at the 5-vesicle stage; the cerebellum develops from the dorsal anterior metencephalon (rhombomere 1). At the pontine flexure, the fourth ventricle forms, and rhombic lips develop on its edges and, rostrally, later converge to the midline to form the vermis, whereas more caudally, they move laterally to give rise to the hemispheres.[85] During this time, a transient posterior outpouching (Blake's pouch), which communicates with the fourth ventricle but not the subarachnoid cisterns, develops; it later regresses with opening of the foramen of Magendie.

Clues to these disorders are found with assessment of the cerebellum and brainstem and a search for any posterior fossa cysts. The **cerebellum** should be examined for the presence and location of any hypoplasia in the vermis, hemispheres, or both. For example, if there is hypoplasia affecting the cerebellar **hemispheres** more severely than the vermis, the so-called "dragon-fly" pattern (best seen with coronal images on brain MRI), then pontocerebellar hypoplasia is present. On the other hand, hypoplasia of the **inferior vermis** more than cerebellar hemispheres may be isolated or may be part of a more complex malformation, such as Dandy-Walker malformation. Any **brainstem** hypoplasia should be looked for, which is best noted on a mid-sagittal image. The **superior cerebellar peduncles** should be examined on sagittal images to see if they are more horizontal and thickened than normal; if so, the midbrain should be assessed on an axial image to look for a molar tooth sign as seen in Joubert syndrome. The presence or absence of the **vermis** should be noted and whether the cerebellar hemispheres are contiguous, particularly in the presence of aqueductal stenosis; vermian hypoplasia/aplasia with fusion of cerebellar hemispheres occurs in rhomboencephalosynapsis. The size of the **fourth ventricle** and patency of the **cerebral aqueduct** should be checked; a small **fourth ventricle** may be seen with aqueductal stenosis, which may occur in isolation or as part of other posterior fossa malformations, such as rhomboencephalosynapsis. Inferiorly **displaced vermis** into foramen magnum is present in Chiari malformations. The location of any **posterior fossa cysts** should be noted and whether they communicate with the fourth ventricle or subarachnoid space. The size of the **posterior fossa** should be noted. The **angle of the tentorium** should be assessed, particularly in the presence of a posterior fossa cyst.

▶ Molar Tooth–Associated Malformations (Joubert Syndrome)

Imaging

Joubert syndrome is an inherited congenital cerebellar ataxia characterized by a midbrain-hindbrain malformation and variable organ involvement. The obligatory hallmark is the molar tooth sign. Examination of the midbrain on brain

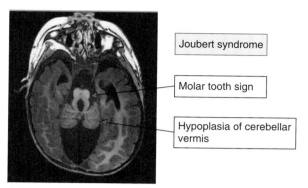

▲ Figure 8–20. Molar tooth–associated malformations.

imaging is an important step in assessing for this malformation. On axial images, the molar tooth appearance of the midbrain results from horizontalized, thickened, and elongated superior cerebellar peduncles; an abnormally deep interpeduncular fossa at the level of the isthmus and upper pons; and vermis hypoplasia (Figure 8–20). Other abnormalities also may be seen on imaging, including Dandy-Walker malformation, ventriculomegaly, occipital cephalocele, polymicrogyria, and periventricular nodular heterotopia.

Embryology

Neuropathology studies show hypoplasia of the cerebellar vermis and brainstem. There is absence of decussation of the superior cerebellar peduncles and the pyramidal tracts, suggesting defective axon guidance. The pathogenic basis of this disorder relates to the dysfunction of the cilium, an immotile organelle that protrudes from the cell surface with different functions, including the detection and transduction of external signals for regular tissue maintenance, polarity, and proliferation.[86]

Etiology

Joubert syndrome is genetically heterogeneous, with 39 causative genes noted to date (Online Mendelian Inheritance in Man [OMIM] 213300).[87] Inheritance is autosomal or X-linked recessive. Features in Joubert syndrome are shared with other ciliopathies, such as Meckel syndrome and Bardet-Biedl syndrome.[86]

Assessment/Outcome

Joubert syndrome is clinically heterogeneous, with neurologic signs and variable multiorgan involvement, mainly of the retina, kidneys, liver, and skeleton. Neurologic issues include cognitive delay, hypotonia, ataxia, abnormal eye movement (including oculomotor apraxia, nystagmus, and strabismus), and abnormal breathing with episodes of apnea and/or tachypnea. Evaluation and regular monitoring for

extra–central nervous system defects are needed, such as defects of the eye (retinal defects), kidney (nephronophthisis or cystic dysplastic kidneys), and liver (fibrosis). Prognosis for survival is based on the severity of breathing dysregulation and the severity of other organ system involvement (renal and liver).[86,88]

▶ Dandy-Walker Malformation

Imaging

In Dandy-Walker malformation, imaging (most apparent on sagittal sequences) will show the characteristic hypoplasia of vermis (especially the inferior portion) with upward/anticlockwise rotation, an enlarged fourth ventricle, and an enlarged posterior fossa with upward displacement of the tentorium, torcula, and lateral sinuses (Figure 8–21).[89] Hydrocephalus is commonly associated and may not develop until after the newborn period. Other brain malformations should be looked for, such as agenesis of the corpus callosum, heterotopia, cephalocele, and molar tooth–associated malformation.

Embryology/Etiology

A variety of causes have been found for Dandy-Walker syndrome, including chromosomal aneuploidy, genetic syndromes (eg, Coffin-Siris and Meckel-Gruber), rarely single-gene disorders, and acquired causes (congenital infection and alcohol exposure). Almost all cases are sporadic.

Assessment/Outcome

If not detected on fetal imaging, Dandy-Walker malformation typically presents with hydrocephalus, developmental delay, or ataxia. Shunting of hydrocephalus is needed in many patients. There is a high frequency of non–central nervous system anomalies that should be looked for, including congenital heart disease, cleft lip/palate, cephaloceles, and facial hemangiomas (as a component of PHACE syndrome [posterior fossa brain malformations, hemangioma, arterial lesions, cardiac abnormalities, and eye abnormalities]).

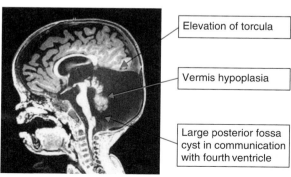

▲ Figure 8–21. Dandy-Walker malformation.

Intellectual disability may occur in 50% of patients; this will be influenced by any associated brain anomalies, timing and adequacy of treatment of hydrocephalus, and complications of shunt treatment (malfunction infections; subdurals). There was a relatively high mortality (25%) in the past due to shunt malfunction or infection, sudden death, associated diseases, uncontrolled hydrocephalus with no shunt, upward herniation after ventriculoperitoneal shunt or cyst shunt failure, and respiratory anomalies, but this has improved.

It is important to differentiate Dandy-Walker malformation from variants and other posterior fossa fluid collections. In Dandy-Walker variant, there is less severe cerebellar vermis hypoplasia, upward rotation of the vermis is absent or less prominent, and the posterior fossa fluid collection is typically smaller. In mega cisterna magna, which is lined by arachnoid, there is enlargement of the cisterna magna, which communicates with the basal subarachnoid space and the fourth ventricle through a mildly widened vallecular. In Blake's pouch cyst, which is lined by ependyma, the cystic cerebrospinal fluid collection in the posterior fossa does not communicate freely with the basal subarachnoid space. Children with mega cisterna magna and Blake's pouch cyst have good neurodevelopmental outcome.

▶ Pontocerebellar Hypoplasia

Imaging

Pontocerebellar hypoplasia (PCH) is a heterogeneous group of autosomal recessive neurodegenerative disorders characterized by hypoplasia of the cerebellum and ventral pons, variable cerebral involvement, microcephaly, severe delay in cognitive and motor development, and seizures. The brain abnormalities are usually present at birth, although microcephaly may not occur until later. Imaging shows hypoplasia affecting the cerebellar hemispheres more severely than the vermis; the flattening of the cerebellar hemispheres with relative preservation of the vermis gives the so-called "dragonfly" pattern, best seen with coronal images of brain MRI (Figure 8–22). A flat ventral pons is noted on mid-sagittal imaging. The cerebral cortex is usually normal initially, but cortical atrophy often develops later.

Embryology

The pathology of PCH, which typically has onset prenatally, results from a failure of development with variable neurodegeneration. As a result, there is hypoplasia with varying severity of atrophy of the cerebellum, inferior olivary and dentate nuclei, and ventral pons, and variable neocortical atrophy.

For a number of subtypes, the pathogenic basis of this disorder relates to the defective formation of subunits (due to mutations in *TSEN54*, and less frequently in *TSEN2*, *TSEN34*, and *TSEN15* genes) of the transfer RNA (tRNA) splicing endonuclease complex, which is needed for cleavage of intron-containing tRNAs. Other subtypes are due to defects in formation of the RNA exosome complex (due to mutations in *EXOSC3* and *EXOSC8* genes) and protein translation (due to mutations in *SEPSECS* and *RARS2* genes).[90]

Etiology

PCH is a heterogeneous group of disorders that have been divided into 17 subtypes.[91] To date, mutations in 25 genes have been reported.[91] Inheritance is autosomal recessive. The most common subtypes are PCH1, caused by mutations in *VRK1*, *EXOSC3*, *EXOSC8*, *EXOSC9*, and *SLC25A46* genes, and PCH2, caused by mutations in *TSEN54*, *TSEN2*, *TSEN34*, *SEPSECS*, *VPS53*, and *TSEN15* genes.

PCH is distinguished by prenatal onset of neurodegeneration, involvement of ventral pons in addition to cerebellar cortex, and autosomal recessive inheritance. Other disorders can also cause cerebellar hypoplasia with variable involvement of the pons, including congenital disorders of glycosylation, mitochondrial disorders, PCHs with neocortical malformations (CASK-related disorders; genes involved in the organization of microtubule, including *TUBA1A*,

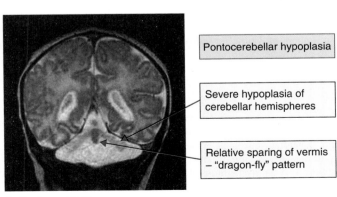

Pontocerebellar hypoplasia

Severe hypoplasia of cerebellar hemispheres

Relative sparing of vermis – "dragon-fly" pattern

▲ **Figure 8–22.** Pontocerebellar hypoplasia.

TUBB2B, *TUBB3*, *TUBB5*, and *TUBA8*; α-dystroglycan–related dystrophies; lissencephaly with cerebellar hypoplasia, including *TUBA1A*, *RELN*, and *VLDLR* genes), and extreme prematurity.[90]

Assessment

Age at onset of PCH varies from the prenatal period to early infancy, with most patients presenting in the neonatal period and the first months of life. The radiologic assessment of PCH begins with defining the pattern and severity of the brain malformation (including cerebellar hemispheres, vermis, brainstem, and neocortex), while the clinical evaluation measures head size and assesses cognitive and motor development; severe impairments typically occur in these areas. Seizures also should be searched for. These clinical neurologic findings are due to dysfunction of the neocortex and basal ganglia; cerebellar symptoms very rarely occur in PCH.[90] Frequent associated clinical problems include dysphagia and aspiration (requiring gavage or gastromy tube), central sleep apnea, gastrointestinal problems (poor gastric emptying, gastroesophageal reflux, and constipation), and autonomic dysfunction. Treatment is symptomatic in all types.[92]

Distinctive features occur in individual PCH subtypes. PCH1 is characterized by muscular hypotonia, weakness, and atrophy due to bulbar and spinal motor neuron loss; PCH2, dystonia, dyskinesias, and episodes of rhabdomyolysis; and PCH4, massive myoclonus, and severe hypertonia. Specific testing is available for most genes.

Outcome

Developmental progress in PCH, if present, is very limited. Many children live only into infancy or childhood, although some affected individuals have lived into adulthood; subtype influences outcome, with better outcome in PCH2. In a natural history study of 33 patients with PCH2, 53% had died before age 11 years.[93]

REFERENCES

1. A general imaging approach to brain malformations. Approach to brain malformations. Accessed June 13, 2022. https://eu-ireland-custom-media-prod.s3-eu-west-1.amazonaws.com/UKMEAEU/eSample/extraits/9780323680318.pdf

2. Tekendo-Ngongang C, Muenke M, Kruszka P. Holoprosencephaly overview. 2000 Dec 27 [Updated 2020 Mar 5]. In: Adam MP, Ardinger HH, Pagon RA, et al, eds. *GeneReviews®* [Internet]. University of Washington, Seattle; 1993-2022.

3. Simon EM, Hevner RF, Pinter JD, et al. The middle interhemispheric variant of holoprosencephaly. *AJNR Am J Neuroradiol.* 2002;23(1):151-156.

4. Lewis AJ, Simon EM, Barkovich AJ, et al. Middle interhemispheric variant of holoprosencephaly: a distinct cliniconeuroradiologic subtype. *Neurology.* 2002;59(12):1860-1865. doi:10.1212/01.wnl.0000037483.31989.b9

5. Hahn JS, Barnes PD, Clegg NJ, Stashinko EE. Septopreoptic holoprosencephaly: a mild subtype associated with midline craniofacial anomalies. *AJNR Am J Neuroradiol.* 2010;31(9):1596-1601. doi:10.3174/ajnr.A2123

6. Kauvar EF, Muenke M. Holoprosencephaly: recommendations for diagnosis and management. *Curr Opin Pediatr.* 2010;22(6):687-695. doi:10.1097/MOP.0b013e32833f56d5

7. Dubourg C, Bendavid C, Pasquier L, et al. Holoprosencephaly. *Orphanet J Rare Dis.* 2007;2:8. doi:10.1186/1750-1172-2-8

8. Solomon BD, Pineda-Alvarez DE, Mercier S, et al. Holoprosencephaly flashcards: a summary for the clinician. *Am J Med Genet C Semin Med Genet.* 2010;154C(1):3-7. doi:10.1002/ajmg.c.30245

9. Golden JA. Towards a greater understanding of the pathogenesis of holoprosencephaly. *Brain Dev.* 1999;21(8):513-521. doi:10.1016/s0387-7604(99)00067-4

10. Levey EB, Stashinko E, Clegg NJ, Delgado MR. Management of children with holoprosencephaly. *Am J Med Genet C Semin Med Genet.* 2010;154C(1):183-190. doi:10.1002/ajmg.c.30254

11. Chadie A, Radi S, Trestard L, et al. Neurodevelopmental outcome in prenatally diagnosed isolated agenesis of the corpus callosum. *Acta Paediatr.* 2008;97(4):420-424. doi:10.1111/j.1651-2227.2008.00688.x

12. Mangione R, Fries N, Godard P, et al. Neurodevelopmental outcome following prenatal diagnosis of an isolated anomaly of the corpus callosum. *Ultrasound Obstet Gynecol.* 2011;37(3):290-295. doi:10.1002/uog.8882

13. Yilmaz MB, Genc A, Egemen E, Yilmaz S, Tekiner A. Pericallosal lipomas: a series of 10 cases with clinical and radiological features. *Turk Neurosurg.* 2016;26(3):364-368. doi:10.5137/1019-5149.JTN.13008-14.0

14. Lubinsky MS. Hypothesis: septo-optic dysplasia is a vascular disruption sequence. *Am J Med Genet.* 1997;69(3):235-236.

15. Webb EA, Dattani MT. Septo-optic dysplasia. *Eur J Hum Genet.* 2010;18(4):393-397. doi:10.1038/ejhg.2009.125

16. Vawter-Lee MM, Wasserman H, Thomas CW, et al. Outcome of isolated absent septum pellucidum diagnosed by fetal magnetic resonance imaging (MRI) scan. *J Child Neurol.* 2018;33(11):693-699. doi:10.1177/0883073818783460

17. Alt C, Shevell MI, Poulin C. Clinical and radiologic spectrum of septo-optic dysplasia: review of 17 cases. *J Child Neurol.* 2017;32(9):797-803. doi:10.1177/0883073817707300

18. Signorini SG, Decio A, Fedeli C, et al. Septo-optic dysplasia in childhood: the neurological, cognitive and, neuro-ophthalmological perspective. *Dev Med Child Neurol.* 2012;54(11):1018-1024. doi:10.1111/j.1469-8749.2012.04404.x

19. Cemeroglu AP, Coulas T, Kleis L. Spectrum of clinical presentations and endocrinological findings of patients with septo-optic dysplasia: a retrospective study. *J Pediatr Endocrinol Metab.* 2015;28(9-10):1057-1063. doi:10.1515/jpem-2015-0008

20. Greene NDE, Copp AJ. Neural tube defects. *Annu Rev Neurosci.* 2014;37:221-242. doi:10.1146/annurev-neuro-062012-170354

21. Jessell TM, Sanes JR. Patterning the nervous system. In: Kandel ER, Schwartz JH, Jessell TM, Siegelbaum SA, Hudspeth AJ, eds. *Principles of Neural Science.* 5th ed. McGraw Hill Medical; 2013:1165-1186.

22. Ben-Amitai D, Davidson S, Schwartz M, et al. Sacral nevus flammeus simplex: the role of imaging. *Pediatr Dermatol.* 2000;17(6):469-471. doi:10.1046/j.1525-1470.2000.01824.x

23. Kriss VM, Desai NS. Occult spinal dysraphism in neonates: assessment of high-risk cutaneous stigmata on sonography. *AJR Am J Roentgenol.* 1998;171(6):1687-1692. doi:10.2214/ajr.171.6.9843314

24. Liptak GS, Dosa N. Myelomeningocele. *Pediatr Rev.* 2010;31(11):443-450. doi:10.1542/pir.31-11-443

25. Ou X, Glasier CM, Snow JH. Diffusion tensor imaging evaluation of white matter in adolescents with myelomeningocele and Chiari II malformation. *Pediatr Radiol.* 2011;41(11):1407-1415. doi:10.1007/s00247-011-2180-6

26. Centers for Disease Control and Prevention. 5 ways to lower the risk of having a pregnancy affected by a neural tube defect. Accessed June 13, 2022. https://www.cdc.gov/ncbddd/birthdefects/5-ways-to-lower-the-risk.html

27. MRC Vitamin Study Research Group. Prevention of neural tube defects: results of the Medical Research Council Vitamin Study. *Lancet.* 1991;338(8760):131-137.

28. Verity C, Firth H, French-Constant C. Congenital abnormalities of the central nervous system. *J Neurol Neurosurg Psychiatry.* 2003;74(suppl 1):i3-8. doi:10.1136/jnnp.74.suppl_1.i3

29. Adzick NS, Thom EA, Spong CY, et al. A randomized trial of prenatal versus postnatal repair of myelomeningocele. *N Engl J Med.* 2011;364(11):993-1004. doi:10.1056/NEJMoa1014379

30. Battibugli S, Gryfakis N, Dias L, et al. Functional gait comparison between children with myelomeningocele: shunt versus no shunt. *Dev Med Child Neurol.* 2007;49(10):764-769. doi:10.1111/j.1469-8749.2007.00764.x

31. Chadduck W, Adametz J. Incidence of seizures in patients with myelomeningocele: a multifactorial analysis. *Surg Neurol.* 1988;30(4):281-285. doi:10.1016/0090-3019(88)90300-x

32. Noetzel MJ, Blake JN. Prognosis for seizure control and remission in children with myelomeningocele. *Dev Med Child Neurol.* 1991;33(9):803-810. doi:10.1111/j.1469-8749.1991.tb14964.x

33. Wilkins-Haug L, Freedman W. Progression of exencephaly to anencephaly in the human fetus—an ultrasound perspective. *Prenat Diagn.* 1991;11(4):227-233. doi:10.1002/pd.1970110404

34. Medical Task Force on Anencephaly. The infant with anencephaly. *N Engl J Med.* 1990;322(10):669-674. doi:10.1056/NEJM199003083221006

35. Dickman H, Fletke K, Redfern RE. Prolonged unassisted survival in an infant with anencephaly. *BMJ Case Rep.* 2016;2016:bcr2016215986. doi:10.1136/bcr-2016-215986

36. Da Silva SL, Yasser Jeelani Y, Dang H, et al. Risk factors for hydrocephalus and neurological deficit in children born with an encephalocele. *J Neurosurg Pediatr.* 2015;15(4):392-398. doi:10.3171/2014.10.PEDS14192

37. Achar SV, Dutta HK. Sincipital encephaloceles: a study of associated brain malformations. *J Clin Imaging Sci.* 2016;6:20. doi:10.4103/2156-7514.183040

38. Patterson RJ, Egelhoff JC, Crone KR, Ball WS Jr. Atretic parietal cephaloceles revisited: an enlarging clinical and imaging spectrum? *AJNR Am J Neuroradiol.* 1998;19(4):791-795.

39. Hoving EW, Vermeij-Keers C. Frontoethmoidal encephaloceles, a study of their pathogenesis. *Pediatr Neurosurg.* 1997;27(5):246-256. doi:10.1159/000121262

40. Morón FE, Morriss MC, Jones JJ, Hunter JV. Lumps and bumps on the head in children: use of CT and MR imaging in solving the clinical diagnostic dilemma. *Radiographics.* 2004;24(6):1655-1674. doi:10.1148/rg.246045034

41. Matos Cruz AJ, De Jesus O. Encephalocele. In: *StatPearls* [Internet]. StatPearls Publishing; 2021.

42. Hockley AD, Goldin JH, Wake MJ. Management of anterior encephalocele. *Childs Nerv Syst.* 1990;6(8):444-446. doi:10.1007/BF00302090

43. Lo BW, Kulkarni AV, Rutka JT, et al. Clinical predictors of developmental outcome in patients with cephaloceles. *J Neurosurg Pediatr.* 2008;2(4):254-257. doi:10.3171/PED.2008.2.10.254

44. Jessell TM, Sanes JR. Differentiation and survival of nerve cells. In: Kandel ER, Schwartz JH, Jessell TM, Siegelbaum SA, Hudspeth AJ, eds. *Principles of Neural Science.* 5th ed. McGraw Hill Medical; 2013:1187-1208.

45. Barkovich AJ, Guerrini R, Kuzniecky RI, Jackson GD, Dobyns WB. A developmental and genetic classification for malformations of cortical development: update 2012. *Brain.* 2012;135(Pt 5):1348-1369. doi:10.1093/brain/aws019

46. Lee J. Malformations of cortical development: genetic mechanisms and diagnostic approach. *Korean J Pediatr.* 2017;60(1):1-9. doi:10.3345/kjp.2017.60.1.1

47. Colombo N, Salamon N, Raybaud C, Özkara C, Barkovich AJ. Imaging of malformations of cortical development. *Epileptic Disord.* 2009;11(3):194-205. doi:0.1684/epd.2009.0262

48. Mirzaa GM, Poduri A. Megalencephaly and hemimegalencephaly: breakthroughs in molecular etiology. *Am J Med Genet C Semin Med Genet.* 2014;166C(2):156-172. doi:10.1002/ajmg.c.31401

49. Keppler-Noreuil KM, Rios JJ, Parker VER, et al. PIK3CA-related overgrowth spectrum (PROS): diagnostic and testing eligibility criteria, differential diagnosis, and evaluation. *Am J Med Genet A.* 2015;167A(2):287-295. doi:10.1002/ajmg.a.36836

50. Harada A, Miya F, Utsunomiya H, et al. Sudden death in a case of megalencephaly capillary malformation associated with a de novo mutation in AKT3. *Childs Nerv Syst.* 2015;31(3):465-471. doi:10.1007/s00381-014-2589-y

51. Evans DG, Ladusans EJ, Rimmer S, et al. Complications of the naevoid basal cell carcinoma syndrome: results of a population based study. *J Med Genet.* 1993;30(6):460-464. doi:10.1136/jmg.30.6.460

52. Evans DG, Farndon PA. Nevoid basal cell carcinoma syndrome. 2002 Jun 20 [Updated 2018 Mar 29]. In: Adam MP, Ardinger HH, Pagon RA, et al, eds. *GeneReviews®* [Internet]. University of Washington, Seattle, 1993-2022. https://www.ncbi.nlm.gov/books/

53. Johnson RL, Rothman AL, Xie J, et al. Human homolog of patched, a candidate gene for the basal cell nevus syndrome. *Science.* 1996;272(5268):1668-1671. doi:10.1126/science.272.5268.1668

54. Farndon PA, Del Mastro RG, Evans DG, Kilpatrick MW. Location of gene for Gorlin syndrome. *Lancet.* 1992;339(8793):581-582. doi:10.1016/0140-6736(92)90868-4

55. Ewing AD, Cheetham SW, McGill JJ. Microdeletion of 9q22.3: a patient with minimal deletion size associated with a severe phenotype. *Am J Med Genet A.* 2021;185(7):2070-2083. doi:10.1002/ajmg.a.62224

56. Smith MJ, Beetz C, Williams SG, et al. Germline mutations in SUFU cause Gorlin syndrome-associated childhood medulloblastoma and redefine the risk associated with PTCH1 mutations. *J Clin Oncol.* 2014;32(36):4155-4161. doi:10.1200/JCO.2014.58.2569

57. Evans DG, Oudit D, Smith MJ, et al. First evidence of genotype-phenotype correlations in Gorlin syndrome. *J Med Genet.* 2017;54(8):530-536. doi:10.1136/jmedgenet-2017-104669

58. Tan MH, Mester J, Peterson C, et al. A clinical scoring system for selection of patients for PTEN mutation testing is proposed on the basis of a prospective study of 3042 probands. *Am J Hum Genet.* 2011;88(1):42-56. doi:10.1016/j.ajhg.2010.11.013

59. Jansen LA, Mirzaa GM, Ishak GE, et al. PI3K/AKT pathway mutations cause a spectrum of brain malformations from megalencephaly to focal cortical dysplasia. *Brain*. 2015;138(Pt 6):1613-1628. doi:10.1093/brain/awv045

60. Blümcke I, Thom M, Aronica E, et al. The clinicopathological spectrum of focal cortical dysplasias: consensus classification proposed by an ad hoc Task Force of the ILAE Diagnostic Methods Commission. *Epilepsia*. 2011;52(1):158-174. doi:10.1111/j.1528-1167.2010.02777.x

61. Parrini E, Ramazzotti A, Dobyns WB, et al. Periventricular heterotopia: phenotypic heterogeneity and correlation with Filamin A mutations. *Brain*. 2006;129(Pt 7):1892-1906. doi:10.1093/brain/awl125

62. Lu DS, Karas PJ, Krueger DA, Weiner HL. Central nervous system manifestations of tuberous sclerosis complex. *Am J Med Genet C Semin Med Genet*. 2018;178(3):291-298. doi:10.1002/ajmg.c.31647

63. Barkovich AJ, Kuzniecky RI. Gray matter heterotopia. *Neurology*. 2000;55(11):1603-1608. doi:10.1212/wnl.55.11.1603

64. Carabalona A, Beguin S, Pallesi-Pocachard E. A glial origin for periventricular nodular heterotopia caused by impaired expression of Filamin-A. *Hum Mol Genet*. 2012;21(5):1004-1017. doi:10.1093/hmg/ddr531

65. Online Mendelian Inheritance in Man. OMIM # 300049. Periventricular nodular heterotopia 1; PVNH1. Accessed June 13, 2022. https://www.omim.org/entry/300049

66. Yilmaz S, Gokben S, Serdaroglu G, et al. The expanding phenotypic spectrum of ARFGEF2 gene mutation: cardiomyopathy and movement disorder. *Brain Dev*. 2016;38(1):124-127. doi:10.1016/j.braindev.2015.06.004

67. Dobyns WB, Truwit CL. Lissencephaly and other malformations of cortical development: 1995 update. *Neuropediatrics*. 1995;26(3):132-147. doi:10.1055/s-2007-979744

68. Abdel Razek AAK, Kandell AY, Elsorogy LG, Elmongy A, Basett AA. Disorders of cortical formation: MR imaging features. *AJNR Am J Neuroradiol*. 2009;30(1):4-11. doi:10.3174/ajnr.A1223

69. Fry AE, Cushion TD, Pilz DT. The genetics of lissencephaly. *Am J Med Genet C Semin Med Genet*. 2014;166C(2):198-210. doi:10.1002/ajmg.c.31402

70. Sicca F, Kelemen A, Genton P, et al. Mosaic mutations of the LIS1 gene cause subcortical band heterotopia. *Neurology*. 2003;61(8):1042-1046. doi:10.1212/wnl.61.8.1042

71. Gleeson JG. Classical lissencephaly and double cortex (subcortical band heterotopia): LIS1 and doublecortin. *Curr Opin Neurol*. 2000;13(2):121-125. doi:10.1097/00019052-200004000-00002

72. Kumar RA, Pilz DT, Babatz TD, et al. TUBA1A mutations cause wide spectrum lissencephaly (smooth brain) and suggest that multiple neuronal migration pathways converge on alpha tubulins. *Hum Mol Genet*. 2010;19(14):2817-2827. doi:10.1093/hmg/ddq182

73. Barkovich AJ. MRI analysis of sulcation morphology in polymicrogyria. *Epilepsia*. 2010;51(suppl 1):17-22. doi:10.1111/j.1528-1167.2009.02436.x

74. Barkovich AJ, Kuzniecky RI, Jackson GD, et al. A developmental and genetic classification for malformations of cortical development. *Neurology*. 2005;65(12):1873-1887. doi:10.1212/01.wnl.0000183747.05269.2d

75. Severino M, Geraldo AF, Utz N, et al. Definitions and classification of malformations of cortical development: practical guidelines. *Brain*. 2020;143(10):2874-2894. doi:10.1093/brain/awaa174

76. McBride MC, Kemper TL. Pathogenesis of four-layered microgyric cortex in man. *Acta Neuropathol*. 1982;57(2-3):93-98. doi:10.1007/BF00685375

77. Inder TE, Huppi PS, Zientara GP, et al. The postmigrational development of polymicrogyria documented by magnetic resonance imaging from 31 weeks' postconceptional age. *Ann Neurol*. 1999;45(6):798-801. doi:10.1002/1531-8249(199906)45:6<798::aid-ana16>3.0.co;2-u

78. Richman DP, Stewart RM, Hutchinson JW, Caviness VS Jr. Mechanical model of brain convolutional development. *Science*. 1975;189(4196):18-21. doi:10.1126/science.1135626

79. Stutterd CA, Leventer RJ. Polymicrogyria: a common and heterogeneous malformation of cortical development. *Am J Med Genet C Semin Med Genet*. 2014;166C(2):227-239. doi:10.1002/ajmg.c.31399

80. Stutterd CA, Dobyns WB, Jansen A, et al. Polymicrogyria overview. 2005 Apr 18 [updated 2018 Aug 16]. In: Adam MP, Ardinger HH, Pagon RA, et al, eds. *GeneReviews® [Internet]*. University of Washington, Seattle; 1993–2022.

81. Curry CJ, Lammer EJ, Nelson V, Shaw GM. Schizencephaly: heterogeneous etiologies in a population of 4 million California births. *Am J Med Genet A*. 2005;137(2):181-189. doi:10.1002/ajmg.a.30862

82. Barkovich AJ, Kjos BO. Schizencephaly: correlation of clinical findings with MR characteristics. *AJNR Am J Neuroradiol*. 1992;13(1):85-94.

83. Barkovich AJ, Kjos BO. Nonlissencephalic cortical dysplasias: correlation of imaging findings with clinical deficits. *AJNR Am J Neuroradiol*. 1992;13(1):95-103.

84. Packard AM, Miller VS, Delgado MR. Schizencephaly: correlations of clinical and radiologic features. *Neurology*. 1997;48(5):1427-1434. doi:10.1212/wnl.48.5.1427.

85. Parisi MA, Dobyns WB. Human malformations of the midbrain and hindbrain: review and proposed classification scheme. *Mol Genet Metab*. 2003;80(1-2):36-53. doi:10.1016/j.ymgme.2003.08.010

86. Romani M, Micalizzi A, Valente EM. Joubert syndrome: congenital cerebellar ataxia with the molar tooth. *Lancet Neurol*. 2013;12(9):894-905. doi:10.1016/S1474-4422(13)70136-4

87. Online Mendelian Inheritance in Man. OMIM # 213300 Joubert syndrome 1; JBTS1. Accessed June 13, 2022. https://www.omim.org/entry/213300

88. Brancati F, Dallapiccola B, Valente EM. Joubert Syndrome and related disorders. *Orphanet J Rare Dis*. 2010;5:20. doi:10.1186/1750-1172-5-20

89. Doherty D, Millen KJ, Barkovich AJ. Midbrain and hindbrain malformations: advances in clinical diagnosis, imaging, and genetics. *Lancet Neurol*. 2013;12(4):381-393. doi:10.1016/S1474-4422(13)70024-3

90. Van Dijk T, Baas F, Barth PG, Poll-The BT. What's new in pontocerebellar hypoplasia? An update on genes and subtypes. *Orphanet J Rare Dis*. 2018;13(1):92. doi:10.1186/s13023-018-0826-2

91. Online Mendelian Inheritance in Man. OMIM # 607596. Pontocerebellar hypoplasia, type 1A; PCH1A. Accessed June 13, 2022. https://www.omim.org/entry/60759

92. Rudnik-Schöneborn S, Barth PG, Zerres K. Pontocerebellar hypoplasia. *Am J Med Genet C Semin Med Genet*. 2014;166C(2):173-183. doi:10.1002/ajmg.c.31403

93. Sánchez-Albisua I, Frölich S, Barth PG, Steinlin M, Krägeloh-Mann I. Natural course of pontocerebellar hypoplasia type 2A. *Orphanet J Rare Dis*. 2014;9:70. doi:10.1186/1750-1172-9-70

Autism Spectrum Disorder and Regressive Developmental Disorders

Heather M. Wied, MD, PhD

Shannon M. Standridge, DO, MPH

AUTISM SPECTRUM DISORDER

Autism spectrum disorder (ASD) is a neurodevelopmental disorder characterized by deficits in communication and social interactions, occurring with restricted patterns of behavior or interest.[1] The ASD diagnosis focuses on the presentation of these behaviors and includes both identifying deficits and restrictions and determining their severity, which may range from mild to severe. Signs of ASD typically manifest within the first 2 years of life, but diagnosis may be delayed until a later age, especially with mild symptoms.

▶ General Considerations

In 2013, the fifth edition of the *Diagnostic and Statistical Manual of Mental Disorders* (DSM-5) combined the diagnoses of autistic disorder, Asperger syndrome, and pervasive developmental disorder not otherwise specified under a single diagnosis of ASD.[1]

Since its introduction, there has been an increase in diagnosis of ASD, likely due to greater public awareness of the disorder and recent diagnostic changes. In 2021, the Centers for Disease Control and Prevention's Autism and Developmental Disabilities Monitoring Network reported the prevalence of ASD in US children aged 8 years old to be around 1 in 44.[2] The World Health Organization estimates global prevalence of ASD to be on average about 1 in 160 children.[3] ASD is seen in all racial, ethnic, and socioeconomic levels and is seen more commonly in males compared to females (4:1).

▶ Clinical Findings

ASD symptoms and behaviors are often first observed and noted by parents and family members. Most often, the deficits become clear by the time a child is 2 to 3 years old, and sometimes earlier. Some children with autism present with a regression in their abilities around this age. It is important for physicians to listen to parents' observations and perceptions regarding the child's development and to ask questions that can help identify potential delays.

Deficits in social communication and interaction may present through:

- Poor eye contact
- Lack of joint attention (eg, not pointing at objects of interest)
- Abnormal prosody of speech
- Regression of language
- Not responding to their names
- Preference to play by themselves

Restricted patterns of behavior and/or interest may present as follows:

- Not playing with toys appropriately (eg, always lining toy cars up in a certain order instead of pushing them around)
- Exhibiting an obsessive interest in a specific topic or object (eg, fascination with trains or certain cartoon characters)
- Showing a preference for looking at letters, shapes, or other objects

Physical behaviors will frequently have stereotypies, including:

- Hand flapping
- Rocking
- Looking out of the corners of the eyes
- Other consistent repetitive movements
- Self-injurious behaviors, such as head banging

▶ Diagnosis and Testing

The American Psychiatric Association's DSM-5[1] provides diagnostic criteria widely accepted as the standard for ASD diagnosis. Per the DSM-5, an individual with ASD must present with persistent deficits in 3 contexts of

Table 9–1. Autism spectrum disorder as defined by the American Psychiatric Association's *Diagnostic and Statistical Manual of Mental Disorders, Fifth Edition* (DSM-5).[1]

Deficits in social communication and interaction (all 3 required):	Restricted, repetitive patterns of behavior and interest (2 or more of 4 required):
• Deficits in social-emotional reciprocity • Deficits in nonverbal communicative behaviors used for social interaction • Deficits in developing, maintaining, and understanding relationships	• Stereotyped or repetitive motor movements, use of objects, or speech • Insistence on sameness, inflexible adherence to routines, or ritualized patterns of verbal or nonverbal behavior • Highly restricted, fixated interests that are abnormal in intensity or focus • Hyperreactivity or hyporeactivity to sensory input or unusual interest in sensory aspects of the environment

Note: Deficits and restrictive behaviors can be present at the time of diagnosis or historically experienced.

social communication and interaction, as well as 2 or more of 4 restricted, repetitive patterns of behavior or interest (Table 9–1). These symptoms must start in early development and significantly impair the child's social functioning. The diagnosis can specify the level of support required at 1 of 3 levels depending on severity of deficits and restrictions.

The intellectual abilities of individuals with ASD vary greatly from severe cognitive impairment to a normal or high level of intelligence. Cognitive ability, however, is not a basis for diagnosis, although the majority of those with ASD do experience moderate to severe cognitive impairments. Diagnosis of ASD may specify occurrence with or without intellectual impairment or language impairment.[1]

A preliminary screening tool for ASD is the Modified Checklist for Autism in Toddlers (M-CHAT). The M-CHAT does not specifically screen for ASD but provides a starting point to evaluate general developmental difficulties and determine if further evaluation is needed.

The 2 common diagnostic tools that screen for ASD are the Autism Diagnostic Observation Schedule (ADOS) and the Autism Diagnostic Interview, Revised (ADI-R). These are typically administered as part of a battery of tests to ultimately diagnose ASD.

Additional Testing

Standardized testing of receptive and expressive language skills, motor skills, and cognitive functioning should be performed in children with a concern for ASD. Hearing tests are highly recommended for concerns of language delay to ensure such delays cannot be attributed solely to hearing deficits or general auditory issues. The American College of Medical Genetics recommends a tiered approach to genetic testing in children with ASD.[4] Typically, this begins with a chromosomal microarray, followed by testing for fragile X in males and females with intellectual disability or family history of intellectual disability; *MECP2* gene testing for Rett syndrome in females (and in males if clinical picture is concerning); and *PTEN* sequencing for patients with macrocephaly. Further neurodevelopmental genetic testing may be considered following these genetic tests, including a targeted autism panel or whole-exome sequencing.

As with any concern for speech or developmental delay, a thorough neurologic examination should occur to rule out tumor, stroke, or other neurologic disease that may explain deficits and delays. Abnormalities on neurologic examination may ultimately warrant evaluation with brain magnetic resonance imaging if appropriate.

Prevention

While the causes of ASD remain unknown, it is widely theorized it is due to a combination of genetic and environmental factors. Identified risk factors for ASD include advanced parental age,[5,6] maternal exposure to valproic acid during pregnancy,[7] and certain genetic conditions such as tuberous sclerosis and fragile X syndrome. No causative association has been found between childhood vaccinations and ASD.[8]

Differential Diagnosis

Motor delays, receptive/expressive language delays, and other behavioral delays may all present as discrete conditions independent of ASD. These may be diagnosed as individual conditions if the full constellation of symptoms required for the ASD diagnosis are not present.

Other syndromes that may present similarly to ASD with regression in skills that would require further evaluation and appropriate testing include genetic syndromes such as Rett syndrome; epileptic encephalopathies, such as Landau-Kleffner or electrical status epilepticus in sleep; or metabolic syndromes, such as creatine deficiency syndromes. Other disorders that can present similarly to ASD include anxiety, attention-deficit/hyperactivity disorder, and posttraumatic stress disorder. It is also important to consider further genetic evaluations for co-occurring conditions such as tuberous sclerosis and fragile X syndrome.

Treatment

The basis of treatment for ASD is largely through education and therapy. Standards include applied behavior analysis therapy, specifically intense 1-on-1 therapy,[9] speech therapy, physical therapy, and occupational therapy.

Early recognition, diagnosis, and intervention are the most important factors in optimizing the best outcome for children with ASD. It is imperative that families have access to resources and community support for early intervention once a diagnosis is made. For children with ASD with the cognitive ability to attend school, starting in the classroom can be particularly difficult due to the new environments and the transition away from home.

It is equally important to diagnose and to start medical treatment as necessary for comorbidities in a child with ASD, the most common being attention-deficit/hyperactivity disorder, anxiety, depression, irritability, and aggression. Other frequent comorbidities in children with ASD include restricted diets, gastrointestinal symptoms, obesity, sleep disorders, and epilepsy.

While intellectual function of those with ASD varies, it is most common for individuals to have intellectual disability (IQ <70), academic learning difficulties, and language delays. Increases in irritability and aggression can be common in individuals with ASD, particularly if they have decreased communication and language delays. Some children with ASD may engage in self-injurious behaviors, which must be addressed to prevent physical harm to self and others. A thorough medical and dental examination is advised whenever baseline aggressive or self-injurious behaviors are found to increase in intensity and frequency, as these changes could be an expression of pain or discomfort.

When prescribing medications for those with ASD, consider medicines known to be effective in addressing more than one health need at the same time. For example, an individual with ASD and comorbidities of epilepsy and obesity may benefit from antiepileptic choices such as topiramate or zonisamide, which target epilepsy but are also known to have decreased appetite as a common side effect. Similarly, valproic acid may be an effective treatment for those needing to control both significant self-injurious behavior and epilepsy.

▶ Prognosis

The prognosis for ASD varies, depending greatly on an individual's specific characteristics and the severity and presentation of ASD. Some adults who were diagnosed with ASD as children and had early intervention have done very well and do not continue to demonstrate any significant ASD symptoms and behaviors.[10,11] However, a majority of children diagnosed with ASD often require lifelong dependence on others. The best prognosis occurs with early diagnosis and a focus on the child's abilities starting at an early age. Early diagnosis leads to earlier interventions, which can maximize services to help increase language, communication, and social functioning.

▶ When to Refer or Admit

When a child with a concern for ASD presents to a physician, the child should be referred for neuropsychological testing, including appropriate ADOS and ADI-R testing.

Those with ASD who exhibit severe aggressive behaviors or escalating self-injurious behaviors should be referred to psychiatry. Such severe behaviors may require admission to inpatient psychiatry services for safety.

Referral to appropriate specialties should occur for management of medical conditions or comorbidities not specific to the diagnosis of ASD. For example, an individual with ASD who has been diagnosed with epilepsy should be referred to neurology for epilepsy treatment and management.

▼ OTHER REGRESSIVE DEVELOPMENTAL DISORDERS

There are several neurodevelopmental genetic disorders that may present similarly to autism with developmental regression or autism-related features such as one of the more well-understood syndromes known as Rett syndrome (RTT).

RETT SYNDROME

RTT is a rare neurodevelopmental disorder seen predominantly in girls typically caused by de novo mutations in the X-linked *MECP2* gene encoding for methyl-CpG binding protein 2 (MeCP2) leading to a loss of function.[12,13] Although MeCP2 is ubiquitously present throughout all human tissues, the highest level of this protein is found within the brain and within the neurons.[13,14] When MeCP2 is abnormal, this leads to aberrant functioning of the brain as well as multisystem effects.

▶ General Considerations

RTT, estimated to affect 1 in every 10,000 female births,[15] was originally classified as an ASD in the DSM-4[16] but is no longer considered a mental health disorder and was removed from the DSM-5.[1] As with most neurodevelopmental disorders, there is a variable spectrum of severity of disease in RTT as well as variable time to presentation and to diagnosis. Over the last several years, the median age at time of diagnosis has decreased from 4 years of age to less than 3 years of age,[17] likely resulting from widely available and more frequently used genetic testing, improved clinician recognition, and increasing parental awareness. Several factors contribute to the variability of RTT including X chromosome inactivation pattern, individual genetic differences and comorbidities, environmental contributions, and the specific *MECP2* genetic mutation.[18,19]

Clinical Findings

After a period of normal or near-normal development, the individual then begins to experience the 4 stages of RTT that extend over their lifetime. First, developmental stagnation between 6 and 18 months of age occurs, followed by the regression stage between 1 and 4 years of age with loss of their developmental skills, including loss of purposeful hand use and loss of speech/language skills. Because of other changes, including social withdrawal, decrease or loss of purposeful eye contact, and development of hand stereotypies, a child may be diagnosed with ASD during this stage.[20] The plateau stage follows the regression stage with possible slow improvements in several areas. Not all individuals experience the fourth and last stage, the late motor decline stage, which is marked by loss of walking.[20]

Although RTT is often heterogenic in severity, the hallmark features of RTT include abnormal hand use, abnormal speech/language, presence of hand stereotypies, and impaired gait. Additionally, the level of disability involving multiple other organ systems is highly variable and evolves over time. Other features often seen include:

- Neuropsychiatric changes: anxiety, depression, aggression, pseudobulbar changes of inappropriate laughter or crying
- Neurology: microcephaly, seizures, abnormal movements, autonomic dysfunction, sleep disorders
- Breathing: disorganized breathing, including breath holding and hyperventilation
- Cardiac: prolonged QTc duration
- Gastrointestinal: swallowing dysfunction, dysmotility, constipation, poor nutrition, abnormal growth
- Musculoskeletal: abnormal tone, weakness, small hands and/or feet, scoliosis
- Other: bruxism, drooling, high pain tolerance, intense RTT stare

Diagnosis and Testing

Even with the advances in genetic testing, RTT primarily remains a clinical diagnosis. In 2010, the revised consensus RTT diagnostic criteria were validated (Table 9–2), which simplified the criteria and differentiated between classic and atypical RTT.[21] Atypical RTT is the diagnosis given to individuals who meet 2 or 3 of the major criteria but not all 4 and have regression history followed by stabilization. Even though genetic testing is not required for the diagnosis, a clinician can often confirm the diagnosis with targeted *MECP2* genetic sequencing and deletion/duplication. Additionally, the *MECP2* gene is commonly included on multiple developmental and epilepsy panels, and when pathogenic *MECP2* mutations are found, they can assist the clinician

with the diagnosis. However, in 3% to 5% of individuals who meet clinical criteria for RTT, no *MECP2* mutation will be found and there are individuals who do not meet RTT criteria in whom *MECP2* mutations are found.[19,22] In addition to genetic testing, the clinician may also order brain imaging to evaluate any additional signs or history not explained by the RTT diagnosis.

Additional Testing

In 2020, the Consensus Guidelines on Managing Rett Syndrome Across the Lifespan included surveillance and monitoring recommendations over the lifetime of an individual with RTT.[23] Additional testing is symptomatically driven; for example, an electroencephalogram is ordered for seizure evaluation, a swallow study for choking/difficulty swallowing, or a sleep study to evaluate significant sleep disordered breathing.

Differential Diagnosis

The age and current stage at the time of presentation can alter the differential diagnosis. For example, the differential diagnosis in a 15-month-old child with baseline poor eye contact and mild decreased tone presenting only with speech loss is very likely to include ASD, unlike a presentation in a similar child at 3 years of age in stage 3. Additional consideration and testing may be necessary to differentiate between individuals with more severe or earlier onset of RTT features and those previously classified as atypical RTT now uniquely classified as having CDKL5 deficiency disorders and FOXG1 syndrome. Other differential diagnoses to consider with overlapping features are non-RTT phenotypes such as autism, Angelman syndrome, Pitt-Hopkins syndrome, and nonspecific X-linked intellectual disability.

Treatment

Currently, there are no RTT-specific US Food and Drug Administration–approved medications. However, the sheer volume of both clinical and bench research studies in the past 2 decades is an obvious marker of the drive to not only treat RTT but ultimately cure RTT.[24,25] Until RTT-specific therapeutic discoveries are made, the medical community continues to try to mitigate the diffuse symptoms with least harm to the individuals often by choosing interventions that can benefit multiple symptoms.[26]

For example, medications such as trazodone or clonidine could benefit both sleep onset and overall improvement of hyperactive or agitation behaviors. Gabapentin, an antiseizure medication, might offer sedative benefits for sleep onset in addition to possible improvement in abnormal movements or decrease in neuropathic pain. Topiramate could potentially decrease seizure burden, reduce breathing dysfunction, and mitigate food-seeking behaviors.

Table 9–2. Revised Rett syndrome diagnostic criteria as validated by International Rett Syndrome Expert Panel.

Revised diagnostic criteria for RTT*
1. Partial or complete loss of acquired purposeful hand skills
2. Partial or complete loss of acquired spoken language**
3. Gait abnormalities: Impaired (dyspraxic) or absence of ability
4. Stereotypic hand movements such as hand wringing/squeezing, clapping/tapping, mouthing and washing/rubbing automatisms

Exclusion criteria for typical RTT
1. Brain injury secondary to trauma (peri- or postnatally), neurometabolic disease, or severe infection that causes neurological problems***
2. Grossly abnormal psychomotor development in first 6 months of life#

Supportive criteria for atypical RTT##
1. Breathing disturbances when awake
2. Bruxism when awake
3. Impaired sleep pattern
4. Abnormal muscle tone
5. Peripheral vasomotor disturbances
6. Scoliosis/kyphosis
7. Growth retardation
8. Small cold hands and feet
9. Inappropriate laughing/screaming spells
10. Diminished response to pain
11. Intense eye communication - "eye pointing"

*Because *MECP2* mutations are now identified in some individuals prior to any clear evidence of regression, the diagnosis of "possible" RTT should be given to those individuals under 3 years old who have not lost any skills but otherwise have clinical features suggestive of RTT. These individuals should be reassessed every 6–12 months for evidence of regression. If regression manifests, the diagnosis should then be changed to definite RTT. However, if the child does not show any evidence of regression by 5 years, the diagnosis of RTT should be questioned.
**Loss of acquired language is based on best acquired spoken language skill, not strictly on the acquisition of distinct words or higher language skills. Thus, an individual who had learned to babble but then loses this ability is considered to have a loss of acquired language.
***There should be clear evidence (neurological or ophthalmological examination and MRI/CT) that the presumed insult directly resulted in neurological dysfunction.
#Grossly abnormal to the point that normal milestones (acquiring head control, swallowing, developing social smile) are not met. Mild generalized hypotonia or other previously reported subtle developmental alterations[16] during the first six months of life is common in RTT and do not constitute an exclusionary criterion.
##If an individual has or ever had a clinical feature listed it is counted as a supportive criterion. Many of those features have an age dependency, manifesting and becoming more predominant at certain ages. Therefore, the diagnosis of atypical RTT may be easier for older individuals than for younger. In the case of a younger individual (under 5 years old) who has a period of regression and ≥2 main criteria but does not fulfill the requirement of 5/11 supportive criteria, the diagnosis of "probably atypical RTT" may be given. Individuals who fall into this category should be reassessed as they age and the diagnosis revised accordingly.
Adapted with permission from Neul JL, Kaufmann WE, Glaze DG, et al. Rett syndrome: revised diagnostic criteria and nomenclature. *Ann Neurol.* 2010;68(6):944–950.

Depending on the severity of the disease, individuals with RTT often benefit from procedural types of therapies such as gastrostomy for poor or unsafe oral intake, tendon lengthening and serial casting to improve gait, spinal fusion to reduce and stabilize scoliosis, or placement of a vagal nerve stimulator to reduce seizure frequency.

Individuals with RTT benefit from ongoing physical therapies, occupational therapies, and speech therapies to focus on improving the main diagnostic RTT features directly.

▶ Prognosis

Tarquinio et al[27] recently showed the survival rate for classic and atypical RTT to be greater than 70% at 45 years of age, and the most common cause of death in RTT is a presumed or confirmed cardiorespiratory event, most notably aspiration. This same group also demonstrated the most significant risk factors affecting the mortality rate in classic RTT (Table 9–3); notably, several of the factors are modifiable, suggesting that a constant unwavering drive to improve these factors may lower the mortality risk.[27]

Because of the growing amount of patient data in research and large databases, clinicians can cautiously offer prognostic considerations based on the genotype-phenotype associations. For example, acknowledging individual variability, individuals with the mutations R106X, R168X, R255X, or R270X or deletions or insertions are similarly found to be at higher risk for a more severe RTT disease.[18,19,28]

Table 9–3. Risk factors for mortality in classic Rett syndrome.[27]

Variable	No. of Patients	Hazard Ratio	Confidence Interval	P Value
Inability to walk	882	3.2	1.6-6.5	.00
Number of hospitalizations	892	1.1	1.0-1.2	.00
Microcephaly	819	9.9	1.7-58	.01
Poor global health	913	1.8	1.1-3.10	.02
Seizure severity	892	2.4	1.0-6.8	.03
Unable to babble or use words	819	2.6	1.1-6.5	.03
Degree of rigidity	882	1.3	1.0-1.7	.04
Poor hand use	882	2.6	1.0-6.8	.05
Low weight Z score on Rett syndrome curve	854	2.9	1.0-8.8	.05
Poverty	819	7.4	0.9-60.5	.06
Unable to sit independently	882	1.3	1.0-1.6	.07
Immunity	813	1.4	1.0-1.9	.07
Degree of dystonia	882	1.4	1.0-2.1	.09

▶ When to Refer or Admit

Over the past several years, the proportion of pediatricians making the diagnosis of classic RTT in a child has doubled to nearly 8%, yet there has been no obvious improvement in decreasing the time to diagnosis for either specialists or pediatricians.[17] As is seen with other neurodevelopmental disorders, a reduced time to diagnosis can and often does translate to better outcomes. Regarding pediatricians, there are a few plausible reasons for minimal change in the time to diagnose. One is the time duration between visits when deploying the "watch and wait" surveillance tactic as children have longer intervals between visits as they age.[17] If an RTT feature is observed at 18 months but the clinician has low suspicion of RTT, unless the caregiver calls with concerns, nearly 6 months may pass before the child is observed again. This is in stark contrast to the decreased time between visits with presentation at 9, 12, or 15 months. Second, there are still challenges with recognizing and developing a high suspicion for RTT with presenting features that deviate from those emphasized in the medical literature.

Tarquinio et al[17] demonstrated that the diagnosis was delayed with more subtle regression, the absence of regression of hand use or verbal language, longer delays in gaining or loss of more advanced hand skills (eg, pincher grasp, utensil manipulation), later onset of supportive diagnostic features, unusual hand stereotypies, and presence of a normal head circumference. Tarquinio et al[17] also found that the RTT diagnosis was often suggested even before all diagnostic criteria were present. When pediatricians keep a high index of suspicion for RTT in children who have a more subtle or slightly variable or delayed presentation and have a low threshold to order genetic testing and/or refer to a specialist, this could lead to an earlier diagnosis and earlier therapies.

REFERENCES

1. American Psychiatric Association, DSM-5 Task Force. *Diagnostic and Statistical Manual of Mental Disorders.* 5th ed. American Psychiatric Association; 2013.
2. Maenner MJ, Shaw KA, Bakian AV, et al. Prevalence and characteristics of autism spectrum disorder among children aged 8 years–autism and developmental disabilities monitoring network, 11 sites, United States, 2018. *MMWR Surveill Summ.* 2021;70(11):1-16.
3. Elsabbagh M, Divan G, Koh YJ, et al. Global prevalence of autism and other pervasive developmental disorders. *Autism Res.* 2012;5(3):160-179.
4. Schaefer GB, Mendelsohn NJ, Professional Practice and Guidelines Committee. Clinical genetics evaluation in identifying the etiology of autism spectrum disorders: 2013 guideline revisions. *Genet Med.* 2013;15(5):399-407.
5. Idring S, Magnusson C, Lundberg M, et al. Parental age and the risk of autism spectrum disorders: Findings from a Swedish population-based cohort. *Int J Epidemiol.* 2014;43(1):107-115.
6. Wu S, Wu F, Ding Y, Hou J, Bi J, Zhang Z. Advanced parental age and autism risk in children: a systematic review and meta-analysis. *Acta Psychiatr Scand.* 2017;135(1):29-41.
7. Christensen J, Grønborg TK, Sørensen MJ, et al. Prenatal valproate exposure and risk of autism spectrum disorders and childhood autism. *JAMA.* 2013;309(16):1696-1703.
8. DeStefano F, Shimabukuro TT. The MMR vaccine and autism. *Annu Rev Virol.* 2019;6(1):585-600.

9. Lovaas OI. Behavioral treatment and normal educational and intellectual functioning in young autistic children. *J Consult Clin Psychol*. 1987;55(1):3-9.

10. Anderson DK, Liang JW, Lord C. Predicting young adult outcome among more and less cognitively able individuals with autism spectrum disorders. *J Child Psychol Psychiatry*. 2014;55(5):485-494.

11. Fein D, Barton M, Eigsti IM, et al. Optimal outcome in individuals with a history of autism. *J Child Psychol Psychiatry*. 2013;54(2):195-205.

12. Amir RE, Van den Veyver IB, Wan M, Tran CQ, Francke U, Zoghbi HY. Rett syndrome is caused by mutations in X-linked MECP2, encoding methylCPG-binding protein 2. *Nat Genet*. 1999;23:185-188.

13. Gonazales ML, LaSalle JM. The role of MeCP2 in brain development and neurodevelopmental disorders. *Curr Psychiatry Rep*. 2010;12:127-134.

14. Shahbazian MD, Antalffy B, Armstrong DL, Zoghbi HY. Insight into Rett syndrome: MeCP2 levels display tissue- and cell-specific differences and correlate with neuronal maturation. *Hum Mol Genet*. 2002;11:115-124.

15. Laurvick CL, de Klerk N, Bower C, et al. Rett syndrome in Australia: a review of the epidemiology. *J Pediatr*. 2006;148: 347-352.

16. American Psychiatric Association, DSM-4 Task Force. *Diagnostic and Statistical Manual of Mental Disorders*. 4th ed. American Psychiatric Association; 1994.

17. Tarquinio DC, Hou W, Neul JL, et al. Age of diagnosis in Rett syndrome: patterns of recognition among diagnosticians and risk factors for late diagnosis. *Pediatr Neurol*. 2015;52(6): 585-591.

18. Cuddapah VA, Pillai RB, Shekar KV, et al. Methyl-CpG-binding protein 2 (MECP2) mutation type is associated with disease severity in Rett Syndrome. *J Med Genet* 2014;51:152-158.

19. Neul JL, Fang P, Barrish J, et al. Specific mutations in methyl-CpG-binding protein 2 confer different severities in Rett syndrome. *Neurology*. 2008;70(16):1313-1321.

20. Neul JL. The relationship of Rett syndrome and MECP2 disorders to autism. *Dialogues Clin Neurosci*. 2012;14:253-262.

21. Neul JL, Kaufmann WE, Glaze DG, et al. Rett syndrome: revised diagnostic criteria and nomenclature. *Ann Neurol*. 2010;68:944-950.

22. Wan M, Lees SS, Zhang X, et al. Rett syndrome and beyond: recurrent spontaneous and familial MECP2 mutations at CpG hotspots. *Am J Hum Genet*. 1999;65:1520-1529.

23. Fu C, Armstrong D, Marsh E, et al. Consensus guidelines on managing Rett syndrome across the lifespan. *BMJ Paediatr Open*. 2020;13;4(1):e000717.

24. Katz DM, Bird A, Coenraads M, et al. Rett syndrome: crossing the threshold to clinical translation. *Trends Neurosci*. 2016;39;100-113.

25. Gomathi M, Subramanian P, Balachandar V. Drug studies on Rett syndrome: from bench to bedside. *J Autism Dev Disord*. 2020;50:2740-2764.

26. Ivy AS, Standridge SM. Rett syndrome: a timely review from recognition to current clinical approaches and clinical study updates. *Semin Pediatr Neurol*. 2021;27:100881.

27. Tarquinio DC, Hou W, Neul JL, et al. The changing face of survival in Rett syndrome and *MECP2*-related disorders. *Pediatr Neurol*. 2015;53:402-411.

28. Colvin L, Leonard H, deKlerk N, et al. Refining the phenotype of common mutations in Rett syndrome. *J Med Genet*. 2004;41:25.

Neurocutaneous Disorders

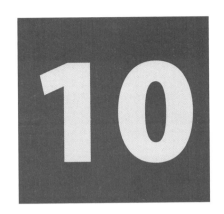

David M. Ritter, MD, PhD
David N. Franz, MD
Darcy A. Krueger, MD, PhD

Neurocutaneous disorders are diverse disorders that affect both the skin and nervous system (Table 10–1). Many either include or increase the risk of tumors as well. A careful history of neurologic symptoms with a thorough skin exam can often point to the diagnosis before genetic testing is obtained. Genetic testing can confirm the diagnosis when uncertain, assist in identifying additional familial cases not previously suspected, and facilitate family counseling and planning. The disorders in this group often result from mutations in 2 common pathways: mammalian target of rapamycin (mTOR, tuberous sclerosis) and Ras-mitogen–activated protein kinase (Ras-MAPK, neurofibromatosis type 1). Although there are several disorders in this category, focusing on a few of these disorders will allow the general pediatrician and pediatric neurologist to start treatment and screening early. Specifically, recent advances in these disorders provide opportunities for targeted therapies in patients.

NEUROFIBROMATOSIS TYPE 1

Neurofibromatosis type 1 (NF1) is an autosomal dominant disorder caused by mutations in the *NF1* gene. It is the most common neurocutaneous syndrome with an incidence of 1 in approximately 3000. Mutations in the *NF1* gene lead to decreased neurofibromin function, a GTPase that inhibits Ras. Loss of neurofibromin function leads to overactivation of the Ras-MAPK pathway and, ultimately, cell overgrowth.

▶ Clinical Findings

Typical findings in NF1 include café-au-lait macules, axillary or inguinal freckling, Lisch nodules, neurofibromas, and optic gliomas. The most readily noticeable skin feature is café-au-lait macules, of which greater than 6 café-au-lait macules will be present. Children with fewer café-au-lait spots should be followed for growth and number of spots, which can increase over time in NF1. Axillary freckling

or cutaneous fibromas in the presence of the café-au-lait spots confirms the diagnosis. However, other rare findings, including vascular lesions or bone lesions (eg, sphenoid dysplasia or tibial bowing/pseudoarthroses), can also be used to diagnose NF1 clinically. In the nervous system, neurofibromas are the hallmark feature. They are benign nerve sheath tumors on peripheral nerves. About one-third of patients can have plexiform neurofibromas, which arrive from nerve fascicules and plexuses. Plexiform neurofibromas may cause significant pain, lead to disfigurement, compromise of the surrounding tissue, and have malignant potential. The presence of optic atrophy and decreased visual acuity early in childhood may suggest an optic glioma. Many patients with NF1 may have several other significant complaints including headaches, attention-deficit/hyperactivity disorder (ADHD), intellectual disability, and chronic pain syndromes. Because NF1 alters the Ras-MAPK pathway, patients remain at higher risk for several types of cancer than the general population including pheochromocytomas, gastrointestinal tumors, brain tumors, and breast cancer.

▶ Diagnosis

Diagnosis is made based on the finding of 2 common features of the disease (Table 10–2) or the presence of 1 feature in the setting of a first-degree relative with an NF1 diagnosis. Genetic testing may help determine if a mutation in *NF1* is present in a patient with café-au-lait macules before the onset of other manifestations.

▶ Screening and Treatment

Skin

There is currently no recommendation for treatment of café-au-lait spots or axillary freckling in NF1. Cutaneous and subcutaneous fibromas may be numerous and disfiguring. Removal by a plastic surgeon or dermatologist may be

Table 10–1. Neurocutaneous syndromes and common features.

Syndrome	Skin Features	Nervous System Features
Neurofibromatosis type 1	Café-au-lait macules and axillary freckling	Neurofibromas, optic pathway gliomas, ADHD
Neurofibromatosis type 2	Café-au-lait macules	Vestibular schwannomas, hearing loss, meningiomas
Schwannomatosis		Schwannomas, chronic pain
Tuberous sclerosis	Ash leaf macules, angiofibromas, ungual fibromas	Cortical tubers, subependymal nodules, SEGAs, seizures, intellectual disability, TAND
Sturge-Weber syndrome	Port-wine stain	Leptomeningeal angioma, seizures
Incontinentia pigmenti	Hypopigmented lesions on lines of Blaschko	Deep subcortical strokes, cerebral dysgenesis, epilepsy
von Hippel-Lindau		CNS hemangioblastomas

ADHD, attention-deficit/hyperactivity disorder; CNS, central nervous system; SEGA, subependymal giant cell astrocytoma; TAND, tuberous sclerosis complex–associated neurologic disorder.

performed if they are causing significant problems. Some skin lesions may cause pruritus that is refractory to topical treatments and antihistamines. Gabapentin may be used to help in these situations. There is no value in counting the number of lesions or measuring them after a diagnosis is made because they carry no predictive value.

Plexiform Neurofibromas

Plexiform neurofibromas vary significantly in number, location, and size. These are usually benign, but malignant transformation is a concern if causing persistent pain or impinging on surrounding tissue and structures. Whole-body magnetic resonance imaging (MRI) is increasingly used to screen for internal plexiform fibromas. Once a plexiform fibroma is identified, a repeat MRI of the dedicated body area where a plexiform neurofibroma exists is recommended if there are any changes in clinical symptoms or if the fibroma

is shown to be growing in size or other concerning features. The frequency of reimaging will depend on the patient's age and level of concern for malignant transformation. Treatment for a malignant peripheral nerve sheath tumor includes resection, chemotherapy, and radiation, but the 5-year survival rate is currently poor. Targeted therapy for malignant peripheral nerve sheath tumors is presently available with selumetinib, a MAPK inhibitor.

Optic Pathway Glioma

These tumors are pilocytic astrocytomas and World Health Organization grade 1. Most occur before 6 years of age. As such, after a diagnosis of NF1, patients should have yearly eye exams with an ophthalmologist familiar with NF1. Yearly MRIs with dedicated sequences of the orbits in all NF1 patients within this age range are performed in some centers. In contrast, others recommend repeated imaging only when there is clinical evidence of progression or other concerning initial imaging features. Treatment of an optic pathway glioma should begin if there is a decrease in visual function, and treatment is with traditional chemotherapy. However, new targeted therapies are being investigated.

Other Neurologic Findings

Moyamoya disease, seizures, headaches, cognitive impairment, and ADHD are more common in NF1 patients than in the general population. Specifically, ADHD occurs in approximately 50% of patients. There are no specific treatments for these issues in NF1. However, with the high prevalence of ADHD and executive function issues, physicians should ensure children are being evaluated for 504 Plans and Individualized Education Plan accommodations

Table 10–2. National Institutes of Health Consensus Development Conference criteria for neurofibromatosis type 1 (NF1).

1. Six or more café-au-lait macules ≥5 mm in prepubertal or ≥15 mm in postpubertal patients
2. Two or more neurofibromas or 1 plexiform neurofibroma
3. Freckling in the axillary or inguinal area
4. Optic glioma
5. Two or more Lisch nodules (iris hamartomas)
6. A distinctive osseous lesion with or without pseudoarthrosis
7. First-degree relative with NF1

Note: Two or more criteria are required to establish the diagnosis of NF1.

in school. There can be areas of hyperintensity in the basal ganglia, brainstem, or cerebellum on T2 brain imaging. Usually, these have no associated clinical symptomatology and may spontaneously disappear in later years. Rarely, these T2 signal abnormalities may represent low-grade gliomas, and patients should be monitored for symptoms.

Other Body Systems

Some optic pathway gliomas can involve the hypothalamus, so attention should be paid to precocious puberty or other growth issues with endocrinology involvement as needed. Many patients may have boney lesions or scoliosis that needs annual monitoring with an orthopedic provider.

Other Tumors

Patients with NF1 are at higher risk for leukemia, pheochromocytoma, and breast cancer, among others. Appropriate, early workup should be done if showing symptoms. If there is a change in blood pressure or heart rate, a pheochromocytoma workup should be completed immediately.

▶ Prognosis

The overall prognosis for patients with NF1 is good, but the increased risk of cancer does decrease average life expectancy by approximately 10 years. Primary care physicians and neurologists can help improve patients' care by probing how their neurofibromas' appearance is altering their interactions with others, advocating for support in school, and responding appropriately to changes in their symptomology. When patients approach reproductive age, having conversations about inheritance and involving a genetic counselor are often needed to help patients understand their future children's risks. Understanding how selumetinib and the development of other targeted therapies may alter the disease course in NF1 will be of great interest in the near future.

NEUROFIBROMATOSIS TYPE 2

Neurofibromatosis type 2 (NF2) is caused by a mutation in the *NF2* gene on chromosome 22, which encodes the protein merlin. Merlin is a scaffolding protein primarily found in neurons and serves upstream regulator of tumor suppressor pathways, including Ras. Inheritance is autosomal dominant, and it has an incidence of approximately 1 in 40,000.

▶ Clinical Findings

The hallmark findings of NF2 are tumors, specifically vestibular schwannomas. Often patients will have bilateral hearing loss, tinnitus, vestibular findings, or brainstem compression

from the vestibular schwannomas. Additionally, cranial nerve tumors, meningiomas, and spinal cord schwannomas are common. Symptoms depend on the tumor's location and involve pain, headaches, weakness, or bowel/bladder incontinence. Most patients will also develop cataracts. An ophthalmologic exam may discover retinal hamartomas, optic disc gliomas, or optic nerve meningiomas. Café-au-lait macules are less frequent and smaller than in NF1, occurring in less than 50% of patients. Another common cutaneous finding is raised, hyperpigmented plaques on the skin.

▶ Diagnosis

Diagnosis is based on clinical findings and subsequent genetic testing. Primarily, this starts with the diagnosis and symptoms of a tumor. There are 4 separate ways to meet the criteria for NF2:

1. Bilateral vestibular schwannoma

2. First-degree relative with NF2 and (a) unilateral vestibular schwannoma or (b) any 2 of the following: meningioma, glioma, neurofibroma, schwannoma, or posterior subcapsular lenticular opacities

3. Unilateral vestibular schwannoma and any 2 of the following: meningioma, glioma, neurofibroma, schwannoma, or posterior subcapsular lenticular opacities

4. Multiple meningiomas and (a) unilateral schwannoma or (b) any 2 of the following: meningioma, glioma, neurofibroma, schwannoma, or posterior subcapsular lenticular opacities

The differential diagnosis for NF2 primarily includes schwannomatosis (see below).

▶ Screening and Treatment

On diagnosis, patients should undergo brain and spine MRIs with and without contrast looking for tumor burden along with ophthalmologic and audiologic evaluations. Genetic testing with a geneticist is indicated, as there is a high rate of mosaicism in NF2 and interpreting genetic testing results at times is challenging.

Screening

MRI of the brain should be done annually to screen for tumor growth, and annual hearing tests should be performed to follow subtle hearing changes.

Tumors

Treatment of NF2 revolves around the treatment of tumors. This primarily includes surgical resection, although there is no clear evidence of a preferred method or timing. Targeted chemotherapy, including monoclonal antibodies and mTOR inhibitors, has been developed and is in testing.

Prognosis

On average, there is a decrease in life expectancy related to atypical meningioma development compared to the general population. Genetic counseling is vital in reproductive years to counsel on the autosomal dominant nature of the disorder.

SCHWANNOMATOSIS

Schwannomatosis is a clinical entity like NF2. Patients have significant pain and are found to have nerve sheath tumors. Unlike NF2, they rarely have vestibular schwannomas but will have schwannomas located elsewhere in the body. Schwannomatosis is autosomal dominant, with most cases familial in nature from mutations in *SMARCB1* and *LZTR1*. Diagnosis should be suspected in any individual with 2 or more schwannomas, no findings of NF1 or NF2, and a lesion confirmed pathologically by histology. The mainstay of treatment is monitoring for schwannomas with regular whole-body MRIs, mainly including short tau inversion recovery sequences to highlight tumors. Treatment is focused on chronic pain treatment and surgical resection if a schwannoma is causing a neurologic deficit. Prognosis is good with no decrease in life expectancy, but many patients suffer from depression and anxiety related to chronic pain.

OTHER DISORDERS OF THE RAS-MAPK PATHWAY

Although not traditionally considered neurocutaneous disorders, it should be appreciated that other genetic disorders affecting the Ras-MAPK pathway frequently have skin and/or neurologic system involvement, as well as other significant clinical findings to be aware of. All, including Noonan syndrome, have a high likelihood of cardiac anomalies or impaired function. Craniofacial abnormalities are also common, including increased likelihood of craniosynostosis and Chiari I malformation. Patients with Noonan syndrome with multiple lentigines, previously referred to as LEOPARD syndrome, have additional characteristic black or dark brown spots on the skin along with intellectual disabilities and speech difficulties. Patients with cardiofaciocutaneous syndrome are characterized by sparse or brittle hair, sparse eyebrows, dystrophic nails, and hyperkeratosis of the skin. Neurologically, cognitive and/or global developmental delays are common, and epilepsy may be present in over 50%.

TUBEROUS SCLEROSIS COMPLEX

Tuberous sclerosis complex (TSC) is caused by mutations in *TSC1* (hamartin) and *TSC2* (tuberin). It is an autosomal dominant condition occurring in 1 in 6000 people resulting in mTOR overactivity. While the disease causes numerous hamartomatous (benign) tumors, TSC is often recognized as the most common single-gene disorder causing autism and epilepsy.

Clinical Findings

Patients are often diagnosed after presenting with seizures early in life and a skin exam finds one of several prototypical skin lesions (eg, hypomelanotic macules, angiofibroma, shagreen patch, confetti lesions) or cardiac rhabdomyomas are found on prenatal ultrasound. However, the spectrum of symptoms in patients is wide-ranging including infants diagnosed with infantile spasms only to be found to have the same mutation that their parent caries who has mild findings. Seizures are often focal seizures, and infants with focal seizures should be monitored closely for the development of infantile spasms and vice versa. Brain findings include tubers, subependymal nodules, and subependymal giant cell astrocytomas (SEGAs). Renal disease is also common, and kidney findings include renal cysts and angiomyolipomas, which may lead to chronic kidney disease and renal hemorrhages. Additionally, patients may develop lesions in their retinas (hamartomas), heart (cardiac rhabdomyomas), lungs (lymphangioleiomyomatosis), liver, and pancreas. Due to their generally benign and slow-growing nature, most tumors in TSC often need no urgent or surgical intervention. Cognitively, patients have a wide range of phenotypes from no issues to severe intellectual disability. Patients may also have autism or carry autism-like phenotypes (eg, anxiety, hyperactivity, stereotypies, communication issues). Finally, TSC-associated neurologic disorder (TAND) is a common finding leading to numerous school problems, social problems, and mental health concerns.

Diagnosis

Diagnosis is made either clinically or genetically. Clinically, if a patient has 2 major features or 1 major and 2 minor features, then a diagnosis is definite (Table 10–3). A possible diagnosis is found from the presence of 1 major feature or 2 minor features. Genetic testing for *TSC1* and *TSC2* is indicated, especially in young children when later features may not have had the opportunity to present themselves but when early intervention, treatment, and screening could have a substantial impact on long-term outcomes.

Screening and Treatment

There are numerous specific options for treatment in TSC, and screening is a lifelong process. Overall care is best performed in a comprehensive center, but the general pediatrician and general neurologist can help ensure all areas are being managed. Over the past 10 years, numerous studies have shown that mTOR inhibitors have activity against nearly every TSC manifestation (SEGA, angiomyolipomas,

Table 10–3. Tuberous sclerosis complex diagnostic criteria.

Major Findings	Minor Findings
Hypomelanotic macules (>3, at least 5 mm)	Confetti skin lesions
Angiofibromas (>3) or fibrous cephalic plaque	Dental enamel pits (>3)
Ungual fibromas (>2)	Intraoral fibromas (>2)
Shagreen patch	Retinal achromatic patch
Multiple retinal hamartomas	Multiple renal cysts
Cortical dysplasia	Nonrenal hamartomas
Subependymal nodules	
Subependymal giant cell astrocytomas	
Cardiac rhabdomyoma	
Lymphangioleiomyomatosis[a]	
Angiomyolipomas (>2)[a]	

[a]Presence of lymphangioleiomyomatosis and angiomyolipomas does not together confirm a diagnosis of tuberous sclerosis complex; other clinic features must be present

retinal hamartomas, cardiac rhabdomyomas, lymphangioleiomyomatosis, epilepsy, angiofibromas, and ungual/subungual fibromas).

Skin

At yearly visits, a skin assessment should be made. Hypopigmented macules generally have no clinical consequence but are an early and easily recognizable manifestation to aid with diagnosis. Angiofibromas appear during childhood and may worsen with sun exposure and, at times, can become bothersome to patients with recurrent bleeding and itching. An oral or topical mTOR inhibitor can help reduce angiofibromas and the irritation. Surgical interventions can be performed for disfiguring angiofibromas. Similar treatment options are available for ungual fibromas, which usually present later in life. Shagreen patches usually show up in the lumbosacral region and do not require any intervention.

Central Nervous System Lesions

Tubers are relatively stable findings in TSC; however, if serving as a focus for seizures, then surgical resection or laser ablation may be indicated. Subependymal nodules should be monitored for growth and transformation into SEGAs. This should be done with MRIs every 1 to 3 years through childhood until 25 years of age. If a patient develops a SEGA, prompt treatment with an mTOR inhibitor will stabilize

the tumor and even cause it to shrink. When missed due to unknown diagnosis or lax screening, SEGAs can obstruct the foramen of Monroe, causing hydrocephalus that is life threatening and requiring immediate surgical resection and the possible need for cerebrospinal fluid diversion via shunting.

Seizures

Prompt recognition and treatment of seizures are crucial. Many patients have localization-related epilepsy; thus, focal antiepileptic agents are a mainstay of therapy (including vigabatrin). Cannabidiol and mTOR inhibitors are approved for epilepsy in TSC. Infants with TSC are at risk for infantile spasms, and any patient presenting with infantile spasms should be further evaluated for a diagnosis of TSC. Vigabatrin is the recommended first-line treatment for infantile spasms in TSC; adrenocorticotropin hormone is reserved for treating infantile spasms not responsive to vigabatrin. Secondary to the high incidence of seizures, infants should be screened at diagnosis with a routine electroencephalogram (EEG) and then every 6 to 8 weeks until a year of life to monitor for changes even if never having reported clinical seizures. Screening EEGs with epileptiform abnormalities should lead to treatment with vigabatrin (and possibly mTOR inhibitors) as seizure control leads to optimal developmental outcomes.

TAND

Screening for TAND-associated symptoms should occur at every visit. Formal screening should occur at routine developmental levels with a focused survey such as the TAND Checklist. Formal neuropsychiatric testing should be performed before starting school to assess for specialized school needs, including Individualized Education Plans.

Kidney

An MRI of the abdomen looking for renal cysts, angiomyolipomas, and other abdominal hamartomas (pancreatic neuroendocrine tumors, splenic hamartomas, ovarian angiomyolipomas, and PEComas) should be performed every 1 to 3 years depending on findings. Renal ultrasounds will miss the other abdominal lesions and often underestimate the severity of renal involvement. Yearly glomerular filtration rates (with cystatin C measurements) and blood pressures should be performed in those with kidney involvement. Angiomyolipomas greater than 3 cm in diameter or that pose a risk for renal dysfunction should be treated with mTOR inhibitors to stabilize their growth and prevent bleeding. If they enlarge or cause renal hemorrhage, treatment is with embolization and corticosteroids. With mTOR inhibitor use, the likelihood of end-stage renal disease and, thus, the need for kidney transplant is reduced. Some patients (1%-3%)

with TSC due to deletion of *TSC2* will also have deletion of nearby *PKD1*, a condition referred to as a contiguous gene syndrome. Such patients may have normal-appearing kidneys at birth but, within the first 2 years of life, will develop rapid cystic replacement of normal kidney tissue. The patients will have early-onset renal hypertension and a gradual reduction in kidney function typically leading to renal transplant within the first 2 decades of life.

Lung

Lymphangioleiomyomatosis (LAM), characterized by cystic disease of the lungs, should be screened for at each visit by assessing dyspnea on exertion and shortness of breath in all patients. However, LAM is most common in adult female patients due to its association with estrogen production. LAM is a form of benign metastasis whereby LAM cells arise in an angiomyolipoma, lymphangioma, or other hamartoma that then spread through the lymphatic system to the lung parenchyma. Once in the lung, LAM cells proliferate, causing decreased gas exchange, restrictive lung disease, and lymphatic obstruction. LAM occurs primarily in females due to estrogen's trophic effects on LAM cells, although less severe forms may occur in up to 20% of male TSC patients. Exogenous estrogen use is discouraged, and continual counseling against smoking is essential for reducing pulmonary complications. Those with severe lymphangioleiomyomatosis may present with pneumothorax after rupture of a bleb or cyst. Following puberty in females, screening high-resolution chest computed tomography scans should be obtained every 5 to 10 years, and vascular endothelial growth factor D (VEGF-D) levels can also be used to assess for risk of LAM. mTOR inhibitors are the treatment of choice for patients with LAM. Pleurodesis procedures are used following pneumothorax to help prevent a recurrence.

Eye

An ophthalmologic exam should be obtained in patients with TSC at diagnosis, and if there are findings, an exam should occur yearly. Retinal hamartomas rarely need intervention unless causing visual problems.

Cardiac

Infants born with rhabdomyomas should have echocardiograms every 1 to 3 years or as clinically indicated to ensure the rhabdomyomas regress over time. In infants with symptomatic rhabdomyomas, an mTOR inhibitor should be started immediately, and successful treatment prenatally has been reported for select situations. Follow-up should be determined by the rate of regression and cardiac function. Patients with TSC are at risk for arrhythmias, and as such, an electrocardiogram every 3 to 5 years should be obtained for screening throughout the patient's life span.

Dental

Dental lesions are common, and regular dental visits should be encouraged. Findings may be treated with surgery if needed.

▶ Prognosis

Life expectancy is average in TSC patients but may be complicated by other issues (eg, intractable epilepsy, polycystic kidneys). While some genotype-phenotype correlations exist, it is not currently possible to predict cognitive development in young children with TSC. Current studies looking at mTOR inhibitors and vigabatrin as early treatments to alter TSC progression are interesting but are ongoing.

STURGE-WEBER SYNDROME

Sturge-Weber syndrome occurs via sporadic somatic mutations in the *GNAQ* gene, which is involved in vascular development. *GNAQ* encodes a G-protein α subunit, and mutations in Sturge-Weber syndrome result in an active subunit. This activation leads to downstream activation of phospholipase C and parts of the ERK pathway. The incidence is approximately 1 in 25,000 births.

▶ Clinical Findings

The hallmark skin finding in Sturge-Weber is a port-wine stain in the distribution of the ophthalmologic branch of the trigeminal nerve. In Sturge-Weber, there is also involvement of the brain, primarily characterized by leptomeningeal angiomas. This results in poor blood flow, gliosis, and brain atrophy. The resulting brain injury can result in migraines, epilepsy, stroke-like episodes, and intellectual disability. Additionally, patients with involvement of both the upper and lower eyelid will be at risk of developing glaucoma in that eye as well.

▶ Diagnosis

Diagnosis is based on the clinical findings. Because the sporadic mutations in Sturge-Weber are somatic and not germline, genetic testing is usually not indicated as tissue from an affected area would have to be sampled to determine if positive.

▶ Screening and Treatment

Screening

The presence of a port-wine stain should prompt screening for Sturge-Weber. Brain MRI and ophthalmologic exams should be performed at that time. Brain MRIs may not show typical findings until 1 year of age.

Skin

The main concern with the port-wine stain is cosmetic issues. Laser treatments have been used but are not necessary.

Neurologic

Symptoms are related to the intracranial findings, and no target therapies exist. Seizures are typically focal in nature, and appropriate antiepileptic drug therapy can be selected. With intractable epilepsy, a hemispherectomy may be considered, especially in young children. Migraines may be treated with regular migraine treatments. For patients with extensive vascular malformations, aspirin therapy should be initiated. However, the reduction of stroke-like symptoms with aspirin treatment remains controversial.

Eye

Frequent ophthalmology evaluations are needed in infancy and early childhood to screen for glaucoma. Patients should then continue with yearly eye exams, even if asymptomatic, throughout their lives.

▶ Prognosis

Intellectual disability and seizure burden are the most significant contributors to prognosis in Sturge-Weber. This appears to have some correlation with intracranial findings. Many patients with port-wine stains and only minor other findings have no sustained issues, whereas those with severe intracranial involvement resulting in intractable epilepsy have an overall worse course.

OTHER NEUROCUTANEOUS SYNDROMES

Several other syndromes present with both cutaneous and central nervous system findings. Incontinentia pigmenti is an X-linked disorder with characteristic skin findings following the lines of Blaschko, and around one-third of patients of have central nervous system involvement including cerebral palsy, deep white matter infarcts, cerebral dysgenesis, microcephaly, and epilepsy. It results from a mutation in *IKBKG* (formerly *NEMO*), and treatment is symptomatic with no formal screening recommendations. von Hippel-Lindau disease is characterized by numerous tumors (including hemangioblastomas in the central nervous system). Occasionally, a nevus or other vascular lesions can be found on the skin. The disease results from a mutation in the *VHL* gene and is autosomal dominant. Treatment revolves around tumor screening, monitoring for bleeding from hemangioblastomas, and surgical resection of tumors.

BIBLIOGRAPHY

Baser ME, Friedman JM, Evans DG. Increasing the specificity of diagnostic criteria for schwannomatosis. *Neurology*. 2006;66:730-732. doi:10.1212/01.wnl.0000201190.89751.41

Baser ME, Friedman JM, Wallace AJ, et al. Evaluation of clinical diagnostic criteria for neurofibromatosis 2. *Neurology*. 2002;59:1759-1765. doi:10.1212/01.wnl.0000035638.74084.f4

Comi AM. Pathophysiology of Sturge-Weber syndrome. *J Child Neurol*. 2003;18:509-516. doi:10.1177/08830738030180080701

De la Torre AJ, Luat AF, Juhász C, et al. A multidisciplinary consensus for clinical care and research needs for Sturge-Weber syndrome. *Pediatr Neurol*. 2018;84:11-20. doi:10.1016/j.pediatrneurol.2018.04.005

Ferner RE, Huson SM, Thomas N, et al. Guidelines for the diagnosis and management of individuals with neurofibromatosis 1. *J Med Genet*. 2007;44:81-88. doi:10.1136/jmg.2006.045906

Franz DN, Agricola K, Mays M, et al. Everolimus for subependymal giant cell astrocytoma: 5-year final analysis. *Ann Neurol*. 2015;78:929-938. doi:10.1002/ana.24523

Franz DN, Krueger DA. mTOR inhibitor therapy as a disease modifying therapy for tuberous sclerosis complex. *Am J Med Genet C Semin Med Genet*. 2018;178:365-373. doi:10.1002/ajmg.c.31655

Gürsoy S, Erçal D. Genetic evaluation of common neurocutaneous syndromes. *Pediatr Neurol*. 2018;89:3-10. doi:10.1016/j.pediatrneurol.2018.08.006

Krueger DA, Northrup H, International Tuberous Sclerosis Complex Consensus Group. Tuberous sclerosis complex surveillance and management: recommendations of the 2012 International Tuberous Sclerosis Complex Consensus Conference. *Pediatr Neurol*. 2013;49:255-265. doi:10.1016/j.pediatrneurol.2013.08.002

Krueger DA, Wilfong AA, Mays M, et al. Long-term treatment of epilepsy with everolimus in tuberous sclerosis. *Neurology*. 2016;87:2408-2415. doi:10.1212/WNL.0000000000003400

Meuwissen ME, Mancini GM. Neurological findings in incontinentia pigmenti; a review. *Eur J Med Genet*. 2012;55:323-331. doi:10.1016/j.ejmg.2012.04.007

Miller DT, Freedenberg D, Schorry E, et al. Health supervision for children with neurofibromatosis type 1. *Pediatrics*. 2019;143:e20190660. doi:10.1542/peds.2019-0660

Minić S, Trpinac D, Obradović M. Incontinentia pigmenti diagnostic criteria update. *Clin Genet*. 2014;85:536-542. doi:10.1111/cge.12223

Neurofibromatosis. Conference statement. National Institutes of Health Consensus Development Conference. *Arch Neurol*. 1988;45:575-578.

Northrup H, Krueger DA, International Tuberous Sclerosis Complex Consensus Group. Tuberous sclerosis complex diagnostic criteria update: recommendations of the 2012 International Tuberous Sclerosis Complex Consensus Conference. *Pediatr Neurol*. 2013;49:243-254. doi:10.1016/j.pediatrneurol.2013.08.001

Plotkin SR, Wick A. Neurofibromatosis and schwannomatosis. *Semin Neurol*. 2018;38:73-85. doi:10.1055/s-0038-1627471

Rosser T. Neurocutaneous disorders. *Continuum (Minneap Minn)*. 2018;24:96-129. doi:10.1212/con.0000000000000562

Stewart DR, Korf BR, Nathanson KL, Stevenson DA, Yohay K. Care of adults with neurofibromatosis type 1: a clinical practice resource of the American College of Medical Genetics and Genomics (ACMG). *Genet Med*. 2018;20:671-682. doi:10.1038/gim.2018.28

Uhlmann EJ, Plotkin SR. Neurofibromatoses. *Adv Exp Med Biol*. 2012;724:266-277. doi:10.1007/978-1-4614-0653-2_20

A General Approach to Pediatric Pain

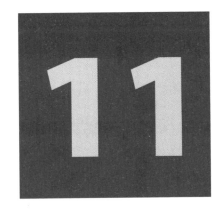

Kenneth R. Goldschneider, MD

Cheryl J. Hartzell, MD

ESSENTIALS OF DIAGNOSIS AND TYPICAL FEATURES

1. Pain is an experience, not just nociceptive stimulation. As such, is it modifiable by a wide range of factors? The biopsychosocial model of pain accounts for this and can be applied to treatment of both acute and chronic pain.

2. Pain is generally classified as primary and secondary, imperfectly correlating with chronic and acute pain, although the two can overlap.

3. Chronic pain is found in children more often than generally believed and can cause significant morbidity and diminishment of quality of life. A functional rehabilitative approach can be used very effectively to restore developmentally appropriate functioning and reduce pain.

GENERAL CONSIDERATIONS

It is most instructive to start with the basic definition of pain, as defined by the International Association for the Study of Pain, most recently revised in 2020: "An unpleasant sensory and emotional experience associated with, or resembling that associated with, actual or potential tissue damage."[1]

Some critical items are noteworthy that will aid and guide assessment and therapy. First is the term *experience*. Pain is not nociception; pain comprises biologic, cognitive, social, and emotional elements. It is for that reason the Biopsychosocial (BPS) Model has been developed for purposes of assessment and treatment of pain. Response to and expression of pain develop over a lifetime and have many influences. The second point is that the manner of expression of pain will vary and does not rely on verbal description or any particular behavior, and the way one person expresses pain may vary tremendously from that of another. Reports of pain need to be respected for what they are, harking back to the age-old expression, "Pain is what the patient says it is." Respecting the patient's right to experience their world as they alone can will promote freer communication (and hence accurate reporting, enhancing the diagnostic process) and generate rapport with the patient and their family in a way that predetermined expectations about what should or should not be painful or "how much is too much" cannot.

The BPS Model of pain was developed to account for the myriad factors that affect pain. Gatchel et al[2] provide a review of the early history of and foundation for this model. The basic premise is that for chronic pain, as for many illnesses, social and psychological factors will affect the experience of pain beyond the stimulus of the biologic insult alone. A simple example would be getting a paper cut on a winning lottery ticket versus the same cut obtained while opening a letter containing bad news. The biologic insult would be the same, yet the person would experience the pain differently based on the extenuating cognitive and emotional situation. While conceived to better explain chronic pain, BPS applies to acute pain as well, as suggested by the example above.

The experience of pain can be grossly divided into 2 basic categories: acute pain and chronic pain. Acute pain is usually associated with tissue damage. It is a signal to protect and repair the injury, resolving as tissue healing completes, usually in a relatively short period of time. Chronic pain may begin with tissue injury but extends beyond the healing phase, ceasing to be a useful marker of injury or disease. The 2 types can overlap, with flares of chronic pain presenting as acute pain. While the distinction between acute and chronic pain is in largest measure temporal, given the difference in pathophysiology of the 2 types, treatment approaches can differ markedly. Furthermore, although acute pain correlates more directly with nociception, negative impacts of biologic, cognitive, emotional, and social influences can still be seen, necessitating the identification and potential treatment of these factors to improve pain outcomes.

PATHOGENESIS

A full discussion of pain pathophysiology exceeds the limits of this chapter, and the reader is referred to several related reviews.[3-6] Pain in the acute phase is often classified in various ways, often depending on the clinical orientation and need of the practitioner. For example, pain can be classified based on site of origin, such as somatic, visceral, or autonomic. Mechanistically, pain can be called nociceptive or neuropathic. The general purpose of acute pain is to alert the organism to a source of injury or other danger to its health and well-being. Chronic pain, now conceptualized as "primary pain,"[7] is classically distinguished from acute pain by duration but differs in some important other ways. Chronic pain exceeds the course of normal healing, no longer serving the productive purpose of protection, and often becomes an impediment to normal functioning. In many cases, there are changes in pain processing, such that ascending nociceptive pathways become emphasized and descending suppressive pathways deemphasized. In such cases, nociceptive or neuropathic pathologies no longer need to be present for pain to be experienced. This situation has long been referred to as central sensitization[8] (CS), although more recently, it has been termed nociplastic pain (NP), with refined diagnostic criteria.[9] The evolution from CS to NP has been recently summarized elsewhere.[10]

CLINICAL FINDINGS

While typical chapters break this section into signs and symptoms, lab findings, and imaging studies, pain assessment does not lend itself to those sorts of clean categories. Assessment of pain is by definition subjective, but a structured and compassionate approach can produce an abundance of useful information. Use of tests and imaging studies is guided by the history and physical and will not find pain but may reveal an organic disease or injury that might cause pain, although often, it will not correlate with the patient's current pain. Thus, for chronic pain, such things are of limited value. Acute pain usually makes its etiology clear (eg, fractured bone, postoperative, infectious), and chronic pain is benefited little by focusing on testing. Acute-on-chronic pain and recurrent acute pain are distinct categories of pain when it comes to testing and imaging. While they are long-term painful conditions, the acute episodes can represent danger and thus require testing and imaging with each episode, as exemplified by sickle cell vaso-occlusive episodes or recurrent acute pancreatitis.

Most practitioners are familiar with the visual or numeric analogue pain scale, usually a scale ranging from 0 to 10 points. While important, intensity of pain is only a small part of the assessment. Table 11–1 illustrates approaches to assessing acute and chronic pain.

Once the pain-targeted assessment is complete, further testing is used judiciously. The approach is analogous to that

Table 11–1. Assessment of pain, general approach.

Acute Pain	Chronic Pain
• Intensity scale (eg, NRS, VAS, FLACC)	• Intensity scale (eg, NRS, VAS, FLACC)
• Description of pain: location, quality (includes context), intensity, timing/course (eg, sudden onset, gradual, waxing/waning, steady), duration	• Description of pain: location, quality (includes context), intensity, timing/course (eg, sudden onset, gradual, waxing/waning, steady), duration
• Associated symptoms, aggravating and alleviating factors	• Associated symptoms, aggravating and alleviating factors
• Past history of pain (with treatment and outcome as indicated)	• Past history of pain
• Effect on recovery (eg, need to mobilize, deep breathe, eat)	• Effect on functioning (eg, ability to complete ADLs, school, hobbies)
	• Meaning of the pain (eg, What do they worry about? How do they think it will affect them long term?)
	• Family history of painful conditions and disability

ADLs, activities of daily living; FLACC, Faces, Legs, Arms, Cry, and Consolability Scale; NRS, Numeric Rating Scale; VAS, Visual Analogue Scale.
NOTE: This table presupposes a standard history of present illness, review of systems, and family and social histories.

for headaches, for which the indication for testing is decided based on suspicion for primary versus secondary headaches. For example, myofascial back pain does not require imaging, but back pain with fever, neurologic changes, or history of cancer may require an extensive workup. While the neurologist will commonly be asked to evaluate neuropathies, headaches, and other sorts of pain related to organic disease, it is critical to remember the definition of pain and that patients are whole people, not hurting body parts. Assessment of the effects on function and interactions with emotional and cognitive factors will be important in the proper care of the patients and are therefore important to be included in the evaluation process. It is critical that this part of the assessment and the information gathered from it are used in a nonpejorative manner, or rapport can be lost and opportunities for therapeutic benefit will diminish. Figure 11–1 shows a simple example the authors use to educate patients and families about the interaction among physical, cognitive, and emotional facets of pain. The simple example highlights the reason for approaching pain along the BPS Model, with attention and importance given to the multiple factors that influence the pain experience.

DIFFERENTIAL DIAGNOSIS

Creating a comprehensive differential diagnosis list for pain can seem to be an all-consuming task, and there are many ways of organizing an approach. One practical approach

Paper cut on a bill

Paper cut on a winning lottery ticket

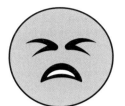 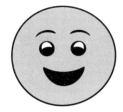

The example is explained as a paper cut (the importance of which is that it is both commonly experienced and an obvious biologic injury) which is experienced very differently depending on the cognitive/emotional context. How much pain is experienced when the cut is obtained when opening a winning lottery ticket versus how much is incurred with the same biological damage when the cut results from opening bad news?

▲ **Figure 11–1.** An example of the interplay among biology and psychology in the pain experience taken from everyday life, so that patients and families can more easily identify with it than with a technical explanation. Plain language examples are helpful in explaining to patients why the biopsychosocial approach is so important in the treatment of pain, especially chronic pain, and that the psychological aspect of pain is both important and perfectly normal. (Reproduced with permission from Natalie Alexander and Kenneth Goldschneider.)

to thinking about the etiologies of pain is summarized in Table 11–2.

COMPLICATIONS

Untreated pain creates a myriad of complications. Early exposure to pain in premature infants can lead to prolonged sensor processing changes, including increases in pain sensitivity, observed weeks to months after the initial exposure to pain.[12] In the acute arena of practice, inadequately treated pain increases the risk for pneumonia and bed sores, decreases mobility, and results in overall slower recovery after acute medical and surgical events.[13] In the acute setting, reliance on opioids alone (an unbalanced treatment regimen) can lead to an overabundance of side effects, such as sedation and constipation, which can slow recovery. There are recent guidelines on the use of opioids for treatment of acute pediatric postoperative pain.[14] Poorly treated acute pain also increases the risk for transformation from acute to chronic pain after surgery, which can be found in up to 20% of studied cases.[15,16] There are also emerging data concerning the economic costs of pediatric pain[17-19] (and the benefits of intensive treatment).

TREATMENT

With the etiologies and influencing factors of pain being as numerous as they are, a full discussion of treatment is not possible here. Regardless of the setting in which pain occurs, the practitioner is reminded to keep the BPS Model in mind to ensure the patient is treated holistically to the greatest extent possible. Especially for chronic pain, psychological approaches should be introduced in a matter of fact manner very early on, as a standard part of treatment. When practitioners introduce psychology only after organic causes have been ruled out, it sends the message that the pain must be psychological in nature, which is usually received poorly by the patient and family. Introducing all modalities upfront sends the message that the patient is being treated as a whole person and not as a hurting body part or as psychosomatic, thereby enhancing rapport and beginning the path back to better health and improved function. For acute pain, it may not be necessary to employ a psychologist, but employing child life workers, recreational therapists, and other means of providing intervention that induce relaxation, anxiety relief, and distraction can be helpful.

An important element of treatment is education. Pain, being both subjective and invisible, can be a hard phenomenon to explain. Primary pain syndromes are particularly difficult to explain because they lack concrete diagnostics to give a straightforward explanation to the layperson. But patients crave information. Therefore, explaining pain is critical in helping patients regain function and in maintaining rapport. There is abundant evidence that this process is not just about giving new information and that replacing prior, poorly phrased concepts, ensuring true understanding, and using language that helps and not hurts are crucial. This is truly the art of medicine, and the cited references provide examples, history, and obstacles related to patient education.[20-23]

Table 11–2. A brief framework for differential diagnoses of pain.

Widespread Pain	Localized Pain
Systemic illnesses	Local trauma or pathology, usually straight forward to diagnose
• Full range from hereditary, toxic/metabolic, infectious to oncologic	• Traumatic, infectious, oncologic, neuropathic
Hypermobility disorders	Complex regional pain syndrome
Generalized primary pain syndromes	Factitious or psychophysical phenomena
• Includes generalized amplified musculoskeletal pain syndrome, fibromyalgia	• Includes functional neurologic disorders
Factitious or psychophysical phenomena	
• Includes functional neurologic disorders	
Practical Tips	**Practical Tips**
1. For factitious and psychophysical phenomena, patient safety needs to be ascertained before entertaining these diagnoses	1. Think about the organs and tissues in the involved area, layer by layer from one side to the other
2. History is critical, and family and social/environmental histories are important	2. Consider referred pain, with pathology located elsewhere
3. Beighton score[11] can be used to explore hypermobility	3. History of migratory pain suggests systemic illness or functional etiology
	4. Review of systems helps to explore if there is pain elsewhere and thereby change the differential list

PROGNOSIS

Acute pain tends to resolve in a time course corresponding to healing of the inciting pathology. Chronic pain has a more variable course. Outcomes of intensive, multidisciplinary treatment are good,[24,25] although no program can boast of 100% success. One concept that is important for predicting and following outcomes in pediatric chronic pain is that improved function virtually always precedes reduction in pain.[24,26] This can be a hard concept for patients, who naturally want the pain to go away before resuming activity, but since the opposite is most frequently found, support and guidance are needed as patients proceed along the path to recovery.

WHEN TO REFER OR ADMIT

Children with acute pain are most often admitted to the hospital or referred for specialty care based on the needs created by the underlying pathology, rather than the pain per se. Chronic pain is best referred to a comprehensive pediatric pain clinic when the effects of the pain manifest as declining function. The multidisciplinary teams that form such clinics are uniquely able to treat patients when functional impairment predominates. Admission to an intensive treatment program is reserved for the most severe cases, with the availability of day programs and inpatient programs varying by location. The following website leads to a listing of pediatric pain and headache programs: http://childpain.org/wp-content/uploads/2021/01/Pediatric-Chronic-Pain-Programs-2021-Update.pdf.

Referrals are made more effective when patients and families are prepared for what to expect. The standard pediatric pain clinic features a multidisciplinary team, which most commonly includes a pain physician, psychologist, and physical therapist, and possibly other disciplines. Many of the established clinics have websites, and it is useful for patients to learn from those sites what to expect and to have processed the concepts, at least partly, prior to arrival. The age cutoff for pediatric care varies from institution to institution, with some cutting off at age 18 years and others at age 21 years, so investigating this ahead of time will save hassle as well.

REFERENCES

1. Raja SN, Carr DB, Cohen M, et al. The revised International Association for the Study of Pain definition of pain: concepts, challenges, and compromises. *Pain.* 2020;161(9):1976-1982. doi:10.1097. PMID: 32694387
2. Gatchel RJ, Peng YB, Peters ML, Fuchs PN, Turk DC. The biopsychosocial approach to chronic pain: scientific advances and future directions. *Psychol Bull.* 2007;133(4):581-624. doi:10.1037/0033-2909.133.4.581
3. Yam MF, Loh YC, Tan CS, Adam SK, Manan NA, Basir R. General pathways of pain sensation and the major neurotransmitters involved in pain regulation. *Int J Mol Sci.* 2018;19(8):2164. doi:10.3390/ijms19082164
4. Marchand S. The physiology of pain mechanisms: from the periphery to the brain. *Rheum Dis Clin North Am.* 2008;34(2):285-309. doi:10.1016/j.rdc.2008.04.003
5. Finnerup NB, Kuner R, Jensen TS. Neuropathic pain: from mechanisms to treatment. *Physiol Rev.* 2021;101(1):259-301. doi:10.1152/physrev.00045.2019
6. Hall RW, Anand KJS. Pain management in newborns. *Clin Perinatol.* 2014;41(4):895-924. doi:10.1016/j.clp.2014.08.010
7. Nicholas M, Vlaeyen JWS, Rief W, et al. The IASP classification of chronic pain for ICD-11: chronic primary pain. *Pain.* 2019;160(1):28-37. doi:10.1097/j.pain.0000000000001390
8. Woolf CJ. Central sensitization: implications for the diagnosis and treatment of pain. *Pain.* 2011;152(3 suppl):S2-S15. doi:10.1016/j.pain.2010.09.030
9. Kosek E, Clauw D, Nijs J, et al. Chronic nociplastic pain affecting the musculoskeletal system: clinical criteria and grading system. *Pain.* 2021;162(11):2629-2634. doi:10.1097/j.pain.0000000000002324
10. Nijs J, Lahousse A, Kapreli E, et al. Nociplastic pain criteria or recognition of central sensitization? Pain phenotyping in the past, present and future. *J Clin Med.* 2021;10(15):3203. doi:10.3390/jcm10153203

11. Kumar B, Lenert P. Joint hypermobility syndrome: recognizing a commonly overlooked cause of chronic pain. *Am J Med.* 2017;130(6):640-647.

12. Walker SM. Long-term effects of neonatal pain. *Semin Fetal Neonatal Med.* 2019;24(4):101005. doi:10.1016/j.siny.2019.04.005

13. Gan TJ. Poorly controlled postoperative pain: prevalence, consequences, and prevention. *J Pain Res.* 2017;10:2287-2298. doi:10.2147/JPR.S144066

14. Cravero JP, Agarwal R, Berde C, et al. The Society for Pediatric Anesthesia recommendations for the use of opioids in children during the perioperative period. *Paediatr Anaesth.* 2019;29(6):547-571. doi:10.1111/pan.13639

15. Rabbitts JA, Fisher E, Rosenbloom BN, Palermo TM. Prevalence and predictors of chronic postsurgical pain in children: a systematic review and meta-analysis. *J Pain.* 2017;18(6):605-614. doi:10.1016/j.jpain.2017.03.007

16. Batoz H, Semjen F, Bordes-Demolis M, Bénard A, Nouette-Gaulain K. Chronic postsurgical pain in children: prevalence and risk factors. A prospective observational study. *Br J Anaesth.* 2016;117(4):489-496. doi:10.1093/bja/aew260

17. Ho IK, Goldschneider KR, Kashikar-Zuck S, Kotagal U, Tessman C, Jones B. Healthcare utilization and indirect burden among families of pediatric patients with chronic pain. *J Musculoskelet Pain.* 2008;16(3):155-164. https://doi.org/10.1080/10582450802161853

18. Lopez Lumbi S, Ruhe AK, Pfenning I, Wager J, Zernikow B. Economic long-term effects of intensive interdisciplinary pain treatment in paediatric patients with severe chronic pain: analysis of claims data. *Eur J Pain.* 2021;25(10):2129-2139. doi:10.1002/ejp.1825

19. Mahrer NE, Gold JI, Luu M, Herman PM. A cost-analysis of an interdisciplinary pediatric chronic pain clinic. *J Pain.* 2018;19(2):158-165. doi:10.1016/j.jpain.2017.09.008

20. Robins H, Perron V, Heathcote LC, Simons LE. Pain neuroscience education: state of the art and application in pediatrics. *Children (Basel).* 2016;3(4):43. doi:10.3390/children3040043

21. Kindelan-Calvo P, Gil-Martínez A, Paris-Alemany A, et al. Effectiveness of therapeutic patient education for adults with migraine. A systematic review and meta-analysis of randomized controlled trials. *Pain Med.* 2014;15(9):1619-1636. doi:10.1111/pme.12505

22. Moseley GL, Butler DS. Fifteen years of explaining pain: the past, present, and future. *J Pain.* 2015;16(9):807-813. doi:10.1016/j.jpain.2015.05.005

23. Beagley L. Educating patients: understanding barriers, learning styles, and teaching techniques. *J Perianesth Nurs.* 2011;26(5):331-337. doi:10.1016/j.jopan.2011.06.002

24. Hechler T, Ruhe A, Schmidt P, et al. Inpatient-based intensive interdisciplinary pain treatment for highly impaired children with severe chronic pain: randomized controlled trial of efficacy and economic effects. *Pain.* 2014;155(1):118-128. doi:10.1016/j.pain.2013.09.015

25. Liossi C, Johnstone L, Lilley S, Caes L, Williams G, Schoth DE. Effectiveness of interdisciplinary interventions in paediatric chronic pain management: a systematic review and subset meta-analysis. *Br J Anaesth.* 2019;123(2):e359-e371. doi:10.1016/j.bja.2019.01.024

26. Lynch-Jordan AM, Sil S, Peugh J, Cunningham N, Kashikar-Zuck S, Goldschneider KR. Differential changes in functional disability and pain intensity over the course of psychological treatment for children with chronic pain. *Pain.* 2014;155(10):1955-1961. doi:10.1016/j.pain.2014.06.008

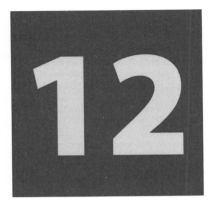

Pediatric Migraine Presentation and Treatment Algorithm

Sharoon Qaiser, MBBS, MD

Antoinette Green, BS

Marielle Kabbouche, MD, FAAN, FAHS

INTRODUCTION

Children are not young adults; thus, we have to take a different approach with caring for this population. Children may have similar pathophysiology as adults, but they respond differently to psychosocial variants and may have some clinical variants that are not present in adults. For example, pain itself is a subjective feeling that is objectively measured with specific pain scales, but this can be challenging to assess in younger children who have difficulties expressing symptoms they are experiencing. Standard pain-related questions may not capture the full picture, as children may have a difference in perception of pain. It is important to note that most of the information collected may be primarily provided by parents or guardians. When taking the history, it is advantageous to direct specific questions to the child at a level they understand. The primary goal is to gather relatively a good history and description of the symptoms using clues or even drawings (this has shown to be a very sensitive tool in younger children). It is the only way to discover what the child is feeling without having the clinical symptoms translated through an interpreter (ie, parents or guardians). Clues could include when a little boy goes into a dark room and stops playing (photophobia) or when a 5-year-old girl draws herself with a hammer hitting her head (throbbing).

This chapter will review key differences in childhood primary headache presentations and summarize different strategies used in treating those headaches including acute, preventive, and behavioral therapies.

HEADACHE CRITERIA

The International Classification of Headache Disorders, Third Edition (ICHD-3) helps to classify different headache disorders including migraine. The diagnostic criteria for children and adolescents are generally similar as adults with few exceptions.[1]

▶ Temporal Criteria

As per the ICHD-3, a migraine lasts between 4 and 72 hours. In children and adolescents, this criterion has been revised to include a shorter duration of headache lasting from 2 to 72 hours. This allowance for a shorter duration of headache has many practical implementations. Time, much like pain, may be very subjective from a younger child's perspective. When asked the duration of headache, they may not be able to accurately describe it. Many children only report headaches to their caregivers when the intensity reaches a moderate or severe level and not necessarily at onset of headache.

▶ Location Criteria

Unilateral location of migraine has been described since antiquity. Pain may not be strictly unilateral in children and adolescents presenting with migraine. ICHD-3 recognizes frontotemporal location of pain in the diagnostic criterion of migraine in adolescents and children. Many younger children report more frontal pain. Location of pain also helps to identify other headache disorders, including occipital neuralgias and trigeminal autonomic cephalgias.

▶ Associated Symptoms

Given the polygenic nature of migraines and the widely distributed genes, children may present with a different phenotype of symptoms as compared to adults. These symptoms may help to aid in diagnosis. Children may have more prominent gastrointestinal symptoms when compared to adults. There are many associated symptoms, but more common symptoms include abdominal pain, lightheadedness, and vertigo. The most common comorbidity in children and adolescents with migraine is an anxiety disorder, which is usually overlooked. A careful assessment during each encounter should be made to identify those who suffer from anxiety and other mood disorders and provide them with resources. In general, migraine in children is a similar disease as in adults but may have different location, temporal characteristics, and associated symptoms. A careful history should clarify subjective terms and should remove any internal and external bias that may be inherent to any childhood disease presentation.

TREATMENT ALGORITHM

According to one survey, 17% of children are sent home more than once from school due to medical ailments and 47% of them have headache. Interestingly, the majority of those with headache do not know what to do when they have a headache.[2] A good treatment algorithm is a triad between children with headaches, their caregivers (including teachers), and healthcare providers. A young child or even an adolescent must learn to identify headache at onset. Caregivers should learn to identify "extra-headache symptoms," and

healthcare providers need to provide the education, treatment plan, and practical steps to remove barriers for treatment. The goal of a robust headache treatment plan is to treat headaches in an outpatient setting and avoid an emergency department visit or inpatient stay. In the following section, we will discuss outpatient treatment algorithms for primary headaches in children, especially migraine.

The treatment approach of migraine has 3 facets:

1. What to do when you have a headache: acute plan

2. What to do to prevent headache and decrease occurrences: preventive plan

3. What to do to avoid a headache: lifestyle changes and behavior measures

Figures 12–1 and 12–2 combine these 3 facets, and we will discuss them individually. We paid special attention in the figures to medication overuse headache and how to approach it while following the algorithm because we must

Evaluation and Treatment Algorithm of Primary Headache in Children and Adolescents

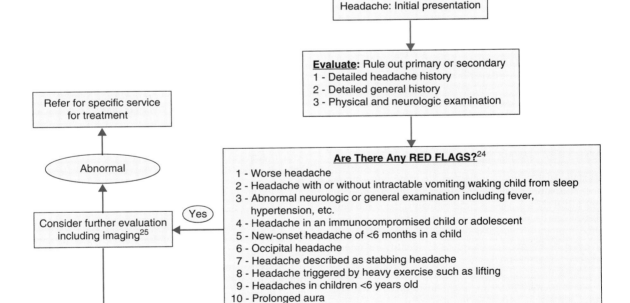

▲ **Figure 12–1.** Headache evaluation algorithm. For any initial encounter with a child or adolescent presenting with a headache, the provider should start with a very detailed history and examination to rule out a possible secondary headache before offering any therapeutic recommendations.

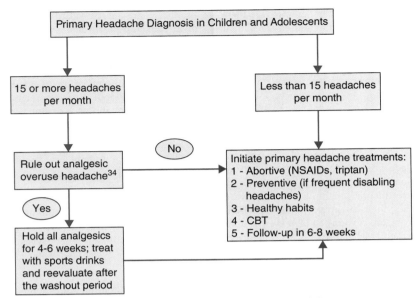

▲ Figure 12–2. Therapeutic algorithm for primary headache in children and adolescents.

identify, treat, and eliminate this common cause of chronic headaches. According to ICHD-3, medication overuse headache is defined as worsening in preexisting primary headache with at least 15 headache days per month in conjunction with taking any single acute medication for pain for more than 15 days per month or a combination of acute medications for more than 10 days per month for at least 3 months.

WHAT TO DO WHEN YOU HAVE A HEADACHE: ACUTE TREATMENT PLAN

Neurogenic edema and vasodilation are important components of the pathogenesis of migraine, and most acute medications target these 2 aspects. Interestingly, after some time, when nociceptive pathways are activated with more central sensitization, these acute medications may not effectively resolve the headache. This helps us to identify an important barrier in acute medication usage—that is, not being able to take medicine at onset of headache either due to poor access or waiting for headache to resolve on its own. Another important barrier is the underdosing of medications. Many over-the-counter medications (ie, nonsteroidal anti-inflammatory drugs [NSAIDs]) may be dosed based on a dose range but not actual per-kilogram dosing standards, which results in poor efficacy and increased risk of medication overuse headache.

The goal of acute treatment is to control the headache in 1 to 2 hours, including the associated symptoms. Thus, the child should be able to return to their typical activity level following administration of acute medications for headache.

▶ NSAIDs

"NSAIDs work in kids—ibuprofen and naproxen sodium."

—*Andrew Hershey: Medscape News 2019 at launch of migraine guidelines*

Hippocrates documented the analgesic properties of willow bark, and the first NSAID, aspirin, was formulated in 1887 with its active ingredient (salicylic acid). NSAIDs are a group of medications that act through the cyclooxygenase pathway and provide analgesic and anti-inflammatory effects. There are many NSAIDs, but ibuprofen and naproxen are the most commonly prescribed NSAIDs in children and adolescents for various conditions. A double-blind, placebo-controlled, crossover study showed that ibuprofen provided better pain control and tolerability in children with migraine when compared to acetaminophen. Hence, acetaminophen is only offered in patients who are unable to tolerate NSAIDs or have contraindications to NSAIDs.[3]

NSAID Type

There is no evidence that any specific NSAID works better than another. Ibuprofen, naproxen, and aspirin are commonly used NSAIDs. Ibuprofen is available in liquid and chewable forms, which may be desirable in younger children. Adolescents aged 16 and older may be offered aspirin as well, preferably not as a combination of over-the-counter medication with caffeine and acetaminophen. Failure of one NSAID should discourage trying other types. A child should be given different options and may make a decision based on previous experience and access.

NSAID Dosing

Anti-inflammatory dosing may be higher than typical antipyretic dosing. The usual recommended dose range is 10 to 15 mg/kg (maximum, 1000 mg). It is important to take the NSAID at headache onset, and each headache should be treated. But treatment should be limited to no more than 3 headaches per week.

NSAID Allowance

A clear NSAID allowance provides better efficacy and decreases the risk of medication overuse headache. If a headache does not resolve in 3 to 4 hours after taking the initial NSAID at onset of the pain, the dose can be repeated once. In children, this regimen may be used to treat up to 3 headaches per week.

NSAIDs and Rapid Hydration

Neurogenic edema and inflammation result in electrolyte imbalance, and rapid hydration with electrolytes may help to provide some relief. It is suggested that every time a child is required to take acute medication (NSAID), they should also take 12 to 36 oz (based on body weight) of noncaffeinated fluid with electrolytes (eg, sports drink) or water with a salty snack. A healthcare provider may help to overcome barriers of access to sports drinks at school.

▶ Triptans

Serotonin receptors are widely distributed in the trigeminovascular system and provide effective targets for serotonergic drugs. Triptans are a class of drugs with action at serotonin receptors 5-HT_{1B} and 5-HT_{1D}, causing vasoconstriction and hence halting the initial cascade of events in the pathogenesis of migraine. Triptans were formulated in the 1990s and have been approved by the US Food and Drug Administration (FDA) for acute treatment of migraine. The American Academy of Neurology and American Headache Society recently published guidelines to treat acute migraine in children that included various triptans as possible treatment options.[4] The triptans can be used when the appropriately dosed NSAIDs are not providing consistent relief. They are usually recommended as a rescue medication.

The best described treatment for migraine is a stratified one: start with education about NSAIDS use (needs to be taken at onset of headaches with sports drinks and repeated in 3-4 hours if no response; use no more than 3 times a week and reevaluate a few weeks later); if some of the headaches are not responding as well as hoped, then a triptan can be added.

Triptan Timing

One of the most important things to consider is that triptans tend to work better if taken at onset of headache due to their mechanism of action; hence, patients and guardians should be educated about timing of taking triptans, and delay in treatment resulting in poor efficacy should not be considered as treatment failure.

Triptan Type and Concomitant Use

There are many types of triptans, and if one triptan does not work, it should not discourage trying a different one. The FDA has approved 4 triptans for children with migraine. Rizatriptan is approved for ages 6 and above, whereas almotriptan, zolmitriptan, and sumatriptan are approved for ages 12 and above. Linder et al[5] conducted a placebo-controlled, double-blind study and provided robust evidence for almotriptan efficacy in adolescents. The combination of sumatriptan and naproxen (Treximet) is approved for acute migraine treatment in adolescents and was found to be superior than sumatriptan or naproxen alone.[6] Other factors involved in choosing a triptan include route (nasal vs oral), allergic reaction to sulfa drugs, access, and choice of prescribing physician.

Triptan Dosing

Like NSAIDs, triptans are usually underdosed and hence do not provide adequate therapeutic response. Dosing is generally weight based, and the maximum dose within the weight range should be offered (Table 12–1).

Triptan Allowance

Triptans can be repeated in 2 hours. A careful well-described plan should be given because there may be confusion regarding timing of triptan use because many children concomitantly use NSAIDs as well. One can treat up to 6 headaches per month using a triptan. We usually recommend treating headache once a week using a triptan to avoid confusion and risk of medicine overuse headache.

Table 12–1. Dosing references for some triptans for acute migraine headache in children and adolescents.

Triptan	Weight <40 kg	Weight >40 kg
Sumatriptan	50 mg 20 mg (nasal)	100 mg 20 mg (nasal)
Almotriptan	6.25 mg	12.5 mg
Zolmitriptan	2.5 mg for both oral and nasal	5 mg for both oral and nasal
Rizatriptan	5 mg	10 mg

In summary, acute headaches should be hit early and hard with NSAIDs plus an electrolyte sports drink, and triptans can be used in selected cases.

WHAT TO DO TO PREVENT HEADACHE: PREVENTIVE TREATMENT

"An ounce of prevention is worth a pound of cure."

—*De Legibus:1240*

▶ Indication

The American Headache Society considers 1 to 2 headache days per week consistently as an indication for daily preventive medication. Other indications include significant disability, emergency department visits, and poor response to acute medication, among others.[7] Powers et al[8] showed that having chronic migraine in adolescence affects quality of life in similar way as pediatric cancer, heart disease, and rheumatoid arthritis. According to one survey, 33% of adolescents with migraine have indications to use daily preventive medication, but only 10% are being offered daily preventive therapy.[9] We recommend daily preventive therapy for all children and adolescents who have 4 or more headache days per month. Other considerations include missed school days, high disability scores (Pediatric Migraine Disability Assessment grade II), and poor response to acute treatment.[10] Once children have better control of daily headaches (<4 per month), they can be weaned off daily preventive therapy.

▶ Evidence

There is consistent evidence for daily preventive medication efficacy in adults for migraine, but results are variable in children. Various previous studies showed some efficacy of commonly used daily preventive medications, but modern more robust studies including the CHAMP trial have failed to show any superiority of common preventive medicines (eg, amitriptyline, topiramate) over placebo.[11] We have observed a consistently high placebo response in all pediatric migraine studies. This highlights the importance of the use of preventive medication along with lifestyle changes. The American Academy of Neurology and American Headache Society published their recent guidelines for migraine prevention in children and list various medications (Table 12–2)[12-18] for prevention of migraine in children with variable evidence.[3]

▶ Types of Preventive Treatment

Migraine is a polygenic neurovascular disease with multifactorial pathogenies; thus, different classes of drugs, including antiepileptics, antidepressants, antihistamines, and antihypertensives, are being used as preventive agents.

Table 12–2. Some preventive medications used in children and adolescents with primary headaches and, specifically, migraine.

Drug	Dose
Antiepileptics	
Topiramate[12,13,a,b]	1-4 mg/kg/d; minimum effective dose is 100 mg/d; typical dose is 50 or 75 mg twice a day
Valproic acid[14,a]	15-30 mg/kg divided twice a day
Zonisamide	100-600 mg/d
Levetiracetam	500-1500 mg twice a day
Antidepressants	
Amitriptyline[15,16,a]	1 mg/kg every night at bedtime
Nortriptyline	10-75 mg every night at bedtime
Antihypertensive	
Propranolol	2-4 mg/kg/d divided twice or three times per day
Antihistamine	
Cyproheptadine[a]	0.25-1.5 mg/kg/d divided twice per day; usually used for younger children ≤6 years of age
Neurotoxins	
Botulinum toxin A[17,18]	155-195 units every 3 months (Food and Drug Administration approved for chronic migraine in adults but not in children and adolescents; only used by headache specialist for intractable cases that failed multiple preventive therapies)

[a]These medications are usually used as first-line preventive treatment. The rest are tried if the initial medications do not result in improvement after 6 weeks with appropriate dosing.

[b]Topiramate is the only preventive medication that has had a placebo-controlled study; it is approved by the Food and Drug Administration for migraine in children and adolescents.

Novel calcitonin gene-related peptide (CGRP) antibodies offer a new target-specific class of drugs that are approved for adults and are being studied in children. At present, the American Headache Society Pediatric Headache Expert Group recommends using CGRP antibodies in postpubertal adolescents in very select cases.[19] These new molecules are not yet FDA approved for the use in the pediatric population (but hopefully, they will be soon), which is why we have not included these novel medicines in our algorithm. Because no preventive therapy is superior, decisions regarding choice of preventive treatment should be made based on comorbidities, personal (patient) choice, physician experience, relative contraindications, blood work, and teratogenicity.

Titration and Dosing

Children report fewer side effects when medicines are titrated slowly. Although there is no study that proves the correct titration process, we recommend an 8- to 12-week titration period, with 2-week intervals between each change to reach the target dose. Family and patients will need to be educated about titration and the goals of preventive medication, as well as the need to reach a full dose to assess effectiveness.

WHAT TO DO TO AVOID HEADACHES: LIFESTYLE CHANGES AND BEHAVIOR MEASURES

The natural history of migraine is variable, but in one prospective study lasting 20 years, it was found that 75% of children with migraine continue to have headaches as adults.[20] This presents migraine as a lifetime ailment (more common in females), highlighting the significance of a healthy lifestyle and behavior measures. Behavior measures should include an evaluation of underlying social triggers and anxiety and possible referral for biofeedback or cognitive behavioral therapy as needed. It is necessary to educate children and their families that this is a major step toward headache improvement.

We suggest the SMART approach, an approach described by Cincinnati Children's Hospital Pediatric Headache Team to simplify the recommended healthy habits when presented to patients and families. The SMART approach is summarized in Table 12–3.

Behavior Measures

Mind and body health have been emphasized in the treatment of chronic pain including migraine in children. There have been a few studies that have shown that behavioral therapy is very effective in preventing headaches in the pediatric population. Powers et al[23] conducted a randomized controlled trial and found that children receiving cognitive behavior therapy along with daily preventive medication (amitriptyline) tend to have better outcome and improved disability score when compared to those who received preventive medication alone. Other useful behavior medicine techniques include biofeedback, progressive relaxation technique, and abdominal breathing technique.

In conclusion, no single preventive measure works absolutely to prevent and treat headache, and the triad of preventive medication, lifestyle changes, and behavior measures should be used as a guide to prevent and treat headaches in children and adolescents.

Table 12–3. The SMART approach.

S: Sleep
- Children 10 and older need 8-10 hours of sleep
- Practice sleep hygiene with regular bed and wake up times
- Keep to a similar schedule over the weekend as well
- Avoid screens before bed

M: Meal
- Eat regular healthy meals without skipping any meals
- Dark green vegetables are rich sources of folate and riboflavin vitamins, which have been used for headache prevention[21]
- Animal products are a rich source of coenzyme Q10[22]
- Dairy products are a source of vitamin D3
- Avoid caffeinated drinks
- Stay hydrated (8-10 glasses of water a day)

A: Activity
- Exercise 40 minutes 3-4 times a week
- Regular cardiopulmonary exercise helps to release β-endorphins, which act as natural painkillers and increase feelings of well-being

R: Relaxation
- Avoid conflicts and minimize stressful situations
- Relaxation apps that are freely downloadable could be helpful tools

T: Avoid proven triggers

REFERENCES

1. Headache Classification Committee of the International Headache Society (IHS). The International Classification of Headache Disorders, 3rd edition (beta version). *Cephalgia.* 2013;33(9):629-808.
2. Buse DC, Scher AI, Dodick DW, et al. The chronic migraine epidemiology and outcomes included the family burden module. *Mayo Clin Proc.* 2016;91(5):596-611.
3. Hämäläinen ML, Hoppu K, Valkeila E, Santavuori P. Ibuprofen or acetaminophen for the acute treatment of migraine in children: a double-blind, randomized, placebo-controlled, crossover study. *Neurology.* 1997;48(1):103-107. https://doi.org/10.1212/WNL.48.1.103
4. Oskoui M, Pringsheim T, Holler-Managan Y, et al. Practice guideline update summary: acute treatment of migraine in children and adolescents. *Neurology.* 2019;93(11):487-499.
5. Linder SL, Mathew NT, Cady RK, Finlayson G, Ishkanian G, Lewis DW. Efficacy and tolerability of almotriptan in adolescents: a randomized, double-blind, placebo-controlled trial. *Headache.* 2008;48(9):1326-1336.
6. Anderson P. FDA okays sumatriptan/naproxen (Treximet) for migraine in teens. Medscape Medical News. Accessed May 15, 2015. http://www.medscape.com/viewarticle/844752
7. Rapoport AM. How to choose a preventive medication for migraine. American Headache Society. Accessed June 16, 2022. https://americanheadachesociety.org/wp-content/uploads/2018/05/Alan_Rapoport_-_Migraine_Prevention_Medications.pdf
8. Powers SW, Patton SR, Hommel KA, Hershey AD. Quality of life in pediatric migraine: characterization of age related effects using Peds QL4.0. *Cephalalgia.* 2004;24:120-127.

9. Lewis DW, Diamond S, Scott D, Jones V. Prophylactic treatment of pediatric migraine. *Headache*. 2004;44(3):230-237.

10. Hershey A, Powers S, Vockell A, LeCates S, Kabbouche M, Maynard M. Development of a patient-based grading system for PedMIDAS. *Cephalalgia*. 2004;24:844-849.

11. Powers SW, Coffey CS, Chamberlin LA, et al. Trial of amitriptyline, topiramate, and placebo for pediatric migraine. *N Engl J Med*. 2017;376:115-124.

12. Lakshmi CV, Singhi P, Malhi P, Ray M. Topiramate in the prophylaxis of pediatric migraine: a double-blind placebo-controlled trial. *J Child Neurol*. 2007;22(7):829-835.

13. Lewis D, Winner P, Saper J, et al. Randomized, double-blind, placebo-controlled study to evaluate the efficacy and safety of topiramate for migraine prevention in pediatric subjects 12 to 17 years of age. *Pediatrics*. 2009;123(3):924-934.

14. Apostol G, Lewis D, Laforet G, et al. Divalproex sodium extended-release for the prophylaxis of migraine headache in adolescents: results of a stand-alone, long-term open-label safety study. *Headache*. 2009;49:45-53.

15. Kacperski J, Kabbouche MA, O'Brien HL, Weberding JL. The optimal management of headaches in children and adolescents. *Ther Adv Neurol Disord*. 2016;9(1):53-68. doi:10.1177/1756285615616586

16. Hershey A, Powers S, Bentii A, deGrauw T. Effectiveness of amitriptyline in the prophylactic management of childhood headaches. *Headache*. 2000;40:539-549.

17. Winner PK, Kabbouche M, Yonker M, Wangsadipura V, Lum A, Brin MF. A randomized trial to evaluate onabotulinumtoxinA for prevention of headaches in adolescents with chronic migraine. *Headache*. 2020;60(3):564-575.

18. Dodick DW, Turkel CC, DeGryse RE, et al. OnabotulinumtoxinA for treatment of chronic migraine: pooled results from the double-blind, randomized, placebo-controlled phases of the PREEMPT clinical program. *Headache*. 2010;50(6):921-936.

19. Szperka CL, VanderPluym J, Orr SL, et al. Recommendations on the use of anti-CGRP monoclonal antibodies in children and adolescents. *Headache*. 2018;58(10):1658-1669.

20. Buse DC, Scher AI, Dodick DW, et al. The chronic migraine epidemiology and outcomes included the family burden module. *Mayo Clin Proc*. 2016;91(5):596-611.

21. Condo M, Posar A, Arbizzani A, Parmeggiani A. Riboflavin prophylaxis in pediatric and adolescent migraine. *J Headache Pain*. 2009;10:361-365.

22. Orr S, Venkateswaran S. Nutraceuticals in the prophylaxis of pediatric migraine: evidence-based review and recommendations. *Cephalalgia*. 2014;34:568-583.

23. Powers SW, Kashikar-Zuck SM, Allen JR, et al. Cognitive behavioral therapy plus amitriptyline for chronic migraine in children and adolescents. *JAMA*. 2013;310(24):2622-2630.

24. Tsze DS, Ochs JB, Gonzalez AE, Dayan PS. Red flag findings in children with headaches: prevalence and association with emergency department neuroimaging: *Cephalalgia*. 2019;39(2):185-196.

25. Medina LS, Pinter JD, Zurakowski D, Davis RG, Kuban K, Barnes PD. Children with headache: clinical predictors of surgical space-occupying lesions and the role of neuroimaging. *Radiology*. 1997;202(3):819-824. https://doi.org/10.1148/radiology.202.3.9051039

Migraine Equivalent or Episodic Syndromes in Children

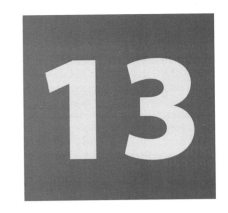

Sharoon Qaiser, MBBS, MD

Antoinette Green, BS

Marielle Kabbouche, MD, FAAN, FAHS

"Migraine is a syndrome and headache is just one symptom."

—Andrew Hershey, MD, PhD, FAHS, FAAN

In recent years, the polygenic nature of migraine has been explored, and up to 39 genes have been associated with migraine.[1] These genes are widely expressed in the entire body and affect all major systems. As a result, children who are diagnosed with migraine in later years may present with different phenotypes in younger years. The 2018 International Classification of Headache Disorders, Third Edition (ICHD-3) guidelines described these different phenotypes as migraine equivalent or episodic syndromes associated with migraine.[2] According to one survey, up to 40% of children diagnosed with episodic syndromes will develop migraine as adults. Types of migraine equivalent or episodic syndromes include the following:

- Infant colic
- Benign paroxysmal torticollis
- Benign paroxysmal vertigo
- Alternating hemiplegia of childhood
- Cyclic vomiting syndrome
- Abdominal migraine

These types are discussed in the following sections.

INFANT COLIC

Before more complex communication skills are developed in infants, crying may be the most important communication skill and may have survival benefits, but inconsolable crying may be a challenging experience for caregivers and may have a secondary cause. According to ICHD-3, infant colic is defined as "recurrent episodes of irritability, fussing or crying from birth to 4 months of age with episodes lasting > 3 hours/day, episodes > 3/days in a week for over 3 weeks, in otherwise healthy infant."[2]

Parents with migraine have a 5-fold risk of having a baby with infant colic, which supports the strong genetic basis of migraine. The pathophysiology of infant colic is not clear, but it is hypothesized that gastrointestinal (GI) inflammation, change in gut bacteria, or feeding techniques may cause GI distress in those who are genetically predisposed.[3] No study has definitively identified the etiologic basis of infant colic. The most important thing to consider is that diagnosis of infant colic requires exclusion of other causes of inconsolable crying. Because risk of shaken baby syndrome is associated with age-related crying, identifying cases of infant colic may help to identify high-risk infants.[4]

BENIGN PAROXYSMAL TORTICOLLIS

The ability of an infant to hold their neck in the first 3 to 4 months of life is considered an important milestone. It helps an infant to observe their surroundings and interact with others and may aid in their posture. According to ICHD-3, benign paroxysmal torticollis is defined as:

- Recurrent episodes of head tilt to either side within the first year of life (most commonly after ability to hold neck) with spontaneous remission in an otherwise healthy infant
- Each episode may last for minutes to days
- These attacks may be associated with any of the following symptoms:
  - Pallor
  - Irritability
  - Malaise
  - Vomiting
  - Ataxia

Historically, nystagmus may be associated with this condition, but it is not listed in the diagnostic criteria. Among all periodic syndromes, this is least prevalent, along with alternating hemiplegia of childhood, with an overall prevalence of less than 1/100,000. A few cases show *CACNA1A* gene mutation, but its link with hemiplegic migraine is not established. This is a diagnosis of exclusion, and other differential diagnoses, including focal dystonia, posterior fossa tumors, gastroesophageal reflux disease, and focal seizures, should be considered. This clinical diagnosis is rare, and because of the pathologic differential, appropriate tests should be done.

BENIGN PAROXYSMAL VERTIGO

Common symptoms like vertigo may be difficult for children to communicate. Children may describe vertiginous symptoms as "feeling strange," "feeling frightful," "a spinning sensation," or "feeling lightheaded." In the past, paroxysmal spells of dizziness in children were thought to be related to vestibular diseases, but in 1988, ICHD included it in their list of migraine equivalent in children.

According to ICHD-3, benign paroxysmal vertigo of childhood is defined as:

1. At least 5 recurrent brief attacks of vertigo that are paroxysmal in nature and resolve spontaneously in a healthy child with normal neurologic exam

2. Each attack may last from minutes to hours without altered conscious

3. Normal documented audiometric and vestibular testing between attacks

4. One of the following symptoms or signs is reported:

   - Nystagmus
   - Ataxia
   - Vomiting
   - Pallor
   - Fearfulness

The pathogenesis of benign paroxysmal vertigo is not completely understood, but it may be an age-related phenotype of migraine. The majority of patients with benign paroxysmal vertigo develop migraine with aura as adults. This presents as only a periodic syndrome that requires diagnostic testing as per ICHD-3. It is a diagnosis of exclusion, and posterior fossa lesions, vestibular etiologies, and seizures should be included in the differential.

ALTERNATING HEMIPLEGIA OF CHILDHOOD

Almost all periodic syndromes are self-limiting or remit and have a benign course expect alternating hemiplegia of childhood. Per ICHD-3, alternating hemiplegia of childhood is defined as "recurrent attacks of alternating hemiplegia with paroxysmal phenomenon with onset before 18 months of age.

This is an encephalopathic, neurodegenerative and progressive disease with strong genetic association with *ATP1A3* gene mutation."[2] Other genes associated with alternating hemiplegia of childhood include *CACNA1A*, *SLC1A3*, and *ATP1A2*.[5] The exact relation of alternating hemiplegia in children with migraine is unknown, but it is clinically related to migraine and has similar genetic mutations as hemiplegic migraine. These known genes affect the Na^+/K^+ pump, and their mutation may lead to channelopathy, which may result in different phenotypes.

More commonly, presentation of symptoms is in late infancy, but a few cases have been reported with onset of symptoms in the neonate period. The most common muscle groups involved are the upper and lower limb girdles, but there is bulbar involvement in some cases that increases the morbidity further due to feeding challenges. Paroxysmal symptoms are associated with hemiplegia and may help to make the diagnosis. The most common paroxysmal symptoms include nystagmus, dystonia, choreoathetosis, ataxia, and autonomic dysfunction. Some of the important differential diagnoses include cerebrovascular disorder, neurodegenerative diseases, metabolic diseases, seizures, and other causes for regression.

CYCLIC VOMITING SYNDROME

Otherwise healthy children with recurrent vomiting may develop migraine later in life. Cyclic vomiting syndrome was described in the literature in the 1800s. In 2004, the ICHD-2 criteria gave the syndrome a specific definition and included cyclic vomiting syndrome as a migraine variant for the first time.[6]

According to ICHD-3, cyclic vomiting syndrome is defined as "at least five attacks of predictable, recurrent attacks of intense nausea and vomiting, lasting more than an hour (up to days) with complete resolution of symptoms in between attacks in an otherwise healthy child."[2] It is important to note that if these symptoms are associated with migraine-defining headache, then it is simply called migraine without aura. One hallmark of cyclic vomiting syndrome is that nausea is persistent and, as opposed to migraine without aura, does not resolve after vomiting. Cyclic vomiting syndrome is a diagnosis of exclusion, may require extensive GI assessment, and may result in diagnostic procedures. Among all periodic syndromes, cyclic vomiting syndrome is associated with significant morbidity including healthcare costs and work loss; one study demonstrated that the annual cost of treatment alone averaged $17,000 per patient.[7] The exact pathogenesis is unknown, but it is postulated that given its cyclic nature higher centers, including the hypothalamus-pituitary-adrenal axis, may be involved in the pathogenesis. Other probable causes include mitochondrial DNA origin and autonomic dysfunction.[8] This debilitating disease is more common in children and often results in diagnostic dilemma.

ABDOMINAL MIGRAINE

"There may be more to the tummy pains than an excuse to miss school."

—Sharoon Qaiser, MD

Nonacute, vague, chronic abdominal pain is a very common complaint in children and may be overlooked. Of 39 genes associated with migraine, many are expressed in the GI system; hence, it is common to have GI symptoms as part of the migraine complex.[2] In 1922, Dr. Brams used the term *abdominal migraine* to describe the cases seen in his practice with recurrent abdominal pain and family history of migraine.[9] In 2004, the ICHD included it in the list of migraine variants and described the diagnostic criteria for abdominal migraine. According to ICHD-3, it is defined as "recurrent paroxysmal attacks of moderate to severe, midline abdominal pain lasting 2-72 hours with associated vasomotor symptoms including anorexia, nausea, vomiting, pallor with complete resolution of symptoms in between attacks in otherwise healthy child."[2]

Many children presenting with recurrent abdominal pain also have headache, and it may be overlooked. In case of recurrent abdominal pain and headache, diagnosis of migraine without aura should be given instead of abdominal migraine. There is no age criterion for abdominal migraine, but children usually present with symptoms around 7 years of age, which coincides with early school years. The exact pathogenesis is unclear, but different hypotheses include immunogenic causes, altered gut motility, and hyperalgesia; however, no hypothesis has explained the higher prevalence in children. Its relation to migraine and presence of vasomotor symptoms are unclear. Abdominal migraine is a diagnosis of exclusion and requires normal GI assessment. This may lead to many unnecessary investigations or procedures.

In conclusion, migraine is a polygenic disease with a wide variety of phenotypes. These phenotypes may present with different symptoms at different ages. Future studies will help to explore the pathogenesis of various migraine variants in children and may help to find targeted specific treatments.

REFERENCES

1. Schurks M. Genetics of migraine in the age of genome wide association studies. *J Headache Pain.* 2012;13(1):1-9.
2. Headache Classification Committee of the International Headache Society (IHS). The International Classification of Headache Disorders, 3rd edition (beta version). *Cephalgia.* 2013;33(9):629-808.
3. Rhoads JM, Fatheree NY, Norori J, et al. Altered fecal microflora and increased fecal calprotectin in infants with colic. *J Pediatr.* 2009;155(6):823-828.
4. Barr RG, Trent RB, Cross J. Age-related incidence curve of hospitalized shaken baby syndrome cases: convergent evidence for crying as a trigger to shaking. *Child Abuse Negl.* 2006;30(1):7-16.
5. Sweney MT, Silver K, Gerard-Blanluet M, et al. Alternating hemiplegia of childhood: early characteristics and evolution of a neurodevelopmental syndrome. *Pediatrics.* 2009;123(3):e534-541.
6. Hammond J. The late sequelae of recurrent vomiting of childhood. *Dev Med Child Neurol.* 1974;16:15-22.
7. Olson AD, Li BUK. The diagnostic evaluation of children with cyclic vomiting: a cost-effectiveness assessment. *J Pediatr.* 2002;141:724-728.
8. Zobel AW, Nickel T, Kunzel HE, et al. Effects of the high affinity corticotrophin-releasing hormone receptor 1 antagonist R121919 in major depression: the first 20 patients treated. *J Psychiatr Res.* 2000;34:171-181.
9. Blitzstein NL, Brams WA. Migraine with abdominal equivalent. *J Am Med Assoc.* 1926;86(10):675-677.

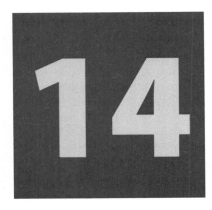

Primary Headache Disorders: Types and Management

Sharoon Qaiser, MD

Marielle Kabbouche, MD, FAAN, FAHS

"Presiding over the entire attack there will be, in du Bois Reymond's words, 'a general feeling of disorder,' which may be experienced in either physical or emotional terms, and tax or elude the patient's powers of description."

—Dr. Oliver Sacks, *Migraine*

Since antiquity, attempts have been made to describe and classify headache disorders. Hippocrates, the father of modern medicine, described headache disorders in his journals. In the second century AD, physicians like Galen of Pergamon and Aretaeus of Cappadocia described different subtypes of headaches including migraine.[1] Despite these attempts, there was no formal classification system until late 20th century. In 1988, the first objective classification system of headache disorders was published by International Headache Society, and it was called the International Classification of Headache Disorders (ICHD). Since its first publication, there have been few revisions to the classification system. The most recent revision of the classification system is ICHD-3, and it was published in 2018, 30 years after the first edition.[2] According to the ICHD-3, primary headache disorders are divided into many types and subtypes. We will use ICHD-3 as a framework for this chapter.[2] It is important to note that a patient may have more than one subtype of primary headache disorder and all individual diagnoses should be given.

TYPES OF PRIMARY HEADACHE DISORDERS

Types of primary headache disorders include the following:

- Migraine
  - Migraine without aura
  - Migraine with aura
  - Migraine with brainstem aura
  - Migraine with motor aura: hemiplegic migraine
  - Migraine with retinal aura: retinal migraine
  - Complications of migraine:
    - Status migrainosus
    - Migraine with persistent aura
    - Migrainous infarction
    - Migraine aura–triggered seizure: migralepsy
- Tension-type headache
- Trigeminal autonomic cephalgia
- Others

MIGRAINE

In children, migraine is the most prevalent headache disorder requiring medical attention. It is estimated that 90% of children seeking medical care for headaches have migraine.[3] ICHD-3 uses the same criteria for migraine in children as in adults with some flexibility. We will describe the criteria and discuss the different subtypes of migraine. It is important to note that a patient may have more than one subtype of migraine and should be given all diagnoses. If a patient with a diagnosis of migraine has 15 or more headache days per month (any kind of headache) or 8 or more migraine-defining days per month for at least 3 months, the patient is considered to have chronic migraine. It is important to obtain a good history because medication overuse headaches (described in a later section) are a common cause of chronic migraine.

▶ Migraine Without Aura

Migraine is described as a paroxysmal primary headache disorder involving the trigeminovascular system and cascades of events involving various neurotransmitters, resulting in neurogenic inflammation. There are 38 genes found to be associated with migraine.[4] A total of 5 headaches with migraine features are required to make the diagnosis.

Duration

In children, a migraine attack (untreated) may last from 2 to 72 hours as compared to 4 to 72 hours in adults. This is important because children report shorter duration headaches. It is important to confirm the duration of untreated attacks because effective acute medication may resolve the headache within 2 hours.

Location

Historically, migraine is considered a hemicranial disorder, but in children and adolescents, it is mostly noticed on both sides.[2] Common locations include the frontal, bifrontal, and frontotemporal regions. The least reported site is the occipital region, and this is usually considered a red flag for further investigations.[2]

Associated Features

According to ICHD-3, there should be either nausea or vomiting or light or sound sensitivity during a migraine-defining headache. Children may not know how to explain nausea; hence, decreased appetite may be an indirect clue for nausea. Likewise, going to a dark quiet room to rest may be a clue for photophobia or phonophobia. Other features include sensitivity to smell; ringing in ears; difficulty thinking, concentrating, talking, or walking; fatigue; spinning sensation; and lightheadedness, among many others. Due to the complex pathways of the trigeminal system and relation to the autonomic system, autonomic features are commonly present during migraine attacks. These autonomic features include nasal stuffiness, watery eyes, and facial flush and may be mistaken for "sinus headaches." Central sensitization during a migraine attack may result in allodynia, and direct questions should be asked to inquire whether nonpainful stimulus causes pain (eg, wearing a ponytail, brushing hair, wearing a hat, clothes, or head gear).

Characterization of Pain

In the past, throbbing pain was considered a hallmark of acute migraine attack, but according to ICHD-3, it is not a requirement to make the diagnosis. Many children and adolescents complain of throbbing pain, but others describe the pain as dull, achy, pulsating, pressing, sharp, or squeezing, and throbbing may only be present during severe attacks. Letting children draw how their headache feels may help characterize the pain better and may also characterize the associated features. According to one study, it was found that when children describe their headache by drawing, it increases the sensitivity of the migraine diagnosis.[5]

According to ICHD-3, pain can be moderate to severe, and many children rate their pain as moderate.[2] An objective numeric pain scale that ranges from 1 to 10 (or the Faces Pain Scale for younger children) should be used, and the child should be encouraged to rate least painful, most painful, and average-intensity headaches.

▶ Migraine With Aura

Almost one-third of patients with migraine experience warning signs before or with onset of headache, usually called auras.[2] Cortical spreading depression is a wave of spreading depolarization followed by repolarization and is thought to be involved in the pathogenesis of migraine with aura.[6] Children may not recognize their auras until asked about them directly; hence, a good history should include direct questions regarding warning signs before headaches. According to ICHD-3, a patient with migraine headaches only needs 2 lifetime episodes of aura for diagnosis of migraine with aura. Aura symptoms start slowly and must last for at least 5 minutes; this differentiates it from other paroxysmal phenomena (eg, seizures) in which aura are much briefer and may last for seconds or less than 5 minutes. According to ICHD-3, the aura usually lasts between 5 and 60 minutes, but in some cases, it may last longer (up to 72 hours). Aura mostly precedes the headache, but in some cases, both aura and headache occur at the same time. A few patients may complain of aura without headache as well.[2]

There are many types of auras, and one can have more than one type of aura. Visual aura is the most common aura (90%); other types include sensory, dysphasic, motor, brainstem, and retinal aura. Children usually describe visual auras as bright spots, dark spots, or scintillating scotoma and less commonly as zigzag lines.[6] Children may have difficulty explaining their aura, and it may be helpful to ask them to draw their aura symptoms, especially visual aura. Dysphasic aura is not common but can be mistaken for stroke, seizure, or other neurologic emergencies. It is important to take a detailed history of aura symptoms because there is an increased risk of cardiovascular events in young women with migraine with aura when compared to controls.[7] This independent risk of stroke increases exponentially if other risk factors (eg, smoking) are present as well.[7]

▶ Migraine With Brainstem Aura

In the past, the term *basilar migraine* was used to describe migraine with brainstem aura; this term is no longer used because it falsely implied the migraine was a purely vascular disease, which would discourage use of the usual acute migraine medicines (eg, triptans). ICHD-3 includes various aura symptoms related to brainstem aura, such as vertigo, ataxia, tinnitus, hyperacusis, speech difficulties, visual changes, confusion, and decreased conscious (Glasgow Coma Scale score of 13).[2] Brainstem aura is more common in adolescent girls.[2] These symptoms may get worse with anxiety and hyperventilation; hence, careful history should include this possibility. Although ataxia is present, brainstem aura does not result in motor symptoms (weakness), and presence of motor symptoms may point toward a different diagnosis.

Hemiplegic Migraine: Migraine With Motor Aura

Migraine with motor aura or hemiplegic migraine is a rare subtype of migraine, but the usual age of onset of symptoms is in adolescence; hence, it is important to include in the differential of acute neurologic deficit in adolescents.[2,8] According to ICHD-3, motor weakness of hemiplegic migraine may last up to 72 hours, even after resolution of headache and, in some cases, for weeks with full recovery in between attacks. Children may mistake sensory symptoms for paresis; hence, a good history must differentiate between these 2 symptoms. According to one survey, almost 90% of children with hemiplegic migraine also had visual and sensory aura.[8] Hemiplegic migraine is divided into 2 subtypes: sporadic and familial. About one-third of cases are sporadic, with no first- or second-degree relatives with hemiplegic migraine. Familial subtype is more common and has a distinct genetic basis. Based on the genetic mutation, it is further subdivided into the following 4 categories[2]:

Familial hemiplegic migraine 1: *CACNA1A* gene mutation

Familial hemiplegic migraine 2: *ATP1A2* gene mutation

Familial hemiplegic migraine 3: *SCN1A* gene mutation

Familial hemiplegic migraine 4: Unknown genetic mutation

These genetic mutations are also seen in other diseases with different phenotypes (eg, spinocerebellar ataxia type 6, episodic ataxia type 2, early infantile epileptic encephalopathy). The diagnosis of hemiplegic migraine requires extensive neuraxis investigations including cerebrospinal fluid assessment and neuroimaging, but per ICHD-3, genetic testing is not required to make the diagnosis.

Retinal Migraine: Migraine With Retinal Aura

ICHD-3 defines retinal migraine as paroxysmal "monocular" visual symptoms lasting 5 to 60 minutes in temporal relation to the attack migraine.[2] The visual symptoms may be positive or negative (eg, loss of vision, scotomata, scintillations). This form of aura is rare, and most of the time, much more common homonymous visual auras are mistaken for pure retinal monocular symptoms. It is important to let the child or adolescent draw their visual symptoms to determine whether they are purely monocular. This is a rare subtype of aura and requires further investigation.

Complications of Migraine

Status Migrainosus

Migraine lasts from 2 to 72 hours, but in a few cases, it may last longer. An attack of migraine lasting more than 72 hours is called status migrainosus. Status migrainosus is the most common cause for inpatient admission related to intractable migraine.[9] Around 6% of children and adolescents who present to the emergency department (ED) for intractable migraine and status migrainosus require hospitalization.[9] It may be difficult to calculate the duration of attack of migraine in children, and the ICHD-3 criteria provide some flexibility in addressing this problem. If headache returns after 12 hours of remission or after sleep, it is considered continuation of the same headache. It is important to differentiate medication overuse headache from status migrainosus because both have different management.

Migrainous Infarction

According to ICHD-3, if aura persists for more than 1 hour with radiologically proven ischemic changes in the appropriate brain area, it is called migrainous infarction. This is a rare complication and usually not seen in children.[2] Based on our current understanding of migraine, vasoconstriction seen during cortical spreading depression of migraine stays under the threshold of infarction, but it is unclear how this leads to infarction in rare cases.[10] There are no current guidelines regarding imaging during aura, and this diagnosis may be difficult to establish.

Migraine Aura–Triggered Seizure: Migralepsy

In 1960, Lennox and Lennox[11] published case series of children with migraine who had migraine-defining headaches followed by convulsive seizures and used the term *migralepsy* to describe this phenomenon. According to ICHD-3, migraine aura–triggered seizure is defined as a clinical epileptic seizure (with or without electroencephalogram [EEG] findings) in temporal relation with migraine with aura or within 1 hour of resolution of headache. Cortical spreading depression during aura may be related to seizure, but this is not clear. It is a poorly understood phenomenon, and it is not clear whether migraine or epilepsy is the primary pathology. In the past, due to concern for aura-triggered seizures, it was common to perform EEG testing in migraine with aura patients; however, this practice is no longer recommended due to lack of evidence.[2]

TENSION-TYPE HEADACHE

Although migraine is the most common type of headache requiring medical attention, tension-type headache is the most prevalent type of headache syndrome with over 80% prevalence.[3] According to ICHD-3, tension-type headache is a primary headache disorder lasting from 30 minutes to 7 days with or without pericranial tenderness. Pain is usually described as nonpulsating band-like pain, but it is not required to make the diagnosis. Pain intensity ranges from mild to moderate and does not affect activity. Patients may report photophobia or phonophobia but not nausea or vomiting. Tension-type headache is categorized based on frequency: infrequent episodic (<12 headaches per year), frequent episodic (1-14 headache days per month), and chronic (≥15 headache days per month). The most common symptoms differentiating it from migraine include lack of nausea or vomiting, no effects on activity level, and mild to moderate intensity. However, in practice, it may be difficult to distinguish tension-type headache from migraine, and patients with perceived tension-type headache may have migraine without aura or probable migraine.

TRIGEMINAL AUTONOMIC CEPHALGIA

Trigeminal autonomic cephalgia (TAC) is a group of primary headache disorders that are classically described as strictly unilateral headaches with ipsilateral craniofacial autonomic symptoms. Trigeminal parasympathetic reflex is responsible for the unique autonomic features. TAC headaches are poorly understood, but the posterior hypothalamus may play an important role in the pathogenesis.[12] TAC headaches are rare in children, with a prevalence of less than 0.1/100,000, but the VAGA epidemiology study showed a prevalence in adolescents closer to that in adults (0.9 vs 1.0, respectively).[13] Different TAC headaches are divided based on duration of symptoms, which last from seconds to months. There is overlap among various TAC subtypes. It is important to note that over 50% of patients with TAC also have migraine.[13]

▶ Types of TAC

Types of TAC in ascending order based on time duration (Figure 14–1) are as follows:

- Short-lasting unilateral neuralgiform headache with conjunctival injection and tearing (SUNCT syndrome) or short-lasting unilateral neuralgiform headache attacks with cranial autonomic features (SUNA)
- Paroxysmal hemicrania
- Cluster headache
- Hemicrania continua

▶ Craniofacial Autonomic Features

There are many craniofacial autonomic features, but the most common include conjunctival injection, lacrimation, nasal congestion/runny nose, eyelid edema, facial sweating, miosis, and ptosis. These symptoms are strictly ipsilateral to the site of pain; if bilateral, then it may be a different type of primary headache (eg, migraine). Sense of restlessness and agitation are hallmarks of TACs and are included in the diagnostic criteria of TACs.[2]

▶ Short-Lasting Unilateral Neuralgiform Headache Attacks (SUNCT/SUNA)

SUNCT/SUNA, as the name implies, are brief attacks of strict unilateral headache lasting from 1 second to 10 minutes. SUNCT is associated with lacrimation and conjunctival injection, and SUNA can have any type of craniofacial autonomic features. SUNCT/SUNA headaches are rare in children, and our understanding is limited to case reports only. It may be important to differentiate SUNCT/SUNA from trigeminal neuralgia: V1 distribution of pain attacks, prominent autonomic features, and lack of a refractory period help to differentiate SUNCT/SUNA from trigeminal neuralgia.

▶ Paroxysmal Hemicrania

Paroxysmal hemicrania is unique, along with hemicrania continua, in its response to indomethacin. Headache attacks in paroxysmal hemicrania last from 2 to 30 minutes with strict unilateral location and ipsilateral craniofacial autonomic features. Based on time duration, there may be an overlap with SUNCT/SUNA and cluster headache; hence, indomethacin may be trialed in overlapping cases.

▶ Cluster Headache

Cluster headaches are the most prevalent among all TAC subtypes, with an overall perveance of 0.9% in adolescents.[13] Pain attacks are strictly unilateral, and the most common locations are orbital, supraorbital, and temporal. Headaches last from 15 to 180 minutes and may come in clusters. There

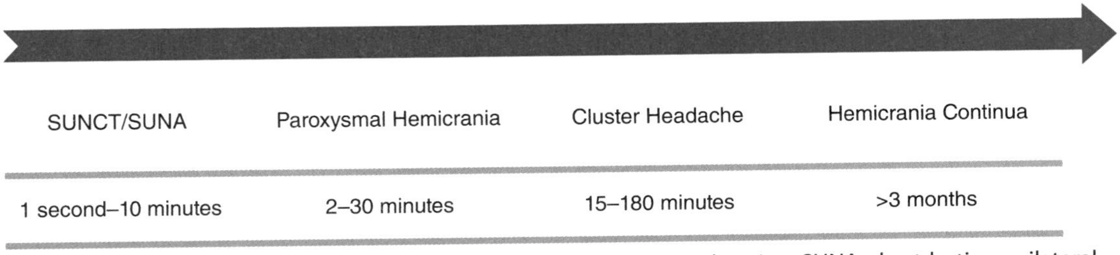

SUNCT/SUNA	Paroxysmal Hemicrania	Cluster Headache	Hemicrania Continua
1 second–10 minutes	2–30 minutes	15–180 minutes	>3 months

▲ **Figure 14–1.** Trigeminal autonomic cephalgia types according to time duration. SUNA, short-lasting unilateral neuralgiform headache attacks with cranial autonomic features; SUNCT, short-lasting unilateral neuralgiform headache with conjunctival injection and tearing.

is no male predominance seen in children as compared to adults.[13] Pain is described as severe or very severe, and pain is associated with restlessness (as compared to migraine, which is associated with lying down in a dark room).

Hemicrania Continua

Hemicrania continua is another indomethacin-responsive headache, along with paroxysmal hemicrania. Responsiveness to indomethacin helps to diagnose and treat this subtype of TAC. Headache is strictly unilateral and lasts for more than 3 months continuously with some intermittent remission lasting for 24 hours. It is rarely seen in children and poorly understood.

OTHER HEADACHES

There are other types of primary headaches (eg, hypnic, sexual activity headache, nummular headache), but they are rarely seen in children and are not included in this chapter.

TREATMENT APPROACH FOR PRIMARY HEADACHE DISORDERS

Headache is the most common ailment resulting in missed school days, with 50% of children reporting headache as a cause when they are sent home from school.[14] It is estimated that migraine-related ED visits cost $700 million annually in treatment costs alone.[15] This calls for a robust treatment approach for primary headache disorders. Since migraine is the most common primary headache disorder in children requiring treatment, we will focus on the treatment approach for migraines in this section.

The migraine treatment approach has multiple facets (eg, acute treatment, preventive treatment, mental health, cognitive measures) (Figure 14-2). These facets are interlinked, interdependent, and work best if incorporated completely in the management plan.

Acute Plan

The majority children and adolescents do not know what to do when they have headache.[14] There are many barriers to a robust acute treatment plan (eg, choice and timing of acute medicine, tendency to treat only "severe" headaches, limited and timely access in school, underreporting or undermining of headaches). A good robust acute plan should resolve the headache within 2 hours while avoiding risk of medication overuse headaches.

Most medicines used for acute treatment of migraine attack act at one of the aspects of migraine pathogenesis (ie, neurogenic edema and vasodilation of vessels, trigeminovascular system pathways, and neurotransmitters including neuropeptides). The acute plan is further divided into a home/school plan and inpatient plan (see Figure 14-2). We will discuss each briefly.

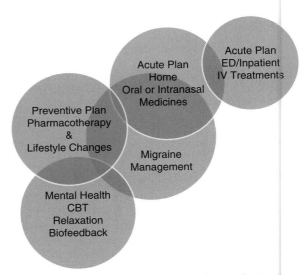

▲ **Figure 14-2.** Different interacting facets of migraine management in children. CBT, cognitive behavioral therapy; ED, emergency department; IV, intravenous.

HOW TO TREAT HEADACHES AT HOME, SCHOOL, OR WORK

"Hit it early; hit it hard."

The 4 important components of acute headache are described below.

Timing

Most medicines for acute migraine attack tend to work better if taken at onset of headache or as early as possible during the course of the headache. It is not clear why, but central sensitization and activation of more complex pathways are suggested to explain this.[16] Few medicines (triptans) work at sites affecting events in the earlier course of pathogenesis of migraine (ie, vascular changes).[17] Hence, it is suggested that all acute medicines must be taken at onset of headache or earlier in the course (eg, migraine with aura as aura usually precedes the headache). This must be emphasized when making an elaborate acute plan involving patients, parents, teachers, and caregivers. It assures the availability of acute treatment when needed.

Dosing

According to the American Academy of Pediatrics headache review, underdosing was a common cause of treatment failure in acute headaches.[18] Since many acute headache medicines are available over the counter, caregivers may use the dose ranges given on the label, which may not be the desired dose. Correct timing and dosing are important components of the acute treatment plan.

Allowance

A common cause of chronic headaches is acute medicine overuse. It is important to clearly state the allowed frequency of each type of acute medicine. Some acute medicines may be used more frequently than others (eg, nonsteroidal anti-inflammatory drugs [NSAIDs] may be used more frequently than triptans). However, each acute medicine has the potential to cause medication overuse headache; hence, clear allowance of each medicine should be explained to both children/adolescents and their caregivers.

Electrolyte Hydration

Neurogenic inflammation and edema are important components of migraine; hence, good hydration with electrolytes is a helpful adjunct therapy. It is advised that at onset of headache, a child should take 24 to 36 oz (based on age and weight) of an electrolyte noncaffeinated drink (eg, sports drinks) or water with a salty snack. This may be another barrier to treatment because children may not have access to sports drinks in school or when they are away from home.

NSAIDs

Neurogenic inflammation is an important component of the pathogenesis of migraines; hence, NSAIDs have an important role in the treatment of migraine. NSAIDs act through the cyclooxygenase pathway to provide analgesic and anti-inflammatory effects. Willow bark was used as a treatment for headache during antiquity, and its active ingredient salicylic acid was extracted in 1887 to formulate the first NSAID, aspirin. There are many types of NSAIDs. The most common oral NSAIDs used in children for various conditions include ibuprofen and naproxen. Adolescents over 14 may be offered aspirin as well. It is not clear if one NSAID is superior to another. A pediatric, double-blind, placebo-controlled, crossover study comparing acetaminophen and ibuprofen for treatment of acute migraine found that ibuprofen was superior to acetaminophen in achieving pain control and was equally tolerated in children.[19]

The most common NSAIDs (ibuprofen, naproxen, and aspirin) are dosed at 10 to 15 mg/kg/dose (maximum, 1000 mg). It is suggested to take the NSAID of choice at onset of headache; the dose may be repeated once per headache in 3 to 4 hours, but overall use should be limited to 3 headaches per week.

Triptans

Triptans are serotonin agonists acting at the serotonin 5-HT_{1B} and 5-HT_{1D} receptors, causing vasoconstriction and modulation of the trigeminovascular system. Triptans

Table 14–1. Dosing references for US Food and Drug Administration–approved triptans in children and adolescents with acute migraine.

Triptan	Weight <40 kg	Weight >40 kg
Sumatriptan	50 mg 20 mg (nasal)	100 mg 20 mg (nasal)
Almotriptan	6.25 mg	12.5 mg
Zolmitriptan	2.5 mg for both oral and nasal	5 mg for both oral and nasal
Rizatriptan	5 mg	10 mg

were the first class of drugs specifically formulated to treat acute attacks of migraine. The American Headache Society and American Academy of Neurology have approved various triptans to treat acute migraine headaches in adolescents and children.[20] They can be used when NSAIDs are ineffective, not tolerated, or contraindicated. Due to their potential to cause medication overuse headache, they are limited to treat no more than 9 headaches per month. Headache experts usually recommend once-a-week usage. It is important to take the triptan at onset of headache, and it may be repeated in 2 hours. There are many triptans available, and failure or intolerance to one type should not discourage the patient and physician from trying other types. The US Food and Drug Administration (FDA) has approved 4 triptans for children with migraine: rizatriptan (ages 6 and above), almotriptan, zolmitriptan, and sumatriptan (ages 12 and above). In a placebo-controlled, double-blind study, almotriptan was found to be superior in adolescents for treatment of acute migraine.[21] The combination of sumatriptan plus naproxen was found to be superior than use of either drug alone.[22] It is not clear which triptan is superior in children and adolescent. Factors to be considered before choosing a triptan include route (nasal vs oral), cost, coverage, sulfa allergies, patient preference, and choice of physician. Commonly used triptans in children and their dosing are listed in Table 14–1. A triptan can be used as a rescue medication if the NSAID has not controlled the headache (taking it 30 minutes to an hour into the headache if there is no improvement with the NSAID) or at onset in combination with the NSAID. The latter is used for patients who are known to have some headaches that are refractory to NSAIDs alone. The 2 medications taken together will act at 2 different pathways of migraine attack and may help to resolve headaches refractory to NSAIDs alone.

Novel Acute Therapies: Gepants

A recent advancement in the treatment of migraine includes drugs targeting calcitonin gene-related peptide (CGRP).

CGRP is a neuropeptide thought to play an integral role in the pathogenesis of migraine. CGRP monoclonal antibodies provide a good parenteral treatment option for migraine prevention, but recently, a novel, oral small molecule binding at the CGRP receptor has been studied; this class of novel drugs is called the gepants.[23] The gepant ubrogepant was studied recently in a placebo-controlled trial and found to be effective in acute treatment of migraine in adults; trials in children and adolescents are currently being initiated.[23] As a result of the study, ubrogepant was approved in adults for acute treatment of migraine. Although there are currently no pediatric studies, in the future, ubrogepant may be a good oral medicine along with NSAIDs and triptans to treat acute migraine attacks.

EMERGENCY DEPARTMENT AND INPATIENT TREATMENT

▶ Intravenous Treatments for Acute Migraine

Oral and intranasal acute treatments play an important role in migraine, but once they fail, children require intravenous (IV) treatments for acute intractable migraine. According to one survey, 60% of children who presented to the ED for acute migraine had already taken oral medicines and hence required IV treatment.[24] It was also noted that 8% to 12% of children who presented to the ED for IV treatment did not respond and required hospitalization for further management.[24,25] We do not have guidelines supported by robust evidence to treat acute migraine using IV medicines in children, and most data are extrapolated from adult studies. We will review most common IV treatment options for children and adolescents.

Dopamine Antagonists

Widely distributed dopamine receptors in the central nervous system may provide an important target site for dopamine antagonist drugs. It is not clear how dopamine affects the pathogenesis of migraine, but it may play a modulatory role in nociception, central processing of pain, and interaction with other neurotransmitters. Commonly used dopamine antagonists include prochlorperazine, chlorpromazine, and metoclopramide. Various studies have proven the safety, tolerability, and efficacy of IV prochlorperazine in the treatment of acute migraine attacks.[26-30] In one pediatric, double-blind, placebo-controlled study comparing prochlorperazine and ketorolac, it was observed that 86% of children responded to prochlorperazine within 2 hours.[29] In another retrospective study by Kabbouche et al,[27] it was found out that 95% of children reported feeling better after 3 hours. In one pediatric, retrospective, observational study comparing prochlorperazine and chlorpromazine, it was found that chlorpromazine was similar in efficacy to prochlorperazine

but associated with more side effects including hypotension and cardiac side effects.[30] In another retrospective pediatric study comparing metoclopramide and prochlorperazine, it was found that prochlorperazine was superior to metoclopramide in preventing revisits.[26]

Currently, prochlorperazine (along with ketorolac and IV bolus) is considered part of the "migraine cocktail" and has good efficacy, tolerability, and safety. The usual recommended dose is 0.15 mg/kg (maximum, 10 mg). The most common side effects include akathisia and dystonic reactions. Side effects usually respond to oral or IV diphenhydramine, but diphenhydramine is reserved for treatment purposes not for premedication purposes because it may reverse the antidopaminergic effects and make prochlorperazine less effective. While assessing side effects, total cumulative dose of all dopamine antagonists should be considered because patients may have received other drugs in a similar category for acute migraine.

IV NSAID: Ketorolac

The importance and role of oral NSAIDs were described earlier in the treatment of acute migraine attack, but an IV NSAID is reserved for cases that do not respond to oral treatment. IV ketorolac, a NSAID, is the most common IV NSAID used for treatment of acute migraine. There are many adult studies showing superiority of IV NSAID over placebo in treating acute migraine attacks. There is one pediatric, double-blind, placebo-controlled, crossover study comparing prochlorperazine, ketorolac, and placebo.[29] It was found that ketorolac (60%) was superior to placebo in achieving headache freedom at 2 hours but less efficacious when compared to prochlorperazine (86%). There were no side effects reported in the ketorolac group.

Based on the current level of evidence, ketorolac (0.5 mg/kg; maximum, 30 mg), IV bolus, and prochlorperazine (0.15 mg/kg; maximum, 10 mg) compose the "migraine cocktail" for children with acute migraine.

IV Hydration/Bolus

Children and adolescents who present to the ED with intractable migraine usually have low hydration because of decreased appetite, nausea, vomiting, and other factors. A dehydrated body may increase the risk of side effects from IV NSAIDs and other medicines given for intractable migraine. More than 50% of children who present to the ED for acute migraine get a secured IV line.[24] As a result, IV fluid bolus is considered part of the "migraine cocktail." There is no robust evidence of efficacy of IV bolus. There is one single-blinded, randomized, parallel-group pediatric study.[31] In this study, one group had expectation of concurrent treatment and the other group had no expectations of concurrent treatment. Both groups were given a normal saline (10 mL/kg) IV bolus and assessed after 30 minutes. It was found that 17.8% of children had pain relief in the hydration-alone group after 30 minutes. This study had 2 limitations: A smaller fluid bolus than in clinical practice was used (10 vs 20 mL/kg), and children were assessed earlier than in other studies (30 minutes vs 2 hours).

At present, it is suggested to include an IV fluid bolus along with ketorolac and prochlorperazine ("migraine cocktail") in the ED or infusion center setting.

IV Dihydroergotamine

Dihydroergotamine (DHE) is derived from ergotamine tartrate and has been used for intractable migraine in its current form since 1926.[32] Ergot interacts with serotonin, dopamine, and adrenergic receptors, modulates the trigeminovascular system, and plays an important role in treating acute migraine.[32] In its IV form, DHE is reserved for intractable migraine not responding to usual IV treatments and status migrainous (acute migraine attack lasting >72 hours). IV DHE is usually given in the inpatient setting. There are various studies proving its efficacy and tolerability in children.[33-35] Kabbouche et al[33] conducted a retrospective study in children aged 6 to 18 and found that DHE was effective and safe.[33] It was found that 75% of children with either status migrainosus or failed usual IV treatment were headache free after up to 14 DHE doses. In a similar study, it was found that most children responded after the fifth dose and a second group responded after the tenth dose. These 2 time points in the treatment may be important to evaluate overall clinical course (Figure 14–3).

Usual dose is 0.5 mg/dose every 8 hours for children 6 to 10 years old (or <25 kg) and 1 mg/dose every 8 hours for children older than 10 years (or >25 kg) for up to a 15-mg total dose of DHE.[33] The goal of treatment is either headache freedom or return to baseline. It has been observed that patients may benefit from an extra dose of DHE after being headache free.[33] In DHE-naïve patients, the first dose is divided into 2 doses 30 minutes apart for better tolerability.[33]

Nausea and vomiting are the most common side effects and are observed in 91% of patients receiving DHE.[33] Due to this concern, patients are premedicated with nausea medicines. It is important to consider the side effect profile of various antiemetics (eg, dopamine antagonists, serotonin modulators, prokinetics). Patients should be assessed before each dose, and if they are tolerating DHE well, they may not require premedication prior to each dose.

Usual contraindications to DHE include hemiplegic migraine, migraine with prolonged aura, hypertension, cerebral vascular disease, cardiovascular disease, hypoperfusion syndromes, and vasculopathies.

At present, DHE in selected patients is the most effective treatment for status migrainosus and intractable migraine not responding to usual IV treatments.

One dose of DHE can still be tried in the ED if a patient fails the "migraine cocktail" (IV fluid bolus, ketorolac, and prochlorperazine). According to expert opinion, based on clinical practice at the Cincinnati Children's Hospital Medical Center, 30% of children presenting with status migrainosus may benefit from a single dose of DHE in the ED. DHE should not be used in the first 24 hours after a triptan, and reciprocally, a triptan should not be used for 24 hours after the last dose of DHE. (This recommendation is based on expert opinion alone; there is no evidence of adverse effects or interactions.)

Valproic Acid Continuous Infusion

Due to the role of cortical spreading depression in the pathogenesis of migraine, various IV antiepileptics have been used for acute migraine attack. Different adult studies have shown variable results for IV valproic acid bolus for acute migraine. Recently, there has been some interest in continuous infusion of valproic acid to treat intractable migraine not responding

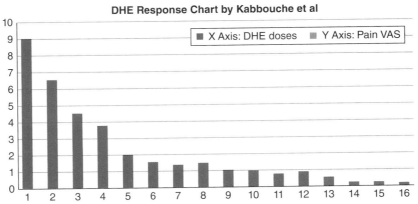

DHE Response Chart by Kabbouche et al

■ X Axis: DHE doses ■ Y Axis: Pain VAS

▲ **Figure 14–3.** Dihydroergotamine (DHE) doses and temporal relation. VAS, visual analog scale.

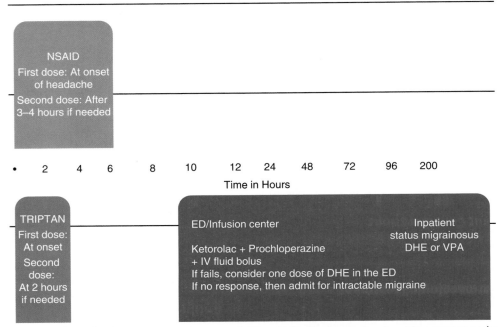

▲ **Figure 14–4.** Timeline of various acute treatment modalities. DHE, dihydroergotamine; ED, emergency department; IV, intravenous; NSAID, nonsteroidal anti-inflammatory drug; VPA, valproic acid.

to usual IV medicines and status migrainosus. Cook et al[36] published their retrospective study showing tolerability and safety of continuous IV infusion of valproic acid in children, and it was implied that continuous IV infusion may provide steadier levels of valproic acid and hence better clinical response. Zafar et al[37] conducted another retrospective study in children with status migrainosus and found out 76% of children had a greater than 50% reduction in their pain score after 24 hours with no serious side effects. Usual recommended dose of valproic acid is a 20-mg/kg load followed by continuous infusion of 1 mg/kg/h for 24 to 48 hours.[37]

At present, based on clinical evidence, it is suggested to use valproic acid infusion for 24 to 48 hours in children with contraindication to, intolerability of, or poor response to DHE for status migrainosus or intractable migraine not responding to usual IV treatments (Figure 14–4).

Novel IV Treatments: IV CGRP Antibodies

CGRP is a neuropeptide associated with the pathogenesis of migraine. Many CGRP monoclonal antibodies have recently been formulated to treat migraine.[38-41] Eptinezumab is the only CGRP monoclonal antibody available in IV form and may be used in acute migraine.[41] Eptinezumab is currently been trialed in an adult, double-blind, placebo-controlled study, called the RELIEF study, to determine its ability to abort acute migraine attacks.[42] We do not have evidence at

the time of publication of this chapter of the efficacy and safety of eptinezumab in children, but pediatric studies will be conducted soon. In the future, specific IV CGRP antibodies may provide an effective treatment option for intractable migraine.

PREVENTIVE TREATMENTS

In children, chronic migraine has similar morbidity as cancer and cardiac and rheumatic diseases.[43] According to the American Headache Society, the presence of 1 to 2 headache days per week consistently is considered an indication for daily preventive therapy.[44] We recommend daily preventive medication for any child with 4 or more headache days per month or for children who show consistently poor response to acute treatment, have frequent ED visits, or have significant disability. Children can be weaned off therapy once they show consistent improvement (eg, <4 headache days per month). There is good evidence for efficacy of preventive medicines in adults, but there is a lack of evidence in adolescents and children. In the placebo-controlled, double-blinded CHAMP trial, 2 common daily preventive treatments (amitriptyline and topiramate) were studied. It was found that both medicines were as effective as placebo.[45] This highlights the importance of combining all treatment arms (ie, robust acute plan, preventive plan, lifestyle changes, and mental health). We will briefly discuss the most common daily preventive treatments as suggested by the American Headache Society guidelines.[44] We can divide daily preventive treatments into 2 categories: pharmacologic and nonpharmacologic.

Pharmacologic Treatment

- Antiepileptics
  - Topiramate, valproic acid, levetiracetam, zonisamide
- Antidepressants
  - Amitriptyline
- Antihypertensives
  - Propranolol
- Antihistamines
  - Cyproheptadine
- Neurotoxins
  - Botulinum toxin A
- CGRP monoclonal antibodies
  - Erenumab, fremanezumab, galcanezumab

Nonpharmacologic Treatment

- Neuromodulation devices
- Cognitive measures

Important Considerations

The following should be considered when choosing preventive therapy.

1. Since we do not have class A evidence for efficacy of any preventive agent, the choice of preventive agent should be tailored based on side effect profile, age, teratogenicity, patient choice, labs, and physician experience.

2. All medicines need to be titrated slowly for better compliance and tolerability; it may take 8 to 12 weeks to reach target dosing. Once at target dose, the patient needs to continue treatment for least 8 weeks before assessing efficacy.

3. If one preventive medicine does not help or has side effects, a different medicine should be trialed. One should not hesitate to try different medicines within the same class (eg, different antiepileptics).

Antiepileptics

The cortical spreading depression is important in the pathogenesis of migraine, and antiepileptics may modulate cortical spreading depression and play a role in prevention of migraine. Topiramate is the only FDA-approved migraine prevention therapy in adolescents. Other antiepileptics used for migraine prevention in children include valproic acid (long-acting formulation), zonisamide, and levetiracetam.

There is no evidence of superiority of any of the antiepileptics, but topiramate is the most common and usually the first-line antiepileptic used for migraine prevention. See Table 14–2 for dosing and side effects of the most common antiepileptics used for migraine prevention.[46-50]

Antidepressants

Serotonin receptors provide an important target site for different migraine therapies. Amitriptyline, a tricyclic antidepressant, is the most common antidepressant used for migraine prevention in children. In one open-label prospective study in 190 children, it was found that amitriptyline was effective in 84% of children in achieving a greater than 50% reduction in headache days with good tolerability. Other options include nortriptyline and serotonin-norepinephrine reuptake inhibitors (eg, venlafaxine, duloxetine) as per adult studies, but these agents have not been tested in children. At present, amitriptyline is considered a first-line medicine in children for prevention of migraine along with topiramate. See Table 14–2 for dosing and side effects of amitriptyline.[51,52]

Antihypertensives

The trigeminovascular system has many calcium and adrenergic receptors that may provide target sites for different antihypertensives. β-Blockers and calcium channel blockers are the most commonly used antihypertensives for migraine prevention in adults and children. Propranolol is the only β-blocker (nonselective) studied in children and adolescents for migraine prevention with some evidence. There is some evidence of efficacy of 2 calcium channel blockers for migraine prevention in children (ie, flunarizine and cinnarizine). Both are not available in the United States at the time of publication of this book. See Table 14–2 for dosing and side effects of propranolol.[53-55]

Antihistamines

First-generation antihistamines are unique in their interaction with serotonin and cholinergic receptors, which may help in their role in migraine prevention. Cyproheptadine is the most common antihistamine agent used for migraine prevention and periodic syndrome in children (usually <6 years old). There is no class A evidence, but it is considered a first-line migraine prevention treatment in younger children.[56] Another closely related antihistamine, pizotifen, is used in other parts of the world for migraine prevention in children but is not available in the United States. See Table 14–2 for dosing and side effects of cyproheptadine.

Neurotoxins

Onabotulinum toxin A, known by its trade name Botox, was approved by the FDA in 2010 for chronic migraine in adults. The PREEMPT trial was performed to calculate dosing and

Table 14–2. Preventive medicines for migraine in children.

Drugs	Dosing	Common Side Effects
Antiepileptics		
Topiramate[46,47,a]	1-4 mg/kg/d; minimum effective dose is 100 mg/d; typical dose is 50 or 75 mg twice a day	Decreased appetite, tingling, tiredness, fatigue, word-finding difficulty, acidosis, risk of nephrolithiasis, glaucoma
Valproic acid[48]	15-30 mg/kg divided twice a day	Teratogenicity with neural tube defects, thrombocytopenia, liver function test derangement, weight gain, drowsiness, alopecia, tremor
Zonisamide[49]	100-600 mg/d	Similar side effect profile as topiramate
Levetiracetam[50]	500-1500 mg twice a day	Drowsiness, fatigue, behavior changes, anxiety, agitation, depression, emotional lability
Antidepressant		
Amitriptyline[51,52,a]	1 mg/kg once daily at nighttime	Agitation, fatigue, sleep disturbance, anticholinergic effects, behavior changes, increased risk of suicide in major depression, weight gain, QT interval prolongation
Antihypertensive		
Propranolol[53]	2-4 mg/kg/d divided twice or 3 times a day	Fatigue, insomnia, hypotension, bronchoconstriction, depression, anticholinergic effects
Antihistamine		
Cyproheptadine[56,a]	0.25-1.5 mg/kg/d divided twice a day; usually used for younger children ≤6 years of age	Sedation, sleep disturbance, increased appetite, weight gain, tiredness, fatigue, drowsiness
Neurotoxin		
Botulinum toxin A[57-60,b]	155-195 units intramuscular at 31 injection sites, as per PREEMPT, every 12 weeks	Injection site reactions are most common; less common side effects include muscle weakness in the muscle groups being injected (eg, ptosis, blurred vision, neck weakness)
CGRP monoclonal antibodies[61-63,b]		
Erenumab	70-140 mg subcutaneous injection/month	Injection site reactions, constipation[c], allergic reactions
Fremanezumab	225 mg subcutaneous injection/month or every 4 months	Allergic reactions, injection site reactions
Galcanezumab, subcutaneous injection	Initial loading dose 240 mg followed by 120 mg/month	Allergic reactions, injection site reactions, immunogenicity

[a]Most common drugs; usually used as first-line treatment.
[b]These are currently approved by the US Food and Drug Administration only for adults but may be used by headache specialists in adolescents who fail multiple therapies.
[c]Manufacturer recently changed the warning of constipation with serious complications requiring hospitalization.

provides a framework for injection sites. Usual recommendations are to give 155 units of onabotulinum toxin A at 31 injection sites at 12-weeks interval. A few experts give up to 185 units per treatment. A retrospective trial by Kabbouche et al[59] showed improvement in headache frequency and morbidity score in adolescents between the first and third treatments. A recent open-label, placebo-controlled trial in 10 children (ages 13-17) showed no significant superiority over placebo after the first treatment, but based on previous studies, more than one treatment may be required to see results. At present, onabotulinum toxin A may be used by headache experts in selected postpubertal adolescents who fail multiple preventive treatments or are not candidate for oral treatment.[57-60]

CGRP Antibodies

As discussed earlier, CGRP is a neuropeptide that plays an important role in pathogenesis of migraine, and antibodies against molecules or receptors may provide target-specific treatment. CGRP antibodies are monoclonal antibodies, mostly given parenterally, targeted to receptors or proteins.

CGRP monoclonal antibodies are approved by the FDA in adults for migraine prevention. Erenumab was the first CGRP antibody approved by the FDA, followed by fremanezumab and galcanezumab.[61,62] Ongoing trials are studying the efficacy, tolerability, and safety of various CGRP antibodies in children, but it may be some years before we have concurrent evidence and FDA approval in children. Because it is considered a potential target-specific treatment for migraine prevention, the American Headache Society Expert Group has provided class IV evidence for CGRP antibody use in children. Similar dosing is used as in adults (see Table 14–2). According to the expert group, a child must have the following indications for CGRP antibodies:[63]

1. Headache frequency: >8 headache days per month

2. Pediatric Migraine Disability Assessment score: >30

3. Previous treatment: failure of >2 preventive treatments (pharmacologic, nutraceutical, and/or nonpharmacologic)

4. Postpubertal adolescent (a few cases may be prepubertal as well)

5. No evidence of recent disturbance of blood-brain barrier (eg, infections, surgeries) or cardiovascular disease

In conclusion, currently, we suggest using CGRP monoclonal antibodies in select postpubertal adolescents (excluding younger children who are part of drug studies) before more concurrent data are available on use in younger children. We suggest using the same dosing guidelines as per adults until we have more pediatric-specific dosing. See Table 14–2 for dosing and side effects.

▶ Neuromodulation

Modulation of the central and peripheral nervous systems via electric, magnetic, or chemical stimulation is called neuromodulation. In ancient times, people used electric eels for chronic pain, which may have worked based on a similar principle. Neuromodulation devices can be invasive or noninvasive. The FDA has approved various noninvasive neuromodulation devices in adults for migraine treatment, such as transcutaneous supraorbital neurostimulator, single-pulse transcranial magnetic stimulator (sTMS), and noninvasive vagal nerve stimulator. So far there is no FDA-approved device to be used specifically in children, but various studies have proven their safety and tolerability in children. Gilbert et al[64] evaluated the safety of sTMS by reviewing 28 studies including 850 children; no adverse effects were reported. Irwin et al[65] conducted an open-label, prospective study evaluating the feasibility and tolerability of sTMS in adolescent with migraine and reported excellent tolerability and feasibility. Currently, there have been no studies in children to assess efficacy. In conclusion, adult studies have shown some efficacy of neuromodulation in migraine management, and pediatric studies have shown excellent tolerability with no side effects.

Table 14–3. The SMART approach.

S: Sleep
- Children age 10-12 and adolescents need 8-10 hours of sleep
- Practice sleep hygiene with regular bed and wake up times
- Keep to a similar schedule over the weekend as well
- Avoid screens before bed

M: Meal
- Eating regular healthy meals without skipping any meals.
- Dark green vegetables are rich source of folate and riboflavin, vitamins that have been used for headache prevention[66]
- Animal products are a rich source of coenzyme Q10[67]
- Dairy products are a source of vitamin D_3
- Avoid caffeinated drinks
- Stay hydrated (8-10 glasses of water a day)

A: Activity
- Exercise for 40 minutes 3-4 times a week
- Regular cardiopulmonary exercise helps to release β-endorphins, which act as natural painkillers and increase feeling of well-being

R: Relaxation
- Avoid conflicts and minimize stressful situations
- Relaxation apps that are freely downable could be helpful tools

T: Avoid proven triggers

LIFESTYLE AND BEHAVIOR MEASURES

The polygenic nature of migraine determines its long clinical history. In high-prevalence groups (eg, women), migraine remains prevalent until age-related hormone changes. This means that what we do every day has a huge impact on overall management of migraine. Following a healthy lifestyle and avoiding triggers have a huge physical and mental benefit that goes beyond migraine management. At the Cincinnati Children's Hospital, headache experts teach children and their caregiver about the SMART headache plan. This is simple approach to a healthy lifestyle that helps manage headaches. The SMART approach is described in Table 14–3.

COGNITIVE MEASURES AND MENTAL HEALTH

Children and adolescents with migraine have a high prevalence of anxiety disorders.[68] Mental health and cognitive measures are important components of migraine management. There are many effective cognitive measures (eg, recognizing underlying social triggers, biofeedback, relaxation techniques, cognitive behavior therapy). Powers et al[69] conducted a randomized controlled trial in children aged 10 to 17. Children received amitriptyline alone, cognitive behavior therapy alone, or both amitriptyline and cognitive behavior therapy. The study found that those who received both amitriptyline and cognitive behavior therapy had better outcomes.[69] Blume et al[70] conducted a retrospective study and found that children aged 8-18 receiving biofeedback sessions for chronic migraine had better outcomes compared to those who did not receive biofeedback.[70] In conclusion, incorporating various aspects of migraine management results in better outcomes.

REFERENCES

1. Koehler PJ, Van de Wiel TW. Aretaeus on migraine and headache. *J Hist Neurosci.* 2001;10(3):253-261.
2. International Headache Society. The International Classification of Headache Disorders 3rd Edition. Accessed June 18, 2022. https://ichd-3.org/
3. Lateef TM, Merikangas KR, He J, et al. Headache in a national sample of American children: prevalence and comorbidity. *J Child Neurol.* 2009;24(5):536-543.
4. Gormley P, Anttila V, Winsvold BS, et al. Meta-analysis of 375,000 individuals identifies 38 susceptibility loci for migraine. *Nat Genet.* 2016;48:856-866.
5. Stafstrom CE, Rostasy K, Minster A. The usefulness of children's drawings in the diagnosis of headache. *Pediatrics.* 2002;109(3):460-472.
6. Eriksen MK, Thomsen LL, Olesen J. The Visual Aura Rating Scale (VARS) for migraine aura diagnosis. *Cephalalgia.* 2005; 25(10):801-810.
7. Kurth T, Bubes V, Buring J. Relative contribution of migraine with aura to cardiovascular disease occurrence in women. *Neurology.* 2013;80:S40.001.
8. Lykke Thomsen L, Kirchmann Eriksen M, Faerch Romer S, et al. An epidemiological survey of hemiplegic migraine. *Cephalalgia.* 2002;22(5):361-375.
9. Kabbouche MA, Linder SL. Management of migraine in children and adolescents in the emergency department and inpatient setting. *Curr Pain Headache Rep.* 2005;9(5):363-367.
10. Kurth T, Diener HC. Migraine and stroke: perspectives for stroke physicians. *Stroke.* 2012;43(12):3421-3426.
11. Lennox WG, Lennox MA. *Epilepsy and Related Disorders.* Little, Brown; 1960.
12. Bussone G. Strictly unilateral headaches: considerations of a clinician. *Neurol Sci.* 2014;35(suppl 1):71-75.
13. Sjaastad O, Bakketeig LS. The rare, unilateral headaches. VAGA study of headache epidemiology. *J Headache Pain.* 2007;8(1):19-27.
14. Buse DC, Fanning KM, Reed ML, et al. The chronic migraine epidemiology and outcomes included the family burden module. *Mayo Clin Proc.* 2016;91(5):596-611.
15. Insinga RP, Ng-Mark DS, Hanson ME. Costs associated with outpatient, emergency room and inpatient care for migraine in the USA. *Cephalgia.* 2011;31(15):1570-1575.
16. Goadsby PJ. Pathophysiology of migraine. *Ann Indian Acad Neurol.* 2012;15(suppl 1):S15-22. doi:10.4103/0972-2327.99993
17. Eiland LS, Hunt MO. The use of triptans for pediatric migraines. *Paediatr Drugs.* 2010;12(6):379-389.
18. Blume HK. Pediatric headache: a review. *Pediatr Rev.* 2012;33(12):562-576. https://doi.org/10.1542/pir.33-12-562
19. Hamalainen ML, Hoppu K, Valkeila E, Santavuori P. Ibuprofen or acetaminophen for the acute treatment of migraine in children: a double-blind, randomized, placebo-controlled, crossover study. *Neurology.* 1997;48(1):103-107. https://doi.org/10.1212/WNL.48.1.103
20. American Academy of Neurology. Practice guideline update: acute treatment of migraine in children and adolescents. Accessed June 18, 2022. https://www.aan.com/Guidelines/Home/GuidelineDetail/966
21. Linder SL, Mathew NT, Cady RK, Finlayson G, Ishkanian G, Lewis DW. Efficacy and tolerability of almotriptan in adolescents: a randomized, double-blind, placebo-controlled trial. *Headache.* 2008;48(9):1326-1336.
22. Anderson P. FDA okays sumatriptan/naproxen (treximet) for migraine in teens. Medscape Medical News. Accessed May 15, 2015. http://www.medscape.com/viewarticle/844752
23. Lipton RB, Dodick DW, Ailani J, et al. Effect of ubrogepant vs placebo on pain and the most bothersome associated symptom in the acute treatment of migraine. The ACHIEVE II randomized clinical trial. *JAMA.* 2019;322(19):1889-1898.
24. Richer LP, Laycock K, Millar K, et al. Treatment of children with migraine in emergency departments: national practice variation study. *Pediatrics.* 2010;126:e150.
25. Kabbouche MA, Linder SL. Management of migraine in children and adolescents in the emergency department and inpatient setting. *Curr Pain Headache Rep.* 2005;9(5):363-367.
26. Bachur RG, Monuteaux MC, Neuman MI. A comparison of acute treatment regimens for migraine in the emergency department. *Pediatrics.* 2015;135:232-238.
27. Kabbouche MA, Vockell A-LB, LeCates SL, Powers SW, Hershey AD. Tolerability and effectiveness of prochlorperazine for intractable migraine in children. *Pediatrics.* 2001;107:e62-e62.
28. Trottier ED, Bailey B, Dauphin-Pierre S, Gravel J. Clinical outcomes of children treated with intravenous prochlorperazine for migraine in a pediatric emergency department. *J Emerg Med.* 2010;39:166-173.
29. Brousseau DC, Duffy SJ, Anderson AC, Linakis JG. Treatment of pediatric migraine headaches: a randomized, double-blind trial of prochlorperazine versus ketorolac. *Ann Emerg Med.* 2004;43:256-262.
30. Kanis JM, Timm NL. Chlorpromazine for the treatment of migraine in a pediatric emergency department. *Headache J Head Face Pain.* 2014;54:335-342.
31. Richer L, Craig W, Rowe B. Randomized controlled trial of treatment expectation and intravenous fluid in pediatric migraine. *Headache.* 2014;54(9):1496-1505.
32. Schaerlinger B, Hickel P, Etienne N, Guesnier L, Maroteaux L. Agonist actions of dihydroergotamine at 5-HT2B and 5-HT2C receptors and their possible relevance to antimigraine efficacy. *Br J Pharmacol.* 2003;140(2):277-284. doi:10.1038/sj.bjp.0705437
33. Kabbouche MA, Powers SW, Segers A, et al. Inpatient treatment of status migraine with dihydroergotamine in children and adolescents. *Headache.* 2009;49(1):106-109.
34. Eller M, Gelfand AA, Riggins NY, et al. Exacerbation of headache during dihydroergotamine for chronic migraine does not alter outcome. *Neurology.* 2016;86(9):856-859.
35. Linder SL. Treatment of childhood headache with dihydroergotamine mesylate. *Headache J Head Face Pain.* 1994;34:578-580.
36. Cook AM, Zafar MS, Mathias S, et al. Pharmacokinetics and clinical utility of valproic acid administered via continuous infusion. *CNS Drugs.* 2016;30(1):71-77. doi:10.1007/s40263-015-0304-5
37. Zafar MS, Stewart AM, Toupin DN, et al. Continuous intravenous valproate as abortive therapy for pediatric status migrainosus. *Neurologist.* 2018;23(2):43-46.

38. Bigal ME, Edvinsson L, Rapoport AM, et al. Safety, tolerability, and efficacy of TEV-48125 for preventive treatment of chronic migraine: a multicentre, randomised, double-blind, placebo-controlled, phase 2b study. *Lancet Neurol.* 2015;14(11):1091-1100. doi:10.1016/s1474-4422(15)00245-8

39. Tepper S, Ashina M, Reuter U, et al. Safety and efficacy of erenumab for preventive treatment of chronic migraine: a randomised, double-blind, placebo-controlled phase 2 trial. *Lancet Neurol.* 2017;16(6):425-434. doi:10.1016/s1474-4422(17)30083-2

40. Ashina M, Saper J, Cady R, et al. Eptinezumab in episodic migraine: a randomized, double-blind, placebo-controlled study (PROMISE-1). *Cephalgia.* 2020;40(3):241-254.

41. Kudrow D, Lipton R, Silberstein S, et al. Eptinezumab for prevention of chronic migraine: results of 2 infusions in the phase 3 PROMISE-2 (Prevention of Migraine via Intravenous Eptinezumab Safety and Efficacy–2) trial (P2.10 006). *Neurology.* 2019;92(15):6-16.

42. ClinicalTrials.gov. A study to evaluate the efficacy and safety of eptinezumab administered intravenously in participants experiencing acute attack of migraine (RELIEF). Accessed June 18, 2022. https://clinicaltrials.gov/ct2/show/NCT04152083

43. Powers SW, Patton SR, Hommel KA, Hershey AD. Quality of life in pediatric migraine: characterization of age related effects using Peds QL4.0. *Cephaligia.* 2004;24:120-127.

44. American Headache Society. How to choose a preventive medication for migraine. Accessed June 18, 2022. https://americanheadachesociety.org/wp-content/uploads/2018/05/Alan_Rapoport_-_Migraine_Prevention_Medications.pdf

45. Powers SW, Coffey CS, Chamberlin LA, et al. Trial of amitriptyline, topiramate, and placebo for pediatric migraine. *N Engl J Med.* 2017;376:115-124.

46. Lakshmi CV, Singhi P, Malhi P, Ray M. Topiramate in the prophylaxis of pediatric migraine: a double-blind placebo-controlled trial. *J Child Neurol.* 2007;22(7):829-835.

47. Lewis D, Winner P, Saper J, et al. Randomized, double-blind, placebo-controlled study to evaluate the efficacy and safety of topiramate for migraine prevention in pediatric subjects 12 to 17 years of age. *Pediatrics.* 2009;123(3):924-934.

48. Apostol G, Lewis D, Laforet G, et al. Divalproex sodium extended-release for the prophylaxis of migraine headache in adolescents: results of a stand-alone, long-term open-label safety study. *Headache.* 2009;49:45-53.

49. Pakalnis A, Kring D. Zonisamide prophylaxis in refractory pediatric headache. *Headache.* 2006;46(5):804-807.

50. Miller GS. Efficacy and safety of levetiracetam in pediatric migraine. *Headache.* 2004;44(3):238-243.

51. Kacperski J, Kabbouche MA, O'Brien HL, Weberding JL. The optimal management of headaches in children and adolescents. *Ther Adv Neurol Disord.* 2016;9(1):53-68.

52. Hershey A, Powers S, Bentii A, deGrauw T. Effectiveness of amitriptyline in the prophylactic management of childhood headaches. *Headache.* 2000;40:539-549.

53. Forsythe WI, Gillies D, Sills MA. Propranolol ("Inderal") in the treatment of childhood migraine. *Dev Med Child Neurol.* 1984;26:737-741.

54. Orge F, De Simone R, Marano E, Nolano M, Orefice G, Carrieri P. Flunarizine in prophylaxis of childhood migraine.

A double-blind, placebo-controlled, crossover study. *Cephalalgia.* 1988;8:1-6.

55. Ashrafi MR, Salehi S, Malamiri RA, et al. Efficacy and safety of cinnarizine in the prophylaxis of migraine in children: a double-blind placebo-controlled randomized trial. *Pediatr Neurol.* 2014;51:503-521.

56. Johnson A, Bickel J, Lebel A. Pediatric migraine prescription pattern at a large academic hospital. *Pediatr Neurol.* 2014;51:706-712.

57. Diener HC, Dodick DW, Aurora SK, et al. PREEMPT 2 Chronic Migraine Study Group. OnabotulinumtoxinA for treatment of chronic migraine: results from the double-blind, randomized, placebo-controlled phase of the PREEMPT 2 trial. *Cephalalgia.* 2010;30(7):804-814.

58. Allergan. 191622-103 BOTOX® (botulinum toxin type a) purified neurotoxin complex as headache prophylaxis in adolescents (children 12 to < 18 years of age) with chronic migraine. 2017. Accessed June 18, 2022. https://clinicaltrials.gov/ct2/show/NCT01662492

59. Kabbouche M, O'Brien H, Hershey AD. OnabotulinumtoxinA in pediatric chronic daily headache. *Curr Neurol Neurosci Rep.* 2012;12(2):114-117.

60. Winner PK, Kabbouche M, Yonker M, et al. A randomized trial to evaluate OnabotulinumtoxinA for prevention of headaches in adolescents with chronic migraine. *Headache.* 2020;60(3):564-575.

61. Goadsby PJ, Reuter U, Hallstrom Y, et al. A controlled trial of erenumab for episodic migraine. *N Engl J Med.* 2017;377:2123-2132.

62. US Food and Drug Administration. FDA approves new treatment for adults with migraine. Accessed June 18, 2022. https://www.fda.gov/news-events/press-announcements/fda-approves-new-treatment-adults-migraine

63. Szperka CL, VanderPluym J, Orr SL, et al. Recommendations on the use of anti-CGRP monoclonal antibodies in children and adolescents. *Headache.* 2018;58(10):1658-1669.

64. Gilbert DL, Garvey MA, Bansal AS, et al. Should transcranial magnetic stimulation research in children be considered minimal risk? *Clin Neurophysiol.* 2004;115(8):1730-1739.

65. Irwin S, Qubty W, Allen IE, et al. Transcranial magnetic stimulation for migraine prevention in adolescents: a pilot open-label study. *Headache.* 2018;58(5):724-731.

66. Condo M, Posar A, Arbizzani A, Parmeggiani A. Riboflavin prophylaxis in pediatric and adolescent migraine. *J Headache Pain.* 2009;10:361-365.

67. Orr S, Venkateswaran S. Nutraceuticals in the prophylaxis of pediatric migraine: evidence-based review and recommendations. *Cephalalgia.* 2014;34:568-583.

68. Peres MFP, Mercante JPP, Tobo PR, Kamei H, Bigal ME. Anxiety and depression symptoms and migraine: a symptom-based approach research. *J Headache Pain.* 2017;18(1):37.

69. Powers SW, Kashikar-Zuck SM, Allen JR, et al. Cognitive behavioral therapy plus amitriptyline for chronic migraine in children and adolescents. *JAMA.* 2013;310(24):2622-2630.

70. Blume HK, Brockman LN, Breuner CC. Biofeedback therapy for pediatric headache: factors associated with response. *Headache.* 2012;52(9):1377-1386.

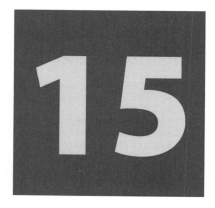

Secondary Headaches in Children and Adolescents

Marielle Kabbouche, MD, FAAN, FAHS

When a patient presents to the office with a chief complaint of headache, the main concern is to differentiate between primary and secondary pathology because the evaluation and treatment pathway are affected by that initial determination.

During the visit, red flags can easily be identified by the following: a detailed history of the headache, including any previous headache, localization, acute changes, age of onset, severity, duration, triggers, and associated symptoms; family history; medications; medical history; and a detailed physical and neurologic examination. When appropriately done, the gathered information helps the provider to not only classify the presenting headache but also guide the clinical decision making.[1]

The red flags[2] or concerning symptoms in children and adolescents are summarized as follows:

1. New-onset headache (<6 months)
2. Worst headache ever
3. Persistent occipital headache
4. Headache when waking the child from sleep
5. Intractable vomiting
6. Abnormal vital signs and/or physical examination (eg, fever, papilledema, abnormal neurologic examination, including neck stiffness)
7. Sudden change in headache pattern
8. No family history of headache
9. A child younger than 6 years old with a history that does not fit all the International Classification of Headache Disorders, Third Edition (ICHD-3) criteria of headache
10. Changes in mental status
11. Prolonged aura

This chapter will summarize secondary headaches that can present to a pediatric neurology office, including headaches due to a central nervous system (CNS) vascular abnormality such as hemorrhages (eg, intracranial, subarachnoid, subdural), headaches associated with genetic disorders in childhood and adolescence (eg, mitochondrial encephalopathy, lactic acidosis, and stroke-like episodes [MELAS], cerebral autosomal dominant arteriopathy with subcortical infarcts and leukoencephalopathy [CADASIL]), headache occurring with intracranial pressure changes (idiopathic increase of cerebrospinal fluid [CSF] pressure and low-pressure headaches), headache secondary to inflammatory processes (infectious or noninfectious), and headache due to space-occupying lesions or congenital anomalies such as neoplasms and Chiari I malformation.[3,4] Headache related to trauma and concussion will be reviewed in Chapter 16 in detail.[3,4]

SECONDARY HEADACHE AS A SYMPTOM OF A VASCULAR PATHOLOGY SUCH AS HEMORRHAGE OR VASCULAR DISSECTION

Intracerebral, subarachnoid, and acute subdural hemorrhages and cervical arterial dissection are causes of secondary headache. Headache in any CNS hemorrhage is acute, very intense, and associated with other neurologic symptoms, including nuchal rigidity, mental status changes, motor or sensory deficits, and more specific neurologic abnormalities related to the localization of the hemorrhage. The headache usually occurs in close temporal relation to other intracranial hemorrhage symptoms and improves with the stabilization of the hemorrhage. It is usually described as a thunderclap headache that is worst on the day of onset and is localized to the site of the hemorrhage. The headache can be an early feature of hemorrhage, especially in cerebellar hemorrhage. As soon as an intracranial hemorrhage is suspected, imaging and neurosurgical evaluation are needed urgently because delay in the diagnosis could be clinically catastrophic. A noncontrast computed tomography (CT) scan of the head is the initial test due to its sensitivity to blood in the CNS, followed by further evaluation to identify the underlying cause of the hemorrhage. Patients will need to be admitted to the intensive care unit and evaluated by the neurosurgical team. A noncontrast CT of the brain depicts a CNS bleed in 99% of cases in the first 6 hours after onset, 98% at 12 hours, and 93% at 24 hours, decreasing to 50% at 7 days.[5] When the CT results are nondiagnostic, lumbar puncture is essential: Xanthochromia is present in all cases of aneurysmal subarachnoid hemorrhage when CSF is collected between 12 hours and 2 weeks after the onset of symptoms.[5] Magnetic resonance imaging (MRI) is not indicated as an initial diagnostic test; however, it may be needed for further evaluation of the underlying cause such as dissection or vascular malformation.

Headache can be the only early manifestation of a cervical arterial dissection; thus, headache is considered the inaugural symptom of a dissection since it is frequently present as the initial symptom even without neck pain in 33% to 86% of cases.[6,7] According to the ICDH-3 criteria, the headache in vascular dissection is usually unilateral to the dissection and severe but can have the same features of a primary headache such as migraine headache. The clinician should look for subtle signs in the history such as a history of trauma, neck manipulation, tinnitus, or Horner syndrome. The diagnosis of an arterial dissection is based on good imaging, including MRI/magnetic resonance angiography, CT angiography, and possibly angiography depending on the case.

GENETIC DISORDERS AND HEADACHE IN CHILDREN AND ADOLESCENTS

A few vascular genetic disorders in childhood are associated with headache, including mitochondrial encephalopathy, lactic acidosis, and stroke-like episodes (MELAS) and cerebral autosomal dominant arteriopathy with subcortical infarcts and leukoencephalopathy (CADASIL).

In MELAS, headache is only one symptom in a variety of multiorgan manifestations, including myopathy, severe encephalopathy, dementia, seizures, hearing loss, and lactic acidosis. The headaches usually occur as recurrent migraine-like attacks with or without aura and associated with stroke-like episodes. The headache is more severe during the stroke-like episode and is present in 54% to 91% of patients with MELAS; vomiting is frequently present too. The mitochondrial mutation in the *MT-TL1* gene occurs in 80% of individuals with MELAS syndrome. Several mechanisms can interact to result in the multiorgan phenotype of MELAS syndrome, including impaired mitochondrial energy production, microvasculature angiopathy, and nitrous oxide deficiency. Management of MELAS syndrome is largely symptomatic and should involve a multidisciplinary team. Several supplements, including antioxidants and cofactors, are being used in MELAS syndrome. Valproic acid, metformin, and dichloroacetate should be avoided.[8,9]

In CADASIL, the headache is usually migrainous, hemiplegic, or accompanied by prolonged aura, hence the inclusion of prolonged aura as a red flag for secondary headache. The diagnosis is made by screening for *NOTCH-3* mutations, by a simple skin biopsy with immunostaining of NOTCH-3 antibodies, or with electron microscopy to assess for extracellular granular osmiophilic material within the arterial media.

CADASIL is an autosomal dominant disease due to mutations of the *NOTCH-3* gene. It is characterized clinically by recurrent small deep infarcts, subcortical dementia, mood disturbances, and in one-third of cases, attacks typical of migraine with aura where aura are prolonged and often hemiplegic motor aura. The MRI is always abnormal, with striking white matter changes on T2-weighted images.[10]

HEADACHE SECONDARY TO INTRACRANIAL PRESSURE CHANGES: IDIOPATHIC INCREASED INTRACRANIAL PRESSURE AND LOW-PRESSURE HEADACHE

Increased intracranial pressure (IIH) is suspected when a patient presents with new-onset headache, head pain associated with tinnitus, visual changes such as diplopia secondary to sixth cranial nerve palsy, and decreased acuity from papilledema.[11,12] The headache may take the features of migraine and be insidious with photophobia and phonophobia. Patients often have other comorbidities such as obesity and use daily medications such as retinoid treatment for acne. The diagnosis is made by a detailed history as well as a good neurologic examination showing the papilledema (a few cases of IIH without papilledema have been reported).[13] When suspected, imaging studies are needed, including an MRI of the brain and magnetic resonance venography, the latter to rule out any venous thrombosis that could be the cause of decreased fluid resorption with subsequent IIH. A spinal tap will show an elevated pressure above 250 to 280 cm H_2O depending on age and weight.[14] The CSF pressure should be measured by a lumbar puncture performed while patient is in the lateral decubitus position without sedating medications (sedatives can falsely give a higher CSF pressure reading). The MRI of the brain may show some secondary signs of increased pressure such as an empty sella turcica, tension of the perioptic subarachnoid space, flattening of the posterior sclerae, and protrusion of the optic nerve sheath secondary to the presence of papilledema.[15]

Low-pressure headache or orthostatic headache is due to low CSF pressure. This can occur spontaneously or secondary to a leak from a spinal tap or a trauma. The headache with low CSF pressure has a specific orthostatic feature; it worsens in the sitting or standing position and improves when laying down. It can be associated with neck pain, tinnitus, changes in hearing, photophobia, and nausea. The headache improves markedly after normalization of the CSF pressure such as after a successful sealing of the CSF leak with a blood patch.

MRI of the brain in low-pressure headache is usually normal but may show parenchymal enhancement, and a spine MRI may show the presence of extradural CSF.

Causes of a low CSF pressure can be secondary to a spinal tap, as mentioned earlier, or due to a spontaneous leak that can be seen in patients with connective tissue anomalies.

SECONDARY HEADACHES DUE TO INFECTION OR INFLAMMATION OF THE CNS

Headache is a frequent and often initial symptom in febrile illnesses in children and adolescents, such as viral illnesses, sinus diseases, and some bacterial illnesses such as streptococcal tonsillitis (ie, strep throat). Rarely, a headache can be part of other systemic illnesses, CNS inflammatory diseases, and infections.

In CNS infections, the headache is a primary symptom, is usually diffuse and all over the head, and can be associated with an ill feeling, fatigue, neck stiffness, and even photophobia. Evaluation of the underlying infection is essential, and treatment of the infection improves the headache markedly. If a CNS infection is suspected, imaging followed by a spinal tap with opening pressure and CSF studies are necessary for evaluation and treatment guidance.

Inflammatory disorders of the CNS will present with a headache that follows the same pattern as the CNS infections and is described as diffuse pain in the head that may be associated with irritability, neck stiffness, and photophobia. The headache improves with treatment of the underlying disorder.

HEADACHE DUE TO SPACE-OCCUPYING LESIONS OR CONGENITAL ANOMALIES SUCH AS CHIARI I MALFORMATION

Other headaches that can present in childhood include those caused by space-occupying lesions, CNS neoplasms, and Chiari I malformations. Postconcussive headache is a headache that occurs with a history of trauma and will be discussed in Chapter 16.

Space-occupying lesions can be associated with a headache, but headache is rarely the initial symptom. Neurologic abnormalities are usually present prior to a headache, starting with signs of increased pressure and focal abnormalities on examination.

In Chiari I malformation, the description of the headache is occipital, not persistent; it is triggered by cough and the Valsalva maneuver and is associated with other symptoms such as numbness in the upper extremities due to a possibility of a syrinx in the spine, trouble swallowing, and unsteadiness.[16] The MRI shows a tonsillar hernia of 5 mm or greater with or without crowding.[17] If crowding is present, the symptoms may be more prominent. An MRI of the brain with a cine will help in evaluating the anatomy of the Chiari malformation as well as the CSF flow. An MRI of the spine is recommended to evaluate for the presence of any syrinx. If diagnosed clinically and on imaging, a referral to neurosurgery is recommended for evaluation and follow-up. If the crowding is not severe, CSF flow is acceptable, and the patient does not have any prominent symptoms, the neurosurgeon may opt for close observation with frequent MRI instead of surgery. It is important to remember that due to the high prevalence of migraine in this population, patients with Chiari I malformation can still have migraine headaches. These patients usually can differentiate between the 2 types of headaches, and a good medical history will help in managing both.

In conclusion, the main goal when evaluating a patient presenting with a chief complaint of headache is to differentiate between a primary and secondary headache. This is a major step that is essential to guide further testing, treatment, and referral.

REFERENCES

1. Lewis DW, Ashwal S, Dahl G, et al. Quality Standards Subcommittee of the American Academy of Neurology; Practice Committee of the Child Neurology Society. Practice parameter: evaluation of children and adolescents with recurrent headaches: report of the Quality Standards Subcommittee of the American Academy of Neurology and the Practice Committee of the Child Neurology Society. *Neurology*. 2002;59(4):490-498.
2. Medina LS, Pinter JD, Zurakowski D, Davis RG, Kuban K, Barnes PD. Children with headache: clinical predictors of surgical space-occupying lesions and the role of neuroimaging. *Radiology*. 1997;202(3):819-824.
3. Abend NS, Younkin D, Lewis, DW. Secondary headaches in children and adolescents. *Semin Pediatr Neurol*. 2010;17:123-133.
4. Headache Classification Committee of the International Headache Society. The International Classification of Headache Disorders 3rd Edition (ICHD-3). *Cephalalgia*. 2018;38(1):1-211.
5. Dubosh NM, Bellolio MF, Rabinstein AA, Edlow JA. Sensitivity of early brain computed tomography to exclude aneurysmal subarachnoid hemorrhage. A systematic review and meta-analysis. *Stroke*. 2016;47:750-755.
6. Maruyama H, Nagoya H, Kato Y, et al. Spontaneous cervicocephalic arterial dissection with headache and neck pain as the only symptom. *J Headache Pain*. 2012;13(3):247-253.
7. Villella V, Molinaro I, Granata G, Finucci A, Granata M. Secondary headache due to bilateral dissection of vertebral arteries. *J Headache Pain*. 2015;16(suppl 1):A129.
8. Hirano M, Pavlakis SG. Mitochondrial myopathy, encephalopathy, lactic acidosis, and strokelike episodes (MELAS): current concepts. *J Child Neurol*. 1994;9:4-13.
9. Sproule DM, Kaufmann P. Mitochondrial encephalopathy, lactic acidosis, and strokelike episodes: basic concepts, clinical phenotype, and therapeutic management of MELAS syndrome. *Ann N Y Acad Sci*. 2008;1142:133-158.
10. Di Donato I, Bianchi S, De Stefano N, et al. Cerebral autosomal dominant arteriopathy with subcortical infarcts and leukoencephalopathy (CADASIL) as a model of small vessel disease: update on clinical, diagnostic, and management aspects. *BMC Med*. 2017;15:41.

11. Mollan SP, Davies B, Silver NC, et al. Idiopathic intracranial hypertension: consensus guidelines on management. *J Neurol Neurosurg Psychiatry*. 2018;89:1088-1100.

12. Jensen RH, Radojicic A, Yri H, et al. The diagnosis and management of idiopathic intracranial hypertension and the associated headache. *Ther Adv Neurol Disord*. 2016;9(4):317-326.

13. Favoni V, Pierangeli G, Toni F, et al. Idiopathic intracranial hypertension without papilledema (IIHWOP) in chronic refractory headache. *Front Neurol*. 2018;9:503.

14. Wall M. Idiopathic intracranial hypertension. *Neurol Clin*. 2010;28:593-617.

15. Bidot S, Saindane AM, Peragallo JH, Bruce BB, Newman NJ, Biousse V. Brain imaging in idiopathic intracranial hypertension. *J Neuroophthalmol*. 2015;35(4):400-411.

16. Meadows J, Guarnieri M, Miller K, Haroun R, Kraut M, Carson BS. Type I Chiari malformation: a review of the literature. *Neurosurg Quart*. 2001;11(3):220-229.

17. Atchley TJ, Alford EN, Rocque BG. Systematic review and meta-analysis of imaging characteristics in Chiari I malformation: does anything really matter? *Childs Nerv Syst*. 2020;36(3):525-534.

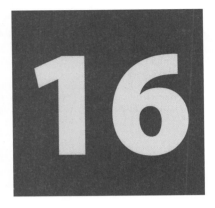

Posttraumatic Headache

Joanne Kacperski, MD, FAHS

Ankita Ghosh, MD

INTRODUCTION

Traumatic brain injury (TBI) is one of the most common injuries in the pediatric age group. It is estimated that as many as half a million children younger than 15 years sustain TBIs that require hospital-based care in the United States each year, with the majority of these injuries being mild in severity.[1] A national cross-sectional study in the United States estimated that 1 of every 220 pediatric patients seen in emergency departments (EDs) receives a diagnosis of mild TBI (mTBI).[2] Headaches are the most common symptom after an mTBI and often occur with a constellation of physical, cognitive, emotional, and behavioral signs and symptoms.[3]

POSTTRAUMATIC HEADACHES

Headache after an mTBI, referred to as posttraumatic headache (PTH), is one of the most common and disabling symptoms after a head injury. Headache has been reported in as many as 86% of high school and college athletes who have suffered from head trauma.[4] Eisenberg et al[5] reported that 85% of pediatric patients presented to a pediatric ED with headache following an mTBI.[5] Kuczynski et al[6] reported that 11% of pediatric patients who presented to a university hospital ED with mTBI continued to report headache 2 weeks after injury. Headaches may affect a child's ability to function and participate in school and extracurricular activities, which can cause disability and impair their quality of life.[3]

▶ Definition

The International Classification of Headache Disorders, Third Edition (ICHD-3) classifies PTHs as a secondary headache type defined as acute if lasting less than 3 months and persistent if lasting more than 3 months after injury. The classification for acute and persistent PTH (PPTH) is summarized in Tables 16–1 and 16–2. Although the ICHD-3 criteria state that PTHs begin within 7 days after injury to

the head or after regaining consciousness, this 7-day cutoff is arbitrary, and some experts believe that headaches may develop after a longer interval.[7]

▶ Risk Factors

Predictive factors for the development of PTH in the pediatric population may include age, sex, prior history of headaches, and family history.[8] Some studies suggest that females are more likely to endorse both preinjury and postinjury headaches consistent with migraine.[9] In a study of 400 patients from a pediatric concussion clinic, although 90% of females versus 79% of males reported PTH, females also demonstrated a longer duration of symptoms compared to males (median recovery time of 80 days vs 34 days, respectively),[10] indicating that the role of sex remains uncertain. Prior headache history may also play a role in the development of PTH. In a pediatric study, 51% of children with persistent PTH at 3 months after mTBI had a preexisting history of headaches and 31% had headaches fulfilling the ICHD-3 criteria for migraine or probable migraine prior to the injury. Furthermore, 56% of the children with persistent PTH also had a positive family history of migraine.[6] Chronic pain, nonsteroidal anti-inflammatory drug (NSAID) use prior to injury, and a family history of headache have also been associated with increased risk of developing PTH.[8] Patients with prior mTBI, preexisting anxiety and/or depression, maladaptive coping styles, or medication overuse headaches seem to be at higher risk for persistent PTH.[11,12] Also of note, a 2019 trial indicated that the only risk factor for the development of PTH was a personal past history of a primary headache disorder and that, in 90% of patients, the PTH was phenotyped as migraine.[13]

▶ Pathophysiology

It is presumed that TBI causes cellular and axonal injury, which can induce excessive glutamate release. Glutamate

Table 16–1. International Classification of Headache Disorders, Third Edition (ICHD-3) definition of acute headache attributed to traumatic injury to the head.

5.1 Acute headache attributed to traumatic injury to the head
A. Any headache fulfilling criteria C and D
B. Traumatic injury to the head[a] has occurred
C. Headache is reported to have developed within 7 days after one of the following:
1. The injury to the head
2. Regaining of consciousness following the injury to the head
3. Discontinuation of medication(s) that impair(s) ability to sense or report headache following the injury to the head
D. Either of the following:
1. Headache has resolved within 3 months after the injury to the head
2. Headache has not yet resolved, but 3 months have not yet passed since the injury to the head
E. Not better accounted for by another ICHD-3 diagnosis

5.1.2 Acute posttraumatic headache attributed to mild traumatic injury to the head
A. Headache fulfilling criteria for 5.1
B. Injury to the head fulfilling none of the following:
1. Associated with none of the following:
a) Loss of consciousness for >30 minutes
b) Glasgow Coma Scale (GCS) score <13
c) Posttraumatic amnesia[b] lasting >24 hours
d) Altered level of awareness for >24 hours
e) Imaging evidence of traumatic head injury, eg, intracranial hemorrhage and/or brain contusion
2. Associated immediately following the head injury with one or more of the following symptoms and/or signs:
a) Transient confusion, disorientation, or impaired consciousness
b) Loss of memory for events immediately before or after the head injury
c) 2 or more other symptoms suggestive of mild traumatic brain injury: nausea, vomiting, visual disturbances, dizziness and/or vertigo, impaired memory, and/or concentration

[a]Traumatic injury to the head is defined as a structural or functional injury resulting from the action of external forces on the head. These include striking the head with an object or the head striking an object, penetration of the head by a foreign body, forces generated from blasts or explosions, and other forces yet to be defined.
[b]The duration of posttraumatic amnesia is defined as the time between head injury and recovery of memory of current events and those occurring in the last 24 hours.
Data from Headache Classification Committee of the International Headache Society (IHS). The International Classification of Headache Disorders, 3rd ed. (Beta version) *Cephalalgia*. 2013;33(9):629–808.

Table 16–2. International Classification of Headache Disorders, Third Edition (ICHD-3) definition of persistent posttraumatic headaches.

5.2 Persistent headache attributed to traumatic injury to the head
A. Any headache fulfilling criteria C and D
B. Traumatic injury to the head[a] has occurred
C. Headache is reported to have developed within 7 days after one of the following:
1. The injury to the head
2. Regaining of consciousness following the injury to the head
3. Discontinuation of medication(s) that impair(s) ability to sense or report headache following the injury to the head
D. Headache persists for >3 months after the injury to the head
E. Not better accounted for by another ICHD-3 diagnosis

5.2.2 Persistent headache attributed to mild traumatic injury to the head
A. Headache fulfilling criteria for 5.2
B. Head injury fulfilling both of the following:
1. Associated with none of the following:
a) Loss of consciousness for >30 minutes
b) Glasgow Coma Scale (GCS) score <13
c) Posttraumatic amnesia[b] lasting >24 hours
d) Altered level of awareness for >24 hours
e) Imaging evidence of traumatic head injury, eg, intracranial hemorrhage and/or brain contusion
2. Associated immediately following the head injury with one or more of the following symptoms and/or signs:
a) Transient confusion, disorientation, or impaired consciousness
b) Loss of memory for events immediately before or after the head injury
c) 2 or more other symptoms suggestive of mild traumatic brain injury: nausea, vomiting, visual disturbances, dizziness and/or vertigo, impaired memory, and/or concentration

[a]Traumatic injury to the head is defined as a structural or functional injury resulting from the action of external forces on the head. These include striking the head with an object or the head striking an object, penetration of the head by a foreign body, forces generated from blasts or explosions, and other forces yet to be defined.
[b]The duration of posttraumatic amnesia is defined as the time between head injury and recovery of memory of current events and those occurring in the last 24 hours.
Data from Headache Classification Committee of the International Headache Society (IHS). The International Classification of Headache Disorders, 3rd ed. (Beta version) *Cephalalgia*. 2013;33(9):629–808.

accumulation in turn causes influx of calcium ion, accumulation of lactate, and oxidative stress, resulting in microtubule collapse and structural axonal damage.[14] Injury to the trigeminal neuronal pathways leads to headaches and allodynia. TBI can also cause muscle strain and ligamentous injury, which can lead to neuralgic pain.[15]

Phenotypes

Despite being classified as a secondary headache type, headache attributed to mTBI often presents with clinical features seen in other primary headache disorders. Like other secondary headache types, PTH has no defining or identifying features. Prospective studies of PTH have found that migraine is the most common phenotype in adults and children. In one study of 378 participants older than 16 years of age admitted for acute inpatient rehabilitation following mTBI, migraine was the most frequent headache phenotype after injury (38%). Probable migraine was suspected in up to 25% of patients, tension-type headache in 21%, and cervicogenic headache in 10%.[9]

Evaluation

Assessment of pediatric PTH is similar to the assessment of a primary headache disorder. Evaluation should exclude other secondary causes of headache, including the possibility of a structural source such as intracranial hemorrhage, cerebral edema, stroke, traumatic dissection (carotid or vertebral), or acute cervical/thoracic neck injury.[8] The history should include evaluation of prior head injuries, preinjury symptoms (eg, preexisting headaches or migraines, anxiety, depression, sleep disturbance), risk factors (eg, family history, learning disabilities), details regarding the injury, current symptoms (eg, location, quality, associated symptoms), and the progression of symptoms after injury. It is important to ask about other postconcussion symptoms such as dizziness, nausea, sleep disturbances, mood changes, and cognitive changes and assess for medication overuse.[15] Thorough general and neurologic examinations should be completed, including fundoscopy to rule out papilledema and head and neck exam to evaluate for neuralgias.[16]

Computed tomography and magnetic resonance imaging are not necessary to establish the diagnosis of mTBI or PTH in children and are not recommended during the acute evaluation unless there are risk factors for intracranial injury or clinical concern for significant injuries that could result in intracranial hemorrhage or a cervical spine injury.[15,17]

Treatment

Acute Therapies

The goal of acute treatment in children with PTH should be a consistent response with minimum side effects and a rapid return to normal function. The treatments should be properly dosed and used as quickly as possible, while minimizing the potential for medication overuse. Patients should have the ability to receive these treatments in the school or at home, without missing school or social activities. To avoid the development of medication overuse headache (MOH), abortive medications should be used no more than 3 days per week. When prescribed, migraine-specific drugs, particularly the triptans, should be used fewer than 9 times per month.[17] Thus, the clinician should make every effort to classify the headache type because this may have treatment implications.[18]

The initial outpatient treatment strategy should include over-the-counter medications, including ibuprofen and acetaminophen. Ibuprofen (10 mg/kg) is considered safe and effective, and acetaminophen (15 mg/kg) is probably just as effective. Naproxen sodium (10 mg/kg) has been effective and routinely recommended in adults as a reasonable option for acute migraine with good response to a similar previously used NSAID and is often tried in children with acute migraine, often when ibuprofen is ineffective. Aspirin (10 mg/kg) can be considered in adolescents 16 years and older but not in younger patients due to concerns for Reye syndrome.[17] Consistent with migraine management in pediatrics, opioids should be avoided due to lack of evidence for efficacy and concern for abuse and MOH and/or chronification.[17,18]

Triptans may be administered to patients whose headaches phenotype to migraine. Caution should be used in the very acute setting of mTBI because of the theoretical risk of vasospasm, which may exacerbate hypoperfusion in children who may have an underlying vascular injury to the brain. Imaging should be done prior to triptan administration in any child with headache and persistent altered mental status or focal neurologic findings.[18] Once vascular injury is ruled out, triptans should be taken at the onset of headache and can be repeated 2 hours later if needed. The dosage maximum per day and per week differs for each of the 7 triptan medications, but all should be limited to no more than 9 days per month to avoid MOH. Adverse effects of triptan use include tightness of the chest, throat, or jaw, which is often brief and transient.[6]

Preventive Treatments

There are no accepted guidelines to aid the clinician on the timing or initiation of preventive therapy. Some have argued that earlier initiation of such agents could potentially decrease the likelihood of developing persistent PTH.[19] Prophylaxis should be limited to those children whose headaches occur with sufficient frequency and/or severity to warrant a daily preventive medication and should be considered if acute treatments are ineffective, poorly tolerated, contraindicated, or overused. The goals of treatment should be outlined at onset. Medications should be titrated to goal dose slowly.

Delayed onset of preventive medication effect, often up to 6 to 8 weeks after initiation, must be highlighted to families. A treatment goal of having fewer than 3 to 4 headaches per month for a sustained period of 4 to 6 months is recommended prior to discontinuing therapy.[17,19] Few medications have been studied for PTH in a systematic way, and most are extrapolated from the migraine literature. There are no placebo-controlled randomized trials of how children with PTH respond to pharmacologic treatment strategies used for primary headache.

Nonpharmacologic Treatments

Nonpharmacologic treatments have established good evidence in children and adolescents with chronic headaches.[20] The US Headache Consortium found that cognitive behavioral therapy was supported by Grade A evidence for the prevention of migraine.[21] Lifestyle modifications are often discussed with patients, including hydration, sleep hygiene, and a well-balanced diet.

REFERENCES

1. Bazarian JJ, McClung J, Shah MN, Cheng YT, Flesher W, Kraus J. Mild traumatic brain injury in the United States, 1998-2000. *Brain Inj.* 2005;19(2):85-91.
2. Meehan WP 3rd, Mannix R. Pediatric concussions in United States emergency departments in the years 2002 to 2006. *J Pediatr.* 2010;157(6):889-893.
3. Powers SW, Andrasik F. Biobehavioral treatment, disability, and psychological effects of pediatric headache. *Pediatr Ann.* 2005;34(6):461-465.
4. Guskiewicz KM, Weaver NL, Padua DA, Garrett WE. Epidemiology of concussion in collegiate and high school football players. *Am J Sports Med.* 2000;28:643-650.
5. Eisenberg MA, Meehan WP, Mannix R. Duration and course of post-concussive symptoms. *Pediatrics.* 2014;133(6):999-1006.
6. Kuczynski A, Crawford S, Bodell L, Dewey D, Barlow K. Characteristics of post-traumatic headaches in children following mild traumatic brain injury and their response to treatment: a prospective cohort. *Dev Med Child Neurol.* 2013;55:636-641.
7. Headache Classification Committee of the International Headache Society. The International Classification of Headache Disorders, 3rd edition (beta version). *Cephalalgia.* 2013;33(9):629-808.
8. Blume HK. Headaches after concussion in pediatrics: a review. *Curr Pain Headache Rep.* 2015;19(9):1-11.
9. Lucas S, Hoffman JM, Bell KR, Walker W, Dikmen S. Characterization of headache after traumatic brain injury. *Cephalalgia.* 2012;32(8):600-606.
10. Bramley H, Heverley S, Lewis MM, Kong L, Rivera R, Silvis M. Demographics and treatment of adolescent posttraumatic headache in a regional concussion clinic. *Pediatr Neurol.* 2015;52(5):493-498.
11. Morgan CD, Zuckerman SL, Lee YM, et al. Predictors of post-concussion syndrome after sports-related concussion in young athletes: a matched case-control study. *J Neurosurg Pediatr.* 2015;15(6):589-598.
12. Kjeldgaard D, Forchhammer H, Teasdale T, Jensen RH. Chronic post-traumatic headache after mild head injury: a descriptive study. *Cephalalgia.* 2014;34:191-200.
13. Lane R, Davies P. Post traumatic headache (PTH) in a cohort of UK compensation claimants. *Cephalalgia.* 2019;39(5):641-647.
14. Barkhoudarian G, Hovda DA, Giza CC. The molecular pathophysiology of concussive brain injury: an update. *Phys Med Rehabil Clin N Am.* 2016;27:373-393.
15. Pinchefsky E, Dubrovsky AS, Friedman D, Shevell M. Part I: evaluation of pediatric post-traumatic headaches. *Pediatr Neurol.* 2015;52:263-269.
16. Blume HK. Posttraumatic headache in pediatrics: an update and review. *Curr Opin Pediatr.* 2018;30(6):755-763.
17. Kacperski J, Arthur T. Management of post-traumatic headaches in children and adolescents. *Headache.* 2016;56(1):36-48.
18. Wilson MB, Krolczyk SJ. Pediatric post-traumatic headache. *Curr Pain Headache Rep.* 2006;10(5):387-390.
19. Pinchefsky E, Dubrovsky AS, Friedman D, Shevell M. Part II: management of pediatric post-traumatic headaches. *Pediatr Neurol.* 2015;52(3):270-280.
20. Blume HK, Brockman LN, Breuner CC. Biofeedback therapy for pediatric headache: factors associated with response. *Headache.* 2012;52(9):1377-1386.
21. Campbell JK, Penzien DB, Wall EM. Evidenced-based guidelines for migraine headache: behavioral and physical treatments. US Headache Consortium. 2000. Accessed June 20, 2022. http://www.aan.com/professionals/practice/pdfs/gl0089.pdf

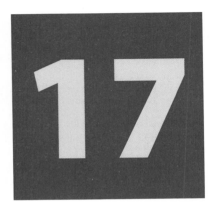

Pediatric Musculoskeletal Pain

Cheryl J. Hartzell, MD

Kenneth R. Goldschneider, MD

ESSENTIALS OF DIAGNOSIS AND TYPICAL FEATURES

▶ Pain related to the musculoskeletal system is common in the pediatric age range. The differential diagnosis list is long; etiologies range from inflammatory and oncologic to primary muscular, hypermobility, overuse, and trauma.

▶ Physical therapy is the cornerstone of treatment of all types of musculoskeletal pain, with appropriate modifications needed for patients with hypermobility disorders.

▶ Trigger point injections are the most frequently performed interventions for myofascial pain and are of low complexity and morbidity. More invasive procedures, such as epidural steroid injections, sacroiliac joint injections, and facet injections, are indicated for specific diagnoses, and patients should be referred to those specially trained to perform them.

INTRODUCTION

Pain related to the musculoskeletal (MSK) system is frequent in the pediatric age range. A longitudinal study within the Prevention and Incidence of Asthma and Mite Allergy (PIAMA) birth cohort study of nearly 4000 adolescents found that the prevalence of MSK pain from age 11 to 20 years ranged from 17.4% to 37.9% in girls and 14.2% to 22.1% in boys.[1] Persistent pain, defined as pain lasting longer than 1 month, was found among 16.5% of girls and 5.1% of boys.[1] Although it is not uncommon for pain to start in a localized area, among the various types of MSK pain, diffuse idiopathic pain syndromes, including juvenile fibromyalgia[2] and benign hypermobility syndrome,[3] are the most common

diagnoses, with the most frequent area of pain being the neck and back.[4,5] In this chapter, we review the clinical findings, pathogenesis, differential diagnoses, and approach to treatment of MSK pain.

CLINICAL FINDINGS

▶ Symptoms and Signs

Diffuse idiopathic MSK pain, a diagnosis of exclusion, is the most common diagnosis of noninflammatory MSK pain. As such, a well-explored pain history is paramount in delineating potential causes, focusing the physical exam, and identifying red flags to determine indicated testing/imaging or further consultations (Box 17–1). Often the pain will develop insidiously in a localized area with no definable injury or illness. As discomfort and pain intensify, pain will become constant with periods of exacerbations. Pain is described in a multitude of ways, including deep, dull, aching, or sharp and shooting in nature. The patient may have radicular pain with electric shock–like pains or numbness and tingling in their extremities, often not in a dermatomal pattern. Patients may report intermittent joint swelling, erythema, color changes, or stiffness, especially of the hands. Various factors will exacerbate the pain, including excessive physical activity or prolonged immobility, psychosocial stressors, changes in mood, poor sleep, and illness.

Pain hypersensitivity is common, leading to pain with light touch (allodynia), pain with nonnociceptive movement, and hypervigilance to avoidance of pain-associated activities (kinesiophobia). Biomechanical malalignment, as seen with joint hypermobility, provides a good example of how pain develops and amplifies from everyday movement. Poor proprioception is common, especially in patients with hypermobility disorders and in those who have altered their body mechanics in response to pain. For instance, the patient is often unaware of how they naturally hyperextend

Box 17–1. Red flag symptoms and physical exam findings of musculoskeletal pain that may indicate further evaluation with laboratory studies or imaging or referral to additional providers.

Red Flags
Unexplained fever
Weight loss
History of neoplasm
Chronic steroid use
Swelling, redness, or warmth of a joint
Morning stiffness
Pain improves with activity
Radicular pain not responding to conservative treatment
Neurologic changes: trouble walking, footdrop, weakness in extremities, loss of reflexes, sensory changes, saddle anesthesia
Urinary retention
Bowel function changes
Joint instability
Night pain, pain waking patient from sleep
Constant pain

their elbows with simple actions such as reaching and lifting or how they stand with their knees hyperextended. These repetitive, daily mechanical alterations lead to a cycle of pain activation: excessive movement of joints → stress on joint surfaces → repetitive microtrauma → overuse injury → overactivation of pain systems and central sensitization.

As pain intensifies, avoidance of activity will occur, leading to progressive muscle deconditioning, diffuse pain amplification, and perpetuation of functional disability. Changes in mood including irritability, anger, depressed mood, and anxiety may occur and can progress to mimic agoraphobia. Patients will commonly try to avoid leaving the security of their home to go out into an environment they cannot control or from which they cannot retreat if pain flares. Low mood is thought to be more a reaction to the pain disability, rather than primary depression, but can be severe and may require treatment. Patients frequently have significant sleep disturbances due to pain, including delayed sleep, frequent awakenings, and daytime napping, all contributing to amplification of pain and functional disability.

A substantial number of patients will have difficulty obtaining accommodations at school, leading to significant school truancy, including leaving school early due to pain, and potentially resulting in enrollment in online or homebound learning. Concomitant withdrawal from sports, school, and social activities and separation from the family at home with a substantial amount of time spent alone lead to further functional disability and worsening quality of life.

Lab Findings

Laboratory studies may be indicated to rule out systemic diagnoses, as indicated by history, physical, or red flags or if clinical presentation is not definitive. In amplified MSK pain disorders, blood counts, chemistry and liver panels, erythrocyte sedimentation rate, and C-reactive protein are typically normal. A positive antinuclear antibody (ANA) test does not necessarily indicate the presence of a rheumatologic disorder, as up to 20% to 30% of the general population is positive for ANA.[6]

Vitamin deficiencies have been shown to be potential contributors to MSK pain. While evidence regarding dietary supplementation remains limited, potential benefits of vitamin supplementation may outweigh the low risk of this conservative treatment. Animal studies have shown anti-inflammatory and antinociceptive effects of vitamin B_{12} (cobalamin), with clinical trials demonstrating effectiveness in treating low back pain and neuralgia.[7] Vitamin C (ascorbic acid) is essential for enzymatic activity necessary to maintain stable collagen cross-links, a principal determinant of ligament, tendon, and bone quality, and is an antioxidant. A study examining cross-sectional data from the US National Health and Nutrition Examination Survey in 2003 to 2004 from 4742 adults with chronic pain found statistically significant associations between suboptimal vitamin C concentrations and presence of pain in the neck, back, or below the knee or arthritis.[8]

Vitamin D affects muscle strength, size, and neuromuscular performance.[9] The association between vitamin D deficiency, MSK pain, and nonspecific back pain has been demonstrated in a multitude of studies.[9-11] One study of 174 adult patients with chronic muscle pain, widespread pain, or arthritis found that 71% of patients had vitamin D deficiency and 21% had vitamin D insufficiency, with only 8% having sufficient vitamin D levels.[12] Low vitamin D levels are also associated with central hypersensitivity with increased mechanical pain and somatic symptoms.[10-12]

Imaging Studies

The primary role of any imaging study is to identify an underlying systemic disease. In the absence of red flag symptoms or physical exam findings, imaging is usually not appropriate. Spine imaging, in particular, has proven to poorly correlate findings to those with pain versus without pain.[4] According to the American College of Radiology Appropriateness Criteria for Low Back Pain 2021 update, in the absence of red flags, imaging is usually not appropriate in patients with acute (0-4 weeks), subacute (4-12 weeks), and chronic (>12 weeks) low back pain with or without radiculopathy.[13] These recommendations are based on adult studies, and although they are a helpful guide, practitioners tend to pursue imaging more aggressively in pediatric patients to avoid missing an underlying malignancy, structural defect, or other cause of harm. Imaging may be considered in patients who have failed

6 weeks of conservative treatment if diagnostic uncertainty remains. It is important to note that these recommendations were based off of adult studies. Imaging is more commonly indicated for children and young adults who likely do not have natural degeneration and thus have a potentially higher likelihood of underlying pathology.

Electromyography is a procedure to test the integrity of spinal nerve roots, peripheral nerves, and skeletal muscles.[14] Diagnostic utility is questionable in patients with localized pain or weakness in a nonanatomic distribution and/or without neuromuscular deficits, almost always yielding a negative result.[14]

PATHOGENESIS

Full coverage of the pathophysiology of MSK pain is beyond the scope of this chapter. However, a few special situations merit mention. Given the increasing awareness and identification of patients with pain and joint hypermobility, the pathophysiology in this setting is an important discussion. Approximately 3% of the population is estimated to have joint hypermobility and an estimated prevalence of hypermobile Ehlers-Danlos syndrome of 1 in 5000, although both are thought to be underestimations.[3,15] Similar to fibromyalgia, studies support the key mechanism of pain due to hypermobility to involve central sensitization and less neuropathic pain.[16,17] Joint laxity results in greater joint range of motion, leading to biomechanical overloading, repetitive microtrauma within and around joints, and chronic soft tissue injury. Biomechanical alterations and malalignment lead to stress on supporting joints, joint and muscle fatigue, and further injury, resulting in overactivation of the pain system and manifesting as arthralgias and diffuse MSK pain.[3,16,17] Additionally, patients with hypermobility tend to have poor proprioception, the ability to sense position of their joints, placing them at greater risk for joint injuries.

Myofascial trigger points are a common contributor to MSK pain. Trigger points are discrete, localized, taut bands of skeletal muscles, mostly found in the neck and upper and lower back, but they may occur in any skeletal muscle.[18,19] They are painful on compression and may produce a referred pain, numbness, tingling, or motor dysfunction. They differ from tender points in that tender points occur in specific locations, are symmetrically located, and do not cause referred pain.[18]

DIFFERENTIAL DIAGNOSIS

The differential diagnosis for MSK pain is extensive (Table 17–1), reinforcing the need to start with a thorough history and physical examination to rule out red flag symptoms and physical exam findings (see Box 17–1). The multidisciplinary approach to MSK pain may include the need to refer to other providers, such as orthopedics, rheumatology, or pain specialists, for further assessment, especially in the presence of red flags. Amplified MSK pain disorders, psychologically related pain, and functional neurologic disorders are diagnoses of exclusion.

Table 17–1. A framework for differential diagnoses for musculoskeletal pain.

Widespread musculoskeletal pain disorders	Diffuse idiopathic musculoskeletal pain
	Hypermobility spectrum disorders (eg, collagen deficiencies and Ehlers-Danlos syndrome)
	Fibromyalgia
Nonrheumatologic joint disorders	Femoroacetabular impingement
	Slipped capital femoral epiphysis
	Legg-Calvé-Perthes disease
	Osgood-Schlatter disease
	Sever disease
	Nursemaid's elbow
Inflammatory disorders	Juvenile idiopathic arthritis
	Rheumatoid arthritis
	Inflammatory bowel disease–associated arthropathy
	Systemic lupus erythematosus
	Myositis
Regional disorders	Complex regional pain syndrome
	Bursitis
	Epicondylitis
	Tendonitis/tendon injury
	Osteoid osteoma
	Peripheral neuropathies (hereditary and acquired)
Spine-related disorders	Compressive disk disorders (eg, disk herniation)
	Diskitis
	Facet arthropathy
	Radiculopathy
	Localized infection (eg, Pott disease)
Nutritional or metabolic disorders	Vitamin or mineral deficiency (B_1, B_{12}, D, calcium, folic acid, iron, magnesium)
	Hypothyroidism
Infectious disorders	Postviral myopathy or arthropathy
	Infectious arthritis (eg, septic hip, gonorrhea arthritis)
Psychological disorders	Anxiety
	Depression
	Disordered sleep
	Functional neurologic disorders
Oncologic disorders	Primary bone or muscle tumors
	Metastatic disease
	Avascular necrosis (secondary to treatment)

Table 17–2. Approach to treatment of musculoskeletal (MSK) pain, framed within the Biopsychosocial Model of pain.

Treatment	Description
Physical/occupational therapy	*Mainstay of treatment* for MSK pain. Goals of therapy are tailored to the patient, addressing: • *Biomechanical realignment* to remove stress on joints → prevent future injury; strengthening and building endurance of muscles supporting joints → improve joint stability; proprioception training → control range of motion. • *Aquatic physical therapy:* Provides the benefits of physical therapy in a warm water environment, adding to muscle relaxation and joint unloading. • *Transcutaneous electrical nerve stimulation (TENS) unit*: Uses low-voltage electric current to relieve pain.
Orthotics	*Pes planus* is common and often overlooked. Malalignment starting with pronation or supination of the feet leads to stress on proximal joints, causing ankle, knee, hip, and back pain. Consider evaluation and treatment by physical therapist or orthotics specialist.
Pain psychology	*Psychoeducational* approach aimed at: • *Cognitive restructuring:* Identifying dysfunctional thoughts and impact on pain and function. • *Utilizing techniques* (eg, diaphragmatic breathing, mindfulness, meditation) to decrease pain amplification and improve pain coping and function.
Aerobic exercise program	Utilizing *low-impact activity* such as yoga, pilates, recumbent bike, or swimming; goal is at least 30 minutes most days of the week.
Medications	*Adjunct*, not main therapy, with goal to decrease pain to a level that allows for improved functioning. • *Daily medications:* To modulate pain signaling, decrease sensitization, hyperalgesia, or allodynia. These may include neuropathic medications (gabapentin, pregabalin), tricyclic antidepressants (amitriptyline, nortriptyline), and serotonin reuptake inhibitors (duloxetine). • *Muscle relaxants:* Target muscle spasms, which commonly contribute to MSK pain but may be difficult for the patient to identify and describe. These may include methocarbamol, cyclobenzaprine, or tizanidine. • *Nonsteroidal anti-inflammatory drugs:* Target inflammation occurring from joint microtrauma or muscle injury. Formulations include oral or topical. • *Acetaminophen:* Essential as-needed treatment to add to a multimodal treatment regimen.
Myofascial trigger point injections	*Most frequent procedure* performed for MSK pain and most effective in quickly relieving acute myofascial trigger point pain.[18,19] Purpose is to break up the muscle bundle to allow relaxation of muscle and decrease inflammation. Dry needling has been shown to be as effective as injecting local anesthetic with dry needling; however, it resulted in more intense soreness.[18]
Interventional procedures	Invasive procedures, such as epidural steroid injections and steroid joint injections such as sacroiliac, facet, or extremity joint injections, are indicated for specific diagnoses, and patients should be *referred to a pain specialist* for further evaluation and treatment.
Vitamin supplementation	*Low-risk treatment* and potential *alternative* for patients wanting natural treatments. Vitamin deficiencies shown to be potential contributors to MSK pain are deficiencies of vitamin D, vitamin C, and vitamin B_{12}. (See Lab Findings section.)
School accommodations	Assist patient to *remain in school*. Examples include: • Ability to stand or walk when needed • Separate books for at school and home to prevent need to carry heavy backpacks • Extended time to walk between classes • Water bottle, access to bathroom • Modifications in physical education classes • A quiet place to practice pain psychology techniques in times of stress
Alternative and holistic therapies	• Acupuncture/acupressure • Massage therapy: most effective when combined with stretching • Osteopathic manipulative treatment

COMPLICATIONS

Untreated or persistent MSK pain holds the same risk of complications as discussed in Chapter 11, A General Approach to Pediatric Pain. Continued activity with poor biomechanics and alignment can lead to overuse injury and place the patient at risk for more serious MSK injuries.

TREATMENT

The gold standard of care for treatment of chronic pain is the *multidisciplinary approach* (Table 17–2), which is based on the Biopsychosocial Model of pain, discussed in Chapter 11, involving at its core a pain provider, pain psychologist, and physical therapist. Other specialists may include massage therapists, yoga instructors, physiatrists, psychiatrists, acupuncturists, and others. Given its efficacy, it can be applied to both acute and chronic pain. The goal is to target factors found to be significantly associated with and modulate pain, including poor sleep hygiene, fatigue, worrying/anxiety/mood disturbances, and injury (most commonly due to sports).[1,4] Above all, the most important treatment is that of education and support to the patient and their family.

PROGNOSIS

Overall, the resolution of MSK pain occurs in the majority of pediatric patients,[1] with acute MSK pain resolving within the natural course of healing according to the injury. Early intervention utilizing a multidisciplinary team, including a physical therapist and pain psychologist, has been demonstrated as the most efficacious approach.[20] Previous prospective studies have shown that poor prognostic factors in preadolescents with persistent or recurrent MSK pain into adolescence included untreated preadolescent pain, hypermobility, psychosomatic symptoms (eg, headache, abdominal pain), and sleep disturbances.[5,21,22] Depression, especially in adolescent females, is significantly associated with recurrent MSK pain.[5,22-24] The multitude of psychosocial risk factors for MSK pain underscores the need for a well-developed multidisciplinary approach and team to address all factors that modulate pain.

REFERENCES

1. Picavet HSJ, Gehring U, van Haselen A, et al. A widening gap between boys and girls in musculoskeletal complaints, while growing up from age 11 to age 20: the PIAMA birth Cohort study. *Eur J Pain.* 2021;25(4):902-912.
2. Connelly M, Weiss JE; for the CARRA Registry Investigators. Pain, functional disability, and their association in juvenile fibromyalgia compared to other pediatric rheumatic diseases. *Pediatr Rheumatol Online J.* 2019;17(1):72.
3. Kumar B, Lenert P. Joint hypermobility syndrome: recognizing a commonly overlooked cause of chronic pain. *Am J Med.* 2017;130(6):640-647.
4. Jones GT, Macfarlane GJ. Epidemiology of low back pain in children and adolescents. *Arch Dis Child.* 2005;90(3):312-316.
5. El-Metwally A, Salminen JJ, Auvinen A, et al. Prognosis of non-specific musculoskeletal pain in preadolescents: a prospective 4-year follow-up study till adolescence. *Pain.* 2004;110(3):550-559.
6. Pisetsky DS. Antinuclear antibody testing: misunderstood or misbegotten? *Nat Rev Rheumatol.* 2017;13(8):495-502.
7. Buesing S, Costa M, Schilling JM, et al. Vitamin B12 as a treatment for pain. *Pain Physician.* 2019;22(1):E45-E52.
8. Dionne CE, Laurin D, Desrosiers T, et al. Serum vitamin C and spinal pain: a nationwide study. *Pain.* 2016;157(11):2527-2535.
9. Wintermeyer E, Ihle C, Ehnert S, et al. Crucial role of vitamin D in the musculoskeletal system. *Nutrients.* 2016;8(6):319.
10. Wu Z, Malihi Z, Stewart AW, et al. The association between vitamin D concentration and pain: a systematic review and meta-analysis. *Public Health Nutr.* 2018;21(11):2022-2037.
11. Haddad HW, Mallepalli NR, Scheinuk JE, et al. The role of nutrient supplementation in the management of chronic pain in fibromyalgia: a narrative review. *Pain Ther.* 2021;10(2):827-848.
12. von Kanel R, Muller-Hartmannsgruber V, Kokinogenis G, et al. Vitamin D and central hypersensitivity in patients with chronic pain. *Pain Med.* 2014;15(9):1609-1618.
13. Expert Panel on Neurological Imaging, Hutchins TA, Peckham M, et al. ACR Appropriateness Criteria(R) Low Back Pain: 2021 update. *J Am Coll Radiol.* 2021;18(11S):S361-S379.
14. Lazaro RP. Electromyography in musculoskeletal pain: a reappraisal and practical considerations. *Surg Neurol Int.* 2015;6:143.
15. Tinkle B, Castori M, Berglund B, et al. Hypermobile Ehlers-Danlos syndrome (a.k.a. Ehlers-Danlos syndrome type III and Ehlers-Danlos syndrome hypermobility type): clinical description and natural history. *Am J Med Genet C Semin Med Genet.* 2017;175(1):48-69.
16. Di Stefano G, Celletti C, Baron R, et al. Central sensitization as the mechanism underlying pain in joint hypermobility syndrome/Ehlers-Danlos syndrome, hypermobility type. *Eur J Pain.* 2016;20(8):1319-1325.
17. Benistan K, Martinez V. Pain in hypermobile Ehlers-Danlos syndrome: new insights using new criteria. *Am J Med Genet A.* 2019;179(7):1226-1234.
18. Alvarez DJ, Rockwell PG. Trigger points: diagnosis and management. *Am Fam Physician.* 2002;65(4):653-660.
19. Borg-Stein J, Iaccarino MA. Myofascial pain syndrome treatments. *Phys Med Rehabil Clin N Am.* 2014;25(2):357-374.
20. Liossi C, Johnstone L, Lilley S, et al. Effectiveness of interdisciplinary interventions in paediatric chronic pain management: a systematic review and subset meta-analysis. *Br J Anaesth.* 2019;123(2):e359-e371.
21. Wurm M, Anniko M, Tillfors M, et al. Musculoskeletal pain in early adolescence: a longitudinal examination of pain prevalence and the role of peer-related stress, worry, and gender. *J Psychosom Res.* 2018;111:76-82.
22. Pourbordbari N, Riis A, Jensen MB, et al. Poor prognosis of child and adolescent musculoskeletal pain: a systematic literature review. *BMJ Open.* 2019;9(7):e024921.
23. Rees CS, Smith AJ, O'Sullivan PB, et al. Back and neck pain are related to mental health problems in adolescence. *BMC Public Health.* 2011;11:382.
24. Stanford EA, Chambers CT, Biesanz JC, et al. The frequency, trajectories and predictors of adolescent recurrent pain: a population-based approach. *Pain.* 2008;138(1):11-21.

Introduction to Seizures, Epilepsy, and Seizure Mimics

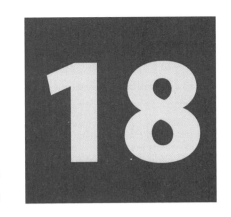

Nan Lin, MD

Colleen Buhrfiend, MD

INTRODUCTION TO SEIZURES AND EPILEPSY

Seizures are relatively common; approximately 1 in 10 people will have a seizure, but not all patients go on to develop epilepsy, typically only 1 in 26.[1] There is a bimodal distribution of seizures, with the highest incidence in the very young (<12 months old) and in the adult population older than 65 years. The incidence of pediatric epilepsy has a wide range between 41 and 187 per 100,000 and can vary by country.[2]

The International League Against Epilepsy (ILAE) has put together continually revised consensus operational and guideline criteria for definitions and classifications of seizures and epilepsy for children and adults, with the most recent update in 2017.[3] By definition, a seizure is a hyperactivation of neuronal brain cells characterized by abnormal synchronized misfiring. A seizure can broadly be classified in a few ways that are helpful for diagnostic and management steps. The first is if there is a temporal association with a provoking factor (eg, caused by a stroke, metabolic derangement such as hypoglycemia, or drug/medication intoxication) as compared to unprovoked where no clear cause is found. A seizure can also be defined by its suspected location of onset, such as focal (originating in one part of the brain), generalized (diffuse or rapid bisynchronized), or unknown (eg, if not witnessed). A third method of seizure classification is based on the reported features (or semiology) seen; that is, if there are motor (eg, tonic or generalized tonic-clonic [GTC]) or nonmotor (eg, an aura) features. ILAE has a website (epilepsydiagnosis.org) that is a very helpful resource for physicians for further review and is highly recommended as a reference for clinicians at any level of learning. Clues regarding seizure onset and type are based first and foremost upon the patient's report and the primary eyewitness account of the events. It is paramount to ask the patient about the events because internal sensory changes such as déjà vu may not be seen. In addition, it is important to ask the primary eyewitness about the seizure because stories can change if related to

another reporter. If events reoccur, we also advise families to obtain videos on a cell phone to review with the provider, but the patient's safety and privacy should be prioritized.

Features that are highly suspicious or suggestive of an epileptic seizure include events that are consistently stereotyped, events arising out of sleep or that are nocturnal, clear tonic-clonic movements, lacerations on the lateral aspects of the tongue (for motor seizures), evolution over time if not treated, and a concordant postictal phase with the seizure. Features such as urinary or bowel incontinence are suggestive but not specific for an epileptic seizure. Preceding paroxysmal events should be explicitly asked about because often the first presentation is the one witnessed but may not be the first seizure the patient has experienced.

Per the ILAE, epilepsy is a condition where a patient is prone to have reoccurring seizures, and the operational definition is currently (1) 2 or more unprovoked seizures separated by 24 hours or (2) 1 seizure with a greater than 60% chance of reoccurrence or (3) as part of an epilepsy syndrome. Epilepsy syndromes by age will be discussed in the next few chapters. Risk factors for developing epilepsy after the first lifetime seizure are listed in Table 18–1, but this is by no means an exhaustive list nor are these risk factors definitive in themselves. Note that most of the time, in otherwise healthy children, no risk factors or definitive cause of epilepsy or the seizure is identified.

A clinician's immediate approach to an acute seizure in the emergency department (ED) involves stabilizing the patient, securing the airway, breathing, and circulation, and performing a glucose check (succinctly summarized as the ABCDs [D for dextrose]). After the initial evaluation in the ED, a thorough neurologic exam should be conducted with focus on vital signs, mental status, and evaluating for any residual deficits after the seizure. Management of status epilepticus will not be discussed here, but a general overview for acute, self-resolving seizures is provided. Labs should be considered in appropriate clinical cases such as

Table 18–1. Risk factors for developing epilepsy.

Complications during pregnancy or birth that affect brain development such as hypoxic-ischemic encephalopathy
Presence of global developmental delay or intellectual disability
Congenital brain malformation such as focal cortical dysplasia
Brain injuries such as those resulting from a moderate-to-severe brain trauma, stroke, infections (eg, meningitis, encephalitis), or autoimmune process
Family history of epilepsy
Autism spectrum disorder
Abnormal electroencephalogram

Table 18–2. Seizure safety measures.

Place the patient down and on the ground away from dangerous objects
Place the patient on their side (does not matter if it is the left or right side; if patient has a ventriculoperitoneal [VP] shunt, place them on the opposite side from their VP shunt)
Do not place anything in their mouth; the person cannot swallow their tongue during a seizure
Do not hold down the person during the seizure
Time the duration of the seizure for when to give the rescue medication
Stay with the person after a seizure for at least 10 minutes to monitor their breathing and color

persistent altered mental status or signs of electrolyte imbalance (eg, significant gastrointestinal losses in the very young) but are not necessarily warranted if the patient is back to their baseline without any deficits or without any preexisting history that places them at increased risk.[4,5] Neuroimaging should be performed urgently if there is a history or exam suggestive of a structural etiology or increased intracranial pressure; presence of any neurologic deficits, encephalitis, or meningitis; persistent altered mental status; young age of patient (<6 months old); or history of prior neurosurgical interventions.[6] While neuroimaging in the ED setting will likely start with a computed tomography of the head with the rapid actionability of the information and short duration required to obtain the results, magnetic resonance imaging (MRI) of the brain is the preferred imaging modality for best visualization of detailed structures that may reveal a structural, traumatic, or metabolic cause that led to the seizure. Lumbar puncture should also be considered when there is concern for infections such as meningitis or encephalitis, and in some cases, neuroimaging should be obtained before lumbar puncture is done. For an overview of acute seizures in pediatric patients and adults, please see the review articles by Romantseva and Lin[7] and Moosavi and Swisher.[8]

Finally, most patients with isolated self-resolving seizures will not necessarily require inpatient care, but all patients should be referred to a child neurologist as outpatients. Seizure safety and seizure precautions should be reviewed with every patient and are key to reduce and prevent injury, morbidity, and mortality. Although not exhaustive, Table 18–2 is a starting point for discussions on how to keep the patient safe. Table 18–3 lists precautions in patients with seizures. A key precaution is the restriction on driving to reduce the risk of injury associated with seizure during driving for appropriate age groups. Please note the Epilepsy Foundation has many of these resources listed on their website, and this information should be provided as a resource for patients. Furthermore, the Epilepsy Foundation provides a free

Table 18–3. Seizure precautions.

Seizure Precaution	Comments
No driving No operating heavy machinery or power tools alone	Individual states have different BMV/DMV-required periods of seizure freedom, ranging from 3 to 12 months (some do not specify, such as Ohio). Not all states have mandated physician reporting. Please refer to each state's laws.
No bathing alone	Showers are fine. The risk here is submersion during the seizure or postictally with concern for drowning. For prevention of falls, encourage installation of nonslipping/nonskidding mats on bathtub or shower floors. Swimming with supervision can be considered.
No cooking independently with an open fire or open source of heat	Cooking with supervision can be considered, but the risk here is sustaining burns. Encourage use of microwaves.
Furniture padding in the house can be considered	Padding sharp edges and securing loose furniture in the household may help reduce injury in case of abrupt fall.
No standing in high places without railing or fall support	This is more for younger patients who are active; climbing on playgrounds should be supervised. For adults with jobs such as roofing, a switch of jobs should be strongly considered.

BM, Bureau of Motor Vehicles; DMV, Department of Motor Vehicles.
Note: We strongly encourage continued employment (unless it meets any of the above concerns), continued attendance in school, and involvement in sports. Neither seizure nor epilepsy should be a limit to these activities.

seizure first aid certification course for families and patients. We also strongly encourage all caregivers and families to learn cardiopulmonary resuscitation.

Most seizures resolve within 5 minutes. If not, in the ED, intravenous (IV) lorazepam is the first-line medication and is given at 0.1 mg/kg (maximum, 4 mg) for motor seizures lasting longer than 5 minutes. This dosing can be repeated if the seizure persists after 5 minutes after initial benzodiazepine rescue, keeping a close eye on airway status. If there is no IV access, intramuscular midazolam at 0.2 mg/kg (maximum, 10 mg) or rectal diazepam dosed by weight/age can be given. To abort seizures in the outpatient setting, rectal diazepam is approved by the US Food and Drug Administration (FDA) for patients age 2 years or older with a discrete seizure lasting more than 5 minutes and is dosed by weight (maximum, 20 mg). Since 2019 and 2020, though, intranasal midazolam and diazepam, respectively, have been approved by the FDA as seizure abortives for clusters of seizures. Anecdotally, these intranasal benzodiazepines are used off-label for seizures lasting longer than 5 minutes given ease of use compared to rectal diazepam.

With regard to epilepsy diagnosis, the first question for the child neurologist is the following: Was this event an epileptic seizure? Seizure mimics are common (see next section). The second question when determining whether the event was an epileptic seizure is: Was this truly the first event of the patient's lifetime? Asking the patient directly about prior stereotyped sensory changes at times reveals that prior seizures have occurred that were not witnessed or reported. Typically, seizure reoccurrence is greatest within the first 2 years, with the risk between 30% and 40%.[9] Antiseizure medication initiation will typically be done after 2 unprovoked seizures and is strongly considered after the first event if the electroencephalogram (EEG) or brain MRI is abnormal or a genetic/structural etiology is found (eg, tuberous sclerosis), although this is tailored to the individual. Discussion of antiseizure medication is beyond the scope of this chapter, but typically, seizure types are targeted with specific medications, balancing against side effects. Side effects of antiseizure medications are generally mild, but the side effects of medication should be discussed with every patient and family.

Currently, there are only a few FDA-approved seizure detection or seizure alert devices, with only one approved for both pediatric patients and adults—the Embrace Empatica, which is a watch that detects seizures. We hope and expect to see more in the future, particularly for nonmotor seizures. For an excellent review of current seizure alert or detection devices on the market, please see the review by Bruno et al.[10] None of these devices has been shown to reduce the risk of sudden unexplained death in epilepsy (SUDEP). A thorough discussion of pros and cons should be had with the primary child neurologist regarding cost (many of these devices not only include initial up-front purchase but also require an ongoing subscription fee), seizure sensitivity and specificity

(particularly for the individual patient's seizure types), false alarm rates, and impact on lifestyle before ordering one of these devices. Limitations of the device should also be discussed as there is no "perfect" seizure detection device. A nocturnal listening device such as a baby monitor or alarm is often recommended.

The most important risk factor for SUDEP is the continued presence of GTCs; in an elegant, nationwide, case-controlled, population-based study done in Sweden in 2020, the presence of GTCs in the preceding year alone was associated with a 27-fold increased risk of SUDEP.[11] Other risk factors found in the same study and in the 2019 North American SUDEP Registry were presence of nocturnal GTCs, living alone or in an unsupervised sleep environment, medication nonadherence, sleep deprivation, excessive alcohol use, and drug use.[11,12] Of note, non-GTC seizures in sleep (eg, focal seizures or absence seizures) were not associated with increased risk of SUDEP in the Swedish study. Therefore, the primary care provider and child neurologist should encourage patients to avoid drugs and limit excessive alcohol use, get consistent sleep, adhere to medications, and closely report any antiseizure medication side effects. Socioeconomic determinants of health will likely also play a role, and a multidisciplinary team approach is best for working with patients and their families.

SEIZURE MIMICS

Newborns, infants, and children can have paroxysmal nonepileptic movements or spells that can mimic seizures. It is important to be knowledgeable about these events to avoid excessive diagnostic testing and inappropriate treatment with antiepileptic medications. This section briefly summarizes many of the common paroxysmal nonepileptic events in the neonatal period, infancy, and childhood.

In general, paroxysmal nonepileptic events can be differentiated from seizures in that they (1) may be elicited by a trigger and (2) are often suppressible or interruptible. However, there may be some cases where an EEG is required to capture the event to clarify the diagnosis.

▶ Neonatal Period

Jitteriness or tremor is common in the neonate and reported to occur in up to 44% of healthy full-term newborns, with onset from 8 to 72 hours of life.[13,14] In the majority of cases, the tremor markedly decreases within the first 3 to 14 days but may last as long as 12 months.[15] The tremor is defined as a rhythmical oscillatory movement around a joint and can be further characterized by low amplitude and high frequency (fine tremor) or high amplitude and low frequency (coarse tremor). In some infants, the tremor occurs during stimulation and wakefulness; in others, it can occur during wake and sleep.[15] Jitteriness is usually provoked by stimuli and can be suppressed by restraining or repositioning the involved limb.[14,15] In addition, there are no associated abnormal eye movements or autonomic changes, differentiating tremors from neonatal seizures. If the newborn demonstrates a fine tremor, has a normal perinatal history, and a normal neurologic exam, then further diagnostic workup beyond a serum glucose level is not required. However, if the tremor is coarse and does not diminish after the third day of life, is not suppressible, or is associated with red flags in the maternal or perinatal history, then further investigation may be warranted. In such cases, consider the possibility of maternal substance abuse, including cannabis; neonatal withdrawal; hypoglycemia; calcium and other electrolyte derangements; hypoxic-ischemic insults; central nervous system infections; or sepsis. Reports of vitamin D deficiency in neonates have been associated with neonatal jitteriness.[16] The majority of neonates with jitteriness have normal developmental outcomes. Parents should be aware that jittery newborns are more difficult to console and may be less visually attentive, and parents often benefit from being taught behavioral techniques aimed at consoling the newborn and attracting visual attention.[14]

Myoclonus is characterized by a brief, rapid movement of a limb due to muscle contraction. It can occur in a single body part or may be generalized. It differs from tremor in that it is of high amplitude and is irregular. Myoclonus can come from the cortex, brainstem, or spinal cord. Epileptic myoclonus is uncommon in the neonate but can occur. If the myoclonic events are seizures, they should not be triggered. Benign neonatal sleep myoclonus begins in the first weeks of life, may be provoked by a stimulus, and often involves bilateral synchronous jerks of upper extremities, usually during quiet sleep and never while awake.[14,15] It is common for the jerks to occur in transition from sleep to wake as one might expect in some epilepsies. Although often bilateral, the jerks can be focal or multifocal, may move from one limb to the other, and may be synchronous or asynchronous. They can occur in clusters and can last for up to 30 to 60 minutes, mimicking seizures. The movements will stop when the infant is awoken. An EEG is often needed to clarify the nature of the events. The EEG is normal in myoclonus. Of note, in some cases, restraining the myoclonus can actually make it worse, unlike jitteriness.

Another paroxysmal movement that begins in the neonatal period is hyperekplexia, which is defined as an exaggerated startle that is longer, more intense, and does not habituate.[17] These episodes are easily triggered by external stimuli (auditory, visual, or tactile). The startle is characterized by head retraction, blinking, and tonic flexion of the extremities and trunk. Newborn exam demonstrates diffuse hypertonicity and hyperreflexia with paucity of movements. Startle responses can cause apnea, increasing the risk of sudden death. Clonazepam is often an effective treatment, and if the startle is sustained, flexing the head/neck and legs toward the torso can be lifesaving.[17] The hypertonia

and hyperreflexia resolve after the first year of life, but the startle episodes persist into adulthood and are often associated with traumatic falls, elicited by unexpected stimuli. The EEG is normal. The startle events can be triggered by tapping the nose. This condition can be acquired (metabolic or central nervous system structural defects) or hereditary. At this time, there are 3 genes associated with hereditary hyperekplexia; the genetic defects cause a dysfunction of glycine inhibitory transmission in the pontine reticular formation.[18]

▶ Infancy

There are many movements that mimic seizures in infancy and childhood. Benign myoclonus of early infancy is a misleading term given the many different presentations associated with the condition. Fernández-Alvarez[15] suggested that the movements be known as *benign polymorphous movement disorders of infancy* (BPMDI). Caraballo et al[19] reported that the main movements actually consist of myoclonus, spasms, tonic contractions, shuddering, atonia, or a combination of these movements. Fernández-Alvarez[15] characterized the main features of BPMDI as having the following features in common: abrupt onset, may occur in clusters, not associated with alteration in consciousness, can occur frequently throughout the day, often triggered by excitement, changes in posture, irritability, onset usually between 4 and 7 months, associated with normal development and neurologic exam, and usually resolve by 2 years of age but can rarely continue into childhood.[15,19] The following can be classified under the rubric of BPMDI:

- Benign spasms of infancy are typically characterized by spasms of the head, neck, shoulder, trunk, and upper extremities; usually last longer than myoclonic jerks with a duration of 1 to 2 seconds; and often occur in clusters, while awake, and frequently at meal time.[15,20] They are not associated with impairment in consciousness or distress. They present in the first year of life, usually between 4 and 7 months. They can be difficult to distinguish from epileptic spasms. Infants have normal development and neurologic exams. Epileptic spasms are important to recognize because immediate treatment can improve developmental outcomes. A video electroencephalogram is often required to differentiate between the 2 types of spasms. The movements typically decrease in frequency within 3 months and usually stop at around 18 to 24 months of life. No treatment is required, and normal developmental outcome is expected.

- Shuddering attacks are characterized as a brief shiver or tremor-like activity of the head, trunk, neck, and upper extremities. They may be associated with facial grimacing or eye blinking and are brief, lasting 5 to 15 seconds, without alteration in consciousness or distress. An EEG is usually not needed; however, a home video of the event can aid in the diagnosis.[15,20]

- Nonepileptic head drops (negative myoclonus) and myoclonus begin between 4 and 7 months and can be difficult to differentiate from myoclonic epileptic seizures. Again, normal development and neurologic exam are the rules. The patients will often need an EEG to evaluate for electrographic changes associated with myoclonic seizure disorders.

Other paroxysmal movements involve dystonic posturing and include benign paroxysmal torticollis in infancy, paroxysmal tonic upgaze of childhood, and paroxysmal tonic downgaze of newborns and infancy.[15] Benign paroxysmal torticollis of infancy is characterized by cervical dystonia or sustained posture of the head and neck. The neck is often tilted with the ear toward one shoulder and the chin rotated to the opposite shoulder. Sometimes there is curvature of the trunk. The infant can remain in this position for minutes to days. Sometimes the head tilt is to the left; other times, it is to the right. Onset is often before 3 months of age, and attacks are variable but typically occur 1 to 2 times a month.[15] Resolution is usually by 3 to 5 years of age.[21] They tend to occur in the morning upon waking, and certain movements can trigger them. They are often accompanied by irritability, ataxia, and autonomic symptoms including vomiting and pallor. The condition is thought to be related to migraines, and there is often a family history of migraines. The events usually resolve by 5 years of age; however, the child often develops migraines later in life. Rare genetic variants in *CACNA1A* and *ATP1A2* have been reported.[21,22] EEG and MRI of the brain and spine are normal in this condition. Developmental outcome is normal. Treatment is not usually necessary.

Sandifer syndrome is defined as abnormal posturing as a result of gastroesophageal reflux disease; hiatal hernia may also be present.[23] The typical presentation is characterized by arching of back, neck, and trunk in an opisthotonic position, but other postures can present such as torticollis.[20] The posturing does not usually occur in extremities, but jerks of the extremities have been reported. The posture is believed to occur in an effort to reduce the pain caused by acid reflux into the esophagus. Apnea, staring, and head and eye deviation may occur, mimicking seizures.[24] Infants are usually irritable. EEG is normal during the event. Treating reflux is an effective treatment.

Infancy to Childhood

Breath-holding spells are common in children, reported to occur in 0.1% to 4.6% of children.[25] They initially present between 6 and 18 month of age and resolve at about 5 years of age. Neonatal onset is rare. There is a family history in 20% to 35% of cases, and several genetic syndromes are associated with severe spells.[11] The spells are classified as cyanotic or pallid based on discoloration of the child's face. Cyanotic breath-holding spells are precipitated by anger; the child is upset, often crying, and then forcefully exhales followed by breath-holding.[25] The infant becomes cyanotic, limp, or sometimes rigid, and loss of consciousness is brief. Prolonged apnea can precipitate a generalized seizure. The spells end with an inhalation and return of color. The entire episode lasts 10 to 60 seconds. Pallid breath-holding is triggered by pain or fear, characterized by a quick gasp and then the child becomes pale. If the duration of unconsciousness exceeds 45 seconds, there may also be seizure-like activity (eg, posturing, clonic motor movements). Following the event, the child returns to baseline. Breath-holding spells do not occur during sleep and always have a preceding trigger, and after the event, there is no confusion or drowsiness. These features help to distinguish the event from seizures. The mechanisms are thought to be multifactorial and include dysregulation of the autonomic nervous system, delayed myelination of brainstem, and iron deficiency.[25] If the patient is iron deficient, replacement is recommended. The spells do not impact development. Counseling parents on the benign nature of the condition is important.

Staring spells are common and can be mistaken for partial or absence seizures. Bye et al[26] reported that staring is the most common nonepileptic spell in those undergoing diagnostic EEG. They often occur in children with developmental delay, autism spectrum disorder, intellectual disabilities, attention-deficit disorder, sleep disorders, anxiety, and learning disabilities.[26] The majority of staring spells are noted to occur in children who are idle or watching TV. Staring spells can be attributed to slow cognitive processing, inattention, poor sleep, or mood disorders. Staring spells can be distinguished from seizures in that they are interruptible by external stimuli. Limb jerks, eye flickering, and urinary incontinence are not typically seen. Parents should clap or touch or tickle their children in addition to calling their name, as the parent's voice is often not enough to break the staring spell. If the spells are interruptible, they are not seizures and an EEG is not required. If it is unclear, an EEG can help aid in the diagnosis.

Tics and Stereotypies

Tics and stereotypies differ from seizures in that there is no alteration in consciousness, the episodes are interruptible (in the case of tics, for a brief period of time), and in the case of tics, the children continue on with their activities. For further information, please refer to Chapter 5.

REFERENCES

1. Hauser WA, Beghi E. First seizure definitions and worldwide incidence and mortality. *Epilepsia.* 2008;49(suppl 1):8-12.
2. Camfield P, Camfield C. Incidence, prevalence and aetiology of seizures and epilepsy in children. *Epileptic Disord.* 2015;17:117-123.
3. Scheffer IE, Berkovic S, Capovilla G, et al. ILAE classification of the epilepsies: position paper of the ILAE Commission for Classification and Terminology. *Epilepsia.* 2017;58(4):512-521.

4. Hirtz D, Berg A, Bettis D, et al. Practice parameter: treatment of the child with a first unprovoked seizure: report of the Quality Standards Subcommittee of the American Academy of Neurology and the Practice Committee of the Child Neurology Society. *Neurology*. 2003;60:166-175.

5. Krumholz A, Wiebe S, Gronseth GS, et al. Evidence-based guideline: management of an unprovoked first seizure in adults: report of the Guideline Development Subcommittee of the American Academy of Neurology and the American Epilepsy Society. *Neurology*. 2015;84(16):1705-1713.

6. Harden CL, Huff JS, Schwartz TH, et al. Reassessment: neuroimaging in the emergency patient presenting with seizure (an evidence-based review). *Neurology*. 2007;69:1772-1780.

7. Romantseva L, Lin N. Acute seizures-work-up and management in children. *Semin Neurol*. 2020;40:606-616.

8. Moosavi R, Swisher CB. Acute provoked seizures-work-up and management in adults. *Semin Neurol*. 2020;40:595-605.

9. Hauser WA, Rich SS, Lee JR, Annegers JF, Anderson VE. Risk of recurrent seizures after two unprovoked seizures. *N Engl J Med*. 1998;338:429-434.

10. Bruno E, Viana PF, Sperling MR, Richardson MP. Seizure detection at home: do devices on the market match the needs of people living with epilepsy and their caregivers? *Epilepsia*. 2020;61:S11-S24.

11. Sveinsson O, Andersson T, Mattsson P, Carlsson S, Tomson T. Clinical risk factors in SUDEP: a nationwide population-based case-control study. *Neurology*. 2020;94:e419-e429.

12. Verducci C, Hussain F, Donner E, et al. SUDEP in the North American SUDEP Registry: the full spectrum of epilepsies. *Neurology*. 2019;93:E227-E236.

13. Parker S, Zuckerman B, Bauchner H, et al. Jitteriness in full-term neonates: prevalence and correlates. *Pediatrics*. 1990;85:17-23.

14. Armentrout DC, Caple J. The jittery newborn. *J Pediatr Health Care*. 2001;15:147-149.

15. Fernández-Alvarez E. Transient benign paroxysmal movement disorders in infancy. *Eur J Paediatr Neurol*. 2018;22:230-237.

16. Collins M, Young M. Benign neonatal shudders, shivers, jitteriness, or tremors: early signs of vitamin D deficiency. *Pediatrics*. 2017;140:e20160719.

17. Praveen V, Patole S, Whitehall J. Hyperekplexia in neonates. *Postgrad Med J*. 2001;77:570-572.

18. Balint B, Thomas R. Hereditary hyperekplexia overview. In: *GeneReviews®* [Internet]. University of Washington, Seattle; 1993–2022. Accessed June 21, 2022. https://pubmed.ncbi.nlm.nih.gov/20301437/

19. Caraballo RH, Capovilla G, Vigevano F, et al. The spectrum of benign myoclonus of early infancy: Clinical and neurophysiologic features in 102 patients. *Epilepsia*. 2009;50:1176-1183.

20. Ghossein J, Pohl D. Benign spasms of infancy: a mimicker of infantile epileptic disorders. *Epileptic Disord*. 2019;21:585-589.

21. Danielsson A, Anderlid BM, Stödberg T, et al. Benign paroxysmal torticollis of infancy does not lead to neurological sequelae. *Dev Med Child Neurol*. 2018;60:1251-1255.

22. Blumkin L. Paroxysmal torticollis of infancy: a benign phenomenon? *Dev Med Child Neurol*. 2018;60:1196-1197.

23. Moore DM, Rizzolo D. Sandifer syndrome. *JAAPA*. 2018;31:18-22.

24. Sheikh S, Stephen TC, Sisson B. Prevalence of gastroesophageal reflux in infants with recurrent brief apneic episodes. *Can Respir J*. 1999;6:401-404.

25. Leung AKC, Leung AAM, Wong AHC, Hon KL. Breath-holding spells in pediatrics: a narrative review of the current evidence. *Curr Pediatr Rev*. 2019;15:22-29.

26. Bye AME, Kok DJM, Ferenschild FTJ, Vles JSH. Paroxysmal non-epileptic events in children: a retrospective study over a period of 10 years. *J Paediatr Child Health*. 2000;36:244-248.

Febrile Seizures

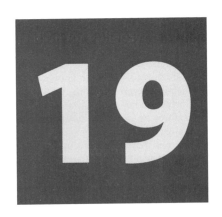

19

Gewalin Aungaroon, MD
Marie Clements, MD

ESSENTIALS OF DIAGNOSIS

▶ A febrile seizure is defined as a seizure occurring in the setting of fever (temperature ≥100.4°F or 38°C by any method), without other cause (eg, central nervous system infection, epilepsy), in children 6 through 60 months of age.[1]

▶ Febrile seizures are categorized as simple or complex. Complex febrile seizures are characterized by 1 or more of the following features: (1) semiology focality, (2) duration of more than 15 minutes, or (3) more than 1 seizure in 24 hours.

▶ The prognosis is excellent in children with simple febrile seizures, and additional neurologic investigations are typically not indicated. However, children with complex febrile seizures or febrile status epilepticus often require further evaluation.

GENERAL CONSIDERATIONS

Febrile seizures are common, occurring in 2% to 5% of children.[1,2] The peak incidence is around 2 years of age, with the vast majority of first-time febrile seizures occurring before 3 years of age.[2] Febrile seizures represent a typically benign, self-limited condition with an excellent prognosis. This chapter will discuss the diagnosis, complications, and management of febrile seizures, with careful attention paid to identifying instances in which further workup is necessary to differentiate febrile seizures from alternate diagnoses. Seizures in the setting of fever occurring in children less than 6 months of age are generally managed differently and will not be discussed here.

PREVENTION

Many have questioned whether prophylactic antipyretic medication can be used in the setting of febrile illness to prevent seizure recurrence in children with a history of febrile seizures. A meta-analysis of randomized controlled trials showed no benefit to antipyretics in seizure prevention during future febrile episodes when compared to placebo.[3]

DIFFERENTIAL DIAGNOSIS

1. **Intracranial infection:** In children who have a decreased level of consciousness or who are not returning to their baseline mental status after a seizure and in those who have meningeal signs on an exam, intracranial infection as the source of fever and cause of subsequent seizure (eg, meningitis, encephalitis, or intracranial abscess) should be considered.

2. **Shaking chills/rigors:** Tremulous movements occur commonly with fevers and can be mistaken for a seizure.

3. **Epilepsy:** Fever can lead to a decreased seizure threshold in children with epilepsy. Therefore, a seizure in the setting of a fever may be the first presentation of a child's underlying epilepsy. Genetic epilepsy with febrile seizures plus (GEFS+) is typically inherited with autosomal dominance and variable penetrance, and therefore, a history of family members with variable presentations of seizures is commonly present. GEFS+ is caused by various genetic mutations, predominantly *SCN1A* mutation but also mutations in several other genes such as *SCN2A*, *SCN1B*, *GABRG2*, and *GABRD*.[4] GEFS+ shows marked phenotypic heterogeneity within families. The most common manifestation is febrile seizures, which sometimes recur well beyond 5 to 6 years of age (febrile seizure plus).

About one-third of patients develop afebrile generalized tonic-clonic seizures in childhood with remission in adolescence. The remaining one-third may have a variety of generalized or focal epilepsies. Severe myoclonic epilepsy of infancy (SMEI), also known as Dravet syndrome, is at the most severe end of the GEFS+ spectrum. SMEI begins during infancy, typically at 5 to 6 months, with prolonged seizures or febrile status epilepticus, which may be generalized or unilateral clonic seizures. Non–fever-related seizures may be the first manifestation in some children with this diagnosis. Early development and electroencephalogram (EEG) studies are normal, and the diagnosis of febrile seizure is typically given at this stage. Around 1 to 4 years of age, other seizure types emerge, such as myoclonic, atonic, atypical absence, and focal seizures, which tend to be treatment resistant. Temperature-sensitive seizures are common; seizures can be triggered by a warm bath, a fever from an acute illness, or immunization. By 2 years of age, EEG background and interictal abnormalities develop, coinciding with developmental plateau and subsequent regression. Ataxia and pyramidal signs develop later in the childhood stage. Seizures are typically difficult to control and cognitive outcomes are generally poor.[5,6]

COMPLICATIONS

Complications from febrile seizures are rare. In a small subset of patients, the febrile seizure is prolonged and does not self-resolve. Febrile status epilepticus (FSE) is defined as a single febrile seizure (or cluster of febrile seizures without a return to baseline mental status in between) lasting longer than 30 minutes. FSE is unlikely to stop spontaneously and typically requires one or more abortive medications.[7] Complications including respiratory and hemodynamic compromise commonly occur, at times necessitating intubation, ventilation, and/or other medical interventions. Data have shown evidence of hippocampal injury in some children following FSE, particularly if the seizure was focal.[8,9] This injury may lead to hippocampal sclerosis and subsequent temporal lobe epilepsy. The incidence of this potential complication is not well established.

TREATMENT

Most febrile seizures are brief, self-resolving, and do not require treatment with antiseizure medication. Supportive care for seizures, fevers, and concurrent illnesses is recommended. A rescue benzodiazepine medication for prolonged or cluster of seizures is commonly considered. Rectal diazepam is approved by the US Food and Drug Administration for children 2 years of age or older, intranasal diazepam for those greater than 6 years, and intranasal midazolam for those greater than 12 years. If the seizure continues, a second dose of benzodiazepine may be used.[10] For seizures that do not abort after adequate benzodiazepine administration, this may be followed by a loading dose of antiseizure medication (typically levetiracetam, valproic acid, or fosphenytoin).[10,11] In cases where the seizure remains resistant to treatment, escalation to midazolam, pentobarbital, propofol, ketamine, or thiopental can be considered.[10]

Generally, febrile seizures are not treated with preventive antiseizure medication. Given the excellent prognosis and self-limited nature of this condition, the potential risks and side effects of antiseizure medications usually do not outweigh the benefits.[12] In lieu of daily antiseizure medication, studies have also investigated treating children with intermittent medication, given only when fevers are detected. While oral diazepam administration during fever can substantially reduce seizure recurrence. Its use is frequently accompanied by adverse effects, including ataxia, agitation, and lethargy.[13] Additionally, there is concern that administering this medication could mask signs of central nervous system infection. Therefore, while this treatment may be used in select cases, it is not considered the standard of care for children with febrile seizures.[12]

PROGNOSIS

About one-third of children with a first febrile seizure will have an additional febrile seizure. Risk factors for recurrent febrile seizures include younger age at first seizure onset, family history of febrile seizure, and lower temperature of fever at the time of seizure.[2]

The majority of children will outgrow their febrile seizures. Those with simple febrile seizures have a slightly increased risk of developing epilepsy compared to the general population.[14] However, complex febrile seizures increased the risk of epilepsy by 5% to 10%, with a higher chance in those with focal or prolonged febrile seizures.[14-16] Other risk factors for the development of epilepsy include younger (6 months to 1 year) or older (3-5 years) age at febrile seizure onset, family history of epilepsy, developmental delay, cerebral palsy, and low Apgar scores.[17]

Children with a history of febrile seizures have similar long-term cognitive outcomes to their healthy counterparts in terms of development, behavior, attention, school performance, and intelligence.[18,19] This is unaffected by the recurrence rate of febrile seizures.[18]

WHEN TO REFER

Simple febrile seizures can often be managed by the patient's primary care provider. Children with complex febrile seizures, especially those with a history of FSE, developmental delay, or abnormal neurologic examination, should be referred to a pediatric neurologist.

WHEN TO WORK UP AND WHEN TO ADMIT

Children presenting to an emergency department with a simple febrile seizure who have returned to their neurologic baseline and a reassuring physical exam, typically do not require diagnostic testing or admission.[1] If indicated, laboratory testing may be used to identify the source of fever.[1] The patient's family should be educated on febrile seizures and their potential for recurrence. A rescue benzodiazepine medication may be considered.

If a child is seen in the emergency department soon after their seizure, there may be a postictal period during which the child is sleepy or has a decreased level of consciousness. In these cases, a period of observation is recommended to ensure proper recovery of their mental status. Further workup and/or admission may be indicated in children who remain altered or those with prolonged, multiple, or focal febrile seizures.

Lumbar puncture is not universally recommended for children presenting with a febrile seizure. Studies have shown that fever and seizures are rarely the sole indications of intracranial infection in children.[1] In a large multicenter study, for children who had no physical exam findings suggestive of meningitis or encephalitis, no bacterial meningitis or herpes simplex virus meningoencephalitis was found.[20] Lumbar puncture should be performed in unimmunized or underimmunized children (specifically those lacking in *Haemophilus influenzae* type B or *Streptococcus pneumoniae* immunization), especially those under 1 year of age, in children who appear ill, and in those with meningeal signs (eg, neck stiffness, Kernig or Brudzinski signs).[1] This should also be considered in children currently or recently on antibiotics, as antibiotic pretreatment can mask physical exam findings of intracranial infection.[1]

A nonurgent EEG and magnetic resonance imaging (MRI) may be considered in children with a focal component to their febrile seizures to assess for focal abnormalities. More urgent neuroimaging is indicated in children with a focal neurologic deficit following a seizure.

REFERENCES

1. Subcommittee on Febrile Seizures; American Academy of Pediatrics. Neurodiagnostic evaluation of the child with a simple febrile seizure. *Pediatrics*. 2011;127(2):389-394. doi:10.1542/peds.2010-3318
2. Verity CM, Butler NR, Golding J. Febrile convulsions in a national cohort followed up from birth. I—Prevalence and recurrence in the first five years of life. *Br Med J (Clin Res Ed)*. 1985;290(6478):1307-1310.
3. Rosenbloom E, Finkelstein Y, Adams-Webber T, Kozer E. Do antipyretics prevent the recurrence of febrile seizures in children? A systematic review of randomized controlled trials and meta-analysis. *Eur J Paediatr Neurol*. 2013;17(6):585-588.
4. Zhang YH, Burgess R, Malone JP, et al. Genetic epilepsy with febrile seizures plus: refining the spectrum. *Neurology*. 2017;89(12):1210-1219.
5. Dravet C. The core Dravet syndrome phenotype. *Epilepsia*. 2011;52(suppl 2):3-9.
6. Genton P, Velizarova R, Dravet C. Dravet syndrome: the long-term outcome. *Epilepsia*. 2011;52(suppl 2):44-49.
7. Seinfeld S, Shinnar S, Sun S, et al. Emergency management of febrile status epilepticus: results of the FEBSTAT study. *Epilepsia*. 2014;55(3):388-395.
8. Shinnar S, Bello JA, Chan S, et al. MRI abnormalities following febrile status epilepticus in children: the FEBSTAT study. *Neurology*. 2012;79(9):871-877.
9. VanLandingham KE, Heinz ER, Cavazos JE, Lewis DV. Magnetic resonance imaging evidence of hippocampal injury after prolonged focal febrile convulsions. *Ann Neurol*. 1998;43(4):413-426.
10. Glauser T, Shinnar S, Gloss D, et al. Evidence-based guideline: treatment of convulsive status epilepticus in children and adults: report of the Guideline Committee of the American Epilepsy Society. *Epilepsy Curr*. 2016;16(1):48-61.
11. Kapur J, Elm J, Chamberlain JM, et al. Randomized trial of three anticonvulsant medications for status epilepticus. *N Engl J Med*. 2019;381(22):2103-2113.
12. Steering Committee on Quality Improvement and Management, Subcommittee on Febrile Seizures. Febrile seizures: clinical practice guideline for the long-term management of the child with simple febrile seizures. *Pediatrics*. 2008;121(6):1281-1286. doi:10.1542/peds.2008-0939
13. Rosman NP, Colton T, Labazzo J, et al. A controlled trial of diazepam administered during febrile illnesses to prevent recurrence of febrile seizures. *N Engl J Med*. 1993;329(2):79-84.
14. Nelson KB, Ellenberg JH. Predictors of epilepsy in children who have experienced febrile seizures. *N Engl J Med*. 1976;295(19):1029-1033.
15. Verity CM, Golding J. Risk of epilepsy after febrile convulsions: a national cohort study [published correction appears in BMJ 1992 Jan 18;304(6820):147]. *BMJ*. 1991;303(6814):1373-1376.
16. Annegers JF, Hauser WA, Elveback LR, Kurland LT. The risk of epilepsy following febrile convulsions. *Neurology*. 1979;29(3):297-303.
17. Vestergaard M, Pedersen CB, Sidenius P, Olsen J, Christensen J. The long-term risk of epilepsy after febrile seizures in susceptible subgroups. *Am J Epidemiol*. 2007;165(8):911-918.
18. Verity CM, Greenwood R, Golding J. Long-term intellectual and behavioral outcomes of children with febrile convulsions. *N Engl J Med*. 1998;338(24):1723-1728.
19. Nørgaard M, Ehrenstein V, Mahon BE, Nielsen GL, Rothman KJ, Sørensen HT. Febrile seizures and cognitive function in young adult life: a prevalence study in Danish conscripts. *J Pediatr*. 2009;155(3):404-409.
20. Guedj R, Chappuy H, Titomanlio L, et al. Do all children who present with a complex febrile seizure need a lumbar puncture? *Ann Emerg Med*. 2017;70(1):52-62.e6.

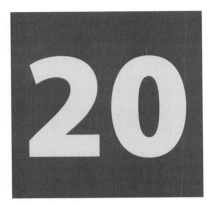

Epilepsy in Infants

S. Katie Ihnen, MD, PhD
Susan L. Fong, MD, PhD

ESSENTIALS OF DIAGNOSIS

▶ Epilepsy in an infant should be considered when seizures are not provoked by an acute, potentially reversible cause.

▶ Epilepsies that present in infancy range from those that are self-limited to others that are marked by significant encephalopathy.

▶ Some epilepsies have specific treatments, and early identification can have management implications.

▶ Initial diagnostic tools include history, exam, laboratory findings, lumbar puncture, neuroimaging, electroencephalography, and genetic testing. Empiric treatment can be diagnostically useful.

▶ Infantile epilepsies include those with presentation as a neonate (<28 days of age) or an infant (28 days to 12 months).

GENERAL CONSIDERATIONS

Seizures affect 1.5 to 3.5 per 1000 full-term newborns and 10 to 130 per 1000 preterm newborns,[1] with the great majority of these seizures being provoked. Clinically subtle seizures are prevalent in neonates, making recognition and treatment challenging.[2] Prognosis for patients with neonatal and infantile epilepsy varies widely. Early seizure identification is crucial, because prompt and sometimes specific treatment can impact long-term prognosis.[3] This chapter will cover epilepsy syndromes with onset in the neonatal period (first 28 days) and during infancy (first 12 months). We will discuss the more common epilepsy syndromes, as well as some rare syndromes that are important due to specific management implications.

PATHOGENESIS

Recent technologic advancements in molecular genetics have led to the identification of numerous pathogenic genetic mutations that are implicated in epilepsy. Although there is significant genotype-phenotype heterogeneity, clinical testing has become increasingly accessible and should be considered early to maximize identification of potentially treatable disorders.

▶ Clinical Findings

A detailed history of the clinical event is helpful, as is any family history including febrile seizures, developmental delay, intellectual disability, and other neurologic diagnoses.

▶ Symptoms and Signs

Onset of seizures in neonates is typically focal; generalized tonic-clonic (GTC) semiology is rare. Motor automatisms may be seen, including oro-buccal-lingual movements and abnormal eye movements. Autonomic changes can be part of seizure semiology, although they are rarely the sole clinical manifestation. As the infant develops and the brain myelinates, seizure semiologies broaden to include generalized types as seen in older patients.

A complete neurologic exam, including mental status and tone, is indispensable. Encephalopathy is an important part of the symptomatology of some epilepsies, and signs include poor feeding, irritability, and abnormal social development. A careful dermatologic exam may raise suspicion for a neurocutaneous disorder.

▶ Laboratory Findings

Lumbar puncture is obligatory in infants under 2 months of age presenting with seizure, as well as older children with seizure and altered mental status. Cerebrospinal fluid (CSF) studies should include cell count, protein, glucose (with concurrent serum glucose), bacterial culture with Gram stain, and basic viral studies. Additional CSF studies may be indicated, including amino acid or neurotransmitter analysis. A complete metabolic panel is recommended, along with a complete blood count if infection is considered. Serum ammonia should be obtained if the patient is encephalopathic. Additional metabolic studies such as lactate, plasma amino acids, urine organic acids, and carnitine/acylcarnitine profile are warranted when a metabolic etiology is on the differential. Consider a toxicology screen if there is possible ingestion. Follow-up of newborn screens should not be overlooked.

▶ Imaging Studies

Head computed tomography is not typically recommended, except in acute cases of suspected trauma or rapidly progressive mass lesion. Head ultrasound may be an appropriate first-line exam for any infant with a patent anterior fontanelle. Brain magnetic resonance imaging (MRI) without contrast is the neuroimaging study of choice for seizures. Due to developmental changes in myelination, repeat imaging after a period of some months may be warranted for infants. Magnetic resonance spectroscopy can be helpful in the evaluation of metabolic etiologies.

▶ Special Tests

Continuous video electroencephalography (EEG) is recommended to confirm or rule out seizures and localize and characterize seizure types, and may aid in diagnosis and management. Specific interictal EEG patterns can be extremely important diagnostically (eg, hypsarrhythmia in association with infantile spasms or burst suppression in neonatal epileptic encephalopathies). Focal slowing may suggest an underlying lesion, whereas generalized slowing may suggest a genetic epilepsy. In neonates with hypoxic-ischemic encephalopathy (HIE), the degree of background abnormality can inform prognosis. Comparison of serial examinations can be used to assess treatment efficacy and be prognostically informative. In all cases, a full neonatal montage is most sensitive, although amplitude-integrated EEG can be useful for screening when continuous EEG monitoring is not available.

Concern for a genetic disorder should prompt evaluation for dysmorphology, organomegaly, and other systemic involvement (eg, cardiac, ophthalmologic, renal). Although genetic epilepsy panels are increasingly becoming standard of care,[4] karyotype and chromosomal microarray may be appropriate first-line tests in patients with syndromic dysmorphology or developmental delay.

DIFFERENTIAL DIAGNOSIS

Several nonepileptic paroxysmal spells can be mistaken for seizures, including normal baby movements, sleep myoclonus, and movement disorders.[5] After ruling out nonepileptic spells, the great majority of seizures in this age group are provoked and result from acute, sometimes treatable insults. Febrile seizures are an important consideration but should *not* be diagnosed in patients younger than 6 months of age. Other important etiologies include HIE, stroke, infection, transient metabolic derangements, ingestion, drug withdrawal, and trauma.

Pediatric epilepsy syndromes are organized primarily by the age of seizure onset, with neonatal syndromes presenting in the first 28 days of life and infantile syndromes presenting in the first year of life. Epilepsy in neonates and infants varies from self-limited ("benign") to highly encephalopathic ("malignant"). Although advances in genomic technologies continue to challenge existing diagnostic classifications, traditional syndromic classifications continue to be clinically helpful.[6]

▶ Epilepsy in the Neonatal Period (<28 Days of Life)

Self-Limited Epilepsy Syndromes

In benign familial neonatal epilepsy (BFNE), otherwise healthy infants present in the first 2 to 3 days of life with asymmetric tonic posturing evolving to focal clonic seizures with shifting laterality. Seizures frequently cluster and are often accompanied by apnea. Remission is typically seen within 6 months. Interictal EEG is normal, and seizures respond well to antiseizure medications (ASMs), particularly sodium channel antagonists such as carbamazepine, oxcarbazepine, and phenytoin. Prognosis is good, and development tends to be normal. Positive family history of neonatal seizures is helpful in making the diagnosis as BFNE is often caused by an autosomal dominant mutation in *KCNQ2*.[7]

Epileptic Encephalopathies

Some epilepsy syndromes are hypothesized to reflect widespread cerebral dysfunction, which often leads to intractable seizures and cognitive impairment. This group of syndromes, called epileptic encephalopathies, is heterogeneous in clinical features and etiology.[8] Two primary epileptic encephalopathies have onset in the neonatal period (Table 20–1). Those who survive often progress to infantile epileptic encephalopathies such as West syndrome or Lennox-Gastaut syndrome.[9]

Early infantile epileptic encephalopathy (EIEE; ohtahara syndrome)—In EIEE, seizures start by 3 months but often begin within the first 2 weeks of life. Tonic spasms, the predominant seizure type, are likely to be seen in frequent

Table 20–1. Neonatal epileptic encephalopathies.

	EIEE	EME
Onset	First 3 months, 30% in first 10 days	First few days
Predominant seizure type	Tonic spasms	Myoclonic
EEG	Burst suppression pattern that persists while awake and asleep	Burst suppression pattern, initially accentuated during sleep
Etiology	Structural and genetic > metabolic	Metabolic > structural and genetic
Example etiologies	Hemimegalencephaly, cortical dysplasia, *ARX*, *STXBP1*, *SLC25A22*, *SCN2A*, *CDKL5*, *KCNQ2*	Amino acidopathies (eg, NKH), organic acidemias, urea cycle defects, mitochondrial disorders, defects of the peroxisomes, Menkes disease, pyridoxine dependency

EEG, electroencephalography; EIEE, early infantile epileptic encephalopathy; EME, early myoclonic encephalopathy; NKH, nonketotic hyperglycinemia.

clusters, but focal and myoclonic seizures are also seen. Seizures often prove refractory to treatment. EEG shows an invariant burst suppression pattern through waking and sleeping states (Figure 20–1). Structural brain abnormalities such as hemimegalencephaly and cortical dysplasia may be present, and mutations in a growing list of genes[10] have been implicated (see Table 20–1).

Early myoclonic encephalopathy (EME)—Myoclonic seizures are the predominant type in EME, with onset within the first month of life. Focal clonic and tonic seizures are also seen. EEG shows a burst suppression pattern that is accentuated in sleep early in disease but becomes persistent as disease progresses. EME is often associated with metabolic disorders such as nonketotic hyperglycinemia (NKH), which is caused

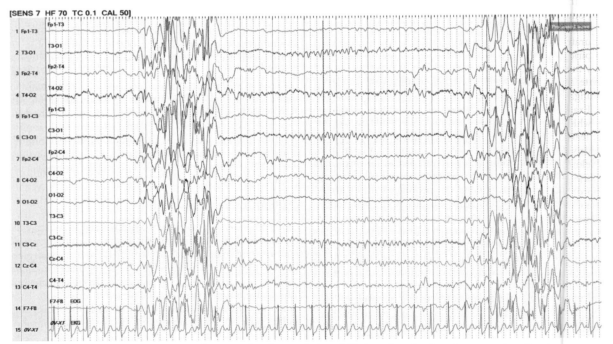

[SENS 7 HF 70 TC 0.1 CAL 50]

▲ **Figure 20–1.** Electroencephalography recording from a 7-day-old infant showing burst suppression. Burst suppression is an interictal finding that is seen in neonatal epileptic encephalopathies, including both early infantile epileptic encephalopathy (EIEE) and early myoclonic encephalopathy (EME). The bursts are high voltage and irregular and separated by periods of very-low-amplitude suppression.

by autosomal recessive or de novo mutation of *GLDC*. In NKH, seizure onset is usually in the first day of life, often with prominent apnea and altered mental status.[11] Mothers sometimes will have noticed hiccups in utero. Diagnosis is made based on elevated CSF glycine. Treatment (sodium benzoate and dextromethorphan) provides only partial relief of the encephalopathy, and mortality is high.

Metabolic, Genetic, and Developmental Disorders

There are many metabolic, genetic, and developmental disorders in which epilepsy may be one important clinical feature. Clues to some of these disorders include the presence of other signs and symptoms in addition to seizures. Metabolic disorders include urea cycle defects, organic acidurias, and amino acid disorders. Urea cycle defects are typically accompanied by hyperammonemia and encephalopathy; the most common of these is X-linked ornithine transcarbamylase deficiency. Organic acidurias present with hyperammonemia, metabolic acidosis, and encephalopathy. Propionic acidemia is one example, in which MRI shows white matter and basal ganglia changes. Maple syrup urine disease is a classic example of an amino acid disorder and presents with seizures in the first week of life. Cerumen is the best place to smell the maple syrup odor.

Some metabolic epilepsies are exceedingly rare but have specific targeted treatments (Table 20–2), making early and accurate diagnosis crucial. Because of clinical overlap, initial empiric treatment for medically refractory neonatal seizures may include a combination of pyridoxine, pyridoxal phosphate, folinic acid, and biotin while awaiting confirmatory testing.[3]

Examples of other genetic and developmental disorders in which neonatal epilepsy may be one important clinical feature include chromosomal anomalies (eg, DiGeorge syndrome, trisomy 13 or 18), malformations of cortical development (eg, polymicrogyria, lissencephaly, hemimegalencephaly, focal cortical dysplasia), neurodegenerative disorders (eg, neuronal ceroid lipofuscinosis), and neurocutaneous disorders (eg, incontinentia pigmenti and tuberous sclerosis complex [TSC]). Collaborating with medical genetics is strongly recommended.

▶ Epilepsy in Later Infancy (28 Days to 12 Months of Life)

Self-Limited Epilepsy Syndromes

Benign familial infantile epilepsy (BFIE)—BFIE is characterized by developmentally normal infants with onset of seizures between 3 and 7 months of age. Seizures classically involve behavioral arrest, staring, automatisms, head and eye deviation, and decreased responsiveness. Autonomic features including apnea and cyanosis may be present.

Seizures can occur in clusters and may evolve into generalized convulsions. Interictal EEG is usually normal. Autosomal dominant mutations in *PRRT2* have been identified in a majority of affected families.[9] Seizures respond well to ASMs commonly used for focal-onset seizures and remit by 3 years. Prognosis for development is favorable, although certain patients later develop paroxysmal movement disorders.

Benign myoclonic epilepsy of infancy—Otherwise healthy infants with benign myoclonic epilepsy in infancy present with onset of seizures between 4 months and 3 years. Myoclonic seizures are often triggered by sensory stimulation and can initially be very subtle. Over time, seizures increase in frequency and severity and may involve altered mental status and falls. EEG typically shows generalized discharges and may demonstrate a photoparoxysmal response (Figure 20–2). A family history of generalized epilepsies or febrile seizures may be present. Prognosis is generally favorable, with some observations of cognitive and behavioral impairments.

Epileptic Encephalopathies

Epilepsy of infancy with migrating focal seizures (EIMFS)—Seizure onset in EIMFS is typically between 2 and 6 months. Seizures may be sporadic at onset but eventually progress to prolonged, multifocal, migrating (within and between hemispheres) focal seizures on EEG. Spasms and tonic and myoclonic seizures may be seen, and status epilepticus is common. Autonomic features such as apnea or bradycardia are present in nearly half of patients. Frequent clinical associations include hypotonia, microcephaly, gastrointestinal dysmotility, and swallowing difficulty. Seizures are quite refractory to traditional therapies including ASMs, corticosteroids, ketogenic diet, and vagal nerve stimulators.[8] *KCNT1* is the most commonly implicated gene, with some case reports of seizure response to quinidine, which reverses the increased conductance of *KCNT1* in vitro.[11] Prognosis is poor, with a high incidence of early death and significant intellectual impairment in survivors.

West syndrome—Infantile spasms typically have onset between 3 and 12 months and are characterized by brief flexor or extensor movements that cluster predominantly during sleep-wake transitions. The triad of infantile spasms, developmental plateau/regression, and hypsarrhythmia on EEG (Figure 20–3) comprise West syndrome. Numerous etiologies have been implicated including congenital and acquired structural abnormalities and mutations in an increasing number of genes. A specific etiology can be determined in approximately 70% to 80% of cases; cortical malformations, HIE, TSC, and trisomy 21 are frequent culprits. Standard therapy is a course of high-dose steroid, either adrenocorticotropic hormone or prednisolone, except in patients with TSC, for whom vigabatrin is used as first-line treatment.

Table 20–2. Metabolic epilepsies with specific targeted treatments.

Disorder	Gene	Treatment	Additional Clues
Pyridoxine-dependent epilepsy	ALDH7A1	Pyridoxine + Lysine-restricted diet + L-Arginine supplements	Encephalopathy Developmental delay High serum pipecolic acid High urine α-aminoadipic semialdehyde
Pyridoxamine 5-phosphate oxidase deficiency	PNPO	Pyridoxal phosphate	Encephalopathy Developmental delay Lactic acidosis High plasma glycine and threonine
Biotinidase deficiency	BTD	Biotin	Developmental delay Skin rash Vision and hearing loss Lactic acidosis, hyperammonemia High CSF lactate and pyruvate
Folinic acid–responsive epilepsy	ALDH7A1	Folinic acid Leucovorin Lysine-free diet	Encephalopathy Apnea Developmental delay
Pyruvate dehydrogenase deficiency	PDHA	Ketogenic diet	Developmental delay Hypotonia Lactic acidosis
Creatine deficiency	GAMT GATM SLC6A8	Creatine monohydrate	Intellectual disability Developmental delay Microcephaly
Molybdenum cofactor deficiency	MOCS1 MOCS2 GPHN	Cyclic pyranopterin	Encephalopathy Cerebral edema Developmental delay
Serine deficiency	PHGDH	L-Serine Glycine	Microcephaly Developmental delay Spastic quadriparesis
Glucose transporter 1 deficiency syndrome	SLC2A1	Ketogenic diet	Progressive microcephaly Ataxia Abnormal eye movements Developmental delay Early-onset absence seizures (<3 years old) Low CSF glucose

CSF, cerebrospinal fluid.

Development is severely affected, and infants often develop intractable epilepsy, including Lennox-Gastaut syndrome. Prompt diagnosis and treatment improve developmental outcomes. Up to a third of patients may die by 3 years.

Dravet Syndrome (Severe Myoclonic Epilepsy in Infancy)—Patients with Dravet syndrome (DS) classically present around 5 to 6 months with a prolonged, hemiclonic or GTC seizure in the setting of fever or following a vaccination. Additional seizures in the setting of fever or environmental hyperthermia accumulate over the first year of life, progressing to later seizures with and without concurrent fever. Myoclonic seizures are prominent, but atypical absence, GTC, focal, and atonic seizures are all seen. Interictal EEG may be normal initially but is typically abnormal by age 2 to 3 years. Developmental stagnation, hypotonia, and

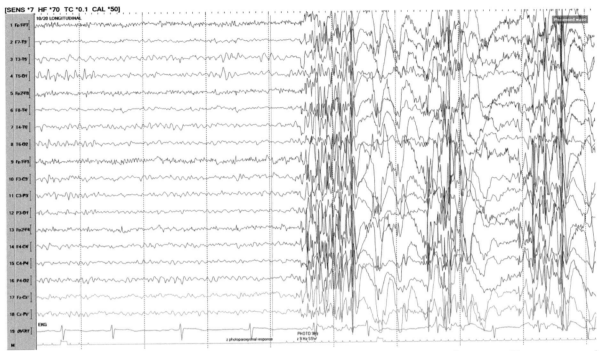

▲ **Figure 20–2.** Electroencephalography (EEG) recording demonstrating photoparoxysmal response. Photoparoxysmal response is an EEG trait characterized by the occurrence of epileptiform discharges in response to intermittent photic stimulation.

ataxia are seen by early preschool years, and a characteristic crouched gait is often seen by adolescence. Mutations in *SCN1A* are found in approximately 80% of patients, although not all *SCN1A* mutations cause DS. Other genes that can cause the DS phenotype include *SCN1B*, *GABRA1*, *GABRG2*, *HCN1*, *STXBP1*, and *PCDH19*. Medical intractability is typical in DS, and polytherapy is commonly employed, often including combinations of valproate, clobazam, stiripentol, ketogenic diet, cannabidiol, and fenfluramine. Sodium channel antagonists such as phenytoin and lamotrigine should be avoided, as they can exacerbate seizures in DS. The rate of sudden unexpected death in epilepsy is particularly high with long-term high mortality.

Hemiconvulsion-hemiplegia-epilepsy syndrome—The typical initial presentation of this rare epilepsy includes a prolonged, unilateral convulsive seizure in the setting of fever between infancy and 4 years of age. Status epilepticus may last days prior to resolution, with subsequent hemiparesis and progressive cerebral hemiatrophy. EEG shows bilateral ictal and interictal abnormalities, although with greater prominence in the affected hemisphere. MRI findings in the acute setting include edema of the affected hemisphere in a nonvascular distribution and increased ipsilateral subcortical

diffusion restriction. Prognosis is quite variable, from resolution of hemiplegia and good development to medically intractable epilepsy and permanent hemiparesis following a variable seizure-free period.

Metabolic, Genetic, and Developmental Disorders

Many of the categories of inborn errors of metabolism mentioned in the neonatal section can alternatively present later in infancy with seizures. Some additional clinically important entities that are especially likely to present between 28 days and 12 months are briefly discussed here. Glutaric aciduria type 1 is an organic aciduria in which infants present at a few months of age in metabolic crisis with opisthotonus and seizures. Macrocephaly is common. MRI shows widened Sylvian fissures and may show subarachnoid blood that may trigger evaluation for nonaccidental trauma. Glucose transporter type 1 (GLUT-1) deficiency presents with microcephaly, movement abnormalities, absence of seizures, and abnormal eye movements. Lumbar puncture reveals very low CSF glucose; ketogenic diet is the preferred treatment. Biotinidase deficiency presents with seizures, lethargy, hypotonia, and rash and is treated with oral biotin.

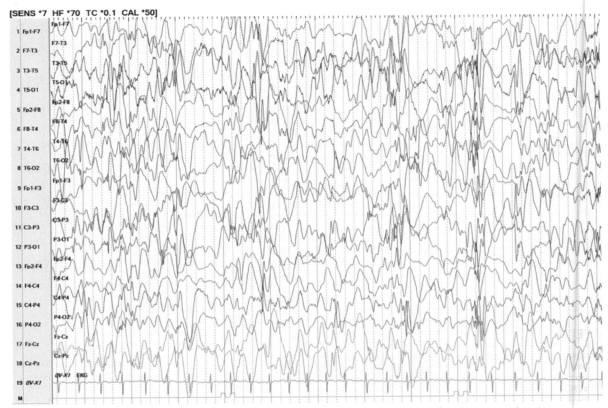

▲ **Figure 20–3.** Electroencephalography recording from an 8-month-old child with infantile spasms showing hypsarrhythmia. Hypsarrhythmia is an interictal finding characterized by a very-high-voltage, disorganized background with multifocal epileptiform discharges.

Phenylketonuria is one of the more common metabolic disorders that is often identified on newborn screen. Disorders such as Angelman, Rett, Prader-Willi, and Wolf-Hirschhorn (4p–) syndromes, creatine deficiency, and defects of serine biogenesis are some examples of other genetic and developmental disorders that are more likely to present after 28 days of age.

COMPLICATIONS

Early-life seizures and ASMs can have detrimental long-term effects on infants with epilepsy. Common comorbidities include developmental plateau/regression, intellectual disability, learning disorders, attention-deficit/hyperactivity disorder, mood disorders, sleep disturbances, impaired bone health, and seizure-related bodily injuries.[5] Sudden unexplained death in epilepsy is a rare complication seen most commonly in patients with uncontrolled nocturnal convulsive seizures. Epilepsy at any age carries a mortality risk, especially in cases of status epilepticus.

TREATMENT

In contrast to the many ASMs that have been approved for adult use, there are significantly fewer options approved for children younger than 2 years of age. Consequently, off-label use of ASMs in infants is common.[2] In the acute setting, commonly used ASMs in neonates and infants include phenobarbital, fosphenytoin, and levetiracetam. For maintenance therapy, levetiracetam, topiramate, zonisamide, and oxcarbazepine are common choices.[12] Valproic acid is typically avoided due to increased risk of fulminant hepatic failure in children under 2 years of age. Some neonatal epilepsies require specific targeted treatments, including ketogenic diet for diagnoses such as GLUT-1 DS and pyruvate dehydrogenase deficiency.[13]

PROGNOSIS

Prognosis is variable and depends on the specific diagnosis and underlying etiology. Approximately one-third of patients with epilepsy will become medically intractable. Infants who show poor response to ASMs, have abnormal brain imaging, show bilateral epileptiform activity on EEG, and/or experience status epilepticus are especially high risk for persistent epilepsy. Cumulative seizure burden is associated with worse developmental outcomes.[2]

WHEN TO REFER

Neonates with concern for seizures should always be admitted for thorough evaluation and treatment. With older infants, clinical judgment and parental concern usually jointly determine whether workup for a concerning event can safely be done as an outpatient. Neonates and infants diagnosed with epilepsy should be followed by pediatric neurologists. Referral to a pediatric epilepsy center with dietary and surgery specialists should be considered as soon as an epilepsy is deemed medically intractable (inadequately responsive to trials of 2 appropriately selected and dosed medications), even in an infant.

REFERENCES

1. Spagnoli C, Falsaperla R, Deolmi M, Corsello G, Pisani F. Symptomatic seizures in preterm newborns: a review on clinical features and prognosis. *Ital J Pediatr.* 2018;44(1):115. doi:10.1186/s13052-018-0573-y

2. Pressler RM, Lagae L. Why we urgently need improved seizure and epilepsy therapies for children and neonates. *Neuropharmacology.* 2020;170:107854. doi:10.1016/j.neuropharm.2019.107854

3. Phitsanuwong C. Genetic and metabolic neonatal epilepsies. *Pediatr Ann.* 2021;50(6):e245-e253. doi:10.3928/19382359-20210518-01

4. Lee EH. Epilepsy syndromes during the first year of life and the usefulness of an epilepsy gene panel. *Korean J Pediatr.* 2018;61(4):101-107. doi:10.3345/kjp.2018.61.4.101

5. Fine A, Wirrell EC. Seizures in children. *Pediatr Rev.* 2020;41(7):321-347. doi:10.1542/pir.2019-0134

6. Scheffer IE, Berkovic S, Capovilla G, et al. ILAE classification of the epilepsies: position paper of the ILAE Commission for Classification and Terminology. *Epilepsia.* 2017;58(4):512-521. doi:10.1111/epi.13709

7. Pisani F, Percesepe A, Spagnoli C. Genetic diagnosis in neonatal-onset epilepsies: back to the future. *Eur J Paediatr Neurol.* 2018;22(3):354-357. doi:10.1016/j.ejpn.2018.02.006

8. Hussain SA. Epileptic encephalopathies. *Continuum (Minneap Minn).* 2018;24(1, child neurology):171-185. doi:10.1212/CON.0000000000000558

9. Pearl PL. Epilepsy syndromes in childhood. *Continuum (Minneap Minn).* 2018;24(1, child neurology):186-209. doi:10.1212/CON.0000000000000568

10. Pavone P, Corsello G, Ruggieri M, Marino S, Marino S, Falsaperla R. Benign and severe early-life seizures: a round in the first year of life. *Ital J Pediatr.* 2018;44(1):54. doi:10.1186/s13052-018-0491-z

11. Cornet MC, Sands TT, Cilio MR. Neonatal epilepsies: clinical management. *Semin Fetal Neonatal Med.* 2018;23(3):204-212. doi:10.1016/j.siny.2018.01.004

12. Vossler DG, Weingarten M, Gidal BE. Summary of antiepileptic drugs available in the United States of America. *Epilepsy Currents.* 2018;18(4 suppl):1-26. doi:10.5698/1535-7597.18.4s1.1

13. Kossoff EH, Zupec-Kania BA, Auvin S, et al. Optimal clinical management of children receiving dietary therapies for epilepsy: updated recommendations of the International Ketogenic Diet Study Group. *Epilepsia Open.* 2018;3(2):175-192. doi:10.1002/epi4.12225

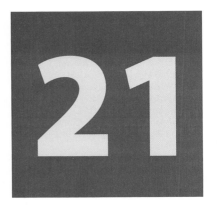

Epilepsy in Children

Gewalin Aungaroon, MD

▶ About a quarter of childhood-onset epilepsy is age related, has characteristic clinical and electroencephalographic features, and has favorable prognoses when properly treated such as childhood absence epilepsy, juvenile absence epilepsy, juvenile myoclonic epilepsy, early-onset childhood occipital epilepsy (Panayiotopoulos type), and benign epilepsy of centrotemporal spikes.

▶ Some epilepsy syndromes in this age group present with worse manifestations and prognoses such as Lennox-Gastaut syndrome, Landau-Kleffner syndrome, and epileptic encephalopathy with continuous spike and wave during sleep.

▶ Early recognition of epilepsy syndromes and their distinction from symptomatic epilepsies can lead to appropriate investigation, treatment, and prognostication.

GENERAL CONSIDERATIONS

This chapter covers common childhood-onset epilepsy syndromes. Other epilepsy diagnoses of various etiologies (eg, cortical dysplasia, tumor, inflammation, metabolic imbalance, mitochondrial encephalopathies) are not discussed in this chapter.

CLINICAL FINDINGS

▶ Childhood Absence Epilepsy

Prevalence

Childhood absence epilepsy (CAE) accounts for 10% to 17% of pediatric epilepsy.[1]

Symptoms and Signs

Age at onset is between 4 and 10 years with a peak at 5 to 7 years. *Typical absence* refers to a characteristic combination of clinical and electroencephalographic (EEG) manifestations. The semiology consists of abrupt transient impairments of consciousness manifested as behavioral pauses that can be accompanied by staring, automatisms (involuntary low-amplitude movement of hands or mouth), and myoclonia lasting from 4 to 20 seconds and occurs frequently throughout the day. Generalized tonic-clonic (GTC) seizures may occur.

EEG Findings

The ictal and interictal discharges are characterized by generalized 3- to 4-Hz spike and slow wave complexes (Figure 21–1).

Imaging

Magnetic resonance imaging (MRI) of the brain shows no pathologic lesions.

Differential Diagnosis

Juvenile myoclonic epilepsy (JME) can present with absence seizures, but the predominant myoclonus and unique EEG features can differentiate the diagnoses. Eyelid myoclonia with absence seizures (Jeavons syndrome) presents with absence seizures associated with predominant eyelid myoclonia and retropulsion of the head. The ictal EEG shows generalized 3- to 6-Hz polyspike-wave complexes provoked by eye closure and photic stimulation.

Absence seizures can also be a part of neurologic manifestations of various disorders such as brain tumors, cortical dysplasia, metabolic disorders, and mitochondrial encephalopathies.

Comorbidities

Cognitive deficits, particularly attention-deficit/hyperactivity disorder and anxiety disorders, may present.[2-4]

Treatment

The first-line antiseizure medications include ethosuximide, valproic acid, and lamotrigine.[5] Carbamazepine and oxcarbazepine can cause worsening in absence seizures.

Prognosis

Seizure remission usually occurs in adolescent years with a higher rate in patients without GTC seizures (78% vs 35%).[6-9]

▶ Juvenile Absence Epilepsy

Juvenile absence epilepsy (JAE) and CAE have an overlap in the age of onset and symptoms and have a relatively similar prognosis (seizure freedom in 54% of patients).[10]

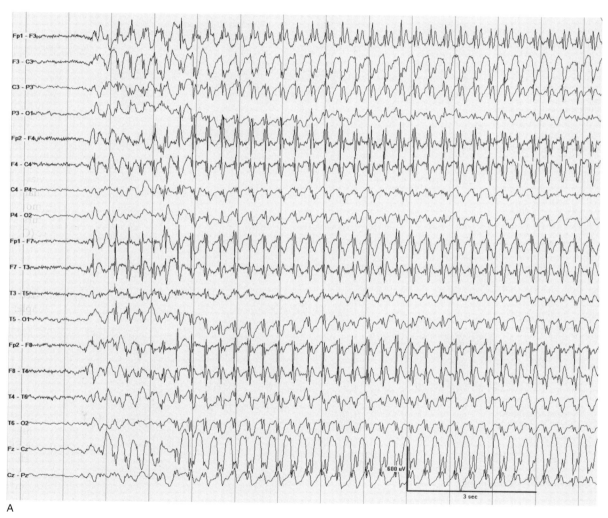

A

▲ **Figure 21–1.** Video electroencephalography (EEG) recording. **(A)** A recording from a 9-year-old male with childhood absence epilepsy with generalized 3-Hz spike-wave complexes associated with an absence seizure. **(B)** A recording from a 16-year-old female with juvenile myoclonic epilepsy with generalized 4-Hz polyspike-wave complexes associated with myoclonia. **(C)** A recording from an 8-year-old male with benign epilepsy of centrotemporal spikes with spikes seen independently in the bilateral centrotemporal region.

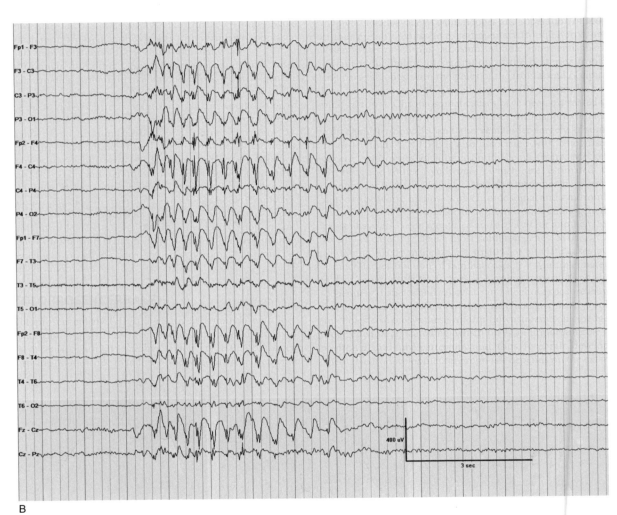

B

▲ **Figure 21–1.** (*Continued*)

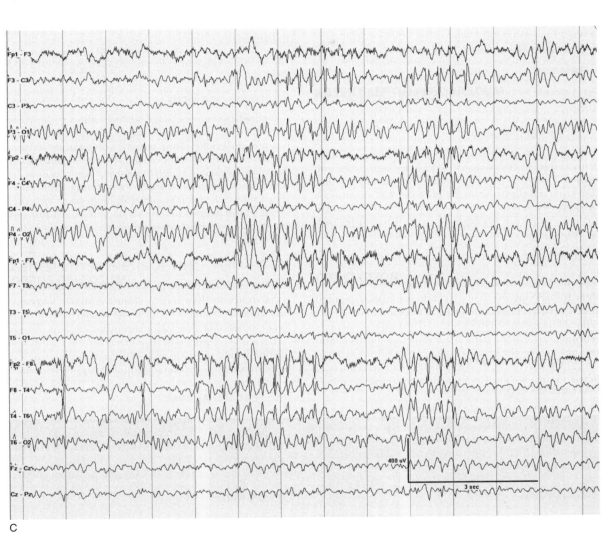

C

▲ **Figure 21–1.** (*Continued*)

The major distinctive considerations include the following. The age of onset is between 7 and 17 years with a peak at 10 to 12 years. Compared to CAE, the occurrence of absence seizure is lower and GTC seizure is higher. Although the treatment of choice is similar to CAE, lamotrigine and levetiracetam should be considered as the first-line therapy in adolescent females due to the risk of valproic acid–related teratogenicity.

▶ Juvenile Myoclonic Epilepsy

Prevalence

JME accounts for 10% of all epilepsy cases in children and adults.

Symptoms and Signs

Age at onset is between 10 and 25 years.[11] Myoclonic seizures are characterized by an abrupt jerk of the head, arms, and shoulders occurring preferentially upon awakening and may cluster over minutes to hours. Absence and GTC seizures are common.

EEG Findings

Interictal EEG shows generalized 4- to 6-Hz polyspike-wave complexes. The ictal EEG is characterized by a burst of high-amplitude 5- to 20-Hz polyspikes followed by a delta wave associated with myoclonia.[11-13] Photic stimulation-induced epileptiform discharges and myoclonia are common.

Imaging

MRI of the brain shows no pathologic lesions.

Differential Diagnosis

Differential diagnosis includes idiopathic generalized epilepsy and other rare diseases including progressive myoclonic epilepsy, especially Lafora disease and Unverricht-Lundborg disease, which also present in adolescence and resemble JME in the early stages.

Comorbidities

Behavioral disturbances and psychiatric disorders can be present.[14-16]

Treatment

Valproic acid is the first-line treatment.[11,17,18] Lamotrigine and levetiracetam should be considered as the first-line therapy in adolescent females with a risk of valproic acid–related teratogenicity.[19] Potential worsening in myoclonus has been reported with some antiseizure medications, especially sodium channel blockers.[20]

Prognosis

Excellent seizure control is achieved in two-thirds of JME patients with proper therapy.[15,21] Antiseizure medication can be withdrawn in 10% to 20% of patients.[22]

▶ Early-Onset Childhood Occipital Epilepsy (Panayiotopoulos Type)

Prevalence

Panayiotopoulos syndrome affects 6% of children with epilepsy.[23-26]

Symptoms and Signs

Age at onset is between 1 and 12 years with a peak at 4 and 5 years.[27] Clinical features include ictal emesis (80%), autonomic manifestations such as pallor and sweating (80%), eye and head deviation (80%), and impairment of consciousness (80%-90%). Focal and generalized tonic-clonic seizures may occur. Seizures predominantly occur during sleep, have a long duration, and commonly evolve into status epilepticus (~50%). Most patients have only a single seizure (45%), some have 2 to 5 seizures (40%), and about 15% have frequent seizures.[27]

EEG Findings

Frequent interictal discharges are seen in the occipital regions and activated by sleep and eye closure. Ictal discharges typically originate from the occipital region and rarely from the extraoccipital area.[28]

Imaging

MRI of the brain shows no pathologic lesions.

Differential Diagnosis

Symptomatic occipital epilepsies should be considered such as celiac disease with occipital calcifications, occipital epilepsy occurring as a result of structural damage due to neonatal hypoglycemia, mitochondrial encephalopathy with lactic acidosis and stroke (MELAS), and basilar migraine.

Comorbidities

Visual processing, visual memory, and verbal memory problems have been reported.[29,30]

Treatment

Carbamazepine, oxcarbazepine, and valproic acid are commonly prescribed. Given the rare occurrence of seizure, antiseizure medication is omitted in some cases. Rectal diazepam has been used to terminate prolonged seizures on an as-needed basis. There is a lack of evidence for intranasal benzodiazepine use in this context.

Prognosis

Seizure remission occurs in 88% of patients and usually within 3 years after onset despite persistent EEG abnormalities.[27]

Late-Onset Childhood Occipital Epilepsy (Gastaut Type)

This is a rare diagnosis with a slightly older but overlapping age of onset and EEG features with Panayiotopoulos syndrome. Core clinical features include visual disturbances with retained awareness with a postictal headache. Ictal vomiting and autonomic symptoms are uncommon. Focal and GTC seizures may present. Duration of seizures is less than 2 minutes, and seizure recurrence is common. Carbamazepine and oxcarbazepine are the typical first-line therapies. The prognosis is highly variable.

Benign Epilepsy With Centrotemporal Spikes and Its Spectrum

Benign epilepsy with centrotemporal spikes (BECTS) has a prevalence of 15% to 20% of all childhood epilepsy.[31] The clinical features include focal seizures with sensorimotor symptoms involving the face and oropharyngolaryngeal muscles, such as vocalization, speech arrest, and salivation with common secondary GTC seizures. Seizures are infrequent and mainly occur during sleep. The interictal EEG is characterized by focal or multifocal spikes, predominantly in the centrotemporal regions, that increase significantly during sleep. Ictal discharges typically localize to the centrotemporal region. Seizures are responsive to antiseizure medication, and seizure remission is achieved in more than 80% of patients and typically by age 14 years.[32,33] Given the benign nature and low seizure burden, antiseizure medication often is not used; however when indicated, carbamazepine, oxcarbazepine, and levetiracetam are the common choices. Neurocognitive deficits, particularly of speech and language, are typically not prominent.

The term *epilepsy with electrical status epilepticus during slow sleep* (ESES) describes an age-limited EEG characterized by a spike-and-wave pattern occupying over 85% of non–rapid eye movement sleep. Wide variations in diagnostic criteria are very common in the literature. ESES is associated with the conditions described below.

In atypical benign epilepsy with centrotemporal spikes (ABECTS), besides the sensorimotor seizures as seen in BECTS, atypical absence, myoclonic, atonic, and GTC seizures are also seen. The EEG shows an atypical morphology and location of epileptiform discharges and an abnormal background.[34] ESES pattern can be seen. Seizures tend to be resistant to antiepileptic medications but usually resolve before adolescence. Neuropsychological deficits are more apparent.[35-37] Landau-Kleffner syndrome is a rare diagnosis characterized by acquired epileptic aphasia with verbal auditory agnosia and various types of seizures.[38] The awake EEG shows epileptiform discharges in the perisylvian region, which may evolve into ESES during sleep.[39,40] Permanent language or cognitive impairments are common. Epileptic encephalopathy with continuous spike and wave during sleep (CSWS) presents at the extreme end of this spectrum. Patients present with global regression of language, cognitive function, and behavior associated with various types of seizures and ESES pattern. Several antiseizure medications, dietary therapy, and surgical interventions have been used for these conditions with variable outcomes.[41,42]

Lennox-Gastaut Syndrome

Prevalence

Lennox-Gastaut syndrome (LGS) accounts for 1% to 10% of childhood epilepsies.

Symptoms and Signs

Age at diagnosis is typically between 3 and 7 years. Core clinical features include (1) multiple seizure types, including tonic, tonic-clonic, atonic, myoclonic, and atypical absence seizures; (2) abnormal EEG; and (3) intellectual disability. LGS often occurs de novo but may also evolve from other severe infantile epileptic disorders, such as West syndrome.[43]

EEG Findings

Slow background with multifocal and generalized epileptiform discharges is seen. Various ictal patterns are seen with different seizure types.

Imaging

MRI findings range from normal to severe pathologic abnormalities of various causes such as cortical dysplasia and tuberous sclerosis.

Differential Diagnosis

Several other conditions may share some characteristics with LGS such as myoclonic-atonic epilepsy, ABECTS, and CSWS.

Comorbidities

Cognitive and behavioral problems, physical disability, and sleep disturbances are common.

Treatment

Seizures in LGS are typically pharmacoresistant. Several antiseizure medications have been used with variable outcomes.[44,45] Cannabidiol and fenfluramine are newer antiseizure medications that have been shown to be efficacious for seizure control in this condition.[46-48] Dietary therapy and surgical interventions are used in pharmacoresistant cases.

Prognosis

Seizures are difficult to control. Neurocognitive deficits are typically permanent.

WHEN TO REFER

Although childhood-onset epilepsy is age-limited, seizures and associated neurocognitive deficits can be challenging to manage in some cases. These patients likely benefit from advanced and comprehensive treatment beyond antiseizure medications such as dietary therapy, epilepsy surgery, and neurocognitive rehabilitation.

REFERENCES

1. Berg AT, Shinnar S, Levy SR, Testa FM, Smith-Rapaport S, Beckerman B. How well can epilepsy syndromes be identified at diagnosis? A reassessment 2 years after initial diagnosis. *Epilepsia.* 2000;41(10):1269-1275. doi:10.1111/j.1528-1157.2000.tb04604.x

2. Caplan R, Siddarth P, Stahl L, et al. Childhood absence epilepsy: behavioral, cognitive, and linguistic comorbidities. *Epilepsia.* 2008;49(11):1838-1846. doi:10.1111/j.1528-1167.2008.01680.x

3. Vega C, Vestal M, DeSalvo M, et al. Differentiation of attention-related problems in childhood absence epilepsy. *Epilepsy Behav.* 2010;19(1):82-85. doi:10.1016/j.yebeh.2010.06.010

4. Glauser TA, Holland K, O'Brien VP, et al. Pharmacogenetics of antiepileptic drug efficacy in childhood absence epilepsy. *Ann Neurol.* 2017;81(3):444-453. doi:10.1002/ana.24886

5. Glauser TA, Cnaan A, Shinnar S, et al. Ethosuximide, valproic acid, and lamotrigine in childhood absence epilepsy. *N Engl J Med.* 2010;362(9):790-799. doi:10.1056/NEJMoa0902014

6. Wirrell EC, Camfield CS, Camfield PR, Gordon KE, Dooley JM. Long-term prognosis of typical childhood absence epilepsy: remission or progression to juvenile myoclonic epilepsy. *Neurology.* 1996;47(4):912-918. doi:10.1212/wnl.47.4.912

7. Trinka E, Baumgartner S, Unterberger I, et al. Long-term prognosis for childhood and juvenile absence epilepsy. *J Neurol.* 2004;251(10):1235-1241. doi:10.1007/s00415-004-0521-1

8. Bouma PA, Westendorp RG, van Dijk JG, Peters AC, Brouwer OF. The outcome of absence epilepsy: a meta-analysis. *Neurology.* 1996;47(3):802-808. doi:10.1212/wnl.47.3.802

9. Callenbach PM, Bouma PA, Geerts AT, et al. Long-term outcome of childhood absence epilepsy: Dutch Study of Epilepsy in Childhood. *Epilepsy Res.* 2009;83(2-3):249-256. doi:10.1016/j.eplepsyres.2008.11.011

10. Trinka E, Baumgartner S, Unterberger I, et al. Long-term prognosis for childhood and juvenile absence epilepsy. *J Neurol.* 2004;251(10):1235-1241. doi:10.1007/s00415-004-0521-1

11. Yacubian EM. Juvenile myoclonic epilepsy: challenges on its 60th anniversary. *Seizure.* 2017;44:48-52. doi:10.1016/j.seizure.2016.09.005

12. Baykan B, Wolf P. Juvenile myoclonic epilepsy as a spectrum disorder: a focused review. *Seizure-Eur J Epilep.* 2017;49:36-41. doi:10.1016/j.seizure.2017.05.011

13. Yacubian EM. Juvenile myoclonic epilepsy: challenges on its 60th anniversary. *Seizure Eur J Epilep.* 2017;44:48-52. doi:10.1016/j.seizure.2016.09.005

14. Wandschneider B, Thompson PJ, Vollmar C, Koepp MJ. Frontal lobe function and structure in juvenile myoclonic epilepsy: a comprehensive review of neuropsychological and imaging data. *Epilepsia.* 2012;53(12):2091-2098. doi:10.1111/epi.12003

15. Gelisse P, Genton P, Thomas P, Rey M, Samuelian JC, Dravet C. Clinical factors of drug resistance in juvenile myoclonic epilepsy. *J Neurol Neurosurg Psychiatry.* 2001;70(2):240-243. doi:10.1136/jnnp.70.2.240

16. de Araujo Filho GM, Yacubian EM. Juvenile myoclonic epilepsy: psychiatric comorbidity and impact on outcome. *Epilepsy Behav.* 2013;28(suppl 1):S74-S80. doi:10.1016/j.yebeh.2013.03.026

17. Hernandez-Vanegas LE, Jara-Prado A, Ochoa A, et al. High-dose versus low-dose valproate for the treatment of juvenile myoclonic epilepsy: going from low to high. *Epilepsy Behav.* 2016;61:34-40. doi:10.1016/j.yebeh.2016.04.047

18. Chowdhury A, Brodie MJ. Pharmacological outcomes in juvenile myoclonic epilepsy: support for sodium valproate. *Epilepsy Res.* 2016;119:62-66. doi:10.1016/j.eplepsyres.2015.11.012

19. Silvennoinen K, de Lange N, Zagaglia S, et al. Comparative effectiveness of antiepileptic drugs in juvenile myoclonic epilepsy. *Epilepsia Open.* 2019;4(3):420-430. doi:10.1002/epi4.12349

20. Thomas P, Valton L, Genton P. Absence and myoclonic status epilepticus precipitated by antiepileptic drugs in idiopathic generalized epilepsy. *Brain.* 2006;129(Pt 5):1281-1292. doi:10.1093/brain/awl047

21. Stevelink R, Koeleman BPC, Sander JW, Jansen FE, Braun KPJ. Refractory juvenile myoclonic epilepsy: a meta-analysis of prevalence and risk factors. *Eur J Neurol.* 2019;26(6):856-864. doi:10.1111/ene.13811

22. Calleja S, Salas-Puig J, Ribacoba R, Lahoz CH. Evolution of juvenile myoclonic epilepsy treated from the outset with sodium valproate. *Seizure.* 2001;10(6):424-427. doi:10.1053/seiz.2000.0530

23. Caraballo R, Cersosimo R, Medina C, Fejerman N. Panayiotopoulos-type benign childhood occipital epilepsy: a prospective study. *Neurology.* 2000;55(8):1096-1100. doi:10.1212/wnl.55.8.1096

24. Kivity S, Ephraim T, Weitz R, Tamir A. Childhood epilepsy with occipital paroxysms: clinical variants in 134 patients. *Epilepsia.* 2000;41(12):1522-1533. doi:10.1111/j.1499-1654.2000.001522.x

25. Ferrie CD, Grunewald RA. Panayiotopoulos syndrome: a common and benign childhood epilepsy. *Lancet.* 2001;357(9259):821-823. doi:10.1016/S0140-6736(00)04192-1

26. Ferrie C, Caraballo R, Covanis A, et al. Panayiotopoulos syndrome: a consensus view. *Dev Med Child Neurol.* 2006;48(3):236-240. doi:10.1017/S0012162206000508

27. Caraballo R, Cersosimo R, Fejerman N. Panayiotopoulos syndrome: a prospective study of 192 patients. *Epilepsia.* 2007;48(6):1054-1061. doi:10.1111/j.1528-1167.2007.01085.x

28. Koutroumanidis M. Panayiotopoulos syndrome: an important electroclinical example of benign childhood system epilepsy. *Epilepsia.* 2007;48(6):1044-1053. doi:10.1111/j.1528-1167.2007.01096.x

29. Hodges SL, Gabriel MT, Perry MS. Neuropsychological findings associated with Panayiotopoulos syndrome in three children. *Epilepsy Behav.* 2016;54:158-162. doi:10.1016/j.yebeh.2015.11.012

30. Kalem SA, Elmali AD, Demirbilek V, et al. Panayiotopoulos syndrome and Gastaut syndrome are distinct entities in terms of neuropsychological findings. *Epilepsy Behav.* 2019;99:106447. doi:10.1016/j.yebeh.2019.106447

31. Blom S, Heijbel J. Benign epilepsy of children with centrotemporal EEG foci: a follow-up-study in adulthood of patients initially studied as children. *Epilepsia.* 1982;23(6):629-632. doi:10.1111/j.1528-1157.1982.tb05078.x

32. Bouma PAD, Bovenkerk AC, Westendorp RGJ, Brouwer OF. The course of benign partial epilepsy of childhood with centrotemporal spikes: a meta-analysis. *Neurology.* 1997;48(2):430-437. doi:10.1212/Wnl.48.2.430

33. You SJ, Kim DS, Ko TS. Benign childhood epilepsy with centrotemporal spikes (BCECTS): early onset of seizures is associated with poorer response to initial treatment. *Epileptic Disord.* 2006;8(4):285-288.

34. Fejerman N. Atypical rolandic epilepsy. *Epilepsia.* 2009; 50(suppl 7):9-12. doi:10.1111/j.1528-1167.2009.02210.x

35. Gobbi G, Boni A, Filippini M. The spectrum of idiopathic rolandic epilepsy syndromes and idiopathic occipital epilepsies: from the benign to the disabling. *Epilepsia.* 2006;47:62-66. doi: 10.1111/j.1528-1167.2006.00693.x

36. Hahn A, Pistohl J, Neubauer BA, Stephani U. Atypical "benign" partial epilepsy or pseudo-Lennox syndrome. Part I: symptomatology and long-term prognosis. *Neuropediatrics.* 2001;32(1):1-8. doi:10.1055/s-2001-12216

37. Doose H, Hahn A, Neubauer BA, Pistohl J, Stephani U. Atypical "benign" partial epilepsy of childhood or pseudo-Lennox syndrome. Part II: family study. *Neuropediatrics.* 2001;32(1):9-13. doi:10.1055/s-2001-12215

38. Kaga M, Inagaki M, Ohta R. Epidemiological study of Landau-Kleffner syndrome (LKS) in Japan. *Brain Dev Jpn.* 2014;36(4):284-286. doi:10.1016/j.braindev.2013.04.012

39. Hughes JR. A review of the relationships between Landau-Kleffner syndrome, electrical status epilepticus during sleep, and continuous spike-waves during sleep. *Epilepsy Behav.* 2011;20(2):247-253. doi:10.1016/j.yebeh.2010.10.015

40. Paetau R. Magnetoencephalography in Landau-Kleffner syndrome. *Epilepsia.* 2009;50:51-54. doi:10.1111/j.1528-1167.2009 .02220.x

41. McTague A, Cross JH. Treatment of epileptic encephalopathies. *CNS Drugs.* 2013;27(3):175-184. doi:10.1007/s40263-013-0041-6

42. Veggiotti P, Pera MC, Teutonico F, Brazzo D, Balottin U, Tassinari CA. Therapy of encephalopathy with status epilepticus during sleep (ESES/CSWS syndrome): an update. *Epileptic Disord.* 2012;14(1):1-11. doi:10.1684/epd.2012.0482

43. You SJ, Kim HD, Kang HC. Factors influencing the evolution of West syndrome to Lennox-Gastaut syndrome. *Pediatr Neurol.* 2009;41(2):111-113. doi:10.1016/j.pediatrneurol.2009.03.006

44. Hancock EC, Cross JH. Treatment of Lennox-Gastaut syndrome. *Cochrane Database Syst Rev.* 2013;2:CD003277. doi: 10.1002/14651858.CD003277.pub3

45. Cross JH, Auvin S, Falip M, Striano P, Arzimanoglou A. Expert opinion on the management of Lennox-Gastaut syndrome: treatment algorithms and practical consideration. *Front Neurol.* 2017;8:505. doi:10.3389/fneur.2017.00505

46. Thiele EA, Marsh ED, French JA, et al. Cannabidiol in patients with seizures associated with Lennox-Gastaut syndrome (GWPCARE4): a randomised, double-blind, placebo-controlled phase 3 trial. *Lancet.* 2018;391(10125):1085-1096. doi:10.1016/S0140-6736(18)30136-3

47. Thiele E, Marsh E, Mazurkiewicz-Beldzinska M, et al. Cannabidiol in patients with Lennox-Gastaut syndrome: interim analysis of an open-label extension study. *Epilepsia.* 2019;60(3):419-428. doi:10.1111/epi.14670

48. Lagae L, Schoonjans AS, Gammaitoni AR, Galer BS, Ceulemans B. A pilot, open-label study of the effectiveness and tolerability of low-dose ZX008 (fenfluramine HCl) in Lennox-Gastaut syndrome. *Epilepsia.* 2018;59(10):1881-1888. doi:10.1111/epi.14540

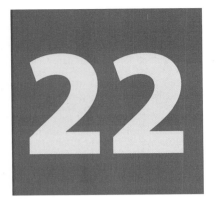

Epilepsy in Adolescents

Katherine Holland, MD, PhD

The incidence of newly diagnosed seizures is lower in adolescents than in younger children. Although focal epilepsy is still the most common epilepsy classification in adolescents, the etiologies of new-onset seizures are slightly different than earlier in childhood. For symptomatic focal seizures, acquired lesions (eg, head trauma, tumors, mesial temporal sclerosis) predominate over congenital or perinatal causes. Similarly, the epilepsy syndromes seen in this age group are different than earlier in childhood. More often, generalized epilepsy syndromes are seen and benign focal epilepsies resolve by this time. Because of the increased incidence of acquired focal epilepsies (over benign focal epilepsy syndromes), neuroimaging is recommended for adolescents with suspected focal-onset seizures and for those in whom the onset cannot be determined.

The effects of epilepsy on daily life are also different in this age group compared to in younger children.[1-3] These effects result from the differences in prognosis in adolescent-onset epilepsy syndromes, the developing self-reliance in this age group, and the sexual maturation that occurs through this period. Each influences the treatment and counseling given to adolescents with epilepsy.

SPECIAL CONSIDERATIONS FOR TEENS

▶ Transitioning to Adulthood

As children mature into adults, they assume responsibility for themselves. Of course, this is also true for children with medical conditions such as epilepsy.[4] As part of the care of an adolescent with seizures, it is important to facilitate this transition. Factors that contribute to successful transitions of care from pediatric to adult providers include an adolescent's comfort with managing medication, obtaining medication refills, and scheduling appointments; knowledge of important epilepsy-related information (eg, seizure frequency); comfort talking to care providers; and some understanding

of health insurance.[5] Encourage adult caregivers to allow the adolescent to progressively take responsibility for their care. Begin by encouraging the patient to be responsible for taking their own medications. A pill reminder box can provide a way for parents to inconspicuously monitor adherence. Address the conversation about care to the adolescent and let them lead the discussion about their care. As time progresses, ask parents to step out of the room while you discuss issues of care with the patient. Because the parents are still legally the people who are responsible for the healthcare decisions, they have to be included, but for older adolescents, try to do so after you have had a chance to discuss issues with the patient (alone) first.

An important part of independence for this age group is driving. Driving laws are not uniform from state to state. Most require a period of seizure freedom before people with epilepsy are allowed to drive, with a median seizure-free period in statute laws of 6 months. Adolescent drivers are already one of the age groups at highest risk for motor vehicle accidents. The increased risk related to epilepsy in this age group is unknown, but people with uncontrolled seizures should not drive.[6] State-specific information is available at the Epilepsy Foundation website (https://www.epilepsy.com/lifestyle/driving-and-transportation/laws).

Peer-to-peer interactions are also increasingly important. They can impact epilepsy in several ways. Experimentation with the use of alcohol or illicit drugs can be a part of some social activities in adolescents. These substances alter the seizure threshold and can also exacerbate medication side effects. For adolescents with a history of prolonged seizures or clustering of seizures, the use of rectal diazepam can be embarrassing. The US Food and Drug Administration has now approved nasal formulations of diazepam and midazolam that can be used instead of rectal diazepam. However, these are considerably more costly and often require prior authorization by insurance. Buccal use of benzodiazepine can also be effective for seizure clusters. These routes of administration can be more prone to abuse, so frequent requests for refills should be questioned.

Employment/Career Counseling

Seizures can potentially limit future career options. This is largely dependent upon seizure control. If seizure control is not sufficient to obtain a driver's license, careers that could place people in hazardous conditions should be avoided. If seizures are well controlled, most professions are open to people with epilepsy. However, in certain circumstances, even a past history of seizures can limit career opportunities. The most commonly restricted option is entry into the military. This is restricted for people with a history of epilepsy, even in cases where seizures are medically controlled. People with seizures beyond the age of 5 years cannot serve unless they have been seizure free for at least 5 years off of all anticonvulsant medications. In addition, they must have a current normal electroencephalogram (EEG). As a result, if an adolescent with a history of well-controlled epilepsy wishes to pursue a military career following high school, early preparation including tapering of anticonvulsant medications is required; unfortunately, usually adolescents do not know if this is the career they want until later in adolescence.

Education

High school environments are less supervised than many elementary and middle schools. This transition can be difficult, especially for those with poorly controlled epilepsy. Students tend to have more teachers, and high school represents a larger community of people. As a result, a large team of people may need to be educated about acute seizure management. If not already in place, a 504 Plan should be considered, and if one is in place, this is a good time to review the plan. In addition to accommodations related directly to seizures, accommodations for epilepsy-related comorbidities (eg, learning disabilities) are important to consider. If a 504 Plan is not in place but could be helpful, anyone (eg, a parent or doctor) can refer a student for an evaluation, but the school district must also have a reason to feel the need for services prior to an evaluation.

After graduation from high school, many young adults with epilepsy attend college. While having epilepsy should not determine which college to attend, there are several things to keep in mind when counseling an adolescent with epilepsy about choosing a school. If seizures are not fully controlled, a good system of transportation in and around campus is important. The availability and quality of health services offered at on-campus health centers, type of coverage offered by the college's insurance or parent's health plan, and easy availability for prescription refills are issues that might influence a choice of college. College students with epilepsy should work in coordination with their neurologist and the college disability office to develop epilepsy-associated accommodations. If a student has a 504 Plan in high school, these accommodations can be applied to a higher education setting. Important considerations to have in place include the ability to take exams at a later date in the event a student has a seizure prior to (or during) an examination, a secure system for delivery of mail-order medications to dormitories, and strategies to mitigate sleep deprivation for people who find this to be a trigger.

Several college scholarship programs are available specifically for people with epilepsy.

Epilepsy and Young Women

There are also special considerations for young women with epilepsy including effects of antiepileptic medication on hormonal methods of contraception, family planning, and interaction of hormones and seizure frequency.

Estrogen, progesterone, and their metabolites can affect neuronal excitability, which clinically can result in cyclical fluctuations in seizure susceptibility. These hormonally regulated patterns begin to become apparent in adolescents. When a reliable pattern of seizure exacerbation is seen during specific times during the menstrual cycle, this is referred to as catamenial epilepsy. The specific definition has varied, so the incidence of catamenial seizures is unclear. Premenstrual exacerbation of seizures is most common, and a catamenial pattern is most commonly seen with focal seizures. Strategies for management of catamenial seizures vary depending on the pattern and degree of seizure exacerbation as well as the regularity of menses. However, the scientific support for some of the proposed strategies is limited.[7]

Many commonly used antiepileptic medications alter the concentrations of endogenous and exogenous reproductive hormones (Table 22–1). This contributes to long-term

Table 22–1. Antiepileptic medications and oral contraceptive efficacy.

May Reduce Efficacy	Unlikely to Reduce Efficacy
Carbamazepine	Benzodiazepines
Eslicarbazepine	Brivaracetam
Felbamate	Gabapentin
Oxcarbazepine	Lacosamide
Perampanel	Levetiracetam
Primidone	Pregabalin
Phenytoin	Tiagabine
Rufinamide	Zonisamide
Topiramate	Valproate
	Vigabatrin

effects of epilepsy on sexual and reproductive health into adulthood, but the immediate and practical implication for adolescent women with epilepsy is the potential for reduced efficacy of oral contraceptives containing a combination of estrogens and progesterone. Emphasizing the use of barrier methods of contraception as a supplement to oral contraceptives is important, especially for adolescent females taking enzyme-inducing antiepileptics. An alternate approach is to recommend using combined oral contraceptives with at least 50 μg of ethinyl estradiol[8] or depot medroxyprogesterone acetate. Also of note is that lamotrigine levels can be reduced by combination oral contraceptive pills.

Counseling adolescent women with epilepsy about potential difficulties that can arise in the event they do become pregnant is also important. These difficulties include (but are not limited to) worsening of seizure control (both because of reduced levels of anticonvulsant medications and because of a reduced seizure threshold) and teratogenic effects of certain antiepileptic drugs (most notably, but not exclusively, valproate). While the majority of women with epilepsy have healthy children, the chances of complications are decreased when pregnancies are planned and a neurologist is involved in management of antiepileptic medications in advance of the pregnancy. Unfortunately, most pregnancies in adolescents are unplanned; however, there are several steps that can mitigate potential complications. Because of its teratogenic effects, the use of valproate in adolescent women, especially as polytherapy, should be avoided,[9] unless this the only antiepileptic drug that can provide adequate seizure control. Although the efficacy and dosing guidelines are unclear, prescription of folic acid (at least 0.4 mg/d) to epileptic women of childbearing age is suggested to reduce the potential teratogenic effects of certain antiepileptic drugs.[10]

Polycystic ovary syndrome (PCOS) is a commonly diagnosed menstrual disorder in women but is more common in women with epilepsy than the general population. Among women with epilepsy, those with a seizure onset in adolescence have the highest incidence of PCOS. The symptoms of PCOS can include irregular menses, hirsutism, severe acne, and weight gain. PCOS is associated with long-term health problems including increased risk for type 2 diabetes and endometrial cancer as well as infertility. PCOS is often associated with the use of valproate but can also occur without valproate exposure. However, this is another reason to avoid initiation of valproate in adolescent females with epilepsy unless no alternate medication is available for adequate seizure control.

COMMON AGE-SPECIFIC EPILEPSY SYNDROMES IN ADOLESCENTS

The majority of epilepsy syndromes with onset in this age group are idiopathic generalized epilepsies (IGEs). As a class of disorders, IGEs represent 15% to 20% of all epilepsies.

They are named for their prototypic seizure type but can have a mixture of different seizure types. In addition, there is some overlap in the clinical and EEG characteristics of these syndromes, so the diagnosis may evolve over time. The development and neurologic examination of the affected people are normal. These syndromes are summarized in Table 22–2 and discussed in more detail in the following sections.

▶ Juvenile Absence Epilepsy

Clinical Manifestations

Juvenile absence epilepsy (JAE) is a generalized epilepsy syndrome that is closely related to childhood absence epilepsy; however, the seizure frequency is lower and age of onset is later. The onset of absence seizures in JAE is around 8 to 12 years of age (range, 8-20 years). The hallmark of JAE is absence seizures. These occur daily but are less frequent and may have milder manifestations than those seen in childhood absence epilepsy (CAE; see Chapter 21). The loss of awareness may be incomplete during some seizures so that affected individual can respond to simple commands but not complex tasks. In addition to absence seizures, the majority of people with JAE also have rare generalized tonic-clonic seizures (GTCs).[11] Typically, the onset of absence seizures occurs prior to the occurrence of GTCs, but the absences may not have been identified as seizures until after a GTC occurs. Although some papers report a low incidence of myoclonic seizures in JAE, the presence of myoclonic seizures is thought to represent juvenile myoclonic epilepsy rather than JAE.

Diagnosis and Ancillary Testing

The diagnosis of JAE relies on a clinical history of absences seizures in a normally developing child along with a characteristic EEG pattern of greater than 2.5-Hz (usually 3-6 Hz) generalized spike-wave or polyspike-wave complexes. The EEG background activity is typically normal; however, intermittent occipital rhythmic delta activity may be present. There is considerable overlap in presentation between CAE and JAE. Clinical features that favor the diagnosis of JAE over CAE include the onset of seizures over the age of 10 years, especially with the presence of GTCs, and an absence seizure frequency of 1 to 2 per day. Other than the EEG, no additional ancillary testing is needed[12]; however, if the EEG has persistent focal features, neuroimaging (and an alternate diagnosis) should be considered.

Treatment

With the exception of CAE (see Chapter 21), there have been no well-controlled clinical trials of treatments for IGEs.[13] Because of its efficacy for both absence and GTC seizures, valproate has been the traditional treatment of choice for JAE. However, some teens with JAE will need to

Table 22–2. Common epilepsy syndromes of adolescents.

Syndrome	Age of Onset (years)	Hallmark Seizure(s)	Description	Seizure Frequency	EEG Features	Common Treatments*	Seizure Prognosis
Juvenile absence epilepsy (JME)	8-20	Absence GTCs	Episodes of staring with altered awareness (usually <10 seconds); loss of awareness may be incomplete About 80% also have GTCs	Several absences per day Infrequent	• Normal background • Generalized 3- to 6-Hz spike and polyspike and wave complexes • Activation with HV	Ethosuximide Valproate Lamotrigine Topiramate	Seizures may remit, but substantial minority continue to have seizures into adulthood
Juvenile myoclonic epilepsy (JME)	8-25	Myoclonic GTCs	Sudden rapid jerks of upper extremities Often following a cluster of myoclonic seizures	Variable Can be precipitated by sleep deprivation, stress, alcohol	• Normal background • Generalized 3.5- to 6-Hz spike and polyspike and wave complexes • May have activation with IPS, HV, and sleep deprivation	Valproate Topiramate Zonisamide Levetiracetam Lamotrigine	Seizures usually controlled on medications; complete remission may occur in some cases, but lifelong treatment common
Epilepsy with GTCs alone (IGE-GTCs)	5-40	GTCs	Infrequent	Can be precipitated by sleep deprivation, stress, alcohol	• Normal background • Generalized 3.5- to 6-Hz spike and polyspike and wave complexes (may only be seen in sleep) • May see activation with IPS	Valproate Topiramate Zonisamide Levetiracetam Lamotrigine	Seizure controlled on medication; complete remission common

*Valproate should not be used as first-line treatment in adolescent women with epilepsy.
EEG, electroencephalogram; GTC, generalized tonic-clonic seizures; HV, hyperventilation; IGE, idiopathic generalized epilepsy; IPS, intermittent photic stimulation.

continue therapy into adulthood[14] and those who will not experience remission cannot be predicted at the time of diagnosis,[14,15] so alternatives to the use of valproate as a first-line therapy for females with JAE should be considered. One alternative is ethosuximide if the patient has only absence seizures; however, if GTCs are also present, other broad-spectrum anticonvulsant medications should be selected. These include lamotrigine, levetiracetam, topiramate, and zonisamide. Because carbamazepine, gabapentin, oxcarbazepine, phenytoin, tiagabine, and vigabatrin may exacerbate seizures in IGE, the use of these agents should be avoided.[16]

Prognosis

The prognosis for seizure control in JAE is generally reported to be good, with the majority of patients becoming seizure free. However, a substantial minority of affected individuals will not enter into remission and may continue to require seizure treatment into adulthood. Although the long-term psychosocial outcomes of JAE have not been well characterized, studies of these outcomes in other IGEs demonstrate higher rates of depression, poor school performance, and unemployment,[17] suggesting that these issues may also be problems for people with JAE even if seizures are controlled.

▶ Juvenile Myoclonic Epilepsy

Clinical Manifestations

This is one of the most common forms of IGE. The onset is between 8 and 25 years of age, and onset peaks in adolescence. The hallmark seizure type is myoclonic seizures characterized by brief sudden jerks typically of the upper extremities. These often occur within an hour of awakening (but can be sporadic). Most people (80%-95%) with juvenile myoclonic epilepsy (JME) also have GTCs, which can be preceded by a cluster of myoclonic seizures. These seizures are often precipitated by stress, sleep deprivation, or alcohol consumption. Approximately one-third of patients also have absence seizures. These are less frequent (not daily) and briefer than those seen with either CAE or JAE. In addition, the associated loss of awareness is minimal. Some affected individuals may initially present with CAE.

Diagnosis and Ancillary Testing

The diagnosis of JME relies on a clinical history of myoclonic seizures in a typically developing teenager along with a characteristic EEG pattern of greater than 2.5-Hz (usually 3.5-6 Hz) generalized spike-wave or polyspike-wave complexes. Bilaterally independent, multifocal fragments of the generalized epileptiform discharges may also be seen. Photoparoxysmal response on an EEG and activation of epileptiform abnormalities by hyperventilation and sleep deprivation can also occur. JME should be suspected in teens with a first GTC, especially if the GTC occurs shortly upon awakening or in the setting a precipitating factor.[18] Often the GTC is the first recognized seizure, but upon further questioning, a history of preexisting myoclonic seizures is present; however, the significance of myoclonus was not recognized by the patient or their family. If the diagnosis of JME is suspected on clinical grounds but a routine EEG is normal, a sleep-deprived EEG may be beneficial. The description of seizures may have some focal features. While this does not preclude the diagnosis of JME, neuroimaging should be done in these cases to exclude a focal lesion. Likewise, although interictal EEGs can have some focal abnormalities (in addition to the generalized discharges), if they are consistently seen in one region, a structural brain abnormality should be considered.

The development of myoclonic seizure can also be seen in progressive myoclonic epilepsy (PME). These disorders are also associated with decline in cognitive performance and development of slowing on the EEG. Because these disorders are rare, evaluation of PME is not indicated in cases of newly diagnosed JME unless there are other clinical suspicions.

Treatment

Treatment recommendations for JME are similar to those for JAE. Valproate has traditionally been considered the first-line therapy, but this should not be used as the first-line treatment for females with JME. Alternatives include topiramate, zonisamide, levetiracetam, and lamotrigine. However, there are reports of lamotrigine-induced exacerbation of myoclonic seizures in some people with JME. Benzodiazepines can also be effective. Carbamazepine, gabapentin, oxcarbazepine, phenytoin, tiagabine, and vigabatrin may exacerbate seizures, and use of these agents should be avoided.[16] In addition to medications, lifestyle changes such as avoiding sleep deprivation, stress reduction, and limited alcohol consumption are also beneficial. Although photosensitivity is often seen on the EEGs of people with JME, only 5% to 15% of people with JME report having visual triggers, so

restrictions on playing video games in adolescents with JME are not necessary unless the patient reports this as a trigger.

Prognosis

Seizures are often well controlled with the appropriate anticonvulsant therapy. Complete remission of seizures off of medication is low (<30%), so many patients will continue therapy indefinitely.[19] Despite the relatively good prognosis for seizure control, people with JME have higher incidences of adverse psychosocial outcomes including unemployment, unplanned pregnancy, and depression.[17]

▶ Idiopathic Generalized Epilepsy With Generalized Tonic-Clonic Seizures Alone

In the past, this syndrome has also been termed *idiopathic generalized epilepsy with generalized tonic-clonic seizures on awakening*. The presence of other seizure types excludes this diagnosis. However, mild absence and myoclonic seizures are not always recognized, so in some cases, this syndrome can be difficult to differentiate from JME and JAE.

Clinical Manifestations

The onset of this syndrome is around 5 to 40 years of age, and it most commonly begins between 11 and 23 years of age. As with the other IGEs, the development, cognition, and neurologic examinations are normal. GTCs are the only seizure type; however, some affected individuals may have a prior history of childhood absence epilepsy. The seizures usually occur within a few hours of awakening and can be triggered by sleep deprivation, alcohol intake, and stress.[20]

Diagnosis and Ancillary Testing

The interictal EEG demonstrates generalized spike-wave discharges and multifocal fragments of generalized discharges. In a portion of patients, the epileptiform abnormalities may be seen only in sleep. As with JME, neuroimaging should be considered if the description of seizures includes focal features or if epileptiform discharges are consistently seen in one region of the brain.

Treatment

Treatment recommendations are similar to those for JME.

Prognosis

Seizures often remit in IGE-GTC.[21] The development of other seizure types (evolution to a different syndrome) is rare. Most patients become seizure free on medications, and long-term follow-up indicates medications may be discontinued following prolonged seizure-free periods in 75% of affected individuals. In contrast to seizure outcome, adverse social outcomes (eg, learning disabilities, mental health problems, unemployment) are relatively common.

REFERENCES

1. Nordli DR Jr. Special needs of the adolescent with epilepsy. *Epilepsia.* 2001;42(suppl 8):10-17.

2. Raty LK, Wilde-Larsson B, Soderfeldt BA. Seizures and therapy in adolescents with uncomplicated epilepsy. *Seizure.* 2003;12:229-236.

3. Raty LK, Wilde Larsson BM, Soderfeldt BA. Health-related quality of life in youth: a comparison between adolescents and young adults with uncomplicated epilepsy and healthy controls. *J Adolesc Health.* 2003;33:252-258.

4. Smith PE Wallace SJ. Taking over epilepsy from the paediatric neurologist. *J Neurol Neurosurg Psychiatry.* 2003;74(suppl 1): i37-i41.

5. Clark SJ, Beimer NJ, Gebremariam A, et al. Validation of EpiTRAQ, a transition readiness assessment tool for adolescents and young adults with epilepsy. *Epilepsia Open.* 2020;5: 487-495.

6. Drazkowski J. An overview of epilepsy and driving. *Epilepsia.* 2007;48(suppl 9):10-12.

7. Harden CL, Pennell PB. Neuroendocrine considerations in the treatment of men and women with epilepsy. *Lancet Neurol.* 2013;12:72-83.

8. Harden CL, Leppik I. Optimizing therapy of seizures in women who use oral contraceptives. *Neurology.* 2006;67: S56-S58.

9. Harden CL, Meador KJ, Pennell PB, et al. Practice parameter update: management issues for women with epilepsy—focus on pregnancy (an evidence-based review): teratogenesis and perinatal outcomes: report of the Quality Standards Subcommittee and Therapeutics and Technology Assessment Subcommittee of the American Academy of Neurology and American Epilepsy Society. *Neurology.* 2009;73:133-141.

10. Harden CL, Pennell PB, Koppel BS, et al. Practice parameter update: management issues for women with epilepsy—focus on pregnancy (an evidence-based review): vitamin K, folic acid, blood levels, and breastfeeding: report of the Quality Standards Subcommittee and Therapeutics and Technology Assessment Subcommittee of the American Academy of Neurology and American Epilepsy Society. *Neurology.* 2009;73:142-149.

11. Obeid T. Clinical and genetic aspects of juvenile absence epilepsy. *J Neurol.* 1994;241:487-491.

12. Camfield C, Camfield P. Management guidelines for children with idiopathic generalized epilepsy. *Epilepsia.* 2005;46(suppl 9): 112-116.

13. Glauser T, Ben-Menachem E, Bourgeois B, et al. Updated ILAE evidence review of antiepileptic drug efficacy and effectiveness as initial monotherapy for epileptic seizures and syndromes. *Epilepsia.* 2013;54:551-563.

14. Bartolomei F, Suchet L, Barrie M, Gastaut JL. Alcoholic epilepsy: a unified and dynamic classification. *Eur Neurol.* 1997;37:13-17.

15. Trinka E, Baumgartner S, Unterberger I, et al. Long-term prognosis for childhood and juvenile absence epilepsy. *J Neurol.* 2004;251:1235-1241.

16. Duron RM, Medina MT, Martinez-Juarez IE, et al. Seizures of idiopathic generalized epilepsies. *Epilepsia.* 2005;46(suppl 9): 34-47.

17. Camfield CS, Camfield PR. Juvenile myoclonic epilepsy 25 years after seizure onset: a population-based study. *Neurology.* 2009;73:1041-1045.

18. Genton P, Thomas P, Kasteleijn-Nolst Trenite DG, Medina MT, Salas-Puig J. Clinical aspects of juvenile myoclonic epilepsy. *Epilepsy Behav.* 2013;28(suppl 1):S8-14.

19. Baykan B, Martinez-Juarez IE, Altindag EA, Camfield CS, Camfield PR. Lifetime prognosis of juvenile myoclonic epilepsy. *Epilepsy Behav.* 2013;28(suppl 1):S18-24.

20. Unterberger I, Trinka E, Luef G, Bauer G. Idiopathic generalized epilepsies with pure grand mal: clinical data and genetics. *Epilepsy Res.* 2001;44:19-25.

21. Camfield P, Camfield C. Idiopathic generalized epilepsy with generalized tonic-clonic seizures (IGE-GTC): a population-based cohort with >20 year follow up for medical and social outcome. *Epilepsy Behav.* 2010;18:61-63.

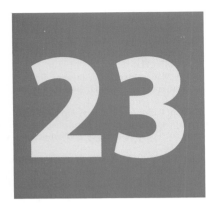

Neurophysiology

Kelly Kremer, MD

INTRODUCTION

An electroencephalogram (EEG) is a test used to detect electrical activity in the brain. It is one test used to help better understand a patient's epilepsy. The EEG signal recorded at the scalp is generated by the summation of neuronal excitatory postsynaptic potentials and inhibitory postsynaptic potentials. Scalp EEG is able to detect radial dipoles from cortical gyri.

DIAGNOSTIC UTILITY OF ELECTROENCEPHALOGRAPHY

Epileptiform activity on EEG is specific but not sensitive for the diagnosis of epilepsy following a paroxysmal event concerning for seizure. The yield of epileptiform abnormalities on initial EEG after a first-time unprovoked seizure or new epilepsy diagnosis in children ranges from 32% to 59%. It has been shown in adults that the sensitivity increases with serial EEGs up to 92% by the fourth EEG.

Interictal epileptiform discharges can be seen in 0.2% to 0.5% of healthy adults and 2% to 4% of healthy children. In one longitudinal study of healthy children, 3.5% were found to have epileptiform discharges. They were followed over 8 to 9 years, and only 5% of them went on to develop epilepsy. All cases were idiopathic generalized epilepsies.

INDICATIONS FOR ELECTROENCEPHALOGRAPHY

▶ Evaluation of First Unprovoked Seizure

Multiple studies have shown that epileptiform discharges or focal slowing on EEG are predictive of seizure recurrence in children who have had their first unprovoked seizure. In one study of children with a single seizure of unknown etiology, 54% of 103 children with an abnormal EEG had seizure recurrence versus 25% of 165 children with a normal EEG.

EEG results should be used in combination with history, neurologic exam, and imaging results to determine the risk for seizure recurrence. EEG can be used to support a diagnosis of seizure and epilepsy and also to help determine seizure type, epilepsy type (focal or generalized), epilepsy syndrome, and seizure recurrence risk. This information can then aid in management and treatment decisions. Therefore, a routine EEG is recommended by the American Academy of Neurology, Child Neurology Society, and American Epilepsy Society after all first unprovoked seizures. EEG abnormalities must be interpreted within the context of each individual patient's presentation, and an EEG should be used to support the clinical diagnosis of seizure, epilepsy, or epilepsy syndrome. An EEG abnormality alone is not sufficient to confirm that an event was an epileptic seizure, nor should a normal EEG be used to exclude the diagnosis. A diagnosis of epilepsy is made either when a patient has had 2 or more unprovoked seizures or when a patient has had a single seizure and has at least a 60% chance of seizure recurrence over the next 10 years.

▶ Determining Epilepsy Type: Focal or Generalized

Generalized interictal epileptiform discharges are frequently seen during a routine EEG in patients who have genetic (idiopathic) generalized epilepsies. Generalized discharges may also be seen in patients who have developmental or epileptic encephalopathies that may be associated with an underlying structural etiology. In genetic generalized epilepsies, normal background activity is seen in conjunction with symmetric, synchronous, typically frontally predominant, generalized spike-and-wave or polyspike-and-wave discharges recurring at 3 Hz or more. Sleep deprivation, photic stimulation, and hyperventilation result in significant activation of interictal epileptiform discharges in genetic generalized epilepsies. In epileptic encephalopathies, diffuse slowing of background activity is seen in conjunction with focal, multifocal, or generalized interictal epileptiform discharges recurring at 2.5 Hz or less.

In focal epilepsies, the EEG may reveal focal slowing and/or focal interictal epileptiform discharges. In adults, the initial EEG showed focal epileptiform discharges in 44% of patients. The yield of EEG in focal epilepsies is related to the epileptogenic zone. Well-localized and lateralized interictal discharges are seen in up to 90% of patients with temporal lobe epilepsy and 60% of patients with frontal lobe epilepsy; however, they are only found in 10% to 15% of patients with parietal lobe epilepsy and 20% of patients with occipital lobe epilepsy. Interictal epileptiform discharges originating in the posterior quadrant are more likely to falsely localize and lateralize.

Identifying the Epileptogenic Zone

Scalp EEG is also used as an initial test to try to identify the epileptogenic zone and irritative zone. There are limitations in recording abnormalities on scalp EEG coming from the insula, frontal-parietal operculum, inferomedial temporal lobe, interhemispheric fissure, orbitofrontal cortex, inferior parietal-occipital cortex, and deep sulcal generators.

Identifying a Specific Epilepsy Syndrome

EEG can also be helpful in identifying a specific epilepsy syndrome, which can aid in treatment decisions. In pediatrics, the epilepsy syndromes most frequently suggested on routine EEG are childhood absence epilepsy (CAE) and benign epilepsy with centrotemporal spikes (BECTS). In CAE, 3-Hz spike-and-wave discharges are seen diffusely with normal background activity. In BECTS, sharp waves and spikes, which are often triphasic, are seen over the right, left, or bilateral centrotemporal head region with a horizontal dipole. These interictal discharges are activated in N1 and N2 sleep.

Determining Whether Therapy Is Effective

EEG can also assist in confirming that antiseizure medication therapy is effective. This is not necessary or recommended in the majority of patients but is beneficial in those who have subtle clinical seizures, particularly absence seizures.

MAXIMIZING YIELD OF ROUTINE ELECTROENCEPHALOGRAPHY

Obtaining both awake and sleep states and including provocative techniques of hyperventilation and photic stimulation are recommended by the American Electroencephalographic Society, American Clinical Neurophysiology Society, and International League Against Epilepsy (ILAE) to increase the yield of routine EEG recordings. Hyperventilation should be included routinely unless there is a medical contraindication (cerebrovascular disease, recent

intracranial hemorrhage, significant cardiopulmonary disease, sickle cell disease or trait, or asthma) or the patient is unable to cooperate. Hyperventilation should be continued for a minimum of 3 minutes. Hyperventilation more frequently provokes generalized seizures, particularly absence seizures and rarely myoclonic seizures. However, one study of patients with focal seizures showed 4.4% had a seizure during hyperventilation. Activation procedures have also been found to precipitate events in patients with psychogenic nonepileptic seizures (PNES).

Photosensitivity is reflected on EEG as a paroxysmal epileptiform response during intermittent photic stimulation. Frequencies of 10 to 20 Hz are most provocative, and therefore, lower flash frequencies should be utilized first. About 5% of patients with epilepsy have a photoparoxysmal response, and the majority of these patients have genetic generalized epilepsy. Photoparoxysmal response can also be found in healthy patients who do not have epilepsy. Epilepsy with eyelid myoclonia (Jeavons syndrome), juvenile myoclonic epilepsy, and genetic generalized epilepsy with generalized tonic-clonic seizures alone are most frequently associated with photosensitivity.

One study that included both children and adults found that an EEG obtained within 24 hours of a seizure was more likely to reveal epileptiform abnormalities (51%) compared to an EEG obtained later (34%). However, EEG interpretation has been found to be more difficult in the immediate postictal period due to diffuse postictal slowing. Therefore, the ideal timing of initial EEG remains unclear.

The reported increased diagnostic yield of sleep-deprived EEG has varied widely (11%-92%). Sleep activation of interictal epileptiform discharges may be seen in about a third of patients with epilepsy and in up to 90% of patients with epilepsies activated by sleep or awakening. This is particularly notable in patients with genetic generalized epilepsies.

ELECTROENCEPHALOGRAPHY IN SPECIAL CIRCUMSTANCES

Status Epilepticus

EEG is highly valuable in assessing for continued electrographic seizures following the resolution of clinical status epilepticus in critically ill patients. In one study of critically ill adults, 48% had continued electrographic seizures and 14% had persistent nonconvulsive status epilepticus following resolution of convulsive status epilepticus.

Neonatal Seizures

Clinician's classification of neonatal seizures based on clinical criteria has been shown to be inaccurate due to multiple factors including subtle or absent clinical manifestations and brief duration of seizures. Nonepileptic paroxysmal movements including tremulousness or jitteriness and myoclonus are also seen frequently in neonates and can be confused for seizures. Therefore, the World Health Organization guideline on neonatal seizures recommends that "where available, all clinical seizures in the neonatal period should be confirmed by electroencephalography."

► Epilepsy Surgery

Scalp EEG recordings have limited spatial resolution, and reliability of localization is higher for convexity foci compared to basal, mesial temporal, or interhemispheric foci; however, its low cost and wide availability increase its utility. While changes are apparent on scalp EEG in 85% to 95% of focal seizures with impairment of consciousness, this is only true for 20% to 30% of focal seizures without impairment of consciousness. This limitation is related to the limited volume of cortex involved in these seizures or the distance from the recording electrodes on the scalp. Localized seizure onsets on scalp EEG are seen more frequently in mesial temporal lobe epilepsy and dorsolateral frontal lobe epilepsy. Parietal and occipital lobe epilepsies are more commonly associated with false localization and lateralization. Approximately one-third of patients with mesial temporal lobe epilepsy have bitemporal spikes on routine scalp EEG, although invasive EEG will demonstrate seizures arising primarily from a single temporal lobe in the majority of cases. In frontal lobe epilepsy, ictal onset is not localizable in more than half of patients. Despite limitations of interictal and ictal scalp EEG, it is recommended as part of the initial evaluation of all patients being evaluated for epilepsy surgery. Intracranial EEG may be required to identify seizure onset with high-frequency oscillations. Intracranial EEG has a higher signal-to-noise ratio and also has high spatial and temporal resolution resulting in improved detection of ictal onset. A focused hypothesis regarding the seizure onset zone is necessary to justify the use of invasive EEG monitoring and create an implantation plan.

► Psychogenic Nonepileptic Seizures

An EEG is recommended by the ILAE as part of the minimum requirements for the diagnosis of PNES. A possible or probable diagnosis of PNES can be established if history and witnessed event (either patient report for possible or clinician review of video for probable) are consistent with PNES and no epileptiform activity is seen on a routine or sleep-deprived interictal EEG. A clinically established or documented diagnosis of PNES requires ictal EEG during a typical event "in which the semiology would make ictal epileptiform EEG activity expectable during equivalent epileptic seizures." It is also important to note that patients may have both PNES and epilepsy, and therefore, each event semiology should be analyzed and classified independently.

OTHER FORMS OF ELECTROENCEPHALOGRAPHY MONITORING

► Long-Term Video EEG/Epilepsy Monitoring Unit

Long-term video EEG monitoring in patients with epilepsy is recommended by the ILAE to clarify seizure type or epilepsy syndrome, quantify seizure frequency, and investigate electroclinical seizure characteristics during epilepsy surgery evaluation. In a study of long-term EEG monitoring in adults, 78% had interictal epileptiform discharges, and of those who had interictal discharges recorded, 96% emerged within 72 hours. In a retrospective review of initial video EEG monitoring in a series of 1000 children suspected to have an epileptic disorder, 32% had successful classification of epilepsy and 22% had successful capture and diagnosis of nonepileptic events, whereas 24% had a normal EEG with no events captured and 22% had an inconclusive EEG (either no habitual events were captured but EEG was abnormal or habitual events were captured but could not be proved or disproved to be epileptic). A specific epilepsy syndrome was diagnosed in 54% of children who had successful classification of epilepsy. The mean monitoring duration was 1.5 days, and 53% of patients had habitual events captured. Longer monitoring improved the rate of successful classification of epilepsy in all age groups.

Antiseizure medications are frequently decreased during video EEG monitoring to increase the likelihood of capturing habitual events. Practices for antiseizure medication reduction are quite variable across epilepsy centers, and standardized protocols do not exist. Studies in adults have shown rapid taper of antiseizure medication in combination with sleep deprivation was safe and reduced time in the epilepsy monitoring unit. Recent proposed ILAE guidelines for the minimum standards for long-term video EEG monitoring recommended that "in patients without a history of status epilepticus or frequent daily seizures a taper of 30-50% daily should be considered."

► Ambulatory EEG

Ambulatory EEG monitoring is less expensive than inpatient video EEG monitoring and also allows assessment of the patient in their home environment with exposure to personal environmental triggers. According to ILAE guidelines, prolonged EEG is recommended when the diagnosis of epilepsy or the classification of epilepsy syndrome remains unclear after routine EEG. In one study of 62 patients that included both children and adults, an ambulatory EEG following a nondiagnostic epilepsy monitoring unit stay provided clinically useful information in 48.4% of cases allowing for the classification of events as epileptic or nonepileptic.

ROLE OF ELECTROENCEPHALOGRAPHY IN PROGNOSIS AND MEDICATION WITHDRAWAL

Estimates of seizure recurrence following antiseizure medication withdrawal vary widely from less than 10% to nearly 70%. Multiple factors are considered when attempting to predict this risk for an individual patient including whether their EEG remains abnormal. In a meta-analysis reviewing relapse following discontinuation of antiepileptic drugs, overall, the risk of relapse was 25% at 1 year and 29% at 2 years. Factors found to be associated with an increased relative risk of relapse included epilepsy of adolescent and adult onset compared to childhood onset, remote symptomatic seizures (seizures in patients who had either static encephalopathy before seizure onset or a prior neurologic insult) compared to idiopathic seizures, and abnormal EEG. The relative risk of recurrence with an abnormal EEG was 1.45. Abnormal EEG in this analysis included any abnormality (epileptiform and nonepileptiform abnormalities were not distinguished).

BIBLIOGRAPHY

American Electroencephalographic Society. Guideline one: minimum technical requirements for performing clinical electroencephalography. *J Clin Neurophysiol.* 1994;11(1):2-5.

Asano E, Pawlak C, Shah A, et al. The diagnostic value of initial video-EEG monitoring in children—review of 1000 cases. *Epilepsy Res.* 2005;66(1-3):129-135. doi:10.1016/j.eplepsyres.2005.07.012

Baldin E, Hauser WA, Buchhalter JR, Hesdorffer DC, Ottman R. Yield of epileptiform electroencephalogram abnormalities in incident unprovoked seizures: a population-based study. *Epilepsia.* 2014;55(9):1389-1398. doi:10.1111/epi.12720

Berg AT, Shinnar S. Relapse following discontinuation of antiepileptic drugs: a meta-analysis. *Neurology.* 1994;44(4):601-608. doi:10.1212/wnl.44.4.601

Camfield PR, Camfield CS, Dooley JM, Tibbles JA, Fung T, Garner B. Epilepsy after a first unprovoked seizure in childhood. *Neurology.* 1985;35(11):1657-1660. doi:10.1212/wnl.35.11.1657

Cavazzuti GB, Cappella L, Nalin A. Longitudinal study of epileptiform EEG patterns in normal children. *Epilepsia.* 1980;21(1):43-55. doi:10.1111/j.1528-1157.1980.tb04043.x

DeLorenzo RJ, Waterhouse EJ, Towne AR, et al. Persistent nonconvulsive status epilepticus after the control of convulsive status epilepticus. *Epilepsia.* 1998;39(8):833-840. doi:10.1111/j.1528-1157.1998.tb01177.x

Fisher RS, Acevedo C, Arzimanoglou A, et al. ILAE official report: a practical clinical definition of epilepsy. *Epilepsia.* 2014;55(4):475-482. doi:10.1111/epi.12550

Fox J, Ajinkya S, Chopade P, Schmitt S. The diagnostic utility of ambulatory EEG following nondiagnostic epilepsy monitoring unit admissions. *J Clin Neurophysiol.* 2019;36(2):146-149. doi:10.1097/WNP.0000000000000559

Hirtz D, Ashwal S, Berg A, et al. Practice parameter: evaluating a first nonfebrile seizure in children: report of the quality standards subcommittee of the American Academy of Neurology, the Child Neurology Society, and the American Epilepsy Society. *Neurology.* 2000;55(5):616-623. doi:10.1212/wnl.55.5.616

International League Against Epilepsy. Proposed guideline: minimum standards for long-term video-EEG monitoring. Accessed June 22, 2022. https://www.ilae.org/guidelines/guidelines-and-reports/proposed-guideline-minimum-standards-for-long-term-video-eeg-monitoring

Jayakar P, Gaillard WD, Tripathi M, et al. Diagnostic test utilization in evaluation for resective epilepsy surgery in children. *Epilepsia.* 2014;55(4):507-518. doi:10.1111/epi.12544

King MA, Newton MR, Jackson GD, et al. Epileptology of the first-seizure presentation: a clinical, electroencephalographic, and magnetic resonance imaging study of 300 consecutive patients. *Lancet.* 1998;352(9133):1007-1011. doi:10.1016/S0140-6736(98)03543-0

LaFrance WC Jr, Baker GA, Duncan R, Goldstein LH, Reuber M. Minimum requirements for the diagnosis of psychogenic nonepileptic seizures: a staged approach: a report from the International League Against Epilepsy Nonepileptic Seizures Task Force. *Epilepsia.* 2013;54(11):2005-2018. doi:10.1111/epi.12356

Martinović Z, Jović N. Seizure recurrence after a first generalized tonic-clonic seizure, in children, adolescents and young adults. *Seizure.* 1997;6(6):461-465. doi:10.1016/s1059-1311(97)80021-0

Salinsky M, Kanter R, Dasheiff RM. Effectiveness of multiple EEGs in supporting the diagnosis of epilepsy: an operational curve. *Epilepsia.* 1987;28(4):331-334. doi:10.1111/j.1528-1157.1987.tb03652.x

Shinnar S, Berg AT, O'Dell C, Newstein D, Moshe SL, Hauser WA. Predictors of multiple seizures in a cohort of children prospectively followed from the time of their first unprovoked seizure. *Ann Neurol.* 2000;48(2):140-147.

Shinnar S, Kang H, Berg AT, Goldensohn ES, Hauser WA, Moshé SL. EEG abnormalities in children with a first unprovoked seizure. *Epilepsia.* 1994;35(3):471-476. doi:10.1111/j.1528-1157.1994.tb02464.x

Stroink H, Brouwer OF, Arts WF, Geerts AT, Peters AC, van Donselaar CA. The first unprovoked, untreated seizure in childhood: a hospital based study of the accuracy of the diagnosis, rate of recurrence, and long term outcome after recurrence. Dutch Study of Epilepsy in Childhood. *J Neurol Neurosurg Psychiatry.* 1998;64(5):595-600. doi:10.1136/jnnp.64.5.595

Tatum WO, Rubboli G, Kaplan PW, et al. Clinical utility of EEG in diagnosing and monitoring epilepsy in adults. *Clin Neurophysiol.* 2018;129(5):1056-1082. doi:10.1016/j.clinph.2018.01.019

Verma A, Radtke R. EEG of partial seizures. *J Clin Neurophysiol.* 2006;23(4):333-339. doi:10.1097/01.wnp.0000228497.89734.7a

Werhahn KJ, Hartl E, Hamann K, Breimhorst M, Noachtar S. Latency of interictal epileptiform discharges in long-term EEG recordings in epilepsy patients. *Seizure.* 2015;29:20-25. doi:10.1016/j.seizure.2015.03.012

World Health Organization. *Guidelines on Neonatal Seizures.* World Health Organization; 2011.

Zivin L, Marsan CA. Incidence and prognostic significance of "epileptiform" activity in the EEG of non-epileptic subjects. *Brain.* 1968;91(4):751-778. doi:10.1093/brain/91.4.751

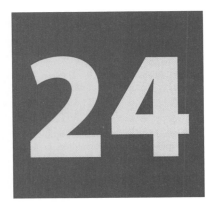

A Review of Magnetoencephalography

Clifford S. Calley, MD
Jeffrey R. Tenney, MD, PhD

INTRODUCTION

Magnetoencephalography (MEG) is a noninvasive method used to directly measure and localize brain activity. Since the first MEG signal was recorded by Bruce Cohen in 1968 using a single sensor, the technique has evolved to include whole-head arrays with over 300 sensors. This allows for greater detection and localization of brain activity due to an improved signal-to-noise ratio and established MEG as a clinically useful technique. As a result, there are now more than 25 MEG centers in the United States alone, with an estimated 750 MEG scans performed in 2016.[1]

PHYSICS AND TECHNICAL REQUIREMENTS

▶ Neuronal Generation of Magnetic Fields and Their Propagation

Individual neurons produce an electrical current when firing, known as an action potential, which is a critical component in neuronal signaling. When neurons fire synchronously, the resulting activity is summated into large-scale electrical currents that can propagate beyond the site of origin and be detected by electrodes on the scalp. However, due to the electrical resistivity of tissues through which the electrical currents must pass (eg, cerebrospinal fluid, dura, skull), the signal intensity is significantly reduced once detected by scalp electrodes.[2,3] This represents the basic concept of electroencephalography (EEG) and is important in understanding the foundational differences between EEG and MEG.

A fundamental component of any electrical current is that it also produces a magnetic field, and the changes in magnetic fields produced by active neurons can also be detected on the scalp, which represent the basic concept of MEG. Unlike electrical fields, however, the properties of magnetic fields are such that intervening tissues offer very little resistance, and this allows for signal detection with minimal distortion or attenuation relative to EEG.[4-6] Another relevant difference between these modalities is that EEG is thought to be sensitive to activity generated by neurons oriented both perpendicular (ie, within the base of sulci and crowns of gyri) and parallel (ie, within gyri) to the scalp, whereas MEG is most sensitive to parallel-oriented neurons (within the walls of the gyri).[6]

▶ Detection of Magnetic Fields by Magnetometers

The intrinsic magnetic flux generated by active neurons is measured by MEG via sensors referred to as superconducting quantum interference devices (SQUIDs), which consist of detection coils capable of sensing extremely small magnetic fluctuations. As a reference of scale, SQUIDs can detect field strengths as small as 10 to 250 femtotesla, or one-billionth the strength of the earth's magnetic field.

SQUIDs can record 1 data point per millisecond and so are equal in temporal resolution to the high sampling rate of EEG. When displayed as a function of time, MEG recordings appear very similar to EEG waveforms (Figure 24–1). Functional magnetic resonance imaging (MRI), as a comparison, has a sampling rate of 1 to 2 seconds. The spatial resolution of MEG is within a few millimeters and far superior to EEG, although research using high-density EEG arrays has sought to improve upon the poor spatial resolution of standard EEG. Regarding sensitivity, about 4 to 6 cm^2 of synchronized neuronal firing is needed for one SQUID to detect this activity, compared to 6 to 10 cm^2 necessary for EEG.[6]

For SQUIDs to detect such small magnetic fluctuations via superconduction, or negligible electrical resistance, they must be supercooled. This is achieved by continuous immersion of the detection coils in liquid helium and consequently contributes to many of MEG's limitations. The liquid helium must be replaced every few days, which adds significantly to operational costs. Newer MEG systems offer the ability

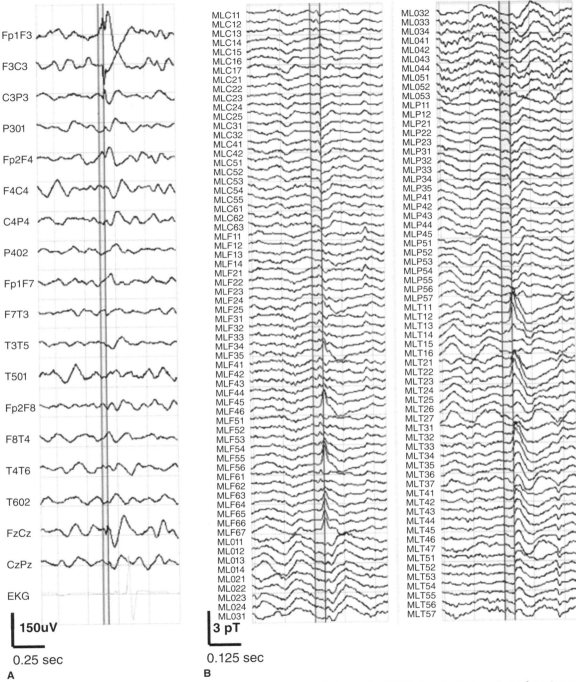

▲ Figure 24–1. Electroencephalogram (EEG) and magnetoencephalography (MEG) signals displayed as a function of time. Raw EEG tracing **(A)** in longitudinal bipolar montage showing a left frontal epileptiform discharge, and raw MEG tracing **(B)** showing the relevant left-sided sensors. The shaded areas show the window used for subsequent source analysis.

to collect and recycle the helium that is continuously lost, thus limiting the need for helium replacement. Due to the need for cooling, the SQUIDs cannot be placed directly on the scalp, which would minimize the distance between source signals and sensors and greatly improve the signal-to-noise ratio. They must be placed into fixed arrays, and this prevents custom placement of sensors to optimally fit individual patients. Some MEG systems allow for the standard MEG sensor array to be exchanged as needed for a smaller array that is optimized for infants. Standard MEG arrays also include numerous sensors (200 to >300), which is another reason MEG offers superior source localization. EEG can also be concurrently recorded as there is room for electrodes between the patient's scalp and the MEG array.

Basics of Shielding and Artifact Reduction

Due to the necessity of magnetometers to detect magnetic fluctuations that are orders of magnitude smaller than those found in the surrounding environment, MEG systems must be operated within a shielded environment, and a magnetically shielded room (MSR) is the most common solution.[7] The cost of construction and the space needed to house the MSR are other reasons why MEG is not more widely available. The location of the MSR must be carefully considered to minimize the electromagnetic noise from the local environment (eg, elevators, MRI machines, medical equipment), as well as sources of noise that may be brought into the MRS including cell phones, dental implants, and implanted medical devices such as vagal nerve stimulators.

Patient movement during MEG data acquisition is a source of artifact due to the inability of sensors to be placed directly on the scalp. This means that the head may move independently from the sensor locations within the MEG array, and even minor adjustments by the patient may render subsequent data unusable. As a result, the patient's head must be carefully secured and made comfortable to minimize movement through the duration of the recording since acceptable recordings typically require less than 5 mm of movement.[7]

This is a significant problem in the pediatric population and not dissimilar to MRI acquisition, where a well-trained staff is necessary to prepare the patient and troubleshoot movement-related problems in real time. When behavioral/environmental tactics fail to adequately minimize movement, some centers rely on pharmacologic sedation to reduce movement, which requires an anesthesiologist to maximize patient safety. In this scenario, the choice of sedation is important to minimize movement but not suppress brain activity or the epileptic spikes of interest.[8]

SOURCE ESTIMATION

Once the data are collected, MEG relies on the use of sophisticated mathematical modeling and a well-trained clinician to guide the analysis.[7,9] Based on the raw MEG signal, specific time points are selected that usually contain noted abnormalities in spontaneous brain activity such as epileptiform discharges or evoked responses that were triggered by the delivery of a stimulus to the patient. Once a time point is selected, computer algorithms process the collected signals from each sensor and provide an estimate of the source signal within the brain, a process commonly referred to as source estimation. Two components are required to proceed with source estimation: a head model and a source model (discussed in further detail below). The result of this process is an estimation of location, strength, and orientation of current at the selected time point, although other estimates are available.

Inverse and Forward Problem

Conceptually, source estimates cannot be definitive as the true source of the signal is not known. This is mostly due to the noninvasive nature of MEG (ie, the separation of the intracranial source signal from the external magnetometers). This limitation can be addressed by approaching the unknown source in 1 of 2 ways: processes described as the "forward" problem and "inverse" problem.[10] Briefly, the forward problem involves estimating the intracranial current sources that produce a given electromagnetic field and then extrapolating the resultant magnetic field. This approach is considered well posed given that the outcome is constrained to one unique solution. However, the inverse problem involves working backward from the recorded magnetic field to estimate all the possible brain sources that could produce such a result. This is considered an ill-posed approach because an infinite number of possible sources could theoretically generate any given result.

Head Modeling

One straightforward way to improve the source estimation is to provide a realistic model of the head. As described earlier, the propagation of currents from an intracranial source to the extracranial sensors is impacted by the tissues through which the currents must pass. Therefore, any information about the conductivity of the intervening space between the source and the sensor can be used in the statistical model to provide more accurate estimations. The 2 most common head models used in MEG are the spherical model and boundary element model (BEM).

Spherical models are the most basic and efficient. Based on patient head imaging or simple external measurements like head circumference, concentric spheres are used to approximate the multiple layers of tissue, with each sphere having its own conductivity approximating that of the corresponding tissue. This model is acceptable for most clinical applications, allows for faster processing, and generates smaller files, which can be stored more efficiently. BEM more closely approximates the patient's head, which is generally derived from the patient's brain MRI. Instead of concentric spheres, BEM uses a process similar to voxel-based morphometry employed in MRI. Each boundary contour between tissues is mapped using parcellated nonoverlapping triangles and assigned an appropriate conductivity for use in the source estimation. This results in significantly improved accuracy relative to spherical modeling but at the expense of processing speed and storage space.

Source Modeling

Once a head model is established, a source model is needed that acts as a simulated current generator that "propagates through" the head model and provides estimates of the true source current. The source model can be set as a single or limited number of current generators, which constrains the source estimation result to a single point within the brain (discrete model), or set as multiple current generators, which allows for a broader estimation of active neurons that contribute to the source current (distributed model). As an example, a clinician may choose a discrete model if they assume that the interictal discharges recorded during the MEG session are focal in origin, as opposed to being generated by a more spatially distributed volume of gray matter.

Discrete modeling is the most common form used in source estimation and is represented best by the equivalent current dipole (ECD) model (Figure 24–2).[10] This widespread acceptance of ECD is likely derived from the preponderance of MEG studies used in epileptic patients to model interictal spikes and thus estimate the seizure-onset zone.

Importantly, the ECD is not a true electrophysiologic product of active neurons but rather a mathematical construct that allows source estimation models to generate a solution to the forward problem that includes a location, orientation, strength, and direction of the source current(s).

Beamformer modeling is another form of source estimation worth mentioning. This involves "tuning" the magnetometers within the MEG array to preferentially record signal from individual voxels sequentially, thus creating "virtual waveforms" that can then be interpreted similar to raw MEG. The voxel locations can be determined a priori by the clinician based on region of interest or simply run as a whole-brain analysis.

CLINICAL APPLICATIONS

Source Localization for Epilepsy

The primary use of MEG is in patients with drug-resistant epilepsy who are undergoing presurgical evaluation and is considered underutilized due to the established evidence of MEG contributing to improved surgical outcomes.[2,3,11,12] This is achieved primarily by providing noninvasive data (phase I testing), which is then used for improved targeting of the seizure onset zone during invasive monitoring (phase II testing).

The MEG data acquired during phase I testing is typically only one modality of a comprehensive presurgical evaluation, which, if indicated, also includes some combination of EEG, positron emission tomography, single-photon

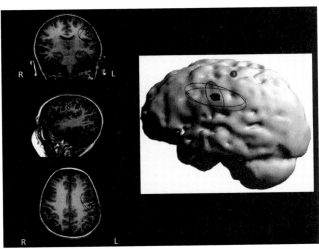

▲ **Figure 24–2.** Example of equivalent current dipole modeling (ECD). Six-year-old girl with intractable localization-related epilepsy. ECD with confidence interval shown superimposed on coronal, sagittal, and axial brain magnetic resonance imaging slices (*left*) and a 3-dimensional reconstruction of the cortical surface (*right*). The purple dot on the 3-dimensional reconstruction indicates the sensory evoked field location via stimulation of the right median nerve. L, left; R, right.

Table 24–1. Comparison of noninvasive source-localizing modalities.

Method	Strengths	Limitations
MEG	• Direct measurement of neuronal activity • Temporal resolution: milliseconds • Spatial resolution: millimeters/centimeters • Magnetic field not attenuated by surrounding tissues • Concurrent use with EEG • Use of evoked potentials to map eloquent cortex	• Cost and maintenance • Need epileptiform activity for localization • Diminished signal from deep structures • Fixed array size • Patient needs to lie still; sometimes needs sedation • Sensitive to artifact
EEG	• Direct measurement of neuronal activity • Temporal resolution: milliseconds • Use of evoked potentials to map eloquent cortex • Portable • Low cost	• Need epileptiform activity for localization • Spatial resolution: centimeters • Diminished signal from deep structures
PET	• Does not require epileptiform activity for localization • Spatial resolution: millimeters • Localization in deep structures	• Indirect measurement of neuronal activity (metabolism) • Temporal resolution: minutes • Radiation exposure via injection and potential associated side effects • Patient needs to lie still; sometimes needs sedation • High cost
SPECT	• Does not require epileptiform activity for localization • Localization in deep structures • SISCOM allows for localization of ictal activity	• Indirect measurement of neuronal activity (blood flow) • Temporal resolution: minutes • Spatial resolution: centimeters • Patient needs to lie still; sometimes needs sedation • SISCOM requires 2 CT scans separated by at least 24 hours, including ictal activity for localization. Ictal activity must be identified within seconds of onset. • Radiation exposure • Short half-life of radioactive tracer requires a limited time window for acquisition • Low cost

CT, computed tomography; EEG, electroencephalogram; MEG, pagnetoencephalography; PET, positron emission tomography; SISCOM, single-photon emission computed tomography coregistered to magnetic resonance imaging; SPECT, single-photon emission computed tomography.

emission computed tomography, functional MRI, and transcranial magnetic stimulation (Table 24–1). These tests can be collected during a single admission at a comprehensive epilepsy center, or the patient can be referred to other centers where desired testing is available. This allows epilepsy surgical centers without MEG to benefit from the modality. The data can be collected and results sent to the managing providers to be used with other acquired modalities.[14] Ordering an MEG should be considered for any patient undergoing phase I testing, and MEG has validated utility in many specific scenarios (Table 24–2).[2,11,12,14-19]

Once the MEG data are collected and analyzed, a report is generated and sent to the ordering physician. This includes examples of epileptic spikes seen on MEG and concurrent EEG, if acquired, and the source localization results that were modeled from the epileptic spikes. A written interpretation of the results is provided by the MEG physician including estimates of confidence in the localization. Digital copies of the data also accompany the report, which can be used by the surgical team to include in their surgical mapping software.

▶ Localization of Eloquent Cortex

Other than its use in localizing the seizure onset zone, MEG can also provide clinically relevant data to aid in the identification of eloquent cortex.[14] This is primarily achieved using evoked potentials, which represent the cerebral processing of a specific sensory modality introduced as a stimulus during the MEG recording. The most common clinical application of evoked potentials is the localization of primary sensory cortex by repeatedly stimulating the median nerve with an electrical current. Stimulation at the wrist travels to the contralateral primary sensory cortex where the resulting neuronal activity can be localized via source estimation much like with epileptiform discharges. This can similarly be achieved with other sensory modalities, and the resultant identification of eloquent cortex can be used during surgical planning including assessing the risks and benefits.

Other commonly tested modalities include auditory, visual, and motor. MEG is also used in a similar fashion for language lateralization. This is done by using specific

Table 24–2. Indications for ordering a presurgical magnetoencephalography (MEG).

• Nonlesional or "MRI-negative" cases, especially if a mesial temporal onset is suspected • Large lesion is seen on MRI • Multilesional cases such as tuberous sclerosis where a primary seizure onset zone is suspected • Evaluation for reoperation due to previous surgical failure	• Intrasylvian or insular seizure onset is suspected • EEG-negative cases where no abnormal discharges are seen • Those with nonlateralized findings on EEG such as bilateral or generalized discharges • Any patient with an imprecise hypothesis for seizure onset

EEG, electroencephalogram; MRI, magnetic resonance imaging.

paradigms to engage a patient's receptive and expressive language skills during an MEG scan and then employing similar source estimation techniques as described above. Importantly, localization of these eloquent cortices by MEG can be ordered for surgical planning in cases other than seizure-focus resection. This is commonly utilized in tumor resection planning.[12]

SUMMARY

MEG is a well-validated clinical tool for defining the zone of irritability and determining the location of eloquent cortices. The results of source analysis are useful for providing targets for subsequent invasive EEG monitoring and neurosurgical planning. It has become a crucial part of presurgical evaluation and leads to improved seizure outcomes for patients with drug-resistant epilepsy.

REFERENCES

1. American Clinical Magnetoencephalography Society. Magnetoencephalography sites across the United States. Accessed June 22, 2022. https://www.acmegs.org/center-directory/
2. Kharkar S, Knowlton R. Magnetoencephalography in the presurgical evaluation of epilepsy. *Epilepsy Behav.* 2015;46:19-26. doi:10.1016/j.yebeh.2014.11.029
3. Pataraia E, Simos PG, Castillo EM, et al. Does magnetoencephalography add to scalp video-EEG as a diagnostic tool in epilepsy surgery? *Neurology.* 2004;62(6):943-948. doi:10.1212/01.wnl.0000115122.81621.fe
4. Goldenholz DM, Ahlfors SP, Hämäläinen MS, et al. Mapping the signal-to-noise-ratios of cortical sources in magnetoencephalography and electroencephalography. *Hum Brain Mapp.* 2009;30(4):1077-1086. doi:10.1002/hbm.20571
5. Leahy RM, Mosher JC, Spencer ME, Huang MX, Lewine JD. A study of dipole localization accuracy for MEG and EEG using a human skull phantom. *Electroencephalogr Clin Neurophysiol.* 1998;107(2):159-173. doi:10.1016/s0013-4694(98)00057-1
6. Malmivuo J, Suihko V, Eskola H. Sensitivity distributions of EEG and MEG measurements. *IEEE Trans Biomed Eng.* 1997;44(3):196-208. doi:10.1109/10.554766
7. Bagić AI, Knowlton RC, Rose DF, Ebersole JS, American Clinical Magnetoencephalography Society Clinical Practice Guideline Committee. American Clinical Magnetoencephalography Society Clinical Practice Guideline 1: recording and analysis of spontaneous cerebral activity. *J Clin Neurophysiol.* 2011;28(4):348-354. doi:10.1097/WNP.0b013e3182272fed
8. Tenney JR, Miller JW, Rose DF. Intranasal dexmedetomidine for sedation during magnetoencephalography. *J Clin Neurophysiol.* 2019;36(5):371-374. doi:10.1097/WNP.0000000000000602
9. Bagić AI, Barkley GL, Rose DF, Ebersole JS, American Clinical Magnetoencephalography Society Clinical Practice Guideline Committee. American Clinical Magnetoencephalography Society Clinical Practice Guideline 4: qualifications of MEG-EEG personnel. *J Clin Neurophysiol.* 2011;28(4):364-365. doi:10.1097/WNO.0b013e3181cde4dc
10. Tenney JR, Fujiwara H, Rose DF. The value of source localization for clinical magnetoencephalography: beyond the equivalent current dipole. *J Clin Neurophysiol.* 2020;37(6):537-544.
11. Bagic A, Funke ME, Ebersole J, ACMEGS Position Statement Committee. American Clinical MEG Society (ACMEGS) position statement: the value of magnetoencephalography (MEG)/magnetic source imaging (MSI) in noninvasive presurgical evaluation of patients with medically intractable localization-related epilepsy. *J Clin Neurophysiol.* 2009;26(4):290-293. doi:10.1097/WNP.0b013e3181b49d50
12. Stefan H, Rampp S, Knowlton RC. Magnetoencephalography adds to the surgical evaluation process. *Epilepsy Behav.* 2011;20(2):172-177. doi:10.1016/j.yebeh.2010.09.011
13. Bagić AI, Knowlton RC, Rose DF, Ebersole JS, ACMEGS Clinical Practice Guideline Committee. American Clinical Magnetoencephalography Society Clinical Practice Guideline 3: MEG-EEG reporting. *J Clin Neurophysiol.* 2011;28(4):362-363. doi:10.1097/WNO.0b013e3181cde4ad
14. Burgess RC, Funke ME, Bowyer SM, et al. American Clinical Magnetoencephalography Society Clinical Practice Guideline 2: presurgical functional brain mapping using magnetic evoked fields. *J Clin Neurophysiol.* 2011;28(4):355-361. doi:10.1097/WNP.0b013e3182272ffe
15. Knowlton RC. Can magnetoencephalography aid epilepsy surgery? *Epilepsy Curr.* 2008;8(1):1-5. doi:10.1111/j.1535-7511.2007.00215.x
16. Knowlton RC, Razdan SN, Limdi N, et al. Effect of epilepsy magnetic source imaging on intracranial electrode placement. *Ann Neurol.* 2009;65(6):716-723. doi:10.1002/ana.21660
17. Ossenblok P, de Munck JC, Colon A, Drolsbach W, Boon P. Magnetoencephalography is more successful for screening and localizing frontal lobe epilepsy than electroencephalography. *Epilepsia.* 2007;48(11):2139-2149. doi:10.1111/j.1528-1167.2007.01223.x
18. Rampp S, Stefan H, Wu X, et al. Magnetoencephalography for epileptic focus localization in a series of 1000 cases. *Brain.* 2019;142(10):3059-3071. doi:10.1093/brain/awz231
19. Yoshinaga H, Nakahori T, Ohtsuka Y, et al. Benefit of simultaneous recording of EEG and MEG in dipole localization. *Epilepsia.* 2002;43(8):924-928. doi:10.1046/j.1528-1157.2002.42901.x

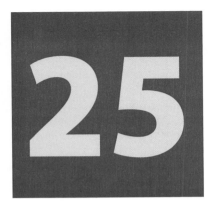

Status Epilepticus

Krista Grande, MD
Katherine Holland, MD, PhD

ESSENTIALS OF DIAGNOSIS AND TYPICAL FEATURES

▶ Status epilepticus is a life-threatening neurologic emergency.

▶ Status epilepticus was traditionally defined as a seizure (or multiple seizures without full recovery of consciousness between seizures) lasting 30 minutes or longer, but the definition has been revised to encourage treatment of prolonged seizures within 5-10 minutes.

▶ Etiology varies by age. The most common cause of status epilepticus in children under 5 years is febrile seizure.

▶ Diagnostic evaluation may include routine blood work, lumbar puncture, neuroimaging, electroencephalogram, and antiseizure medication levels, depending on the circumstances under which status epilepticus occurs.

▶ Several guidelines have been developed for treatment of status epilepticus. First-line treatment involves administration of a benzodiazepine, whereas loading doses of other anticonvulsants are used for seizures that do not terminate with initial benzodiazepine use.

▶ Prognosis is dependent on underlying etiology.

INTRODUCTION

This chapter will cover pediatric status epilepticus, including its epidemiology, etiology, treatment, and outcomes. Special attention will be paid to febrile status epilepticus and neonatal status epilepticus, which have different prognoses and, in the case of neonatal status epilepticus, different treatment.

EPIDEMIOLOGY

Status epilepticus is the most common pediatric neurologic emergency, affecting an estimated 3 to 42 per 100,000 children annually worldwide based on several population-based studies.[1] The true incidence may be higher, as nonconvulsive status epilepticus may go unrecognized or unreported. One study of 236 comatose patients of all ages with no overt signs of seizure showed that 8% of these patients met criteria for status epilepticus on electroencephalogram (EEG).[2] Another study of 550 children in the intensive care unit undergoing EEG monitoring found that 30% of them had electrographic seizures, and of the children with electrographic seizures, 36% had electrographic status epilepticus.[3] In addition, intermittent seizures without return to full consciousness may not initially be recognized as status epilepticus.

Status epilepticus occurs most commonly at the extremes of age. Studies of status epilepticus in children have consistently found that younger children are more susceptible.[4-6] One study that included 364 children aged 1 month to 16 years found that children under the age of 2 years made up almost 50% of cases of status epilepticus in this population.[4] This may be due to increased susceptibility to seizures in the developing brain,[7] a higher incidence of acute symptomatic causes of seizures in young children, or the contribution of febrile status epilepticus to these figures.

CLINICAL FEATURES

Status epilepticus may be classified broadly into convulsive and nonconvulsive status epilepticus based on whether or not there is prominent motor involvement.[8] Convulsive status epilepticus is defined by prominent motor features. The most common type of status epilepticus in children is generalized convulsive status epilepticus, which may be either primarily generalized or focal onset evolving to generalized.[9]

Other types of status epilepticus with prominent motor features, including simple focal motor status epilepticus and myoclonic status epilepticus, while also considered to be convulsive forms of status epilepticus, have different etiologic considerations, treatment, or prognosis and are not discussed here. Nonconvulsive status epilepticus includes absence status epilepticus, focal status epilepticus without motor features with or without impairment of consciousness, and status epilepticus with coma with subtle additional features or without additional features.[8] Most status epilepticus management protocols apply to convulsive status epilepticus. Of note, convulsive status epilepticus may rarely evolve into nonconvulsive status epilepticus. EEG should be considered in patients who do not regain consciousness after cessation of convulsions, as well as in patients with unexplained coma.

In 2015, the International League Against Epilepsy (ILAE) revised its definition of status epilepticus to include 2 time points, t1 and t2.[8] t1 represents the time after which a seizure is considered prolonged due to "failure of the mechanisms responsible for seizure termination or from the initiation of mechanisms that lead to abnormally prolonged seizures,"[8] and t2 is the time point at which long-term consequences can occur. t1 and t2 vary based on type of seizure. For generalized tonic-clonic seizures, t1 is 5 minutes and t2 is 30 minutes. This is because if a seizure continues beyond 5 minutes, it is less likely to self-resolve and has a higher risk of continuing to the point of neurologic injury.[10] In addition, treatment becomes more difficult after this time point. Time points are less clear for other types of status epilepticus, but the ILAE suggests a t1 of 10 minutes and a t2 of 60 minutes for focal seizures with impaired consciousness and a t1 of 10 to 15 minutes for absence seizures.[8] For practical purposes, initiation of treatment is recommended at the t1 time: 5 minutes for generalized convulsive seizures and 10 minutes for focal seizures with impaired awareness.

ETIOLOGY

Status epilepticus in childhood can be classified broadly according to etiology into febrile, acute symptomatic, remote symptomatic, acute on remote symptomatic, idiopathic epilepsy related, cryptogenic epilepsy related, and unclassified status epilepticus.[11] Etiology is highly related to age. Most status epilepticus in children under the age of 5 years occurs in neurologically typical children without a history of seizures.[4] In children younger than 5 years, febrile seizures are the single most common cause of status epilepticus, accounting for 40% of status epilepticus.[6] Acute symptomatic seizures are also common in this age group, particularly in children younger than 1 year. The most common acute symptomatic cause of status epilepticus in children is central nervous system (CNS) infection.[12] In contrast, most status epilepticus in older children occurs in neurologically impaired children with a history of prior seizures.[4] Approximately 10% of children with epilepsy will have at least one episode of status epilepticus following their diagnosis.[13] Risk factors for status epilepticus in children with epilepsy include prior history of status epilepticus, younger age of onset, and symptomatic etiology.[13]

EVALUATION

In 2006, the American Academy of Neurology (AAN) published a practice parameter for the diagnostic evaluation of children with status epilepticus.[12] Of note, this guideline excluded children with febrile status epilepticus and refractory status epilepticus. The authors reviewed data regarding blood culture, lumbar puncture, antiseizure medication levels, metabolic and genetic testing, toxicology, and imaging.

Acute symptomatic causes of status epilepticus are common. Studies have reported an average 6% diagnostic yield of electrolyte and glucose testing.[12] Studies in which blood culture and lumbar puncture were done selectively for evaluation of children with status epilepticus and fever or presumed infection found that 2.5% of children had a positive blood culture and 12.8% had a CNS infection.[12] Based on these data, the authors of the AAN practice parameter concluded that there was insufficient data to recommend either blood culture or lumbar puncture on a routine basis in children with status epilepticus. Ingestion is a rare but important cause of status epilepticus, reported in 1% to 5% of cases, and serum toxicology studies are recommended in children with status epilepticus of unknown etiology.[12]

Imaging may reveal a remote symptomatic etiology of status epilepticus or, less frequently, an acute symptomatic etiology. Imaging abnormalities have been found in a significant percentage of patients presenting with status epilepticus. In a study of 144 children with status epilepticus of at least 20 minutes who had neuroimaging evaluation with either head computed tomography, magnetic resonance imaging, or both as part of their etiologic evaluation, 30% had an imaging abnormality.[14] The most common imaging abnormalities identified in this cohort included cortical dysgenesis and inborn errors of metabolism, followed by remote vascular insults. Ten percent had acute imaging abnormalities. Therefore, neuroimaging should be considered for etiologic evaluation of status epilepticus with an unknown etiology once the child has been stabilized.

When initial evaluation fails to find a cause for status epilepticus, genetic or metabolic testing may be considered, and findings may change management. In a series of 276 children with refractory status epilepticus, 46% of the patients who had an unknown etiology at presentation had an etiology identified at later follow-up, the most frequent of which was genetic (43%).[15] In particular, status epilepticus associated with unexplained neonatal encephalopathy, unexplained developmental delay, and neurologic dysfunction that worsens significantly during acute illness should prompt evaluation for genetic and metabolic disorders. Dravet syndrome is an important cause of childhood status epilepticus, and sodium channel blockers may worsen seizures in this population.[16] Pyridoxine-dependent epilepsy is refractory to typical antiseizure medications but responds to large doses of pyridoxine.[17] In children with epilepsy associated with *POLG* mutations, valproic acid may precipitate acute liver failure.[18]

In children with known epilepsy presenting with status epilepticus, antiseizure medication levels have been reported to be low in an average of 32%,[12] and withdrawal of an antiseizure medication within the prior week has been shown to be an antecedent of status epilepticus.[19] Therefore, it is reasonable to obtain medication levels in this population.

EEG should be considered acutely in cases of suspected nonconvulsive status epilepticus, in children with convulsive status epilepticus who are not returning to baseline, or in cases of suspected nonepileptic events mimicking status epilepticus in order to avoid overtreatment. EEG should also be considered as a diagnostic tool after an episode of status epilepticus because identification of generalized versus focal abnormalities may allow for more targeted antiseizure medication selection.

TREATMENT

A treatment algorithm based on the American Epilepsy Society recommendations is show in Figure 25–1. Treatment of status epilepticus should begin with basic emergency support measures, including hemodynamic and respiratory support, and establishing intravenous access. Once airway, breathing, and cardiovascular status have been initially stabilized, specific antiseizure treatment should be initiated.

Benzodiazepines are first-line treatment for status epilepticus in children and adults. Of the available benzodiazepines, lorazepam, diazepam, and midazolam have intravenous forms. Diazepam is also available in rectal and intranasal formulations, and midazolam is available in buccal, intranasal, and intramuscular formulations. These are easily administered, fast-acting formulations that are suitable for treatment of status epilepticus. Extensive research has been done comparing different benzodiazepines for use in seizures. A meta-analysis of 16 studies including 1821 pediatric patients with status epilepticus found that intravenous lorazepam, intravenous diazepam, and nonintravenous midazolam were more successful in achieving seizure cessation than nonintravenous diazepam.[20] Of the nonintravenous options, a meta-analysis of 16 pediatric studies found that intramuscular midazolam was superior to other options in terms of time to seizure cessation after administration, time to seizure cessation after arrival in the hospital, and time to treatment initiation.[21]

It is important to note, however, that most seizure emergencies occur outside of a medical setting, and although they may be less effective, there is a role for benzodiazepines that can be easily administered by caregivers, including rectal and intranasal formulations. Children with a prior history of seizures or febrile seizure may have abortive benzodiazepines available at home and school. The readily available treatments are nasal or rectal preparations of diazepam and midazolam. The preparations and dosing are listed in Table 25–1. These are especially important for those with a prior history of prolonged seizures as these children are at higher risk for future prolonged seizures. Out-of-hospital administration of abortive treatment begins for convulsive seizures lasting longer than 5 minutes and for clusters of seizures (which is typically done on an individualized basis).

Benzodiazepines are effective in terminating status epilepticus in 40% to 60% of cases.[22] Intravenous lorazepam or diazepam may be repeated once if needed.[22] When benzodiazepines fail to stop a seizure, providers should move on to second-line treatment. Until recently, there were few large trials comparing second-line treatment of status epilepticus in children. In recent years, 3 randomized controlled trials have compared the use of loading doses of common antiseizure medications in cases of status epilepticus in children who have failed to respond to treatment with benzodiazepines. The ConSEPT trial compared the use of phenytoin and levetiracetam in 233 children aged 3 months to 16 years in Australia and New Zealand with status epilepticus. They found that phenytoin was not superior to levetiracetam for second-line treatment of pediatric status epilepticus.[23] Each was effective in termination of the seizure within 5 minutes of administration in approximately 50% of cases, and median time to clinical seizure cessation was similar between the 2 drugs. At 2 hours, approximately 50% in each group maintained seizure control and did not require further anticonvulsant treatment. Additional patients achieved seizure control with administration of the alternative study drug, with a total of 78% of patients in the phenytoin group and 72% of patients in the levetiracetam group achieving seizure control with one or both study drugs at the 2-hour time point. A second trial (EcLiPSE) compared the second-line use of levetiracetam and phenytoin in children in the United Kingdom ages 3 months to 18 years with status epilepticus. EcLiPSE found that median time from randomization to seizure cessation was 35 minutes in the levetiracetam group and 45 minutes in the phenytoin group, which was nonsignificant.[24] ESSETT compared fosphenytoin, levetiracetam, and valproic acid for benzodiazepine-refractory status epilepticus in adult and pediatric patients older than 2 years and found that each medication abolished seizures in approximately half of patients[25] and the treatments had a similar safety profile. An extension of ESSETT found no differences in drug effectiveness or safety among pediatric, adult, and elderly age groups.[26]

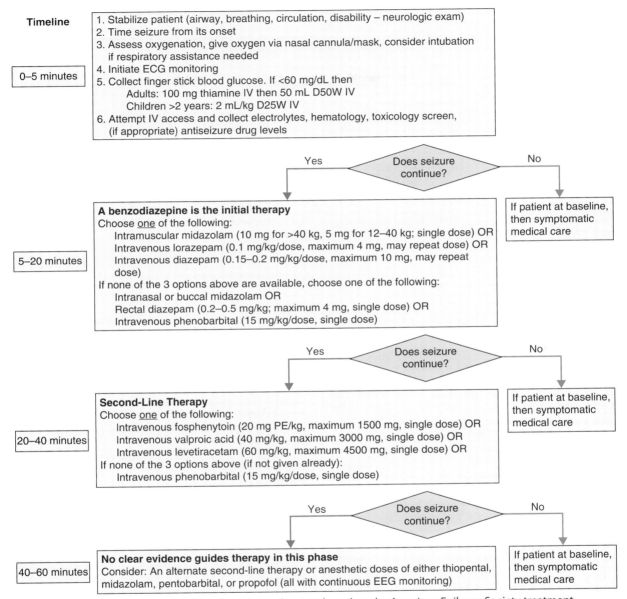

Figure 25–1. A treatment algorithm for status epilepticus based on the American Epilepsy Society treatment guidelines. ECG, electrocardiogram; EEG, electroencephalogram; IV, intravenous; PE, phenytoin equivalent.

If first- and second-line treatment both fail, status epilepticus is considered to be refractory. These cases are treated with general anesthesia based on uncontrolled studies and case series, as no controlled studies have compared treatments for refractory status epilepticus.[27] When anesthetic agents fail to control status epilepticus, it is then considered to be super-refractory. Treatment modalities may include emergency epilepsy surgery, including resective surgery, corpus callosotomy and vagal nerve stimulator placement with rapid uptitration of settings, hypothermia, ketogenic diet, immunomodulatory therapy, and electroconvulsive therapy.[27]

Table 25–1. Dosing for commercially available preparations for treatment of prolonged seizures.

Diazepam rectal gel	Supplied in 2.5-, 10-, and 20-mg delivery systems; dosing adjusted in pharmacy		
Age 2-5 years	0.5 mg/kg		
Age 6-11 years	0.3 mg/kg	Round dose up to nearest 2.5 mg	Maximum dose 20 mg
Age ≥12 years	0.2 mg/kg		
Diazepam intranasal	Supplied in 5 mg and 10 mg doses and dosing packs for 15 mg (two 7.5 mg does) and 20 mg (two 10 mg doses)		
Age 6-11 years (0.3 mg/kg)	Age ≥12 years (0.2 mg/kg)		
10 to <19 kg	14 to <28 kg	One 5-mg device	1 spray in 1 nostril
19 to <38 kg	28 to <51 kg	One 10-mg device	1 spray in 1 nostril
38 to <56 kg	51 to <76 kg	Two 7.5-mg devices	1 spray in each nostril
56 to 74 kg	≥76 kg	Two 10-mg devices	1 spray in each nostril
Midazolam intranasal	Nayzilam spray 5 mg/device		
Age ≥12 years	5 mg	One 5-mg device; may repeat in 5 minutes if seizure continues	

OUTCOME

Status epilepticus carries a risk of death and disability. The estimated mortality of status epilepticus in children ranges from 2% to 11.5%.[28] This estimate is based on studies that primarily defined status epilepticus as continuous or intermittent seizures lasting 30 minutes or longer. Studies conducted before 2000 showed a higher mortality (2.6%-11.5%) than those conducted after 2000 (2.1%-6%).[28] The reason for this is unclear, but it is speculated that it may be at least partially a result of improved emergency treatment. Several studies have shown worse outcomes when treatment is delayed.[29,30] A multicenter, prospective cohort study of 218 pediatric patients with refractory status epilepticus showed that patients who received first-line benzodiazepine treatment after 10 minutes have a higher odds ratio of death compared to those who received timely benzodiazepine administration.[29] In addition, estimates of mortality are higher in developing countries, with a study in sub-Saharan Africa reporting a mortality of 17.5%.[31] This is confounded by the differing etiologies in this population, however, as cerebral malaria, which has a very high mortality, is a common cause of status epilepticus in Africa.

It is difficult to determine the effect of status epilepticus itself on morbidity and mortality. Outcome appears to be primarily related to underlying etiology of status epilepticus. Children with acute symptomatic etiologies of status epilepticus consistently have worse outcomes than those with remote symptomatic or unknown etiologies or those with febrile seizures.[32] Many series have demonstrated a higher mortality in infants under 1 year of age,[33] which is likely because acute symptomatic etiology is more common in this age group.[6] Baseline neurologic impairment is also a risk factor for mortality in children with status epilepticus. In one population-based study of status epilepticus, of children who survived the initial 30 days following status epilepticus, those with a prior neurologic abnormality had a mortality 19 times that of previously healthy children 8 years later.[34] In terms of status epilepticus itself as a contributor to mortality, longer duration of status epilepticus does appear to increase mortality,[35] but again, this may be at least partially a function of underlying etiology.

Morbidity of status epilepticus includes motor, cognitive, and behavioral impairment and future epilepsy. A recent review found that 28% to 34% of children with status epilepticus had long-term cognitive sequelae.[36] Like mortality, risk of morbidity is affected by underlying etiology, age, and duration of status epilepticus. In a series of 276 children with refractory status epilepticus, the only predictor for developing a new neurologic deficit was electroclinical status duration.[15] Of note, as compared to other studies implicating treatment delay in outcome,[29,30] in this cohort of patients, the time to benzodiazepine administration was not predictive of long-term morbidity or of duration of status epilepticus.

In pediatric patients, the risk of subsequent epilepsy following status epilepticus has been reported to range from 5% to 36%.[36] The overall risk is comparable to the risk of seizure recurrence after a single unprovoked seizure, which is reported to be 42% in children.[37] Risk factors for development of epilepsy after status epilepticus include nonfebrile, remote symptomatic, and acute symptomatic etiologies.[36] There is a risk for recurrent status epilepticus. Children with a first episode of status epilepticus have a risk of recurrence that ranges from 10% to 56%.[36]

FEBRILE STATUS EPILEPTICUS

Febrile seizures are the most common cause of childhood seizures, occurring in 2% to 5% of all children.[38] Of those with febrile seizures, 5% develop status epilepticus.[39] Febrile status epilepticus is therefore the leading etiology of status epilepticus in children, accounting for 25% of all status epilepticus in children.[4] Febrile status epilepticus is defined as a febrile seizure lasting 30 minutes or longer or a series of febrile seizures without return to baseline in between within a period of 30 minutes or longer. Compared to those with shorter febrile seizures, children with febrile status epilepticus are more likely to have pre-existing neurological impairments, have a history of neonatal seizures, and have a family history of epilepsy, while they are less likely to have a family history of febrile seizures.[10] Incidence of epilepsy following febrile status epilepticus is lower than for other causes of childhood status epilepticus.[40] However, febrile status epilepticus may be an important cause of temporal lobe epilepsy associated with hippocampal sclerosis in adults. Retrospective studies of adults undergoing temporal lobectomy for intractable temporal lobe epilepsy have shown that a significant proportion of these patients report a history of prolonged seizures in early childhood, particularly febrile seizures.[41,42] FEBSTAT, a prospective study designed to explore this association, found that 11.5% of children with febrile status epilepticus had definite or equivocal increased T2 signal in the hippocampus, compared to no children in the control group of children with simple febrile seizures.[43]

NEONATAL STATUS EPILEPTICUS

Guidelines for treatment of status epilepticus in children are intended to be used for children beyond the neonatal period, as the majority of pediatric studies comparing treatment efficacies do not include neonates.[22] However, neonates have a particularly high risk of status epilepticus. Seizures occur in the neonatal period in 1 to 5 of 1000 live births,[44-46] and status epilepticus may be fairly common in neonates with seizures. In one study of 40 infants with electrographic seizures, 43% of them had status epilepticus.[47] Of note, there is no universally accepted definition of status epilepticus in neonates. The most commonly accepted definition is a continuous seizure lasting longer than 30 minutes or recurrent seizures occurring for greater than 50% of a total EEG epoch, as it is difficult to determine a return to mental status baseline in this population.[48] EEG is critical to the identification of status epilepticus in ill neonates, as most neonatal seizures have no clinical correlate, and other movements may be misidentified as seizures.[49] Furthermore, electroclinical dissociation, in which an antiseizure medication terminates clinical seizure but not electrographic seizure, is common in neonates.[50] Most neonatal seizures and status epilepticus are due to acute neurologic injury, including hypoxic-ischemic encephalopathy, stroke, CNS infection, and electrolyte abnormalities.[51]

Other causes of neonatal seizures and status epilepticus, including neonatal epilepsy syndromes and inborn errors of metabolism, are less common. Seizures have a greater impact on the developing brain and are independently associated with worse outcomes.[52] Neonatal seizures are typically treated aggressively for this reason, and there are no separate guidelines for neonatal status epilepticus. Rather, treatment of neonatal status epilepticus is derived from treatment of neonatal seizures.

REFERENCES

1. Gurcharran K, Grinspan ZM. The burden of pediatric status epilepticus: epidemiology, morbidity, mortality, and costs. *Seizure*. 2019;68:3-8. doi:10.1016/j.seizure.2018.08.021
2. Towne AR, Waterhouse EJ, Boggs JG, et al. Prevalence of nonconvulsive status epilepticus in comatose patients. *Neurology*. 2000;54(2):340-345. doi:10.1212/wnl.54.2.340
3. Abend NS, Arndt DH, Carpenter JL, et al. Electrographic seizures in pediatric ICU patients: cohort study of risk factors and mortality. *Neurology*. 2013;81(4):383-391. doi:10.1212/WNL.0b013e31829c5cfe
4. Shinnar S, Pellock JM, Moshé SL, et al. In whom does status epilepticus occur: age-related differences in children. *Epilepsia*. 1997;38(8):907-914. doi:10.1111/j.1528-1157.1997.tb01256.x
5. Sillanpää M, Shinnar S. Status epilepticus in a population-based cohort with childhood-onset epilepsy in Finland. *Ann Neurol*. 2002;52(3):303-310. doi:10.1002/ana.10286
6. Chin RF, Neville BG, Peckham C, et al. Incidence, cause, and short-term outcome of convulsive status epilepticus in childhood: prospective population-based study. *Lancet*. 2006;368(9531):222-229. doi: 10.1016/S0140-6736(06)69043-0
7. Moshé SL. Epileptogenesis and the immature brain. *Epilepsia*. 1987;28(suppl 1):S3-S15. doi:10.1111/j.1528-1157.1987.tb05753.x
8. Trinka E, Cock H, Hesdorffer D, et al. A definition and classification of status epilepticus—report of the ILAE Task Force on Classification of Status Epilepticus. *Epilepsia*. 2015;56(10):1515-1523. doi:10.1111/epi.13121
9. DeLorenzo RJ, Hauser WA, Towne AR, et al. A prospective, population-based epidemiologic study of status epilepticus in Richmond, Virginia. *Neurology*. 1996;46(4):1029-1035. doi:10.1212/wnl.46.4.1029
10. Shinnar S, Berg AT, Moshe SL, Shinnar R. How long do new-onset seizures in children last? *Ann Neurol*. 2001;49(5):659-664.
11. Chin RF, Neville BG, Scott RC. A systematic review of the epidemiology of status epilepticus. *Eur J Neurol*. 2004;11(12):800-810. doi:10.1111/j.1468-1331.2004.00943.x
12. Riviello JJ Jr, Ashwal S, Hirtz D, et al. Practice parameter: diagnostic assessment of the child with status epilepticus (an evidence-based review): report of the Quality Standards Subcommittee of the American Academy of Neurology and the Practice Committee of the Child Neurology Society. *Neurology*. 2006;67(9):1542-1550. doi:10.1212/01.wnl.0000243197.05519.3d
13. Berg AT, Shinnar S, Testa FM, et al. Status epilepticus after the initial diagnosis of epilepsy in children. *Neurology*. 2004;63(6):1027-1034. doi:10.1212/01.wnl.0000138425.54223.dc
14. Singh RK, Stephens S, Berl MM, et al. Prospective study of new-onset seizures presenting as status epilepticus in childhood. *Neurology*. 2010;74(8):636-642. doi:10.1212/WNL.0b013e3181d0cca2

15. Gaínza-Lein M, Barcia Aguilar C, Piantino J, et al. Factors associated with long-term outcomes in pediatric refractory status epilepticus. *Epilepsia.* 2021;62(9):2190-2204. doi:10.1111/epi.16984

16. Shi XY, Tomonoh Y, Wang WZ, et al. Efficacy of antiepileptic drugs for the treatment of Dravet syndrome with different genotypes. *Brain Dev.* 2016;38(1):40-46. doi:10.1016/j.braindev.2015.06.008

17. van Karnebeek CD, Tiebout SA, Niermeijer J, et al. Pyridoxine-dependent epilepsy: an expanding clinical spectrum. *Pediatr Neurol.* 2016;59:6-12. doi:10.1016/j.pediatrneurol.2015.12.013

18. Wolf NI, Rahman S, Schmitt B, et al. Status epilepticus in children with Alpers' disease caused by POLG1 mutations: EEG and MRI features. *Epilepsia.* 2009;50(6):1596-1607. doi:10.1111/j.1528-1167.2008.01877.x

19. Maytal J, Novak G, Ascher C, Bienkowski R. Status epilepticus in children with epilepsy: the role of antiepileptic drug levels in prevention. *Pediatrics.* 1996;98(6 Pt 1):1119-1121.

20. Zhao ZY, Wang HY, Wen B, Yang ZB, Feng K, Fan JC. A comparison of midazolam, lorazepam, and diazepam for the treatment of status epilepticus in children: a network meta-analysis. *J Child Neurol.* 2016;31(9):1093-1107. doi:10.1177/0883073816638757

21. Arya R, Kothari H, Zhang Z, Han B, Horn PS, Glauser TA. Efficacy of nonvenous medications for acute convulsive seizures: a network meta-analysis. *Neurology.* 2015;85(21):1859-1868. doi:10.1212/WNL.0000000000002142

22. Glauser T, Shinnar S, Gloss D, et al. Evidence-based guideline: treatment of convulsive status epilepticus in children and adults: report of the Guideline Committee of the American Epilepsy Society. *Epilepsy Curr.* 2016;16(1):48-61. doi:10.5698/1535-7597-16.1.48

23. Dalziel SR, Borland ML, Furyk J, et al. Levetiracetam versus phenytoin for second-line treatment of convulsive status epilepticus in children (ConSEPT): an open-label, multicentre, randomised controlled trial. *Lancet.* 2019;393(10186):2135-2145. doi:10.1016/S0140-6736(19)30722-6

24. Lyttle MD, Rainford NEA, Gamble C, et al. Levetiracetam versus phenytoin for second-line treatment of paediatric convulsive status epilepticus (EcLiPSE): a multicentre, open-label, randomised trial. *Lancet.* 2019;393(10186):2125-2134. doi:10.1016/S0140-6736(19)30724-X

25. Kapur J, Elm J, Chamberlain JM, et al. Randomized trial of three anticonvulsant medications for status epilepticus. *N Engl J Med.* 2019;381(22):2103-2113. doi:10.1056/NEJMoa1905795

26. Chamberlain JM, Kapur J, Shinnar S, et al. Efficacy of levetiracetam, fosphenytoin, and valproate for established status epilepticus by age group (ESETT): a double-blind, responsive-adaptive, randomised controlled trial. *Lancet.* 2020;395(10231):1217-1224. doi:10.1016/S0140-6736(20)30611-5

27. Vasquez A, Farias-Moeller R, Tatum W. Pediatric refractory and super-refractory status epilepticus. *Seizure.* 2019;68:62-71. doi:10.1016/j.seizure.2018.05.012

28. Jafarpour S, Stredny CM, Piantino J, Chapman KE. Baseline and outcome assessment in pediatric status epilepticus. *Seizure.* 2019;68:52-61. doi:10.1016/j.seizure.2018.04.019

29. Gaínza-Lein M, Sánchez Fernández I, Jackson M, et al. Association of time to treatment with short-term outcomes for pediatric patients with refractory convulsive status epilepticus. *JAMA Neurol.* 2018;75(4):410-418. doi:10.1001/jamaneurol.2017.4382

30. Cohen NT, Chamberlain JM, Gaillard WD. Timing and selection of first antiseizure medication in patients with pediatric status epilepticus. *Epilepsy Res.* 2019;149:21-25. doi:10.1016/j.eplepsyres.2018.10.014

31. Ahmad S, Ellis JC, Kamwendo H, Molyneux E. Efficacy and safety of intranasal lorazepam versus intramuscular paraldehyde for protracted convulsions in children: an open randomised trial. *Lancet.* 2006;367:1591-1597.

32. Lv RJ, Wang Q, Cui T, Zhu F, Shao XQ. Status epilepticus-related etiology, incidence and mortality: a meta-analysis. *Epilepsy Res.* 2017;136:12-17. doi:10.1016/j.eplepsyres.2017.07.006

33. Raspall-Chaure M, Chin RF, Neville BG, Scott RC. Outcome of paediatric convulsive status epilepticus: a systematic review. *Lancet Neurol.* 2006;5(9):769-779. doi:10.1016/S1474-4422(06)70546-4

34. Pujar SS, Neville BG, Scott RC, Chin RF; North London Epilepsy Research Network. Death within 8 years after childhood convulsive status epilepticus: a population-based study. *Brain.* 2011;134(Pt 10):2819-2827. doi:10.1093/brain/awr239

35. Sánchez Fernández I, Klehm J, An S, et al. Comparison of risk factors for pediatric convulsive status epilepticus when defined as seizures ≥ 5 min versus seizures ≥ 30 min. *Seizure.* 2014;23(9):692-698. doi:10.1016/j.seizure.2014.05.009

36. Sculier C, Gaínza-Lein M, Sánchez Fernández I, Loddenkemper T. Long-term outcomes of status epilepticus: a critical assessment. *Epilepsia.* 2018;59(suppl 2):155-169. doi:10.1111/epi.14515

37. Shinnar S, Berg AT, Moshe SL, et al. The risk of seizure recurrence after a first unprovoked afebrile seizure in childhood: an extended follow-up. *Pediatrics.* 1996;98(2 Pt 1):216-225.

38. Shinnar S, Glauser TA. Febrile seizures. *J Child Neurol.* 2002;17(suppl 1):S44-S52. doi:10.1177/08830738020170010601

39. Berg AT, Shinnar S. Unprovoked seizures in children with febrile seizures: short-term outcome. *Neurology.* 1996;47(2):562-568. doi:10.1212/wnl.47.2.562

40. Pujar SS, Martinos MM, Cortina-Borja M, et al. Long-term prognosis after childhood convulsive status epilepticus: a prospective cohort study. *Lancet Child Adolesc Health.* 2018;2(2):103-111. doi:10.1016/S2352-4642(17)30174-8

41. Cendes F, Andermann F, Dubeau F, et al. Early childhood prolonged febrile convulsions, atrophy and sclerosis of mesial structures, and temporal lobe epilepsy: an MRI volumetric study. *Neurology.* 1993;43(6):1083-1087. doi:10.1212/wnl.43.6.1083

42. French JA, Williamson PD, Thadani VM, et al. Characteristics of medial temporal lobe epilepsy: I. Results of history and physical examination. *Ann Neurol.* 1993;34(6):774-780. doi:10.1002/ana.410340604

43. Shinnar S, Bello JA, Chan S, et al. MRI abnormalities following febrile status epilepticus in children: the FEBSTAT study. *Neurology.* 2012;79(9):871-877. doi:10.1212/WNL.0b013e318266cfcc5

44. Glass HC, Pham TN, Danielsen B, Towner D, Glidden D, Wu YW. Antenatal and intrapartum risk factors for seizures in term newborns: a population-based study, California 1998-2002. *J Pediatr.* 2009;154(1):24-28.e1. doi:10.1016/j.jpeds.2008.07.008

45. Lanska MJ, Lanska DJ, Baumann RJ, Kryscio RJ. A population-based study of neonatal seizures in Fayette County, Kentucky. *Neurology.* 1995;45(4):724-732. doi:10.1212/wnl.45.4.724

46. Saliba RM, Annegers JF, Waller DK, Tyson JE, Mirzahi EM. Incidence of neonatal seizures in Harris County, Texas, 1992-1994. *Am J Epidemiol.* 1999;150(7):763-769. doi:10.1093/oxfordjournals.aje.a010079

47. McBride MC, Laroia N, Guillet R. Electrographic seizures in neonates correlate with poor neurodevelopmental outcome. *Neurology.* 2000;55(4):506-513. doi:10.1212/wnl.55.4.506

48. Abend NS, Wusthoff CJ. Neonatal seizures and status epilepticus. *J Clin Neurophysiol*. 2012;29(5):441-448. doi:10.1097/WNP.0b013e31826bd90d

49. Murray DM, Boylan GB, Ali I, Ryan CA, Murphy BP, Connolly S. Defining the gap between electrographic seizure burden, clinical expression and staff recognition of neonatal seizures. *Arch Dis Child Fetal Neonatal Ed*. 2008;93(3):F187-F191. doi:10.1136/adc.2005.086314

50. Scher MS, Alvin J, Gaus L, Minnigh B, Painter MJ. Uncoupling of EEG-clinical neonatal seizures after antiepileptic drug use. *Pediatr Neurol*. 2003;28:277-280.

51. Tekgul H, Gauvreau K, Soul J, et al. The current etiologic profile and neurodevelopmental outcome of seizures in term newborn infants. *Pediatrics*. 2006;117(4):1270-1280. doi:10.1542/peds.2005-1178

52. Glass HC, Glidden D, Jeremy RJ, Barkovich AJ, Ferriero DM, Miller SP. Clinical neonatal seizures are independently associated with outcome in infants at risk for hypoxic-ischemic brain injury. *J Pediatr*. 2009;155(3):318-323. doi:10.1016/j.jpeds.2009.03.040

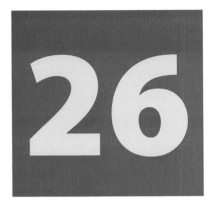

Disorders of Consciousness

Samuel Alperin, MD
Melissa Squires, MD, MPH

INTRODUCTION

Consciousness is defined by 2 components, wakefulness and awareness, requiring arousal (pontine tegmentum and thalamus) and awareness (cerebral and subcortical structure).[1,2] A spectrum of disease states exists for disorders of consciousness (DOC) including coma, vegetative state/unresponsiveness wakefulness syndrome (UWS), minimally conscious syndrome (MCS), emergence from MCS, and locked-in state. Assessment of DOC in children is complicated by age and developmental stage, and more formal diagnostic tools and outcome assessments in children continue to be needed,[3] as DOCs are estimated to affect more than 130,000 children per year in the United States.[4]

DEFINITIONS

See Table 26–1 for definitions of DOCs.

Causes of DOC unique to children can include acute/acquired traumatic brain injury; genetic/perinatal, metabolic, or degenerative causes; status epilepticus; or unknown/undefined causes. One study of over 5000 children with UWS and MCS found that 15.2% had acquired brain injury, 43.2% had perinatal/genetic conditions, and 2.1% had metabolic/degenerative disorders, with about 40% having an undetermined cause.[8]

WORKUP

Diagnosis of DOC should be based on highest level of consciousness obtained via a multimodal approach that includes comprehensive neurologic and behavioral examination, electroencephalography (EEG), and/or neuroimaging.[9,10] History should include timing of symptoms, symptom progression, and possible exposures. Comprehensive neurologic examinations need to be repeated to reduce error due to fluctuations and to assess for trajectory.[3,9] Of note, arousal and responsiveness can fluctuate and can be influenced by external factors like metabolic toxins (renal, hepatic), infections, hemodynamic instability, electrolyte derangements, and medications. Therefore, serial physical and neurologic examinations should be performed to determine persistent findings. Further assessments can be found in Table 26–2.

TREATMENT

Once acute symptoms are stabilized, inpatient rehabilitation is an important component of recovery, both cognitively and physically[9] based on the disabilities and the resulting limitations on activity, rather than on the specific pathologic process. Therapies should be initiated as soon as possible, usually prior to discharge from the hospital. The care for children with DOC includes a multidisciplinary team that consists of child neurologists, physiatrists, speech and language pathologists, therapists (occupational and physical), and neuropsychologists that can help with recovery and ongoing assessment to consider readiness for school reintegration, home accessibility, and other necessary adaptions to the psychosocial environment.[2] The focus should be on recovering function, with the understanding that variable degrees of recovery may be incomplete. Studies have found that a multicomponent neurorehabilitation program resulted in improvement in a majority of individuals who participated in intensive daily activities with physical therapy, occupational therapy, oral therapy, and sensory stimulation.[15]

Studies of pharmacologic treatment of DOC are limited in pediatrics, and there are no established therapies for children with prolonged DOC.[9] Medications that have been explored include dopaminergic drugs (eg, levodopa and amantadine), GABAergic drugs (eg, zolpidem), and serotonin and norepinephrine reuptake inhibitors (eg, methylphenidate).[5,15] Amantadine has thus far shown the most evidence for faster improvement, but at this time, it is used only in those older

Table 26–1. Definitions of disorders of consciousness.

Disorder	Definition	Presentation
Coma	Sustained loss of wakefulness and loss of awareness due to (1) dysfunction of RAS, (2) dysfunction of cerebral hemispheres (both), (3) bilateral thalamic dysfunction, and/or (4) toxic/metabolic causes.[3,5]	Eyes closed, completely unarousable, and nonresponsive to all stimuli except reflex responses. Absent sleep-wake cycles. Requires alteration for at least 4 weeks. May evolve to diagnoses below.
Unresponsive wakefulness syndrome (previously vegetative state)	Arousal with lack of awareness, sleep-wake cycling, Nonpurposeful motor function, respiratory function/without pain sensation.[1,4]	1 month after coma. Eyes may be open without visual fixation. No external evidence of pain. May make sounds, facial expressions, or body movements. Not sustained.
Minimally conscious state (MCS)	Present arousal and partial awareness, sleep-wake cycling.[6] Usually split into MCS, or MCS without depending on presence or absence of receptive/expressive language, respectively.	May follow commands, yes/no, purposeful behaviors (vocalization, reaching objects, visual pursuit, gestures).
Cognitive-motor dissociation	Signs of mental activity based on neuroimaging or electrophysiologic paradigms, but unable to outwardly show this with behavioral signs of consciousness.[7] Differentiated from locked-in syndrome where there are some willful movements (usually vertical eye movements).	Completely unable to move or follow commands with motor activities, but signs of cognition are present when using fMRI or EEG.
Stupor	Appears sleeping.	Arousable *only* when noxious stimulus is applied with eye opening and nonverbal communication.
Obtundation	Aroused but appears drowsy; reduced alertness.	Slowed responses; requires frequent stimuli to stay awake.
Lethargy	Mild sleepiness.	Confusion and sleepiness.
Delirium	Waxing and waning mental status resulting in periods of confusion.[2]	Disoriented, irritable, fearful, with sensory misperceptions (visual or auditory hallucinations).
Confusion	Impaired ability to think and reason clearly.[2]	Awake and alert but not oriented, with difficulty with cognitive processes and making new memories.

EEG, electroencephalogram; fMRI, functional magnetic resonance imaging; RAS, reticular activating system.

than age 16 years. Known side effects of amantadine (estimated in 10%) include aggression, delusions, hallucinations, and emesis.[9]

PROGNOSIS

Functional outcomes after DOC depend on the mechanism of injury, severity of DOC, and duration of depressed levels of consciousness. Most individuals will improve from their initial state of DOC to higher level, although the more depressed the DOC, the lower the likelihood of significant recovery. In children, there is a higher chance of recovery from traumatic causes.[9] At this time, there is no single test or assessment, whether EEG, imaging modality, or neurobehavioral assessment, that is predictive of outcome in both children and adults.[3]

JOURNEY TO A NEW NORMAL

Children recovering from DOC can encounter many different complications, including behavioral and psychiatric issues, seizures, tone abnormalities, and dysautonomia.

Tone often evolves from an initial flaccid/decreased state to that of spasticity (velocity-dependent inappropriately increased tone) and/or rigidity (velocity independent).[2] Interventions include range-of-motion exercises, casting and splinting, oral medications (including benzodiazepines [eg, diazepam or clonazepam], baclofen, or tizanidine), and botulinum toxin injections. Both baclofen toxicity and withdrawal can precipitate serious neurologic sequelae, so dosing must be closely monitored and adhered to (symptoms include altered mental status, hallucinations, high fever, hypertension, muscle rigidity, and seizures).

Table 26–2. Assessment of disorders of consciousness.

Assessment	Component	Comments
Physical exam	Airway/breathing/circulation	HOB up vs HOB down, neutral head position
	Adequate BP	
	GCS score11	
	Assess for raised ICP	CN III (consider pupillometry), Cushing triad
	Signs of seizure	
Laboratory/imaging studies	Glucose, ammonia, chemistry panel, ABG, LFT/RFT, CBC, lactate, pyruvate, toxicology, urinalysis	NB: obtaining studies should *not* delay care
	HCT +/− CTA; current paradigm shift to rapid MRI if feasible and does *not* delay care	
Emergent interventions after airway (where appropriate)	Thiamine and glucose	If concern for Wernicke encephalopathy or thiamine deficiency
Therapeutic agents	Antibiotics and/or acyclovir	Usually empirically treat unless compelling reason to avoid; use age-appropriate agents for likely pathogens
	Specific antidotes if exposure known and appropriate (eg, do *not* use flumazenil for benzodiazepine overdose as it can precipitate difficult-to-manage seizures)	Organophosphate (treat with atropine and pralidoxime), botulism (treat with antitoxin), opiates (treat with naloxone), carbon monoxide (treat with hyperbaric oxygen)
	HTS vs mannitol +/− hyperventilation; NSGY	For ICP management
	Treat seizures	Start with benzodiazepines, then trial second-tier infusions (levetiracetam, valproic acid, and/or fosphenytoin); consider drip as next step (eg, midazolam, ketamine, pentobarbital)
	Reduce cerebral metabolic demands	Watch glucose, temperature management, etc
Urgent investigation	LP, continuous EEG, MRI, additional labs	*Consider* metabolic, thyroid, autoimmune causes
Coma scales	FOUR score[12] and Coma Recovery Scale[13,14]	To assess progression, include aspects of GCS as well as evaluation of brainstem

ABG, arterial blood gas; BP, blood pressure; CBC, complete blood count; CN, cranial nerve; CTA, computed tomography angiography; EEG, electroencephalogram; FOUR, Full Outline of Unresponsiveness; GCS, Glasgow Coma Scale; HCT, head computed tomography; HOB, head of bed; HTS, hypertonic saline; ICP, intracranial pressure; LFT, liver function tests; LP, lumbar puncture; MRI, magnetic resonance imaging; NB, nota bene; NSGY, neurosurgery; RFT, renal function test

A pause or regression in development is often seen in children after brain trauma or with prolonged stay for DOC.[2] Behavioral disturbances can contribute to academic difficulties or vice versa (difficulty concentrating or focusing in class can contribute to worsening behavior). These include agitation, emotional regression, hyperactivity, and impulsivity, especially in younger children; older children tend to have decreased motivation and anhedonia. Behavioral changes can be managed, if necessary, with a variety of medications that include antidepressants, anticonvulsants (eg, valproate, carbamazepine), amantadine, or clonidine. For decreased arousal, inattention, or slow cognition, stimulants can also be helpful. Management with stimulants is similar to that of attention-deficit/hyperactivity disorder,

with no contraindication if patients have comorbid seizures, and treatment can be managed by the primary medical doctor (PMD). Amantadine can be used to treat decreased arousal or concentration difficulties. It is also possible that behavioral and mood changes can be a side effect of medications (eg, depression from levetiracetam or amantadine, delusions/hallucinations from amantadine).

Seizures are common in brain trauma, with about 8% to 10% of children having seizures within the first 7 to 10 days.[2] However, long-term seizure risk (posttraumatic epilepsy) is much lower and mediated by severity of traumatic brain injury and presence of early seizures. Prophylactic treatment with antiseizure medications has not been effective in reducing posttraumatic epilepsy. Treatment for early seizures may only be necessary for a brief period (unless there are multiple focal seizures or follow-up EEG continues to show epileptiform activity). Side effects are not uncommon with antiseizure medications and can include irritability and agitation with levetiracetam or sedation with most other medications (see chapter on treatment of epilepsy). It is important to evaluate sedation in someone recovering from DOC to assess whether it is due to medication side effects, infection, or nonconvulsive status epilepticus.

Autonomic disturbances are also common after brain injury, including fever of central origin and paroxysmal sympathetic hyperactivity.[2] Central fevers present usually in conjunction with other features of dysautonomia (ie, hypertension, tachycardia, tachypnea, dystonia, and rigidity). It is important to rule out other sources of fever, including infection and medication side effects. Treatment for dysautonomia can include gabapentin, bromocriptine, propranolol, labetalol, clonidine, morphine, and midazolam.[2] Often, many of these medications are able to be weaned in the setting of chronic recovery.

CONCLUSION

DOCs are not uncommon in the pediatric population, and there is usually potential for at least some recovery. Quick detection, stabilization, and diagnosis with multimodal assessments are essential to achieve the best possible outcome. Recovery from DOC usually involves a multidisciplinary team and requires vigilant evaluations for complications and strong communication from all team members.

REFERENCES

1. Multi-Society Task Force on PVS. Medical aspects of the persistent vegetative state (1). *N Engl J Med.* 1994;330:1499-1508.
2. Swaiman KF, Ashwal S, Ferriero DM, et al, eds. *Swaiman's Pediatric Neurology: Principles and Practice.* 6th ed. Elsevier; 2018.
3. LaRovere KL, Tasker RC. Defining catastrophic brain injury in children leading to coma and disorders of consciousness and the scope of the problem. *Curr Opin Pediatr.* 2020;32:750-758.
4. Ashwal S. The persistent vegetative state in children. *Adv Pediatr.* 1994;41:195-222.
5. Edlow BL, Claassen J, Schiff ND, Greer DM. Recovery from disorders of consciousness: mechanisms, prognosis and emerging therapies. *Nat Rev Neurol.* 2021;17:135-156.
6. Giacino JT, Ashwal S, Childs N, et al. The minimally conscious state: definition and diagnostic criteria. *Neurology.* 2002; 58:349-353.
7. Schiff ND. Cognitive motor dissociation following severe brain injuries. *JAMA Neurol.* 2015;72:1413-1415.
8. Strauss DJ, Ashwal S, Day SM, Shavelle RM. Life expectancy of children in vegetative and minimally conscious states. *Pediatr Neurol.* 2000;23:312-319.
9. Giacino JT, Katz DI, Schiff ND, et al. Practice guideline update recommendations summary: disorders of consciousness: report of the Guideline Development, Dissemination, and Implementation Subcommittee of the American Academy of Neurology; the American Congress of Rehabilitation Medicine; and the National Institute on Disability, Independent Living, and Rehabilitation Research. *Arch Phys Med Rehabil.* 2018;99:1699-1709.
10. Kondziella D, Bender A, Diserens K, et al. European Academy of Neurology guideline on the diagnosis of coma and other disorders of consciousness. *Eur J Neurol.* 2020;27:741-756.
11. Reilly PL, Simpson DA, Sprod R, Thomas L. Assessing the conscious level in infants and young children: a paediatric version of the Glasgow Coma Scale. *Childs Nerv Syst.* 1988;4:30-33.
12. Wijdicks EFM, Bamlet WR, Maramattom BV, Manno EM, McClelland RL. Validation of a new coma scale: the FOUR score. *Ann Neurol.* 2005;58:585-593.
13. Giacino JT, Kalmar K, Whyte J. The JFK Coma Recovery Scale-Revised: measurement characteristics and diagnostic utility. *Arch Phys Med Rehabil.* 2004;85:2020-2029.
14. Slomine BS, Suskauer SJ, Nicholson R, Giacino JT. Preliminary validation of the coma recovery scale for pediatrics in typically developing young children. *Brain Inj.* 2019;33:1640-1645.
15. Houston AL, Wilson NS, Morrall MC, Lodh R, Oddy JR. Interventions to improve outcomes in children and young people with unresponsive wakefulness syndrome following acquired brain injury: a systematic review. *Eur J Paediatr Neurol.* 2020; 25:40-51.

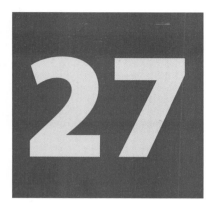

Pediatric Syncope and Related Phenomena

Martha W. Willis, RN, MS, CNP

Amy L. Wiseman, RN, BSN

Ashley McGill, RN, BSN

Karen Leonard, RN, BSN

Heather Wilson, RN, BSN

Cameron Thomas, MD, MS

INTRODUCTION

Syncope is a relatively sudden, brief, self-limited loss of postural tone and consciousness followed by rapid spontaneous recovery without any neurologic sequelae.[1-3] Syncope is a common pediatric problem, representing 1% to 3% of all pediatric emergency department (ED) visits and 6% of hospital admissions. It has an estimated population incidence of 10% to 15%.[4,5] In children and adolescents, syncope is substantially more common in females (65.6% female, 34.4% male). Although syncope can occur in any demographic group throughout the world, in North America, those who seek medical care for this complaint are more likely to be White and have private insurance.[1,5,6] For instance, one study found that 54% of pediatric syncope patients presenting to an East Coast ED were White, whereas 22% were Latino, 16% were Black, and 2% were Asian.[7] Of these pediatric ED patients, 68% had private primary insurance and 32% had public insurance.[7] Syncope, although not a serious illness and typically benign in etiology, can have high healthcare costs. In a study of one cohort, pediatric syncope accounted for $1.1 million dollars of testing over a 2-year period, with an average cost of $2488 per patient.[1] Much of this testing was unnecessary due to the benign nature of syncope. In addition to being common and having high healthcare costs, syncope deserves attention because it significantly impacts quality of life. Pediatric syncope patients are known to have Pediatric Quality of Life Inventory total scores as low as children and adolescents with other chronic illnesses such as diabetes, asthma, obesity, and end-stage renal disease.[6,8-10]

To treat this common condition effectively, while simultaneously being mindful of cost and quality-of-life concerns, a comprehensive history and physical examination should be performed with particular attention given to red flags that signify more serious pathologies masquerading as syncope. In this chapter, we discuss the critical components of this evaluation, the salient red flags and summarize this information in a useful algorithm that has served as the framework for our multidisciplinary syncope clinic. Finally, we discuss treatment and educational tools that can rapidly address symptoms, provide reassurance to families, and reduce unnecessary healthcare utilization.

PATHOPHYSIOLOGY AND TERMINOLOGY

Neurocardiogenic syncope (NCS) is triggered by a fall in systemic arterial pressure created by a combination of increased vagal tone (bradycardia) and decreased sympathetic tone (vasodilation).[1-5] This decreases venous return and, hence, cardiac output, resulting in cerebral hypoperfusion and subsequent syncope. Vasovagal syncope, neurally mediated syncope, vasodepressor syncope, and orthostatic intolerance are synonyms for NCS.

EVALUATION

▶ History

To ensure that syncope is due to benign causes and not indicative of a more ominous health problem, it is imperative to conduct a thoughtful and thorough evaluation considering a broad differential of cardiac, neurologic, psychiatric, and other causes.[5] The foundation of this evaluation is a detailed history of the events and their context. The history of events surrounding syncope can be considered in 3 phases: the prodrome, the event itself, and the signs and symptoms that follow the event.

Prodrome

Consideration of the prodrome includes medical or environmental factors or conditions that contribute to the onset of symptoms as well as any signs or symptoms evident prior to the loss of consciousness (LOC). In many cases of NCS, specific triggers are identified by the patient or family. These may include a rapid change to a more upright position (from sitting or lying to standing), prolonged standing, environmental heat (eg, warm room, standing outside in the sun or heat, or vigorous exercise in a warm environment), and/or recent or concurrent illnesses—particularly ones in which dehydration has occurred.[11] Strong sensory or emotional stimuli or anticipation thereof may also trigger syncopal events. For instance, pain sustained as part of an injury, receiving (or awaiting) an injection or vaccination, or the sight of blood or other unexpectedly gory material may provoke syncopal episodes.[12] Medical conditions may also contribute to the milieu of factors that result in a syncopal event. Patients who have recently started menstruation or who have menorrhagia and/or dysmenorrhea, those who have had recent growth spurts or have experienced rapid weight loss, and patients with psychiatric or gastrointestinal conditions that limit food or fluid intake may all be at increased risk for syncopal events. Finally, strong emotional states or extremes of anxiety, whether alone or accompanied by hyperventilation, may result in or closely mimic syncope.

Signs and symptoms that occur in the prodromal phase can be varied and reflect the duress of the transiently hypoperfused brain. They include, but are not limited to, dizziness, light-headedness, numbness or tingling of extremities, headache, visual changes (including seeing spots, pixels, squiggles, or flashes, or having blurred, blackened, or tunnel vision), auditory changes (muffled hearing or ear ringing), nausea, sensation of warmth, diaphoresis, and pallor.[11] Changes in heart rate (either faster or slower depending on phase of the event) can be perceived and even measured. Loss of postural tone may occur while consciousness is still preserved. Prodromal signs and symptoms may be very brief but are often of sufficient duration to provide a warning period in which the patient can respond to the symptoms in a way that decreases their likelihood of uncontrolled loss of postural tone and/or complete LOC. This is typically achieved by having the patient sit or lay down. Failure to heed these signs or symptoms often culminates in full and uncontrolled loss of postural tone and LOC.

Typical Syncopal Event

The length of time a patient with NCS is typically unconscious will vary from seconds to minutes, although most syncopal events are less than 1 minute in duration.[11] Time distortion, in which observers of the event perceive the duration to be much longer than its actual timed length, is common and can complicate analysis by the medical provider. When querying regarding the duration of LOC, it can be helpful to ask if reported duration is based upon perceived versus recorded time (bystanders or surveillance systems may record or document an actual time). Estimating time based on other factors (ie, how long it took to call 911, time until ambulance arrival, time to get the school nurse) may also be helpful.

During the actual LOC, the patient is completely unaware of their surroundings and unable to see, hear, or respond to what is going on around them. The patient also retains no memory of this phase of the event. The patient often appears pale and/or diaphoretic. Heart rate can vary in this phase, and stress responses of bystanders may make accurate assessment of pulse difficult. Eyes are typically open with various described types of involuntary movements including rolling up/back, roving, or jerking/nystagmoid movement. Extremity movements shortly after LOC are also common, with stiffening and myoclonic jerks occurring in more than 50% of patients in whom syncope is captured or recorded in a controlled environment (eg, tilt-table lab, epilepsy monitoring unit).[13] Although this is referred to as convulsive syncope (due to the movements), it is not a distinct pathophysiologic entity and does not indicate that the event was a seizure, nor does it confer any additional risk of epilepsy. Tongue biting during syncope is occasional and tends to be in the anterior portion of the tongue (lateral tongue biting is more common in seizures).[14] Urinary incontinence is not infrequent and thus should not be considered a reliable marker for distinguishing between syncopal and epileptic events.

After the Event

The return to consciousness may occur in phases. Many patients report a return of auditory capacity prior to fully regaining consciousness. Although they begin to hear what is going on around them, they may initially be unable to respond verbally. During this phase, they may be able to answer questions by nodding, thus demonstrating awareness. Within a couple of minutes of regaining consciousness, patients can converse coherently. Most patients who have experienced a syncopal event report feeling exhausted. This exhaustion may persist for 1 to 2 hours or for the rest of the day. Residual dizziness and headache are also common. Patients recovering from syncope are not confused. They recognize who is around them and where they are, although they might be confused as to how they ended up in their current position (eg, laying on the ground). Although they will be amnestic for the brief period of unconsciousness (and rarely for part of the prodrome), prolonged periods of amnesia that include times where the patient was known to be conscious should prompt consideration of nonsyncopal events. Increased emotionality may be present following the event due to the sudden and often unexpected sequence of events that culminated in LOC. This emotional state may be heightened by the responses of eyewitnesses and bystanders who are often upset themselves at having witnessed such an event (despite syncope's generally benign nature, witnesses often perceive it as a near-death event). Postsyncopal hyperventilation may occur and, in some instances, is severe or prolonged, resulting in hypocarbia, calcium ion fluxes, and eventual carpopedal spasm. Careful history can distinguish this from seizure activity.

▶ Red Flags

What we have outlined in the preceding paragraphs is the history of a typical, benign syncopal event. While benign NCS is overwhelmingly the most common form of syncope, it is important to recognize when atypical features either of history or examination should raise red flags. Red flags herald a potentially more serious pathologic condition. Understanding when red flags should prompt additional focused history and/or lead to additional diagnostic testing is crucial to ruling out serious or even life-threatening medical conditions.

Situational Details

For cardiac concerns, red flags include exertional syncope (syncope during peak exercise) or near-drowning, which may be symptoms of hypertrophic obstructive cardiomyopathy (HOCM), anomalous coronary arteries, or some forms of long QT syndrome. Anomalous coronary arteries and HOCM account for the most frequent causes of sudden cardiac death in young athletes. Males have a higher incidence of sudden cardiac death than females, and recent data suggest that Blacks have a higher occurrence than other groups, although the causes for this difference are not well understood.[2,15,16] Another cardiac red flag is syncope provoked by heightened excitement (eg, riding a roller coaster) or by a startle or scare (eg, someone jumping out at the patient from a hiding spot), which may indicate a type of arrhythmia such as long QT syndrome, atrioventricular nodal reentrant tachycardia, or catecholaminergic polymorphic ventricular tachycardia.

For neurologic concerns, red flags include stiffening or jerking movements beginning prior to loss of tone; bilateral, slow (1-2 Hz), rhythmic jerking lasting more than a few seconds, particularly if followed by prolonged confusion or unconsciousness; and prolonged postictal confusion or focal neurologic finding after an event of any duration or description. Any of these constellations of symptoms more strongly suggest seizure activity. In addition, syncope consistently caused by bending over or forward with head below the waist accompanied by sudden severe headache can suggest acute obstructive hydrocephalus and is a neurosurgical emergency. The presence of vertigo is also a neurologic red flag (distinct from dizziness, particularly if accompanied by nystagmus and/or ataxia). Finally, events accompanied by significant physical injury (suggesting a type or velocity of fall that is atypical for NCS) could portend either neurologic or cardiac causes, and associated symptoms should be considered carefully when determining the best option for referral.

Family History

Several family history factors warrant further cardiac investigation. These include a first-degree relative with a history of a channelopathy (long QT syndrome or Brugada syndrome), cardiomyopathy, or sudden unexplained death before the age of 50 (particularly with a negative autopsy), or any individual with a pacemaker or defibrillator for indications other than atrial fibrillation or following repair of congenital heart defects.

Family history features that raise neurologic concern include first-degree relatives with childhood- or adolescent-onset epilepsy, genetic epilepsies/channelopathies, arteriovenous malformations, cavernous malformations (cavernomas), childhood or young adult strokes, neuromuscular disorders with potential to impact cardiac function, or any neurodegenerative condition.

Physical Exam

Cardiac examination findings that raise a red flag include a high-pitched, crescendo-decrescendo, mid-systolic murmur heard best at the left lower sternal border (characteristic of HOCM) or an unusually loud S_2 best heard in the semi-recumbent position during quiet inspiration and a precordial heave or thrill (suggestive of pulmonary hypertension).[17] Extreme tachycardia greater than 180 bpm should also prompt evaluation by cardiology.

Neurologic examination findings that should prompt additional investigation include any motor or reflex asymmetries, cranial neuropathies, or signs of papilledema on fundoscopic examination.

Diagnostic Tests

Red flags can also arise from a completed electrocardiogram (ECG). For this reason, an ECG is ideally performed prior to or during the evaluation visit. ECG findings that should lead to cardiology referral include QTc interval greater than 460 milliseconds, T-wave inversion, Brugada pattern (incomplete right bundle branch block pattern with ST-segment elevations in leads V_1-V_3),[12,18] pre-excitation (PR interval <120 milliseconds with a delta wave), abnormally high voltage, or first-degree atrioventricular block (PR interval >250 milliseconds).[12,18-20]

▶ Yellow Flags

Whereas red flags connote potentially serious pathologies with implications for health and safety, yellow flags should alert the clinician that the pathology differs from typical syncope and may require different treatments. Although the immediate threat to the patient's safety for yellow flag symptoms is less than for red flag symptoms, the impact on quality of life and overall wellness may still be considerable. Common yellow flags identified in syncope evaluations include syncope when in a seated position, when laying down, or when perceived to be "sleeping." Very frequent syncopal episodes (as many as dozens of discreet episodes daily) would also raise a yellow flag. These types of symptoms raise concern for psychological or psychiatric etiologies. Quite often, the patient's initial event may have been physiologically consistent with NCS, but abnormal stress responses to the inciting event evolve to include very frequent daily episodes that no longer share the inciting physiology. It is common for these episodes to closely resemble and even be confused for NCS events. However, although the appearance of the events may mimic NCS, their frequency does not. A detailed history typically also finds differences in the prodromal phase (eg, less likely to have antecedent dizziness, vision/hearing changes) and in the event itself (eyes are generally closed throughout the event, and patients often report being able to hear but not speak through the duration of symptoms).

DIFFERENTIAL DIAGNOSIS

▶ Cardiac Causes

A practical approach to the evaluation of syncope will distinguish between NCS and other critical causes of syncope. Although NCS is by far the most common cause for LOC in children and adolescents, less common and more dangerous cardiac causes of LOC must be considered. Cardiac causes of syncope are grouped into right or left ventricular outflow tract dysfunction/obstruction and arrhythmias.

Left ventricular outflow tract obstructions are lesions that limit cardiac output resulting in inadequate cerebral blood flow.[5] With physical evaluation, a systolic ejection murmur or evidence of heart failure (eg, edema, hepatosplenomegaly) is often present. Patients presenting with syncope and a new systolic ejection murmur should be referred to cardiology for further evaluation. Right ventricular outflow tract obstruction—obstruction of pulmonary blood flow—rarely causes cardiac syncope. However, in conditions where pulmonary hypertension (PH) develops and progresses, poor pulmonary blood flow can lead to reduced cardiac output and ultimately syncope. Although more common in adults, this sequence of events associated with PH may also present in adolescents or younger children. Although most cardiac conditions that result in outflow obstruction occur de novo, detailed cardiac family history is still worthwhile. Right ventricular hypertrophy on ECG, a systolic ejection murmur, a loud S_2, and a palpable heave can indicate PH.

Patients with a history of syncope can have ventricular tachycardia (VT). This may be idiopathic or a result of congenital or acquired heart disease. VT may also be induced by drug ingestion including illicit drugs, antimicrobials, psychotropic medications, and antiarrhythmics. If the VT is sustained or prolonged, cardiac output is insufficient for cerebral perfusion and syncope occurs.[21] Patients with a family history of sudden death or who present with exertional syncope should have testing for long QT syndrome. The upper limits of normal for calculated QT intervals are 460 milliseconds in females and 450 milliseconds in males.[22] Values that exceed these thresholds should prompt referral to cardiology. Although exertional or peak exercise syncope is very concerning, syncope after completion of exercise can occur due to postexercise vasodilation and hypotension as a normal variant.[23]

▶ Neurologic Causes

Seizure

A seizure is a stereotyped event that might include characteristic movements or LOC accompanied by abnormal (typically hypersynchronized, high-voltage) electrical discharges within a specific cortical region or across the entire surface of the brain. If the patient's presentation has features potentially consistent with seizures, inquiring about other epileptic phenomena may be useful as there are several seizure types that could mimic syncope. In an adolescent who has previously experienced typical neurodevelopment, the most common type of epilepsy that could be confused for syncope would be juvenile myoclonic epilepsy (JME). JME may include several seizure types and other characteristic features. Generalized tonic-clonic seizures are the quintessential seizure associated with JME and may be difficult to differentiate from syncope based on appearance alone. Additional history may help to distinguish the event etiology. In addition to important history about the event and postictal state, asking about morning myoclonus (large-amplitude jerks of extremities typically shortly after awakening that can cause dropping or flinging of held objects); asking about periods of lost time or awareness not associated with loss of tone that might suggest absence seizures; and asking if the event was photoconvulsive (ie, provoked by flashing or flickering lighting [eg, disco, haunted house, high-action movies, certain forms of anime, tree-lined roads on a sunny day]) may reveal additional confirmatory evidence of JME. Other forms of seizure such as atonic or negative myoclonic seizures could mimic the loss of postural tone that occurs in syncope. In such cases, the velocity of the fall can be useful in differentiating events. The loss of tone that occurs with syncope is typically described as a slow collapse or melting to the ground, although it may also begin slowly and gather speed (similar to a felled tree). Atonic events are very sudden—like a lightning strike. There are no prodromal symptoms with atonic seizures, which may also aid in distinguishing syncope from seizure. Focal-onset seizures with impaired awareness followed by a secondarily generalized seizure could also mimic a syncopal event with prodromal period. However, loss of awareness or confusion prior to loss of tone and a confused postictal state would be common for this type of seizure and very unusual for syncope.

Cerebrovascular

At its core, syncope results from a sequence of pathophysiologic events culminating in transient hypoperfusion of the brain. Thus, it should come as no surprise that other events resulting in cerebral hypoperfusion could mimic syncope. Occlusion of either the anterior or posterior cerebral circulations may cause LOC. In children, anterior circulation (carotid) occlusion from medical causes is very uncommon. There are instances in which trauma or injury that involves rapid acceleration or deceleration or severe torsional forces of the head or neck may result in arterial dissection. By disrupting the intimal lining of the vessel, dissection may provoke thrombosis of the vessel. Conceivably, transient occlusions from this or similar mechanisms could cause syncope, although more typically they would result in stroke or transient ischemic attacks with focal neurologic symptoms. Furthermore, in the absence of connective tissue disorders, this type of injury would only result from a degree of trauma that would cause other notable injuries to the brain or body, making pure syncope an unlikely culprit.

Purposeful occlusion of the carotid arteries may occur as part of "The Choking Game" or "Passing Out Challenge" and result in syncope (or even death). This activity occurs most often in adolescence when participants seek a drug-free "high" or sense of euphoria that may occur as cerebral perfusion returns after the hypoperfusion induced by carotid occlusion is relieved. This may be suspected if syncope only occurs when the patient is alone or with certain friends, if occlusive aids (eg, belts, straps, ropes, bandanas) are found where the syncope occurred, or if there is accompanying erythema or abrasion of the neck. In 2015, a survey reported that 7.4% of teenage respondents had participated in strangulation activity.[24] Strangulation or suffocation activities cause cerebral hypoxia and hypoperfusion, increase thoracic pressure, and decrease cardiac output, all of which may culminate in syncope.[25-27] Another variant of this activity occurs when participants employ extreme hyperventilation. When hyperventilation is performed until symptoms of hypocapnia (eg, tingling, light-headedness) occur, it causes cerebral vasoconstriction, and when paired with Valsalva or other vagal maneuvers, it can induce syncope or near-syncope and be used to seek the same "high" as in the purposeful carotid occlusion described earlier.

Vertebrobasilar insufficiency (VBI), inadequate blood flow through the posterior cerebral circulation, can also result in syncope. Furthermore, its associated symptoms, including dizziness, light-headedness, headache, and changes in hearing, often overlap with presyncopal symptoms. However, VBI does have distinguishing characteristics including vertigo, ataxia, or episodic (often vertical) nystagmus prior to LOC. VBI can be mediated by subclavian steal in which occlusion of the proximal subclavian artery leads to retrograde flow in the vertebral artery. This should be strongly considered if there are correlated upper extremity symptoms, such as paresthesia, pain, numbness, or unusual fatigue, or if the neurologic manifestations are provoked by upper extremity exercise.[28] Unilateral time lag when comparing radial pulses or differences in upper extremity blood pressures of greater than 15 mm Hg may be used to confirm suspicions of VBI if they are high (although these vitals and maneuvers are not done routinely on all patients). VBI may also occur with rotational occlusion of the vertebral artery, as in Bow Hunter's Syndrome.

Obstruction of Cerebral Spinal Fluid Circulation

Most obstruction of cerebrospinal fluid (CSF) circulation occurs gradually and is accompanied with the progressive onset of symptoms associated with hydrocephalus including headache, nausea, vomiting, lethargy or irritability, changes in coordination or continence, and vision changes such as double vision, blurry vision, or fixed downward gaze (sunsetting). In rare instances, the onset of hydrocephalus can be hyperacute with explosive symptom onset and sudden loss of postural tone. This unusual sequence of events may be provoked by bending over with the head down, ultimately causing colloid cysts or other tumors that are mobile within the ventricle to fall into a position that obstructs CSF flow into the third ventricle at the foramen of Monro. Although, these events are exceptionally rare, having a high index of concern is essential as these sudden obstructive events can result in rapid neurologic decompensation or even death if not recognized or treated appropriately.[29,30]

Sleep Disorders

Narcolepsy and cataplexy are neurologic conditions to consider when evaluating patients experiencing episodes of LOC. Onset of narcolepsy is usually in the teen years. Those with narcolepsy cannot regulate their sleep-wake cycles. They experience sudden, overwhelming periods of excessive daytime sleepiness and daytime bouts of sleep. Duration of sleep can range from a few seconds to over an hour. It is distinguished from syncope by the prodromal sensation of profound tiredness or need to sleep. Cataplexy is a sudden, brief loss of muscle tone following a strong emotional stimulus (often mirthful). Generally, consciousness is maintained throughout the period of loss of tone.

▶ Psychological Causes

Frequently, recurrent episodes of LOC should lead to further investigation for underlying psychological or psychiatric disorders. Certain psychiatric disorders as described in the *Diagnostic and Statistical Manual of Mental Disorders, 5th edition, Text Revision,* have associated syncope-like events.[31] Functional neurologic disorder, Munchausen syndrome, malingering, panic attacks, anxiety, and depression are specific disorders that can be associated with events that mimic pediatric syncope. Patients with functional neurologic disorder will have multiple events of LOC that may last minutes to hours. During their unresponsiveness, the patient will typically have heart rate and blood pressure values that are normal for age. In contrast to NCS, these events that mimic syncope are infrequently triggered by change of position, prolonged standing, or heat. A component of functional neurologic disorder can be psychogenic nonepileptic spells. These events may share similarities in appearance to generalized tonic-clonic seizures, but, often, characteristic body and eye movements may provide clues to the psychological etiology of these events. For instance, eyes kept closed throughout the event, head shaking side to side, hip or pelvic thrusting, and distractable or entrainable movements might all suggest psychological underpinnings for the symptoms. A complete psychosocial history might disclose anxiety or stressors contributing to this type of syncope-like event, although catastrophic stressors need not be present as a prerequisite to developing these types of disorders. A referral to and treatment by a psychologist experienced in treating functional neurologic symptoms or other psychological disorders will best address this diagnosis.[32] Treatments might include cognitive behavioral therapy, biofeedback, or other coping skills training.

Munchausen syndrome, a self-imposed factitious disorder, and malingering, an intentional exaggeration of symptoms, may manifest with LOC. External incentives, human attention, hospital visits, and medical testing motivate the behavior. In these situations, episodes are often unwitnessed by others, which allows the patient to create their own narrative that draws attention to the patient and facilitates the desired outcome. Skilled psychological evaluation and treatment are necessary for these diagnoses.

Psychological stress increases the frequency of syncope-like events. Panic attacks, anxiety, and depression are caused by mental stress and result in increased occurrence of syncope during stressful situations. Hyperventilation, which frequently accompanies panic attacks and increases heart rate, if prolonged, may result in respiratory alkalosis, uncompensated hypocapnia, and potentially hypotension. This generally results in symptoms such as light-headedness, dizziness, and vision and hearing changes, which may reinforce the sense of panic and perpetuate hyperventilation. Ultimately, this prolonged hyperventilation can result in cerebral vasoconstriction and syncope.

Metabolic Causes

Syncope can be caused by metabolic issues. Anemia, respiratory distress such as sleep apnea or asthma, and congenital heart defects can result in hypoxia. Hypoxia decreases cerebral perfusion, which leads to syncope. Hypoglycemia

induces sympathetic nervous system stimulation. With this abnormal response, vasodilation and bradycardia lead to syncope.

Reflex Causes

The nervous system involuntarily responds causing a vasovagal reaction and resulting in bradycardia and vasodilation. This can occur during micturition, defecation, coughing, fear, anxiety, or intense emotional stress.[33] In hair grooming and stretching syncope, the vagus nerve is stimulated, perhaps in response to input from carotid baroreceptors via the glossopharyngeal nerve. The resultant decrease in heart rate and blood pressure produces LOC.[33,34]

Intoxications

Alcohol intoxication, a rapid rise in alcohol levels, produces dehydration, vasodilation, and hypotension, often leading to syncope.[35] Vaping and marijuana smoking impact the autonomic nervous system.[36] The specific response seems to be dose dependent, with the responses being hypotension, bradycardia, and syncope. It can also affect the cardiovascular system causing arrhythmias and cardiomyopathy.[36]

Breath Holding

Breath-holding spells are events experienced by children in response to a strong or sudden physical or emotional stimulus. Most events occur between the ages of 6 months and 4 years.[37] The prodrome begins with the stimulus, which can be either pain or emotional upset. In reaction to the stimulus, children frequently begin to cry and then stop breathing or bear down (although some children stop breathing without an audible cry first). This sequence of events is then felt to result in a strong vagal stimulus that causes extreme bradycardia or even brief asystole and accompanying LOC. During the unconscious period, children may appear pale (pallid breath holding) or cyanotic. They may be limp or have some stiffening or jerking movements. Consequently, many parents confuse these spells with seizures. Generally, these events are benign and require no further neurologic or cardiac evaluation.[38] Total LOC should be less than 1 minute. If LOC exceeds this duration, then cardiology evaluation for prolonged (and potentially life-threatening) asystole is indicated. With experience (eg, repeated events), some parents find ways to disrupt the sequence of events that results in LOC by blowing in the child's face or placing a cold rag on their face. Breath-holding spells do not occur while the child is asleep.[38]

There is a strong association between iron deficiency and breath-holding spells.[39] For children with frequent spells, serum iron studies may be warranted. Even without true iron deficiency anemia, supplementation with iron has been shown to reduce the frequency of breath-holding events.

Optimal treatment including education regarding the benign nature of the events, preventing iron deficiency caused by excessive milk consumption, and supplementing iron to reduce event frequency can decrease family anxiety and healthcare overutilization.

EVALUATION

A standard approach to the syncopal patient is important and includes a careful and thoughtful history specifically focusing on the cardiac, neurologic, and psychological systems; orthostatic vital signs; physical examination with a focus on the neurologic and cardiac systems; and an ECG to assist in differentiating NCS from serious or potentially life-threatening neurologic or cardiac causes for syncope or loss of postural tone.[40,41] Multiple guidelines for the assessment of NCS have been developed.

Orthostatic vital signs can give an indication of NCS. After the patient has been lying for 3 minutes, the health-care provider obtains a manual heart rate and blood pressure. The patient then stands without support for 3 minutes. A heart rate and blood pressure are then taken and documented. The gold standard for diagnosing NCS is an increase in heart rate of 40 bpm from lying to standing and a decrease in systolic blood pressure of 20 mm Hg from lying to standing according to American College of Cardiology/American Heart Association/Heart Rhythm Society clinical practice guidelines.[42] However, orthostatic vital sign changes may not be observed in many patients suffering from NCS due to many extraneous factors. In every case, a comprehensive event, medical, and family history and a thorough physical examination with emphasis on the cardiac and neurologic examination are imperative to definitively diagnose NCS.[40,43] While a complete neurologic examination is preferred, in many cases, a detailed cranial nerve and fundoscopic examination to rule out signs of increased intracranial pressure and testing of the vestibular system are sufficient to confirm the history and to eliminate serious pathology. Heart rate and rhythm should be obtained, including identification of any heart rhythm abnormalities. Auscultation should be performed specifically listening for any loud or new murmurs or gallops. Palpating the precordium to identify a left or right ventricular heave is also part of a complete cardiac exam. An ECG should be performed to rule out many arrhythmias or other underlying cardiac abnormalities.[5,20,44] An ECG is the gold standard in syncope evaluation and assists in predicting prognosis and risk stratification in syncope patients.[42] Determining treatments and offering anticipatory guidance and education are also important aspects of care.

During initial evaluation, further diagnostic testing, such as blood work and cardiac or neurologic imaging tests, is not recommended and is of low yield.[7] However, should any red flags become apparent in the workup, further tests may be warranted. An echocardiogram should be ordered if a patient is experiencing chest pain with exertion or syncope during peak exercise, has an ECG with abnormal voltage or ST-segment or T-wave changes, an abnormal cardiac examination, or a significant family history of sudden death or cardiomyopathy. In addition, it is recommended that a graded exercise test be completed if the patient had syncope during exercise, chest pain prior to syncope, or a significant physical injury from a sudden fall with a normal echocardiogram (Figure 27–1). A sleep-deprived electroencephalogram is ordered when there is seizure activity with a postictal state or other history concerning for a seizure. A focal neurologic finding following a syncopal event should prompt urgent neuroimaging.

Lab testing is not routinely indicated. However, in cases where specific risk factors exist, thyroid testing, serum iron studies, and glucose monitoring can be considered to treat thyroid disease, iron deficiency anemia, and disorders of glucose homeostasis. Although these are rarely the primary cause of syncope, they are readily treatable disorders, and effective treatment would alleviate the associated syncope. If a urine-specific gravity is obtained and is elevated during an ED visit, hydration can be addressed and discussed. It is not typical to routinely obtain a urine-specific gravity due to the variability of results based on current hydration status and kidney function.

INITIAL TREATMENT

Treatment for NCS begins with education. Once the proper diagnosis has been made, the patient and their family need to understand the diagnosis and how to prevent syncope. The first line of treatment is understanding the triggers and avoiding them. Many patients should change positions slowly and avoid heat and extremely stressful situations. Education should continue by teaching the patient to respond to their prodromal symptoms by sitting down and bending at the waist or lying down and lifting one's legs up (countermaneuver training) until there is a resolution of symptoms. For those who experience syncope in relation to medical events such as intravenous line placement or vaccination, there is evidence that crossing one's legs and activating large muscle groups in the buttocks and thighs combined with a seated or laying position and a postprocedure waiting period can reduce the likelihood of syncopal events.[45] When presyncope resolves, it is recommended that the patient return slowly to an upright position and slowly continue with the previous activity.

Nonpharmacologic treatment for syncope includes volume expansion with aggressive hydration to 80 to 100 oz of fluid daily. This is the best treatment for NCS according to the American College of Cardiology/American Heart Association/Heart Rhythm Society clinical practice guidelines.[42] Increased dietary sodium of 3 to 5 g daily is also recommended to assist in retention of increased hydration. Consider 2 additional salty snacks daily in addition to a regularly

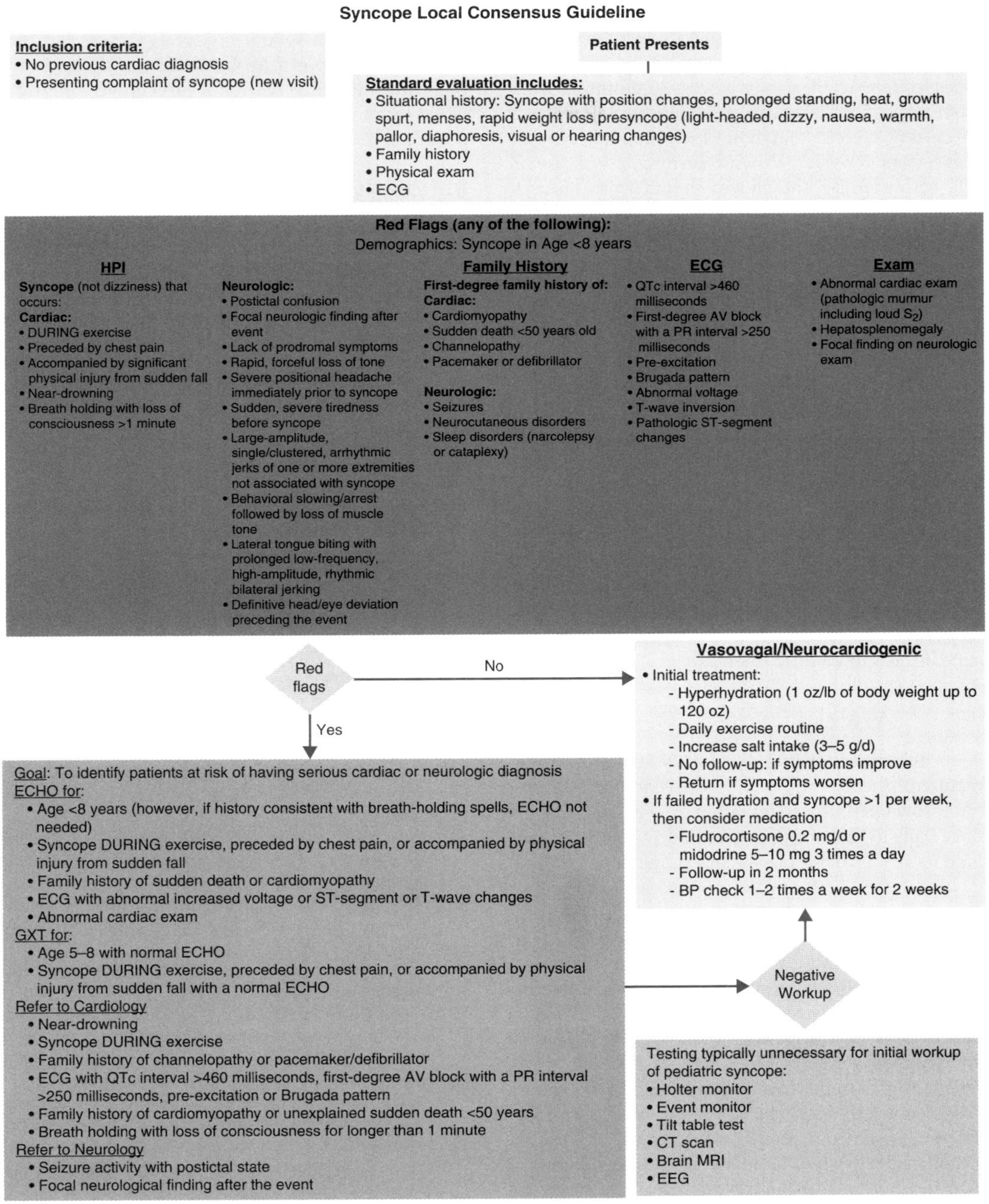

Syncope Local Consensus Guideline

Patient Presents

Inclusion criteria:
- No previous cardiac diagnosis
- Presenting complaint of syncope (new visit)

Standard evaluation includes:
- Situational history: Syncope with position changes, prolonged standing, heat, growth spurt, menses, rapid weight loss presyncope (light-headed, dizzy, nausea, warmth, pallor, diaphoresis, visual or hearing changes)
- Family history
- Physical exam
- ECG

Red Flags (any of the following):
Demographics: Syncope in Age <8 years

HPI

Syncope (not dizziness) that occurs:
Cardiac:
- DURING exercise
- Preceded by chest pain
- Accompanied by significant physical injury from sudden fall
- Near-drowning
- Breath holding with loss of consciousness >1 minute

Neurologic:
- Postictal confusion
- Focal neurologic finding after event
- Lack of prodromal symptoms
- Rapid, forceful loss of tone
- Severe positional headache immediately prior to syncope
- Sudden, severe tiredness before syncope
- Large-amplitude, single/clustered, arrhythmic jerks of one or more extremities not associated with syncope
- Behavioral slowing/arrest followed by loss of muscle tone
- Lateral tongue biting with prolonged low-frequency, high-amplitude, rhythmic bilateral jerking
- Definitive head/eye deviation preceding the event

Family History

First-degree family history of:
Cardiac:
- Cardiomyopathy
- Sudden death <50 years old
- Channelopathy
- Pacemaker or defibrillator

Neurologic:
- Seizures
- Neurocutaneous disorders
- Sleep disorders (narcolepsy or cataplexy)

ECG
- QTc interval >460 milliseconds
- First-degree AV block with a PR interval >250 milliseconds
- Pre-excitation
- Brugada pattern
- Abnormal voltage
- T-wave inversion
- Pathologic ST-segment changes

Exam
- Abnormal cardiac exam (pathologic murmur including loud S_2)
- Hepatosplenomegaly
- Focal finding on neurologic exam

Red flags — No → **Vasovagal/Neurocardiogenic**
- Initial treatment:
  - Hyperhydration (1 oz/lb of body weight up to 120 oz)
  - Daily exercise routine
  - Increase salt intake (3–5 g/d)
  - No follow-up: if symptoms improve
  - Return if symptoms worsen
- If failed hydration and syncope >1 per week, then consider medication
  - Fludrocortisone 0.2 mg/d or midodrine 5–10 mg 3 times a day
  - Follow-up in 2 months
  - BP check 1–2 times a week for 2 weeks

Red flags — Yes ↓

Goal: To identify patients at risk of having serious cardiac or neurologic diagnosis
ECHO for:
- Age <8 years (however, if history consistent with breath-holding spells, ECHO not needed)
- Syncope DURING exercise, preceded by chest pain, or accompanied by physical injury from sudden fall
- Family history of sudden death or cardiomyopathy
- ECG with abnormal increased voltage or ST-segment or T-wave changes
- Abnormal cardiac exam
GXT for:
- Age 5–8 with normal ECHO
- Syncope DURING exercise, preceded by chest pain, or accompanied by physical injury from sudden fall with a normal ECHO
Refer to Cardiology
- Near-drowning
- Syncope DURING exercise
- Family history of channelopathy or pacemaker/defibrillator
- ECG with QTc interval >460 milliseconds, first-degree AV block with a PR interval >250 milliseconds, pre-excitation or Brugada pattern
- Family history of cardiomyopathy or unexplained sudden death <50 years
- Breath holding with loss of consciousness for longer than 1 minute
Refer to Neurology
- Seizure activity with postictal state
- Focal neurological finding after the event

Negative Workup → (to Vasovagal/Neurocardiogenic)

Testing typically unnecessary for initial workup of pediatric syncope:
- Holter monitor
- Event monitor
- Tilt table test
- CT scan
- Brain MRI
- EEG

▲ **Figure 27–1.** Syncope local consensus guideline. This syncope algorithm was developed with dual goals of standardizing care for patients with pediatric syncope and reducing unnecessary healthcare expenditures associated with this diagnosis while ensuring red flags for serious cardiac or neurologic problems are appropriately investigated. AV, atrioventricular; BP, blood pressure; CT, computed tomography; ECG, electrocardiogram; ECHO, echocardiogram; EEG, electroencephalogram; GXT, graded exercise test; MRI, magnetic resonance imaging. (Reproduced with permission from Chris Statile, MD, Cincinnati Children's Hospital Medical Center, Division of Cardiology collaborated in development of original unpublished version of algorithm of which this is a revision.)

balanced meal or a sodium supplement to achieve increased sodium intake. Patients are encouraged to exercise daily to improve their cardiac output. If a patient is deconditioned or has not been exercising, the goal is at least 30 minutes 5 days per week. If the patient is an athlete, they should continue with their current exercise regimen, which should be at least 30 minutes 5 days per week. When returning to exercise or continuing with exercise, the patient should work on progressively prolonged periods of upright posture to encourage orthostatic tolerance. Lower body and core strength training is an important aspect of the exercise regimen to augment venous return and vasomotor responsiveness and thus prevent a rapid drop in blood pressure and resultant cerebral hypoperfusion.[46]

Other nonpharmacologic treatments include full-length compression stockings (30-40 mm Hg), more counter-maneuver training (eg, wall squats for exercise, raise head of bed at night), eating regularly, eating a diet high in protein and sodium, and practicing good sleep hygiene. Avoidance of caffeinated beverages, which cause increased urinary output and decreased blood volume, may also play a role in symptom management. Biofeedback has been shown to be an effective intervention for anxiety and depression, both of which can exacerbate syncope and presyncope.[32] Finally, further reassurance regarding the benign nature of the diagnosis and the expectation of successful treatment are imperative to pediatric NCS patients and their families.

FURTHER TREATMENT

If after 2 to 3 months of consistent and daily implementation of the treatment plan by the patient there is no noted symptomatic improvement, then initiation of fludrocortisone 0.2 mg once daily in the morning or midodrine 5 mg 3 times daily would be appropriate. The patient should have a blood pressure check 1 to 2 times a week for 2 weeks while beginning either medication to evaluate for hypertension.

Fludrocortisone is a mineralocorticoid used to treat orthostatic intolerance. The blood volume is increased as a result of fludrocortisone promoting increased reabsorption of sodium from distal renal tubules. Fludrocortisone is dependent on daily aggressive hydration to be an effective adjunctive treatment for NCS.[47]

Midodrine is a class IIA treatment for neurocardiogenic syncope at 10 mg 3 times a day.[42] As an α_1-agonist, midodrine increases blood pressure and vascular tone.[48] It is not as dependent on aggressive hydration, but aggressive hydration remains an integral part of the treatment plan to facilitate future weaning from medication and to achieve the goal of holistic management of symptoms without medication.

Typically, only one medication is used in the initial medication treatment program. Fludrocortisone has been known to increase compliance due to once-daily dosing. Midodrine seems to be more effective in patients who are challenged with aggressive hydration intake such as patients with gastroparesis, reflux, food avoidance, or other gastrointestinal issues. Follow-up in 2 to 3 months to evaluate the efficacy of the medication intervention is imperative. Referral to cardiology or an autonomic dysfunction center at any point for medication management is acceptable.

REFERENCES

1. Redd C, Thomas C, Willis M, Amos M, Anderson J. Cost of unnecessary testing in the evaluation of pediatric syncope. *Pediatr Cardiol*. 2017;38:1115-1122.
2. Fant C, Cohen A. Syncope in pediatric patients: a practical approach to differential diagnosis and management in the emergency department. *EB Med*. 2017;14(4):1-28.
3. Arthur W, Kaye G. The pathophysiology of common causes of syncope. *Postgrad Med J*. 2000;76:750-753.
4. Chen-Scarabelli C, Scarabelli T. Neurocardiogenic syncope. *Br Med J*. 2004;329(7461):336-341.
5. Anderson J, Willis M, Lancaster H, Leonard K, Thomas C. The evaluation and management of pediatric syncope. *Pediatr Neurol*. 2016;55:6-13.
6. Anderson J, Czosek R, Cnota J, Meganathan K, Knilans T, Heaton P. Pediatric syncope: National Hospital Ambulatory Medical Care Survey Results. *J Emerg Med*. 2012;43(4):575-583.
7. Shanahan K, Monuteaux M, Brunson D, et al. Long-term effects of an evidence-based guideline for emergency management of pediatric syncope. *Pediatr Qual Saf*. 2020;5(6):e361.
8. Hockin B, Heeney N, Whitehurst D, Claydon V. Evaluating the impact of orthostatic syncope and presyncope on quality of life: a systematic review and meta-analysis. *Front Cardiovasc Med*. 2022;9:834-879.
9. Varni J, Limbers C, Burwinkle T. Impaired health-related quality of life in children and adolescents with chronic conditions: a comparative analysis of 10 disease clusters and 33 disease categories/severities utilizing the PedsQL 4.0 Generic Core Scales. *Health Qual Life Outcomes*. 2007;5:43.
10. Anderson J, Czosek R, Knilans T, Marino B. The effect of pediatric syncope on health-related quality of life. *Cardiol Young*. 2012;22(5):583-588.
11. Grubb B. *The Fainting Phenomenon: Understanding Why People Faint and What to Do About It*. 2nd ed. Wiley-Blackwell; 2007.
12. Grubb B, Olshansky B. *Syncope: Mechanisms and Management*. 2nd ed. Blackwell; 2005.
13. Lempert T, Bauer M, Schmidt D. Syncope: a videometric analysis of 56 episodes of transient cerebral hypoxia. *Annal Neurol*. 1994;36(2):233-237.
14. Brigo F, Bongiovanni L, Nardone R. Lateral tongue biting versus biting at the tip of the tongue in differentiating between epileptic seizures and syncope. *Seizure*. 2013;22(9):801.
15. Maron B, Haas T, Ahluwalia A, Murphy C, Garberich R. Demographics and epidemiology of sudden deaths in young competitive athletes: from the United States National Registry. *Am J Med*. 2016;129(11):1170-1177.
16. Maron B, Haas T, Murphy C, Ahluwalia A, Rutten-Ramos S. Incidence and causes of sudden death in U.S. college athletes. *J Am Coll Cardiol*. 2014;63(16):1636-1643.
17. Stanford Medicine 25. Cardiac Second Heart Sounds. 2022. Accessed June 29, 2022. https://stanfordmedicine25.stanford.edu/the25/cardiac.html

18. Sieira J, Brugada P. The definition of the Brugada syndrome. *Eur Heart J.* 2017;38(40):3029-3034.

19. Dovgalyuk J, Holstege C, Mattu A, Brady W. The electrocardiogram in the patient with syncope. *Am J Emerg Med.* 2007;25(6):688-701.

20. Drezner J, Acekreman M, Anderson J, et al. Electrocardiographic interpretation in athletes: the "Seattle criteria." *Br J Sports Med.* 2013;47(3):122-124.

21. Tisdale J, Chung M, Campbell K, et al. Drug induced arrhythmias: a scientific statement from the American Heart Association. *Circulation.* 2020;142:e214-e233.

22. Rautaharju P, Surawicz B, Gettes L, et al. AHA/ACCF/HRS recommendations for the standardization and interpretation of the electrocardiogram: part IV: the ST segment, T and U waves, and the QT interval: a scientific statement from the American Heart Association Electrocardiography and Arrhythmias Committee, Council on Clinical Cardiology; the American College of Cardiology Foundation; and the Heart Rhythm Society: endorsed by the International Society for Computerized Electrocardiology. *Circulation.* 2009;119(10):e241-250.

23. Halliwill J, Buck T, Lacewell A, Romero A. Postexercise hypotension and sustained postexercise vasodilation: what happens after we exercise? *Exp Physiol.* 2012;98(1):7-18.

24. Busse H, Harrop T, Gunnell D, Kipping R. Prevalence and associated harm of engagement in self-asphyxial behaviours ('choking game') in young people: a systematic review. *Arch Dis Child.* 2015;100(12):1106.

25. Ullrich N, Goodkin H. The "choking game" and other strangulation activities in children and adolescents. *Up To Date.* February 2022. Accessed June 29, 2022. https://www.uptodate.com/contents/the-choking-game-and-other-strangulation-activities-in-children-and-adolescents

26. Centers for Disease Control and Prevention (CDC). Unintentional strangulation deaths from the "choking game" among youths ages 6-19 years—United States, 1995-2007. *MMWR Morbid Mortal Wkly Rep.* 2008;57:141.

27. Westendorp R, Blauw GJ, Frölich M, Simons R.. Hypoxic syncope. *Aviat Space Environ Med.* 1997;68(5):410-414.

28. Kikkeri N, Nagalli S. Subclavian steal syndrome. *StatPearls (Internet).* StatPearls Publishing; January 2022.

29. Beaumont T, Limbrick D, Rich K, Wippold F, Dacey R. Natural history of colloid cysts of the third ventricle. *J Neurosurg.* 2016;125:1420-1430.

30. Vazhayil V, Sadashiva N, Nayak N, Prabhuraj A, Shukla D, Somanna S. Surgical management of colloid cysts in children: experience at a tertiary care center. *Child Nerv Syst.* 2018;34:1215-1220.

31. American Psychiatric Association Task Force on DSM-5-TR. *Diagnostic and Statistical Manual of Mental Disorders, Fifth Edition, Text Revision (DSM-5-TR).* 5th ed. American Psychiatric Association; 2022.

32. Schab L. *The Coping Skills Workbook.* Childswork/Childsplay; 1991.

33. Evans W, Acherman R, Kip K, Restrepo H. Hair-grooming syncope in children. *Clin Pediatr.* 2009;48(8):834-836.

34. Stewart J. Common syndromes of orthostatic intolerance. *Pediatrics.* 2013;131(5):968-980.

35. Krzyzlof N, Cooley R, Somers V. Alcohol potentiates orthostatic hypotension: implications for alcohol-related syncope. *Circulation.* 2000;101:398-402.

36. Latif Z, Garg N. The impact of marijuana on the cardiovascular system: a review of the most common cardiovascular events associated with marijuana use. *J Clin Med.* 2020;9(6):1925.

37. Arslan M, Karaibrahimoğlu A, Demirtaş MS. Does iron therapy have a place in the management of all breath-holding spells? *Pediatr Int.* 2021;63(11):1344-1350.

38. Gurbuz G, Perk P, Cokyaman T. Iron supplementation should be given in breath-holding spells regardless of anemia. *Turk J Med Sci.* 2019;49(1):230-237.

39. Hamed S, Gad E, Sherif T. Iron deficiency and cyanotic breath-holding spells: the effectiveness of iron therapy. *Pediatr Hematol Oncol.* 2018;35(3):186-195.

40. Moodley, M. Clinical approach to syncope in children. *Semin Pediatr Neurol.* 2013;20:12-17.

41. Grubb BP, Kanjwal Y, Karabin B, Nasar I. Orthostatic hypotension and autonomic failure: a concise guide to diagnosis and management. *Clin Med Cardiol.* 2008;279-291.

42. Shen W, Sheldon R, Benditt D, et al. 2017 ACC/AHA/HRS guideline for the evaluation and management of patients with syncope. *J Am Coll Cardiol.* 2017;70(5):620-655.

43. Wieling W, Ganzeboom K, Saul J. Reflex syncope in children and adolescents. *Heart.* 2004;90(9):1094-1100.

44. Maron B, Friedman RA, Kligfield P, et al. Assessment of the 12-lead electrocardiogram as a screening test for detection of cardiovascular disease in healthy general populations of young people (12-25 years of age): AHA ACC scientific statement. *J Am Coll Cardiol.* 2014;64(14):1479-1514.

45. McIntyre-Patton L, Wanderski S, Graef D, Woessner L, Baker R. Randomized trial evaluating the effectiveness of a leg crossing and muscle tensing technique on decreasing vasovagal symptoms among pediatric and young adult patients undergoing peripheral IV catheter insertion. *J Pediatr Nurs.* 2018;38:53-56.

46. Gielen S, Schuler G, Adams V. Cardiovascular effects of exercise training. *Circulation.* 2010;122(12):1221-1238.

47. Fludrocortisone: mechanism of action. In Microcmedex (Columbia Basin College Library ed.) (Electronic version). Greenwood Village, CO: Truven Health Analytics. 2022. Accessed March 25, 2022. https://www.micromedexsolutions.com/

48. Midodrine: mechanism of action. In Microcmedex (Columbia Basin College Library ed.) (Electronic version). Greenwood Village, CO: Truven Health Analytics. 2022. Accessed March 25, 2022. https://www.micromedexsolutions.com/

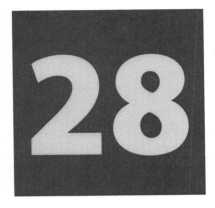

Normal Sleep and the Sleep Evaluation of Pediatric Patients

Rochelle M. Witt, MD, PhD

Wei K. Liu, MD

Thomas J. Dye, MD

NORMAL SLEEP IN CHILDREN

Sleep is the primary brain activity of the youngest children with an estimated 9500 hours (13 months) spent in sleep by the time a child is 2 years old (as compared to 8000 hours awake).[1] The sheer proportion of time young individuals spend in this state suggests its importance in appropriate development. Many have similarly argued that sleep is of particular importance in developing animals.[2-5] Although the functions of sleep are still not well elucidated, roles for sleep in cognition, learning, and memory consolidation are well founded.[4,6-10] It therefore stands to reason that issues of sleep may have developmental consequences, both for typically developing children and those with atypical neurodevelopment.

▶ Sleep Architecture

Sleep is a physiologic, reversible, and recurrent behavioral state of perceptual disengagement from the surrounding environment and relative unresponsiveness to external stimuli.[11] It is dynamic, resulting from the complex interplay of physiologic and behavioral processes that can be broadly segmented into (1) non–rapid eye movement (NREM) sleep, a sleep state characterized by unconscious or bland thoughts, a synchronized electroencephalogram (EEG) dominated by slower frequencies in the delta (0-4 Hz) and theta (4-7 Hz) ranges, and low sympathetic tone; and (2) rapid eye movement (REM) sleep, a dreaming or paradoxical sleep characterized by bursts of fast saccadic eye movements, a low voltage, mixed EEG pattern, variable sympathetic tone, and atonia of all voluntary muscles (except the extraocular muscles and the diaphragm).[12]

Age-Related Changes in Sleep Time, Sleep Architecture, and Sleep Staging

Sleep in most age groups (except infants) is categorized into 4 stages, primarily using EEG characteristics: stage N1, stage N2, stage N3 (deep sleep, delta wave sleep, or slow wave sleep), and stage REM. Stage N1 is typically characterized by slow, conjugate, sinusoidal eye movements of greater than 500 milliseconds. A transition from wakefulness to stage N1 often includes a slowing of background frequencies to low-amplitude, mixed-frequency (predominantly 4-7 Hz) EEG activity. Sharply contoured vertex waves of less than 0.5 seconds may also be present; these waveforms typically appear at 4 to 6 months postterm. Stage N2 is characterized by the presence of K complexes and/or sleep spindles on EEG. A K complex is a well-defined, negative, sharp deflection, usually maximal in amplitude in the frontal derivations, lasting for 0.5 seconds or more. Sleep spindles are trains of 11- to 16-Hz sinusoidal waves whose amplitudes are maximal in central derivation. K complexes are seen in the sleep EEGs of most infants by 3 to 6 months postterm. Sleep spindles may be seen by age 6 weeks to 3 months postterm and are present in all typically developing infants by 2 to 3 months of age.[13] The physiologic significance of these 2 wave types is unclear, but intriguing functions have been proposed. K complexes have been hypothesized to be an index of sleep arousals[14-16] or to protect sleep from disruption.[17-19] Sleep spindles have also been proposed to protect sleep from external perturbations, as higher spindle densities are associated with longer N2 sleep duration. These oscillations also evolve with a characteristic profile that parallels cortical development in postnatal, adolescent, and aging periods, suggesting the significance of sleep spindles in the age-related maturation of involved neural circuits and the processes they subserve.[20] N3 sleep is characterized by the presence of 20% or greater slow wave activity, 0.5- to 2-Hz waves of amplitudes greater than 75 uV measured over the frontal head region. Stage REM is characterized by rapid eye movements (conjugate, irregular, sharply peaked eye movements whose initial deflection is <500 milliseconds) and low chin electromyography (EMG) tone in the setting of low-amplitude, mixed-frequency EEG activity without K complexes or sleep spindles. Although generalized muscle atonia is typical of REM, transient muscle

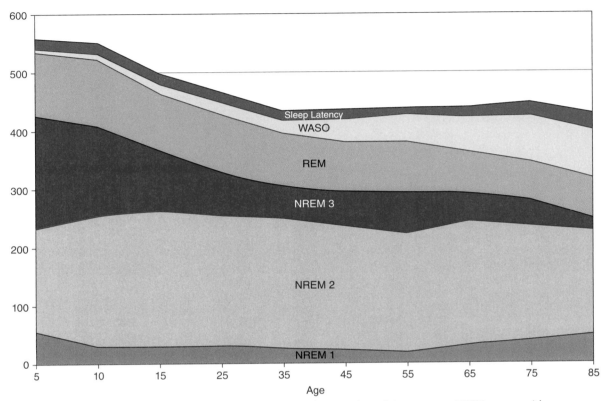

▲ **Figure 28–1.** Age associated changes in daily duration and proportion of sleep stages. NREM, non–rapid eye movement; WASO, wakefulness after sleep onset. (Reproduced with permission from Ohayon MM, Carskadon MA, Guilleminault C, et al. Meta-analysis of quantitative sleep parameters from childhood to old age in healthy individuals: developing normative sleep values across the human lifespan. *Sleep.* 2004;27(7):1255-1273.)

activity (short, irregular bursts of activity <0.25 seconds long often in the chin or anterior tibial EMG derivations) is often superimposed on this low EMG tone. See Figures 28–1 and 28–2 for age-related sleep characteristics.

Developmental Changes in Sleep-Wake Regulation

The 2-process model of sleep-wake regulation (Figure 28–3) describes how the interaction of the homeostatic sleep drive (process S) and endogenous circadian timing (process C) controls sleep and arousal.[21] Initially described by Borbely[22] and later refined by Borbely and others,[23-28] the 2-process model posits that the homeostatic sleep drive accumulates during wake, whereas it dissipates in sleep. The circadian process, generated at the level of the suprachiasmatic nucleus (SCN) by the master circadian pacemaker[29] and whose main markers are body temperature and melatonin, oscillates with a near 24-hour rhythmicity.

There is evidence that both processes undergo maturation from infancy to adulthood. The SCN is still immature at birth and undergoes rapid postnatal development over a few months.[30] The age of emergence and consolidation of the human circadian sleep-wake cycle has not been definitively established. The emergence of 24-hour rest-activity cycling has been seen in the first month of life,[31,32] but the consolidation of this rhythm is thought to occur around the third month of life[33] or the latter half of the first year.[31,34-36] Notably, salient interactions with the environment, as occurs in preterm birth, in breastfeeding, and in photoperiod exposure at birth, can modulate the development of the circadian timing system.[37] EEG markers of sleep homeostasis appear in the first postnatal months. At 2 months of age and thereafter, theta activity (but not delta activity) exhibits a declining trend across consecutive sleep episodes, which could be fit by an exponential function.[38] This behavior is similar to the exponential time course of delta activity, a core feature of the 2-process model of sleep regulation, seen across consecutive sleep episodes in adults.[22,23,39] In adults, the declining trend of EEG power and the increase in its initial level after sleep deprivation extend to the theta and alpha bands, in addition

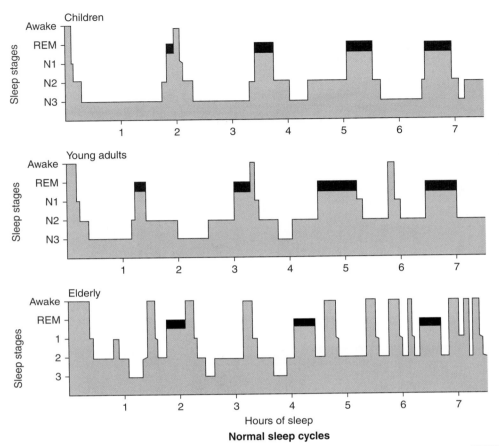

▲ **Figure 28–2.** Changes in sleep architecture (non–rapid eye movement [NREM]–rapid eye movement [REM] cycling) with age: hypnograms demonstrating the normal distribution of sleep stages in healthy children, adults, and the elderly. (Reproduced with permission from Mindell JA, Owens JA. *A Clinical Guide to Pediatric Sleep: Diagnosis and Management of Sleep Problems.* Philadelphia, PA: Lippincott Williams & Wilkins; 2015.)

to the delta band.[39-42] Thus, theta activity during NREM sleep may be a marker of sleep homeostasis during development, when the generators of delta activity are not yet coupled to the mechanisms involved in sleep homeostasis.[38] One theory regarding why process S may factor more prominently in sleep-wake regulation during early infancy as compared to process C is that the large sleep requirement seen in infants necessitates a sleep drive that is relatively insensitive to environmental influences. Additionally, sleep may function to promote long-term memory consolidation and cortical development, and sleep-wake cycling predominantly regulated by process S may be evolutionarily advantageous.[37]

Teens experience maturational changes in their sleep biology, which include a slowing of the accumulation of sleep homeostatic pressure across the waking day[43] and a slowing of the dissipation of sleep homeostatic pressure (late adolescence).[44] Process C is also undergoing maturational changes. A phase delay in the circadian timing system[45,46] and a heightened sensitivity to light[47] occur in adolescence. Psychosocial factors (eg, shifts in roles and responsibilities during the teenage years and social engagements in the evenings),[44,48] sociocultural factors (eg, early school start times), and behavioral practices (eg, later bedtimes, increased technology use, and screen time)[49] conspire with biologic factors to create a "perfect storm" of vulnerability with respect to sleep issues in adolescence.

Circadian preference, a predilection for an early, typical, or late sleep schedule, as well as times preferred for peak cognitive and physical performance and times at which psychological aspects are experienced vary significantly across the life span.

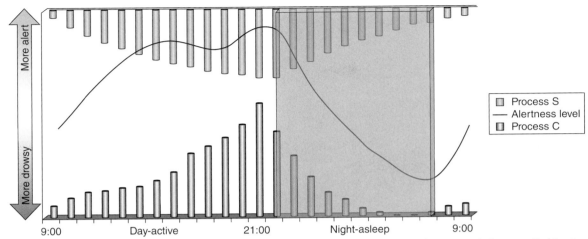

▲ **Figure 28–3.** Two-process model of sleep. A linearly accumulating then dissipating homeostatic (process S) drive to sleep is opposed by a circadian alerting signal that oscillates with a near 24-hour periodicity. (Reproduced with permission from Schneider L. Neurobiology and Neuroprotective Benefits of Sleep. *Continuum (Minneap Minn)*. 2020;26(4):848-870.)

Morningness is more prevalent in young children, but a decrease in this prevalence begins at 1 to 2 and 3 to 4 years of age.[50] Eveningness becomes more common in adolescence, reaching a maximum around 20 years of age. After this time, a shift occurs toward morningness prevalence in the adult population.[51,52] Differences in a single individual's circadian and homeostatic sleep regulation[53] can result in a specific circadian preference that does not respect these general trends.[54]

Sleep Recommendations by Age

While it is clear the amount of sleep required by infants, children, and adults changes with age, the determination of the precise amount necessary has been complicated. The recommended amount of sleep for pediatric populations, according to the Consensus Statement of the American Academy of Sleep Medicine (AASM), states that infants 4 to 12 months of age should sleep 12 to 16 hours per 24 hours (including naps), whereas children between 1 and 2 years old need 11 to 14 hours nightly and adolescents 13 to 18 years of age need 8 to 10 hours of sleep.[55] Based on a review of 864 published articles considering childhood sleep duration, sleeping the recommended durations was associated with improved health outcomes including better attention, behavior, learning, memory, emotional regulation, quality of life, and physical and mental health. The panel that developed the consensus recommendations noted these were intended as a first step to evaluate the published literature on pediatric sleep durations and to encourage an adequate sleep duration for all children, while they acknowledged existing knowledge gaps in that literature.[56,57] Another, differing set of recommendations for daily sleep duration was generated

by a multidisciplinary expert panel convened by the National Sleep Foundation (Figure 28–4). Recommended daily sleep durations were as follows: 14 to 17 hours for newborns, 12 to 15 hours for infants, 11 to 14 hours for toddlers, 10 to 13 hours for preschoolers, 9 to 11 hours for school-aged children, and 8 to 10 hours for teenagers. Seven to 9 hours of sleep are recommended for young adults and adults, and 7 to 8 hours of sleep are recommended for older adults.[58] Clinicians should be aware of this difference when advising families about daily sleep duration.

EVALUATION OF CHILDHOOD SLEEP DISORDERS

▶ History

Like most neurology, sleep medicine relies on the taking of a careful and accurate history to reach diagnoses. A thorough medical history will often reveal comorbid diagnoses in addition to sleep disorders. These include asthma, gastroesophageal reflux disease, allergies, chronic lung disease, sickle cell disease, obesity, prematurity, and pain, as well as neurologic diagnoses of epilepsy, headache, cerebral palsy, developmental delay, attention-deficit/hyperactivity disorder, autism spectrum disorder, neuromuscular disorders, Chiari malformations, and traumatic brain injury. Psychiatric diagnoses, including anxiety, depression, and bipolar disorder, can also adversely impact sleep. A developmental history, behavioral assessment, and assessment of school functioning are key. A social history should include the patient's (if appropriate) and the caregivers' occupation, especially if shift work is involved. A focused family history can identify patients at

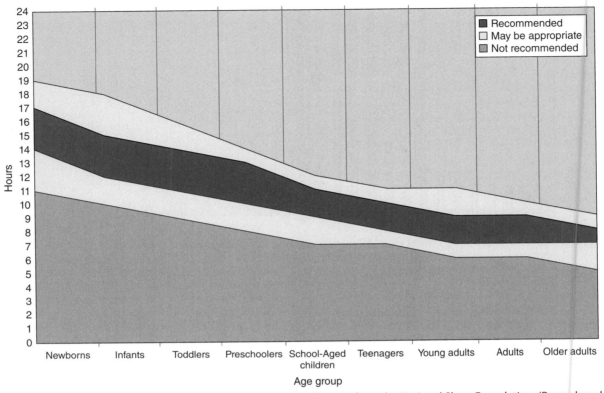

▲ **Figure 28–4.** Sleep duration recommendations across the life span from the National Sleep Foundation. (Reproduced with permission from Hirshkowitz M, Whiton K, Albert SM, et al. National Sleep Foundation's updated sleep duration recommendations: final report. *Sleep Health.* 2015;1(4):233-243.)

increased risk for sleep apnea, narcolepsy, partial arousal parasomnias, restless legs syndrome, and circadian rhythm sleep-wake disorders. Prescribed medications and other substances that affect sleep, including caffeine and alcohol, should be documented.[59]

The basic sleep history details both a patient's nights and their days. Collateral history from caregivers or observers is critical to understanding the symptoms of the pediatric patient with a sleep complaint. A detailing of the patient's bedtime routine can uncover important clues as to the cause of a sleep issue; sleep associations and behaviors, the sleep environment, and activities performed close to the desired bedtime, including screen use, should be recorded. Characterization of sleep initiation, sleep maintenance, and sleep termination on weekdays, weekends, and vacations is important. Nocturnal respiratory symptoms (eg, snoring, witnessed apneas) and abnormal movements (eg, restless legs, periodic limb movements, behaviors consistent with parasomnias and/or nocturnal seizures) should be considered. Daytime symptoms of excessive daytime sleepiness, cataplexy, and sleep paralysis should be noted.[60] A sleep history should also include naps, including their timing, duration, location, and the consistency of napping behavior.

► **Physical Examination**

A physical examination should be performed on all pediatric patients with sleep complaints. The patient's general appearance should be noted, including signs of fatigue and/or sleepiness. The patient's activity level should also be noted, as a sleep-deprived child may be disinhibited and hyperactive in the clinic. Of particular importance is an assessment of a patient's growth, including height, weight, age- and sex-adjusted body mass index, and neck circumference. Craniofacial features should be detailed, and an ear, nose, and throat exam should be performed, because a deviated nasal septum, turbinate hypertrophy, adenotonsillar hypertrophy, oropharyngeal crowding, and a large tongue could all contribute to sleep-disordered breathing. A neurologic examination should also be performed, especially in children with symptoms consistent with a sleep-related movement disorder, excessive daytime sleepiness, atypical parasomnias, and seizures. Myopathies and scoliosis increase the risk of hypoventilation or sleep apnea.

▶ Tools and Tests

Polysomnography

Polysomnography (PSG) is the continuous recording of several physiologic parameters during sleep, generally including a limited EEG; a limited-lead electrocardiogram (ECG); left and right electro-oculograms (EOGs); airflow as determined by a nasal pressure transducer and thermistor; respiratory effort as measured by inductive plethysmometry; gas exchange using pulse oximetry and end-tidal capnometry (carbon dioxide); pulse wave amplitude; EMG of the chin, legs, and intercostals; snore; microphone; respiratory rate; body positioning; and video monitoring. Technical and digital specifications for routine PSGs, as well as standardized scoring rules for the generated data, can be found in *The AASM Manual for the Scoring of Sleep and Associated Events: Rules, Terminology and Technical Specifications*.[13] Ambulatory sleep studies are advised against in children at present because there is insufficient evidence to assess whether certain features typical of sleep in children, including restless sleep, monitoring intolerance, frequency of arousal-based respiratory events needing an EEG for detection, and sleep fragmentation, may affect the validity of an ambulatory sleep study in children.[61]

Indications for a PSG include assessment for obstructive sleep apnea before and after surgical intervention; assessment of sleep-disordered breathing, including central sleep apnea, hypoventilation, and/or sleep-related hypoxemia; titration of noninvasive respiratory support; BRUE (brief resolved unexplained event) assessment with clinical evidence of sleep-disordered breathing; evaluation prior to decannulation (select protocols); assessment of sleep-related movement disorders; evaluation of atypical presentations of potential parasomnias, especially when historical elements suggest possible nocturnal seizure activity; and evaluation of central disorders of hypersomnolence (paired with a multiple sleep latency test [MSLT] the following day).[62-64] The limited EEG montage employed in PSG can also be expanded to a full EEG montage for the evaluation of sleep-related epilepsy or when seizures and parasomnias cannot be differentiated on history alone.[65]

Multiple Sleep Latency Test and Maintenance of Wakefulness Test

The MSLT and the maintenance of wakefulness test (MWT) are objective measures of somnolence and alertness, respectively. In both procedures, several physiologic parameters are continually recorded, including a limited EEG, a limited-lead ECG, left and right EOGs, EMG of the chin, and video monitoring. The MSLT objectively measures one's sleep propensity in nonstimulating, laboratory conditions. A shorter time to sleep onset reflects greater daytime sleepiness. Several measurements of sleep latency at regular intervals across the day (typically, five 20-minute nap opportunities spaced the day (typically, five 20-minute nap opportunities spaced 2 hours apart) are averaged to calculate a mean sleep latency (MSL). The MSL and the number of naps in which REM sleep occurs are criteria used to diagnose narcolepsy types 1 and 2 and idiopathic hypersomnia.[66] Persistent sleepiness after the treatment of other sleep disorders such as obstructive sleep apnea is also assessed by the MSLT.[67]

In contrast, the MWT is an objective measure of the ability to stay awake under nonstimulating conditions.[68] A prolonged sleep latency reflects an increased ability to stay awake in the context of trying to remain awake. Similar to the MSLT, several measurements of sleep latency at regular intervals across the day (typically, four 40-minute nap opportunities) are averaged to calculate the MSL. The MWT evaluates a treatment regimen's ability to adequately control excessive sleepiness and to assess alertness in individuals who must remain awake for safety reasons.[68,69] Data from both tests are scored according to standardized criteria.[13]

Sleep Diary

A sleep diary is a systematic pictorial or graphic log kept prospectively to record daily bedtimes, sleep and wake times (including night wakings and daytime naps), sleep quality, and other factors that may affect sleep (eg, caffeine ingestion). Sleep diaries are typically maintained for 1 to 2 weeks or longer. Indications include assessment for insomnia and circadian rhythm sleep-wake disorders, need for clarification of an unclear history, and postintervention assessment. Sleep diaries are often included in actigraphy studies for verification of times and identifying artifact.

Actigraphy

Actigraphy is a procedure that uses a wristwatch-like device with an accelerometer to record and integrate the occurrence and degree of movement over time to estimate rest-activity cycles as a surrogate for sleep-wake cycles. Many devices also collect ambient light data and surface body temperature data. The devices are typically worn unobtrusively on the wrist or ankle for days or weeks. Actigraphy data are usually combined with sleep diary data. The American Academy of Sleep Medicine commissioned a task force of experts who made the following recommendations for pediatric patients: Clinicians should use actigraphy in the assessment of insomnia disorder (Strength of Recommendation: Conditional), and circadian rhythm sleep-wake disorders (Strength of Recommendation: Conditional). It was also recommended that clinicians use actigraphy to monitor total sleep time prior to testing with the MSLT in adult and pediatric patients with suspected central disorders of hypersomnolence (Strength of Recommendation: Conditional). The task force also recommended that clinicians *not* use actigraphy in place of EMG for the diagnosis of periodic limb movement disorder in adult and pediatric patients (Strength of Recommendation: Strong).[70] Furthermore, the task force notes that actigraphy provides consistent objective data that are often unique from patient-reported sleep logs for some sleep parameters in adult and pediatric patients with suspected or diagnosed insomnia, circadian rhythm sleep-wake disorders, sleep-disordered breathing, and central disorders of hypersomnolence. Finally, the task force indicates that actigraphy is not a reliable measure of periodic limb movements in adult and pediatric patients.[71]

REFERENCES

1. Mindell JA, Owens JA. *A Clinical Guide to Pediatric Sleep: Diagnosis and Management of Sleep Problems*. Lippincott Williams & Wilkins; 2015.
2. Abel T, Havekes R, Saletin JM, Walker MP. Sleep, plasticity and memory from molecules to whole-brain networks. *Curr Biol*. 2013;23(17):R774-R788.
3. Diekelmann S, Born J. The memory function of sleep. *Nat Rev Neurosci*. 2010;11(2):114-126.
4. Frank MG. Sleep and synaptic plasticity in the developing and adult brain. *Curr Top Behav Neurosci*. 2015;25:123-149.
5. Roffwarg HP, Muzio JN, Dement WC. Ontogenetic development of the human sleep-dream cycle. *Science*. 1966;152(3722):604-619.
6. Tononi G, Cirelli C. Sleep and the price of plasticity: from synaptic and cellular homeostasis to memory consolidation and integration. *Neuron*. 2014;81(1):12-34.
7. Kurdziel L, Duclos K, Spencer RM. Sleep spindles in midday naps enhance learning in preschool children. *Proc Natl Acad Sci U S A*. 2013;110(43):17267-17272.
8. Walker MP, Stickgold R. Sleep-dependent learning and memory consolidation. *Neuron*. 2004;44(1):121-133.
9. Clawson BC, Pickup EJ, Ensing A, et al. Causal role for sleep-dependent reactivation of learning-activated sensory ensembles for fear memory consolidation. *Nat Commun*. 2021;12(1):1200.
10. Spruyt K. Neurocognitive effects of sleep disruption in children and adolescents. *Child Adolesc Psychiatr Clin N Am*. 2021;30(1):27-45.
11. Carskadon MA, Dement WC. Monitoring and staging human sleep. In: Kryger MH, Roth T, Dement WC, eds. *Principles and Practice of Sleep Medicine*. Elsevier Saunders; 2011:16-26.
12. Scammell TE, Arrigoni E, Lipton JO. Neural circuitry of wakefulness and sleep. *Neuron*. 2017;93(4):747-765.
13. Berry RB, Quan S, Abreu A. *The AASM Manual for the Scoring of Sleep and Associated Events: Rules, Terminology and Technical Specifications, Version 2.6*. American Academy of Sleep Medicine; 2020.
14. Karadeniz D, Ondze B, Besset A, Billiard M. EEG arousals and awakenings in relation with periodic leg movements during sleep. *J Sleep Res*. 2000;9(3):273-277.
15. MacFarlane JG, Shahal B, Mously C, Moldofsky H. Periodic K-alpha sleep EEG activity and periodic limb movements during sleep: comparisons of clinical features and sleep parameters. *Sleep*. 1996;19(3):200-204.
16. Montplaisir J, Boucher S, Gosselin A, Poirier G, Lavigne G. Persistence of repetitive EEG arousals (K-alpha complexes) in RLS patients treated with L-DOPA. *Sleep*. 1996;19(3):196-199.
17. De Gennaro L, Ferrara M, Bertini M. The spontaneous K-complex during stage 2 sleep: is it the "forerunner" of delta waves? *Neurosci Lett*. 2000;291(1):41-43.
18. Wauquier A, Aloe L, Declerck A. K-complexes: are they signs of arousal or sleep protective? *J Sleep Res*. 1995;4(3):138-143.
19. Amzica F, Steriade M. The functional significance of K-complexes. *Sleep Med Rev*. 2002;6(2):139-149.
20. Fernandez LMJ, Luthi A. Sleep spindles: mechanisms and functions. *Physiol Rev*. 2020;100(2):805-868.
21. Schneider L. Neurobiology and neuroprotective benefits of sleep. *Continuum (Minneap Minn)*. 2020;26(4):848-870.
22. Borbely AA. A two process model of sleep regulation. *Hum Neurobiol*. 1982;1(3):195-204.
23. Daan S, Beersma DG, Borbely AA. Timing of human sleep: recovery process gated by a circadian pacemaker. *Am J Physiol*. 1984;246(2 Pt 2):R161-R183.
24. Borbely AA, Achermann P. Sleep homeostasis and models of sleep regulation. *J Biol Rhythms*. 1999;14(6):557-568.
25. Borbely AA, Achermann P, Trachsel L, Tobler I. Sleep initiation and initial sleep intensity: interactions of homeostatic and circadian mechanisms. *J Biol Rhythms*. 1989;4(2):149-160.
26. Achermann P, Dijk DJ, Brunner DP, Borbély AA. A model of human sleep homeostasis based on EEG slow-wave activity: quantitative comparison of data and simulations. *Brain Res Bull*. 1993;31(1-2):97-113.
27. Edgar DM, Dement WC, Fuller CA. Effect of SCN lesions on sleep in squirrel monkeys: evidence for opponent processes in sleep-wake regulation. *J Neurosci*. 1993;13(3):1065-1079.
28. Dijk DJ, Czeisler CA. Contribution of the circadian pacemaker and the sleep homeostat to sleep propensity, sleep structure, electroencephalographic slow waves, and sleep spindle activity in humans. *J Neurosci*. 1995;15(5 Pt 1):3526-3538.
29. Schwartz MD, Kilduff TS. The neurobiology of sleep and wakefulness. *Psychiatr Clin North Am*. 2015;38(4):615-644.
30. Swaab DF, Hofman MA, Honnebier MB. Development of vasopressin neurons in the human suprachiasmatic nucleus in relation to birth. *Brain Res Dev Brain Res*. 1990;52(1-2):289-293.
31. Jenni OG, Deboer T, Achermann P. Development of the 24-h rest-activity pattern in human infants. *Infant Behav Dev*. 2006;29(2):143-152.
32. Nishihara K, Horiuchi S, Eto H, Uchida S. The development of infants' circadian rest-activity rhythm and mothers' rhythm. *Physiol Behav*. 2002;77(1):91-98.
33. Fukuda K, Ishihara K. Development of human sleep and wakefulness rhythm during the first six months of life: discontinuous changes at the 7th and 12th week after birth. *Biol Rhythm Res*. 1997;28:94-103.
34. Iglowstein I, Jenni OG, Molinari L, Largo RH. Sleep duration from infancy to adolescence: reference values and generational trends. *Pediatrics*. 2003;111(2):302-307.
35. Paavonen EJ, Morales-Muñoz I, Pölkki P, et al. Development of sleep-wake rhythms during the first year of age. *J Sleep Res*. 2020;29(3):e12918.
36. Kleitman N, Engelmann TG. Sleep characteristics of infants. *J Appl Physiol*. 1953;6(5):269-282.
37. Tonetti L. Circadian rhythms in children. In: *Pediatric Sleep Medicine*. Springer; 2021:105-111.
38. Jenni OG, Borbely AA, Achermann P. Development of the nocturnal sleep electroencephalogram in human infants. *Am J Physiol Regul Integr Comp Physiol*. 2004;286(3):R528-R238.
39. Borbely AA, Baumann F, Brandeis D, Strauch I, Lehmann D. Sleep deprivation: effect on sleep stages and EEG power density in man. *Electroencephalogr Clin Neurophysiol*. 1981;51(5):483-495.

40. Aeschbach D, Borbely AA. All-night dynamics of the human sleep EEG. *J Sleep Res.* 1993;2(2):70-81.

41. Dijk DJ, Shanahan TL, Duffy JF, et al. Variation of electroencephalographic activity during non-rapid eye movement and rapid eye movement sleep with phase of circadian melatonin rhythm in humans. *J Physiol.* 1997;505(Pt 3):851-858.

42. Finelli LA, Baumann H, Borbély AA, Achermann P. Dual electroencephalogram markers of human sleep homeostasis: correlation between theta activity in waking and slow-wave activity in sleep. *Neuroscience.* 2000;101(3):523-529.

43. Jenni OG, Achermann P, Carskadon MA. Homeostatic sleep regulation in adolescents. *Sleep.* 2005;28(11):1446-1454.

44. Carskadon MA. Sleep in adolescents: the perfect storm. *Pediatr Clin North Am.* 2011;58(3):637-647.

45. Crowley SJ, Acebo C, Carskadon MA. Sleep, circadian rhythms, and delayed phase in adolescence. *Sleep Med.* 2007;8(6):602-612.

46. Hagenauer MH, Perryman JI, Lee TM, Carskadon MA. Adolescent changes in the homeostatic and circadian regulation of sleep. *Dev Neurosci.* 2009;31(4):276-284.

47. Crowley SJ, Cain SW, Burns AC, et al. Increased sensitivity of the circadian system to light in early/mid-puberty. *J Clin Endocrinol Metab.* 2015;100(11):4067-4073.

48. LeBourgeois MK, Giannotti F, Cortesi F, Wolfson AR, Harsh J. The relationship between reported sleep quality and sleep hygiene in Italian and American adolescents. *Pediatrics.* 2005;115(1 suppl):257-265.

49. Carskadon MA, Acebo C. Regulation of sleepiness in adolescents: update, insights, and speculation. *Sleep.* 2002;25(6):606-614.

50. Randler C, Fassl C, Kalb N. From lark to owl: developmental changes in morningness-eveningness from new-borns to early adulthood. *Sci Rep.* 2017;7:45874.

51. Roenneberg T, Kuehnle T, Pramstaller PP, et al. A marker for the end of adolescence. *Curr Biol.* 2004;14(24):R1038-R1039.

52. Tonetti L, Fabbri M, Natale V. Sex difference in sleep-time preference and sleep need: a cross-sectional survey among Italian pre-adolescents, adolescents, and adults. *Chronobiol Int.* 2008;25(5):745-759.

53. Mongrain V, Paquet J, Dumont M. Contribution of the photoperiod at birth to the association between season of birth and diurnal preference. *Neurosci Lett.* 2006;406(1-2):113-116.

54. Adan A, Archer SN, Hidalgo MP, et al. Circadian typology: a comprehensive review. *Chronobiol Int.* 2012;29(9):1153-1175.

55. Paruthi S, Brooks LJ, D'Ambrosio C, et al. Recommended amount of sleep for pediatric populations: a consensus statement of the American Academy of Sleep Medicine. *J Clin Sleep Med.* 2016;12(6):785-786.

56. Paruthi S, Brooks LJ, D'Ambrosio C, et al. Consensus statement of the American Academy of Sleep Medicine on the recommended amount of sleep for healthy children: methodology and discussion. *J Clin Sleep Med.* 2016;12(11):1549-1561.

57. Paruthi S, Brooks LJ, D'Ambrosio C, et al. Pediatric sleep duration consensus statement: a step forward. *J Clin Sleep Med.* 2016;12(12):1705-1706.

58. Hirshkowitz M, Whiton K, Albertet SM, al. National Sleep Foundation's updated sleep duration recommendations: final report. *Sleep Health.* 2015;1(4):233-243.

59. Rana M, Khatwa U, Kothare S. *Handbook of Pediatric Neurology.* Lippincott Williams & Wilkins; 2013:464-485.

60. Silber MH. Diagnostic approach and investigation in sleep medicine. *Continuum (Minneap Minn).* 2017;23(4):973-988.

61. Kirk V, Baughn J, D'Andrea L, et al. American Academy of Sleep Medicine position paper for the use of a home sleep apnea test for the diagnosis of OSA in children. *J Clin Sleep Med.* 2017;13(10):1199-1203.

62. Aurora RN, Chowdhuri S, Ramar K, et al. The treatment of central sleep apnea syndromes in adults: practice parameters with an evidence-based literature review and meta-analyses. *Sleep.* 2012;35(1):17-40.

63. Aurora RN, Zak RS, Karippot A, et al. Practice parameters for the respiratory indications for polysomnography in children. *Sleep.* 2011;34(3):379-388.

64. Wise MS, Nichols CD, Grigg-Damberger MM, et al. Executive summary of respiratory indications for polysomnography in children: an evidence-based review. *Sleep.* 2011;34(3):389-398.

65. Jain SV, Dye T, Kedia P. Value of combined video EEG and polysomnography in clinical management of children with epilepsy and daytime or nocturnal spells. *Seizure.* 2019;65:1-5.

66. Sateia M, ed. *International Classification of Sleep Disorders.* 3rd ed. American Academy of Sleep Medicine; 2014.

67. Krahn LE, Arand DL, Avidan AY, et al. Recommended protocols for the multiple sleep latency test and maintenance of wakefulness test in adults: guidance from the American Academy of Sleep Medicine. *J Clin Sleep Med.* 2021;17(12):2489-2498.

68. Arand D, Bonnet M, Hurwitz T, et al. The clinical use of the MSLT and MWT. *Sleep.* 2005;28(1):123-144.

69. Wise MS. Objective measures of sleepiness and wakefulness: application to the real world? *J Clin Neurophysiol.* 2006;23(1):39-49.

70. Smith MT, McCrae CS, Cheung J, et al. Use of actigraphy for the evaluation of sleep disorders and circadian rhythm sleep-wake disorders: an American Academy of Sleep Medicine Clinical Practice Guideline. *J Clin Sleep Med.* 2018;14(7):1231-1237.

71. Smith MT, McCrae CS, Cheung J, et al. Use of actigraphy for the evaluation of sleep disorders and circadian rhythm sleep-wake disorders: an American Academy of Sleep Medicine systematic review, meta-analysis, and GRADE assessment. *J Clin Sleep Med.* 2018;14(7):1209-1230.

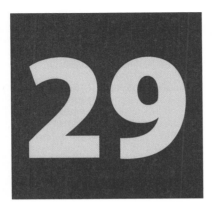

Parasomnias and Sleep-Related Movement Disorders

Wei K. Liu, MD

Rochelle M. Witt, MD, PhD

Thomas J. Dye, MD

RESTLESS LEGS SYNDROME AND PERIODIC LIMB MOVEMENT DISORDER

Diagnostic Essentials

Restless legs syndrome (RLS) is a common sensorimotor neurologic disorder with symptoms in both wakefulness and sleep. It affects 5% to 10% of adults, with up to 38% of adults reporting the onset of symptoms in childhood and 8% to 13% reporting symptoms before age 10.[1] RLS is a clinical diagnosis with 4 essential symptom criteria: (1) an urge to move the legs, usually in association with or due to uncomfortable sensations in the legs; (2) symptoms that begin or worsen during rest or inactivity (ie, sitting or lying down); (3) partial or complete relief of symptoms with movement; and (4) symptoms that are only present or become worse at night (Table 29–1). RLS is a unique clinical entity, and therefore, the symptoms cannot be due to other conditions such as muscle cramps, neuropathies, or positional discomfort.[2,3]

General Considerations

Eliciting the typical symptoms of RLS in children is especially challenging, limited often by the child's ability to describe sensations that cause discomfort but are frequently not painful. As such, special considerations should be made when assessing the quality of RLS symptoms described by children.[3] Common descriptive terms used by children include creepy-crawlies, ants crawling, jittery, worms moving, shock-like feelings, burning, throbbing, tight feelings, fidgety, and itchy bones.[4] Caregivers may report restlessness in bed with limb jerks or leg kicking, difficulty falling or staying asleep, and daytime consequences such as fatigue or behavioral symptoms.

Etiology and Pathogenesis

The pathophysiology of RLS has not been fully elucidated, although brain iron deficiency related to abnormalities of central nervous system iron transport and/or iron storage is thought to be a primary cause.[5,6] Secondary causes of RLS include disorders related to iron metabolism or iron deficiency including chronic renal disease, iron deficiency anemia, and pregnancy. Circadian dysregulation of dopaminergic neurons[7] may explain the treatment response to dopaminergic agents as well as the exacerbation of symptoms seen with antidopaminergic medications (antiemetics, antipsychotics). Pediatric RLS shows a high degree of heritability, with up to 80% children with RLS having one parent with symptoms of RLS.[8] Genome-wide association studies have identified several genetic polymorphisms, including at *BTBD9*, that increase the risk for RLS.[9]

Clinical Findings

RLS is a clinical diagnosis, and all 4 of the typical URGE symptoms (see Table 29–1) are necessary to establish the definite diagnosis in adults. Therefore, polysomnography (PSG) is typically not indicated in this population. However, when the diagnosis is suspected in children but symptomatic history is unclear, supportive criteria (including PSG) can be used to assist in diagnosis (Table 29–2).

The physical exam is generally normal in pediatric RLS, although causes of secondary RLS should be assessed. Evaluation of iron insufficiency should be performed in all children with signs and symptoms of RLS. This includes serum ferritin, iron, total iron-binding capacity (TIBC), and percent transferrin saturation (%TSAT), which should be obtained fasting and in the morning.[10]

Differential Diagnosis

Nocturnal leg cramping can be differentiated from RLS by the typically painful symptoms often localized to the calves. Peripheral neuropathies may mimic some of the symptoms of RLS in terms of a bilateral distribution with worsening of symptoms at nighttime, although they typically are not

Table 29–1. Essential symptoms of restless legs syndrome (URGE).

- **U**rge to move the legs
- **R**elieved with movement
- **G**ets worse when lying down or sitting
- **E**vening and sleep worsen symptoms

improved with activity and may be associated with other exam findings such as weakness or sensory changes. Hypnagogic foot tremor is a 0.3- to 4-Hz rhythmic movement of the feet or toes typically seen during transitions from waking to sleep and generally lacks the sensory symptoms seen in RLS.

Treatment

Treatment of RLS should include both pharmacologic and nonpharmacologic behavioral modifications to address the sensorimotor symptoms and the associated sleep disturbance. Iron supplementation is the initial pharmacologic treatment option in patients with serum ferritin less than 50 ng/mL. Doses of 3 mg/kg/d up to 130 mg of elemental iron are recommended. Absorption is thought to be best when taken once daily (but can be divided twice daily if not tolerated). Vitamin C supplementation can be used to aid absorption. Iron and ferritin values should be followed every 3 months until the serum ferritin reaches 50 ng/mL or greater, after which if levels are supratherapeutic the dose can be tapered off or converted to a multivitamin with iron. Patients should be counseled on the risk of constipation, and a bowel regimen should be considered in children with preexisting constipation. In cases where absorption is inadequate or enteral supplementation is unsuccessful, intravenous iron formulations can be used.[11] Gabapentin or pregabalin given 1.5 hours before typical sleep onset can also be used for patients with refractory symptoms or individuals who cannot tolerate iron supplementation. Dopaminergic agonists such as pramipexole or ropinirole are typically not used in pediatric patients due to the risk of adverse effects but can be considered in severe cases.

Stretching exercises prior to bedtime may provide symptomatic relief of motor restlessness at sleep onset, although strenuous activity should be avoided. Caffeine consumption

Table 29–2. Supportive clinical features of restless legs syndrome (RLS).

- Family history of RLS, particularly first-degree relatives
- Presence of periodic limb movements (during wakefulness or sleep) on polysomnography
- Response to dopaminergic therapy

Table 29–3. Medications that may aggravate symptoms of restless legs syndrome.

- Selective serotonin reuptake inhibitors
- Serotonin-norepinephrine reuptake inhibitors
- Tricyclic antidepressants
- Nicotine
- Diphenhydramine
- Metoclopramide
- Alcohol

should be avoided because it may increase motor restlessness. Certain medications may exacerbate symptoms of RLS (Table 29–3).

Prognosis

Primary pediatric RLS is generally believed to be a chronic condition, although prognosis remains uncertain due to underreporting and limited prospective data. For children with milder cases of RLS, it may have a more waxing and waning or self-remitting course. Cases that come to the attention of sleep physicians are typically moderate to severe, and for these patients, symptoms tend to increase over time into adulthood.

PERIODIC LIMB MOVEMENT DISORDER

Diagnostic Essentials

Periodic limb movements of sleep (PLMS) are a PSG finding typically described as an extension of the toe, dorsiflexion of the ankle, and/or flexion of the knee and hip (similar to unprovoked triple flexion), which occur in a periodic fashion, typically every 20 to 40 seconds, during sleep. The diagnosis of periodic limb movement disorder (PLMD), therefore, is based on the presence of increased PLMS observed on PSG (>5 per hour of sleep in children) and an associated sleep disturbance or daytime dysfunction. Similar to RLS, caregivers may report restlessness in bed with limb jerks or leg kicking as well as sleep disturbances including difficulty falling or staying asleep, daytime fatigue, or behavioral symptoms. Periodic limb movements can also be seen in association with other sleep disorders including RLS, as well as disorders associated with sleep continuity fragmentation such as narcolepsy and sleep apnea, although in these cases, a diagnosis of PLMD is superseded by the primary sleep disorder.

Etiology and Pathogenesis

Considered a separate disorder to RLS in adults, recent studies have suggested that there is an overlap between RLS and PLMD in children, especially those who lack the appropriate developmental language skills to report typical symptoms of RLS. Retrospective studies of children with RLS have reported that a diagnosis of PLMD preceded a diagnosis of RLS in 60% to 78% of children by an average of 4 years.[6,12] Therefore, the pathogenesis of PLMD is likely to overlap with RLS.

Clinical Findings

Diagnosis of PLMD in children requires not only a PSG finding of more than 5 PLMS per hour of sleep but also a clinical complaint of a sleep disturbance or associated daytime dysfunction such as attention difficulties or impulsivity.

Differential Diagnosis

The differential diagnosis of PLMD includes other motor activity seen during PSG such as hypnagogic foot tremor, normal phasic motor activity of rapid eye movement (REM) sleep, and fragmentary myoclonus. Secondary PLMS can also be seen in neurodegenerative conditions or after neurologic injury. Myoclonic seizures can present with similar limb movements but do not occur in a periodic fashion.

Treatment

Treatment of PLMD is similar to treatment of RLS and includes both pharmacologic and nonpharmacologic interventions. Iron supplementation and alpha-2-delta ligands are the mainstays of therapy.

Prognosis

The natural course of PLMD is uncertain because there is scant prospective data on the condition in children. Retrospective data are limited to children with PLMD who then went on to be diagnosed with RLS.

RESTLESS SLEEP DISORDER

Diagnostic Essentials

Restless sleep disorder (RSD) is an emerging pediatric sleep-related movement disorder characterized by restlessness in sleep and the presence of large body movements of the head, limb, or whole body that are not explained by another sleep or medical disorder. The prevalence of RSD is still being established, although it has been reported in up to 8% of all children and adolescents referred to a pediatric sleep center.[11]

General Considerations

Restless sleep is the core complaint provided by the patient or caregiver, although other descriptive terms related to frequent repositioning, disarrayed bedsheets, or movements in sleep may also be used (Table 29–4). Diagnosis requires confirmation of large body movements on PSG.

Table 29–4. Descriptive terms for restless sleep disorder.[11]

- Restless sleeper
- Trashes the bed
- All over the bed
- Beats you up during sleep
- Like a helicopter
- Falls out of bed

Etiology and Pathogenesis

The pathogenesis of RSD is uncertain but may exist along a spectrum of involuntary symptoms of motor restlessness. It is postulated that this may exist on a continuum of abnormalities in iron transport and subsequent dopaminergic dysfunction, similar to RLS/PLMD.[13] Serum ferritin levels in children with RSD were similar when compared to children with RLS in one prospective study.[14] Another retrospective study found that children with non–rapid eye movement (NREM) parasomnias and coexisting RSD had lower mean ferritin levels than children with NREM parasomnias alone.[15]

Clinical Findings

Patients suspected of having RSD should undergo PSG to confirm the presence of large body movements and to exclude other sleep disorders such as RLS/PLMD or parasomnias. Currently, a large body movement index of 5 or more per hour of sleep is supportive of RSD, although studies are ongoing.[13] Serum iron and ferritin levels, TIBC, and %TSAT should be obtained if PSG confirms the diagnosis of RSD.

Differential Diagnosis

The movements in RSD are typically nonrhythmic and nonstereotyped and can involve the limbs, head, or trunk. In comparison, PLMS occur in a repetitive fashion and involve the lower and upper extremities. Stereotyped movements with dystonic motor patterns are more commonly associated with nocturnal/sleep-related seizures. Sleep-related rhythmic movement disorders are a common group of rhythmic movements seen in children and can include head banging/rocking or whole-body rocking, most frequently seen at sleep onset or following a middle-of-night waking.

Treatment

At present, the most effective treatment for RSD is unknown, although expert opinion is to approach RSD in a similar fashion to RLS/PLMD with both pharmacologic and nonpharmacologic interventions.

NON–RAPID EYE MOVEMENT PARASOMNIAS AND DISORDERS OF AROUSAL

Diagnostic Essentials

The NREM parasomnias are a group of sleep-related paroxysmal events characterized by (1) recurrent episodes of arousal from sleep, (2) inappropriate or absent responsiveness to external stimulus, (3) limited or no associated dream imagery, and (4) partial or complete amnesia to the event. They are considered disorders of arousal stemming from incomplete awakening from sleep. Abnormal behaviors during an event can include ambulation, eating, talking, or other complex motor phenomena as well as frequent autonomic activation including tachycardia, diaphoresis, tachypnea, and mydriasis. Disorders of arousal are more likely to occur in the first third of the night, owing to the greater proportion of NREM stage 3 sleep during this period.

General Considerations

Disorders of arousal are further divided into 4 subtypes believed to share a common pathophysiology and clinical findings:

1. Confusional arousals are characterized by awakenings in bed with associated confusion. There is typically a lack of autonomic symptoms. If the patient gets out of bed, then the confusional arousal has transitioned into sleepwalking (somnambulism). Events are typically a few minutes in duration, although they can rarely persist for up to an hour.

2. Sleepwalking is characterized by ambulation out of bed with impairment in awareness following an arousal. Complex motor phenomena frequently occur, although they are typically inappropriate such as urinating in the bathtub, moving objects to inappropriate locations, or opening doors and attempting to leave the house.

3. Sleep terrors are characterized by a cry or scream and are accompanied by autonomic symptoms such as tachycardia, flushing, sweating, or tachypnea. The person is typically unresponsive to caregiver interventions. Children typically do not get out of bed, although sleep terrors in adults can be associated with jumping out of bed or out of the room. Duration is variable, but similar to confusional arousals, they can last from 5 minutes to up to an hour.

4. Sleep-related eating disorder is a condition of dysfunctional eating that occurs during a period of partial arousal. It is similar to the other NREM parasomnias with amnesia of the event but is defined by recurrent episodes of involuntary eating. The food choices are often peculiar, and there is risk for injury associated with cooking or eating behaviors as well as adverse outcomes from consumption of excess calories or toxic substances.

Etiology and Pathogenesis

Disorders of arousal are thought to arise out of an incomplete transition from NREM sleep into wakefulness. NREM stage 3 sleep (also known as slow wave sleep) is associated with a higher arousal threshold. Factors that disrupt sleep (eg, environmental noise, sleep apnea, or sleep-related movement disorders) during this period result in a failure of the brain to transition quickly and completely into wakefulness. Disorders of arousal are common in young children (17% in those aged 3-13 years[16]) with subtypes often overlapping.

Clinical Findings

NREM parasomnias are usually diagnosed clinically, although PSG findings of either a typical event or partial arousals out of NREM sleep can be supportive. Although infrequent NREM parasomnias likely exist on a continuum of normal human physiology, signs or symptoms of sleep disturbance that may be leading to increased arousals should be explored, particularly for frequent parasomnias. If clinically suggested, PSG can be used to evaluate for contributing sleep disturbances such as from sleep-disordered breathing or sleep-related movement disorders.

Differential Diagnosis

Other paroxysmal sleep events and sleep-related epilepsy should be considered. Compared with nocturnal seizures, NREM parasomnias are more likely to be stimulus induced, occur in the first third to first half of the night, and involve semi-purposeful actions or talking and are generally longer in duration but less frequent. Events that are brief and stereotyped, occur multiple times per night, and/or occur immediately upon sleep onset or very late in the sleep phase are atypical for NREM parasomnias. Combined electroencephalography-PSG monitoring can be useful in these circumstances.[17]

Treatment

Behavioral modifications, avoidance of triggers such as sleep deprivation, and conservative treatment of the events with redirection to bed are adequate for most cases of infrequent NREM parasomnia. Environmental modification is essential. Emphasis should be made on removal of bedside objects or furniture that may cause injury, locked storage or removal of firearms or weapons in the home, and locking of windows and doors. A bed or bedroom door alarm can be used to notify caregivers when a patient is out of their room. When clinically suspected, evaluation and treatment of aggravating factors such as sleep-disordered breathing or sleep-related movement disorders should be pursued. Obstructive sleep apnea (OSA) is the most common sleep disorder found in adolescents and young adults who present with disorders of arousal, and OSA treatment generally results in control of parasomnias.[18,19] Treatment of comorbid RLS/PLMD can result in reduction of NREM parasomnia severity.[20]

Pharmacotherapy can be considered when behavioral modifications and sleep behavioral therapy are not adequate and there is also additional history of dangerous or injurious behavior. Benzodiazepines such as a low-dose clonazepam can help limit arousals, although the evidence for its use is conflicting in the literature.[16,19]

▶ Prognosis

Disorders of arousal typically peak in early childhood and decrease through adolescence, with a prevalence between 2% and 4% in adulthood.

RAPID EYE MOVEMENT–RELATED AND OTHER PARASOMNIAS

ESSENTIALS OF DIAGNOSIS AND TYPICAL FEATURES

▶ Although not as common as NREM-related parasomnias in children, REM-related parasomnias still represent a significant cause of disrupted sleep.

▶ Nightmare disorder is characterized by recurrent, dysphoric, well-remembered dreams that often cause awakening and subsequent distress or dysfunction.

▶ Nightmares typically arise from REM during the second half to last third of the sleep episode.

▶ Predisposing factors to recurrent isolated sleep paralysis include sleep deprivation and irregular sleep-wake schedules, and there is also an increased prevalence in those with comorbid anxiety disorders and posttraumatic stress disorder (PTSD).

▶ REM sleep behavior disorder (RBD) is seen infrequently in children, and although its presence may signal narcolepsy, a developmental disorder, or selective serotonin reuptake inhibitor use, it does not have an association with synucleinopathies, as it does in adults.

▶ Sleep enuresis, recurrent involuntary voiding during sleep, affects 6 million children in the United States. Treatment of co-occurring conditions, such as OSA, can lead to resolution of sleep enuresis.

NIGHTMARE DISORDER

▶ General Considerations

Nightmares are disturbing or unpleasant dreams that one recalls when awakening. Nightmare disorder occurs when the frequency and severity of nightmares result in persistent distress or an impairment in functioning. In pediatric populations, nightmare disorder occurs most often in those who have experienced severe psychosocial stressors.[21,22]

▶ Etiology and Pathogenesis

Occasional nightmares occur frequently in children. They usually begin between 3 and 6 years old, with the peak prevalence occurring between 6 and 10 years old. Although the overall prevalence of nightmares is estimated to be between 60% and 75%, frequent dysphoric dreams resulting in persistent distress or an impairment in functioning occur in only 5% of preadolescents.[23] An association between anxiety and nightmares in adolescents has been reported.[24] Medications that affect norepinephrine, serotonin, dopamine, γ-aminobutyric acid, acetylcholine, and histamine have been associated with nightmares. Recovery from a period of insufficient sleep can result in vivid, intense dreams due to REM rebound.

▶ Clinical Findings

A thorough clinical history should include an assessment of nightmare frequency and severity of associated sleep disruptions as well as an assessment of anxiety or a history of abuse or trauma. A sleep diary can be useful in evaluating nightmare patterns or potential triggers. Evaluation by PSG is not routinely performed when nightmare disorder is suspected unless trying to exclude the presence of other parasomnias, nocturnal seizures, or repetitive or stereotyped sleep behaviors. When nightmares have been captured on PSG, awakenings from REM with increased heart rate and respiratory rate are seen, although the autonomic changes are often small.

▶ Differential Diagnosis

The differential diagnosis of nightmare disorder includes nocturnal seizures, sleep terrors, sleep paralysis (hypnogogic or hypnopompic), hypnogogic hallucinations, RBD, nocturnal panic attacks, and sleep-related dissociative disorder.[21]

▶ Treatment

Stress reduction, adequate sleep, and avoidance of frightening and overstimulating images may also help reduce nightmare frequency. Behavioral techniques, including imagery rehearsal therapy, systematic desensitization, relaxation techniques, extinction, and eye movement desensitization, are first-line treatments for nightmare disorder, although recommendations are based on observations from small, nonrandomized case series.[25-28] Medications are rarely indicated for transient nightmares, although clonidine or prazosin can be considered in comorbid PTSD.

Prognosis

Nightmares are typically a transient phenomenon, although they may persist in some children or adolescents, especially if the nightmares are related to a traumatic event.[29] Although half of PTSD cases resolve within 3 months, posttraumatic nightmares can persist throughout life.[21]

SLEEP PARALYSIS

General Considerations

Sleep paralysis is a paroxysmal inability to perform volitional movement in the setting of preserved consciousness. It is a nonspecific and relatively common phenomenon, with prevalence estimated to be at least 8% (and as high as 40%) for a single event.[21,30] Onset is usually during adolescence. Recurrent isolated sleep paralysis is present when repeated episodes of sleep paralysis occur independently of another sleep or neurologic disorder.

Etiology or Pathogenesis

Sleep paralysis is an example of sleep state dissociation in which REM atonia intrudes into wakefulness. This leads to skeletal muscle paralysis (respiration is preserved) and complete inability for volitional movement while transitioning into or out of sleep. The episodes typically last seconds to minutes and are often associated with a profound state of anxiety. Auditory, visual, or tactile hallucinations can accompany the paralysis. Hearing footsteps or crashes, sensing the presence of someone else, or experiencing pressure on the chest are all commonly reported.[31] As a nonspecific phenomenon, sleep paralysis can occur sporadically in the setting of REM sleep deprivation (eg, general sleep deprivation, irregular sleep-wake schedules, following forced awakenings), as part of another sleep disorder or disorder of arousal (eg, narcolepsy, PTSD, anxiety disorders), or in familial forms.[32-36]

Clinical Findings

Although not required for diagnosis, a PSG that captures recurrent isolated sleep paralysis may reveal aspects of REM sleep (eg, REM-related electromyographic atonia) that intrude into conscious wakefulness.[21]

Differential Diagnosis

The differential diagnosis of recurrent isolated sleep paralysis also includes periodic paralysis syndromes, atonic seizures, and cataplexy, although these are not restricted to times of sleep-wake transition. Nocturnal panic attacks can have similar profound anxiety but are not associated with paralysis.[21]

Treatment

Typically, reassurance is the foundation of treatment of recurrent isolated sleep paralysis, given the benign nature of the episodes. Counseling to avoid sleep deprivation and other precipitating factors such as supine sleep is appropriate. Recurrent episodes that cause extreme distress and dysfunction can be treated with REM-suppressing medications, such as low doses of tricyclic agents, clonidine, or clonazepam.[31]

RAPID EYE MOVEMENT SLEEP BEHAVIOR DISORDER

General Considerations

RBD is characterized by loss of normal REM atonia, resulting in recurrent episodes of complex motor behaviors and/or vocalizations during REM sleep. It is very rare in children, although its presence can signal specific comorbid sleep or neurodevelopmental disorders.

Etiology or Pathogenesis

In children, RBD is almost always secondary to another condition, most frequently narcolepsy.[37] Other causes include brainstem abnormalities (eg, pontine glioma, pontocerebellar hypoplasias) or rare conditions such as Smith-Magenis or Moebius syndromes. It is also seen with use of selective serotonin reuptake inhibitors or serotonin-norepinephrine reuptake inhibitors.[38] In adults, RBD can often be seen as a manifestation of α-synucleinopathies (Parkinson disease, multiple system atrophy, or dementia with Lewy bodies), although rarely in children. Secondary causes are thought to be due to degeneration of pontine and/or medullary neurons that normally inhibit spinal motor neurons during REM sleep.

Clinical Findings

A clinical diagnosis of RBD can be made with a history of dream enactment behavior (recollection of dream content that closely corresponds to observed action). The actions can be nonviolent (eg, laughing, crying, gesturing, singing) or violent (eg, punching, kicking, grabbing, jumping from bed), and injuries to self or another in close proximity can occur. However, given the rare nature of RBD in children, the presence of REM sleep without atonia should be confirmed on PSG.

Differential Diagnosis

The differential diagnosis of RBD in children includes sleepwalking, sleep terrors, OSA, sleep-related epilepsy (nocturnal frontal lobe epilepsy), rhythmic movement disorders, sleep-related dissociative disorders, frightening hypnopompic hallucinations, and PTSD.[21]

Treatment

Melatonin and clonazepam are the first-line pharmacologic treatments for RBD. Clonazepam likely works by consolidating sleep, whereas melatonin appears to partially restore REM atonia.[39] The sleep environment should be carefully reviewed to reduce the risk of injury to self or those close by.

Prognosis

RBD prognosis relates to comorbid conditions and precipitating factors. If RBD is medication associated, removal of the offending agent can resolve the RBD.

SLEEP ENURESIS

General Considerations

Sleep enuresis, also known as nocturnal enuresis, is defined by recurrent episodes of urinary incontinence during sleep in children older than 5 years that occur at least twice a week for at least 3 months. It is the most common urinary complaint in pediatrics, with estimated prevalences of 6% to 10% at age 7 and 2% at age 15.[40] The spontaneous cure rate is 15% per year. It can be primary (the child has never achieved a period of dryness at night) or secondary (the incontinence develops after at least 6 months of nighttime dryness).[21] Secondary enuresis is more likely associated with acquired factors, including OSA, diabetes mellitus, sickle cell disease, increased pressure on the bladder (eg, chronic constipation), increased urine output secondary to excessive fluid intake at night, neurologic diseases, and psychological stressors.

Etiology and Pathogenesis

Sleep enuresis can occur during any sleep stage when an urge to urinate fails to trigger an arousal from sleep. Sleep disorders that fragment sleep, such as OSA or PLMD, are associated with sleep enuresis, and impaired arousal has been shown on PSG.[41] There is strong heritability; the prevalence of sleep enuresis when both parents or either parent had sleep enuresis as a child is 77% and 44%, respectively.[40]

Clinical Findings

Given the breadth of possible causes of enuresis, evaluation should include a thorough history and physical examination as well as lab studies when appropriate. A PSG should be performed if signs and symptoms of OSA are present. Among children with OSA, up to 40% have a history of nocturnal enuresis.[42,43]

Differential Diagnosis

Anatomic abnormalities of the urinary tract should be considered, although these are more likely to present with incontinence or abnormal voiding during the day as well.

Treatment

After addressing comorbid conditions, strategies such as bladder training, programmed awakenings, rewarding dry nights, and fluid restriction may be employed. The first-line therapy for primary enuresis is conditioning therapy using an alarm that sounds when the bed or clothing becomes damp. Due to the inherent difficulties arousing the patient from sleep in nocturnal enuresis, the parent will usually need to wake the child once the alarm is triggered. Eventually the child will develop a conditioned arousal response to the preceding sensation of a full bladder.[44,45] Pharmacotherapies include those that increase the bladder's capacity (antimuscarinic medications such as oxybutynin and tolterodine)[46] and those that reduce nocturnal urine output (desmopressin). Patients often have a rapid response to desmopressin therapy, with 70% of children having some positive effect.[44] Tricyclics increase urinary osmolality, decrease detrusor tone, and increase sphincter tone.[47] Children treated with tricyclic antidepressants for sleep enuresis usually see a 25% long-term cure rate with relapses occurring often.[48]

REFERENCES

1. Picchietti MA, Picchietti DL. Restless legs syndrome and periodic limb movement disorder in children and adolescents. *Semin Pediatr Neurol.* 2008;15(2):91-99.
2. American Academy of Sleep Medicine. *International Classification of Sleep Disorders–Third Edition (ICSD-3).* American Academy of Sleep Medicine; 2014.
3. Picchietti DL, Bruni O, de Weerd A, et al. Pediatric restless legs syndrome diagnostic criteria: an update by the International Restless Legs Syndrome Study Group. *Sleep Med.* 2013;14(12):1253-1259.
4. Allen RP, Picchietti D, Hening WA, et al. Restless legs syndrome: diagnostic criteria, special considerations, and epidemiology: a report from the restless legs syndrome diagnosis and epidemiology workshop at the National Institutes of Health. *Sleep Med.* 2003;4(2):101-119.
5. Sun ER, Chen CA, Ho G, et al. Iron and the restless legs syndrome. *Sleep.* 1998;21(4):371-377.
6. Dye TJ, Jain SV, Simakajornboon N. Outcomes of long-term iron supplementation in pediatric restless legs syndrome/periodic limb movement disorder (RLS/PLMD). *Sleep Med.* 2017;32:213-219.
7. Clemens S, Sawchuk MA, Hochman S. Reversal of the circadian expression of tyrosine-hydroxylase but not nitric oxide synthase levels in the spinal cord of dopamine D3 receptor knockout mice. *Neuroscience.* 2005;133(2):353-357.
8. Picchietti D, Allen RP, Walters AS, et al. Restless legs syndrome: prevalence and impact in children and adolescents—the Peds REST study. *Pediatrics.* 2007;120(2):253-266.
9. Lyu S, Xing H, DeAndrade MP, et al. The role of BTBD9 in the cerebellum, sleep-like behaviors and the restless legs syndrome. *Neuroscience.* 2020;440:85-96.
10. Allen RP, Picchietti DL, Auerbach M, et al. Evidence-based and consensus clinical practice guidelines for the iron treatment of restless legs syndrome/Willis-Ekbom disease in adults and children: an IRLSSG task force report. *Sleep Med.* 2018;41:27-44.

11. DelRosso L, Bruni O. Chapter 11: treatment of pediatric restless legs syndrome. In: Clemens S, Ghorayeb I, eds. *Advances in Pharmacology*. Elsevier; 2019:237-253.

12. Picchietti DL, Stevens HE. Early manifestations of restless legs syndrome in childhood and adolescence. *Sleep Med*. 2008;9(7):770-781.

13. DelRosso LM, Jackson CV, Trotter K, Bruni O, Ferri R. Video-polysomnographic characterization of sleep movements in children with restless sleep disorder. *Sleep*. 2019;42(4):zsy269.

14. DelRosso LM, Bruni O, Ferri R. Restless sleep disorder in children: a pilot study on a tentative new diagnostic category. *Sleep*. 2018; 41:8.

15. Senel GB, Kochan Kizilkilic E, Karadeniz D. Restless sleep disorder in children with NREM parasomnias. *Sleep*. 2021;44(7):zsab049.

16. Irfan M, Schenck CH, Howell MJ. NonREM disorders of arousal and related parasomnias: an updated review. *Neurotherapeutics*. 2021;18(1):124-139.

17. Jain SV, Dye T, Kedia P. Value of combined video EEG and polysomnography in clinical management of children with epilepsy and daytime or nocturnal spells. *Seizure*. 2019;65:1-5.

18. Ohayon MM, Priest RG. Night terrors, sleepwalking, and confusional arousals in the general population: their frequency and relationship to other sleep and mental disorders. *J Clin Psychiatry*. 1999;60(4):268-276.

19. Guilleminault C, Kirisoglu C, Bao G, et al. Adult chronic sleepwalking and its treatment based on polysomnography. *Brain*. 2005;128(5):1062-1069.

20. Gurbani N, Dye TJ, Dougherty K, et al. Improvement of parasomnias after treatment of restless leg syndrome/periodic limb movement disorder in children. *J Clin Sleep Med*. 2019;15(5):743-748.

21. Sateia M, ed. *International Classification of Sleep Disorders*. 3rd ed. American Academy of Sleep Medicine; 2014.

22. Secrist ME, Dalenberg CJ, Gevirtz R. Contributing factors predicting nightmares in children: trauma, anxiety, dissociation, and emotion regulation. *Psychol Trauma*. 2019;11(1):114-121.

23. Chen X, Ke ZL, Chen Y, Lin X. The prevalence of sleep problems among children in mainland China: a meta-analysis and systemic-analysis. *Sleep Med*. 2021;83:248-255.

24. Nielsen TA, Laberge L, Paquet J, et al. Development of disturbing dreams during adolescence and their relation to anxiety symptoms. *Sleep*. 2000;23(6):727-736.

25. Krakow B, Sandoval D, Schrader R, et al. Treatment of chronic nightmares in adjudicated adolescent girls in a residential facility. *J Adolesc Health*. 2001;29(2):94-100.

26. Palace EM, Johnston C. Treatment of recurrent nightmares by the dream reorganization approach. *J Behav Ther Exp Psychiatry*. 1989;20(3):219-226.

27. Pellicer X. Eye movement desensitization treatment of a child's nightmares: a case report. *J Behav Ther Exp Psychiatry*. 1993;24(1):73-75.

28. Cavior N, Deutsch AM. Systematic desensitization to reduce dream-induced anxiety. *J Nerv Ment Dis*. 1975;161(6):433-435.

29. Mindell JA, Owens JA. *A Clinical Guide to Pediatric Sleep: Diagnosis and Management of Sleep Problems*. Lippincott Williams & Wilkins; 2015.

30. Sharpless BA, Barber JP. Lifetime prevalence rates of sleep paralysis: a systematic review. *Sleep Med Rev*. 2011;15(5):311-315.

31. Kotagal S. Parasomnias in childhood. *Sleep Med Rev*. 2009;13(2):157-168.

32. Otto MW, Simon NM, Powers M, et al. Rates of isolated sleep paralysis in outpatients with anxiety disorders. *J Anxiety Disord*. 2006;20(5):687-693.

33. Denis D, French CC, Gregory AM. A systematic review of variables associated with sleep paralysis. *Sleep Med Rev*. 2018;38:141-157.

34. Wing YK, Lee ST, Chen CN. Sleep paralysis in Chinese: ghost oppression phenomenon in Hong Kong. *Sleep*. 1994;17(7):609-613.

35. Bell CC, Dixie-Bell DD, Thompson B. Further studies on the prevalence of isolated sleep paralysis in black subjects. *J Natl Med Assoc*. 1986;78(7):649-659.

36. Dahlitz M, Parkes JD. Sleep paralysis. *Lancet*. 1993;341(8842):406-407.

37. Antelmi E, Pizza F, Vandi S, et al. The spectrum of REM sleep-related episodes in children with type 1 narcolepsy. *Brain*. 2017;140(6):1669-1679.

38. Kotagal S. Rapid eye movement sleep behavior disorder during childhood. *Sleep Med Clin*. 2015;10(2):163-167.

39. Boeve BF, Silber MH, Saper CB, et al. Pathophysiology of REM sleep behaviour disorder and relevance to neurodegenerative disease. *Brain*. 2007;130(Pt 11):2770-2788.

40. Bruni O, Novelli L, Finotti E, Ferri R. Sleep enuresis. In: *The Parasomnias and Other Sleep-Related Movement Disorders*. Cambridge University Press; 2010:175-183.

41. Soster LA, Alves RC, Fagundes SN, et al. Non-REM sleep instability in children with primary monosymptomatic sleep enuresis. *J Clin Sleep Med*. 2017;13(10):1163-1170.

42. Brooks LJ, Topol HI. Enuresis in children with sleep apnea. *J Pediatr*. 2003;142(5):515-518.

43. Weissbach A, Leiberman A, Tarasiuk A, et al. Adenotonsilectomy improves enuresis in children with obstructive sleep apnea syndrome. *Int J Pediatr Otorhinolaryngol*. 2006;70(8):1351-1356.

44. Caldwell PH, Deshpande AV, Von Gontard A. Management of nocturnal enuresis. *BMJ*. 2013;347:f6259.

45. Glazener CM, Evans JH, Peto RE. Alarm interventions for nocturnal enuresis in children. *Cochrane Database Syst Rev*. 2005;2:CD002911.

46. Nijman RJ. Role of antimuscarinics in the treatment of non-neurogenic daytime urinary incontinence in children. *Urology*. 2004;63(3 suppl 1):45-50.

47. Norgaard JP, Djurhuus JC, Watanabe H, et al. Experience and current status of research into the pathophysiology of nocturnal enuresis. *Br J Urol*. 1997;79(6):825-835.

48. Bruni O, Miano S. Parasomnias. In: Gozal D, Kheirandish-Gozal L, eds. *Pediatric Sleep Medicine*. Springer; 2021:415-429.

Fetal Neurology

Charu Venkatesan, MD, PhD

Usha Nagaraj, MD

Beth Kline-Fath, MD

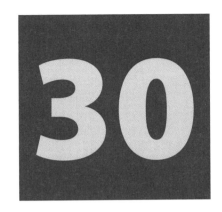

HISTORICAL OVERVIEW

Routine prenatal care includes surveillance for fetal anatomic malformations using ultrasound. Development of ultrasound as an imaging modality began in the 1940s and 1950s, and the first fetal central nervous system (CNS) anomalies were reported in the 1970s. Over the next 2 decades, ultrasound studies described fetal CNS anomalies including Chiari II malformation, agenesis of corpus callosum, and hydrocephalus. In the early 2000s, magnetic resonance imaging (MRI) became an important adjunct to ultrasound both for evaluation of maternal complications and detection of fetal anomalies.[1-3]

There are several advantages to MRI in fetal diagnostics.[4] MRI is not limited by fetal lie, calvarial ossification, maternal obesity, or oligohydramnios. It offers excellent soft tissue contrast and multiplanar visualization of all organs. Limitations include motion artifact from movement of either the fetus or the mother. Typically, MRI scans are not performed in the first trimester due to small fetal size and increased fetal motion. A large study comparing 242 fetal ultrasound and fetal MRI studies showed that MRI changed the diagnosis in about 32% of patients.[5] Large multicenter trials have shown that fetal MRI can have a diagnostic accuracy of 93%, whereas ultrasound was found to have an accuracy of 68%.[6] A study comparing pre- and postnatal findings found that the primary fetal diagnostic classification remained unchanged in 98% of cases.[7] Postnatal MRI identified additional foci of cortical malformations or progression of vascular injury, but these findings did not change the clinical implications that had already been discussed during fetal counseling.

The use of fetal MRI for evaluation of CNS malformations and pediatric neurology consultative services has increased since 2010. Continued efforts at longitudinal studies of outcome of prenatally diagnosed CNS malformations will aid with pregnancy planning, neonatal care, accurate prognostication, and provision of anticipatory guidance. Discussion of the numerous intracranial anomalies is beyond the scope of this chapter. The focus, therefore, will be to provide a brief overview of the more common abnormalities, which include isolated ventriculomegaly, posterior fossa malformations (specifically Dandy-Walker malformation, vermian hypoplasia, and Blake pouch cyst), agenesis/dysgenesis of corpus callosum, congenital aqueductal stenosis, and holoprosencephaly.

ISOLATED VENTRICULOMEGALY

The lateral ventricles begin as primitive cerebral cavities that communicate with each other and the third ventricle and are visible at 13 to 14 weeks of gestation. Ventriculomegaly is the most common CNS anomaly identified by prenatal ultrasound, with an incidence of 1 to 2 cases per 1000 births.[8,9] Ventriculomegaly can be due to hydrocephalus (either obstructive or communicating) or decreased cerebral volume (either congenital or acquired).[10] Fetal ventriculomegaly is defined by a measurement taken at the level of the atrium that is equal to or larger than 10 mm. Mild ventriculomegaly is defined as a measurement of 10 to 12 mm; moderate ventriculomegaly is 12.1 to 15 mm; and severe ventriculomegaly is greater than 15 mm (Figure 30–1). Prognosis, in the absence of other malformations, is related to ventricular size, progression of enlargement, and unilateral versus bilateral ventriculomegaly (worse with bilateral).[9] In cases of mild ventriculomegaly, routine use of MRI is debated; one study found that MRI showed additional findings in 20% of cases but only provided information of clinical value in 1% of cases.[11]

A study evaluating immediate postnatal outcome of 11 fetuses with isolated ventriculomegaly (classified as mild in 6, moderate in 3, and severe in 2 of the 11 fetuses) found that no patients required intubation at delivery or respiratory or feeding support at discharge.[7] Overall, ventriculomegaly resolves in 41%, remains stable in 43%, and progresses in

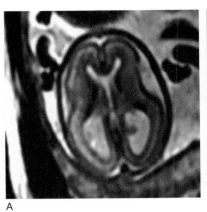 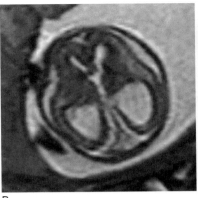 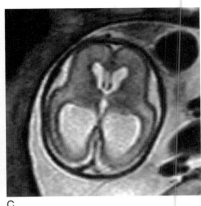

A   B   C

▲ **Figure 30–1.** Axial T2 single-shot fast spin-echo images from fetal magnetic resonance imaging (MRI) of ventriculomegaly of the lateral ventricles measured as mild (**A**), moderate (**B**), and severe (**C**). Gestational ages at fetal MRI were 24, 20, and 25 weeks, respectively.

16% of patients.[12] Mild isolated ventriculomegaly, which can represent a normal variant, has higher rates (about 90%) of stable or regressing ventricular measurements.[13] Associated anomalies can be seen in 56% of patients with moderate and 6% with mild ventriculomegaly; chromosomal anomalies are seen in 3% to 13% of cases, and infections, primarily TORCH (toxoplasmosis, other [syphilis, varicella-zoster, parvovirus B19], rubella, cytomegalovirus, and herpes infections), are evident in 10% to 20% of cases with severe ventriculomegaly.[4,14] Overall, neurodevelopmental outcome is favorable in isolated cases, with upward of 90% of patients with mild, 75% to 85% with moderate, and 63% with severe ventriculomegaly having normal outcome.[15-18] Counseling should discuss possible genetic testing, evaluation for TORCH infections, and need for close postnatal follow-up.

CONGENITAL AQUEDUCTAL STENOSIS

The incidence of congenital aqueductal stenosis (CAS) is 0.5 to 1 per 1000 births.[19] X-linked hydrocephalus is the most common hereditary hydrocephalus, with an incidence of 1 in 30,000 births.[19,20] Etiology includes hemorrhage, genetic syndromes (eg, Walker-Warburg syndrome, VATER syndrome) and maternal exposure (insulin-dependent maternal diabetes, fetal alcohol, and TORCH).[21,22] Mutations in *L1CAM*, a gene encoding a neural cell adhesion molecule, are found in a subset of patients with X-linked hydrocephalus. These patients can have associated anomalies: agenesis of the corpus callosum, absent septum pellucidum, thalamic fusion, small brainstem, and adduction of thumbs.[20] Nine percent of patients with CAS can have rhombencephalosynapsis (RES; fusion of cerebellar hemispheres with absence of vermis).[23] Fifty percent of patients with RES can have associated aqueductal stenosis.[23] One study found that shunting

in CAS with RES groups occurred earlier (average, 6 days of life vs 55 days of life in CAS-only group) and 53% of patients with CAS with RES required feeding assistance versus 20% with CAS only.[24]

CAS carries an overall mortality of 40%.[25] Affected patients typically undergo placement of a ventriculoperitoneal shunt in the neonatal period. The majority of patients typically do not require invasive ventilator or feeding support.[7] When this condition occurs in isolation (about 10% of cases), normal development can be seen in 50% of children.[4] However, overall, normal development is only seen in about 10% of children.[4] Although seizures typically do not occur in the immediate neonatal period, patients with CAS are at high risk for epilepsy. They can also have variable motor and cognitive delays and deficits.

POSTERIOR FOSSA MALFORMATIONS

Malformations involving the posterior fossa can result from genetic or acquired causes and occur in about 1 in every 5000 births.[26] Genetic or syndromic causes include a range of diagnoses including dystroglycanopathies (eg, Walker-Warburg syndrome), ciliopathies (eg, Joubert syndrome), Chiari malformation, pontocerebellar hypoplasia, cerebellar agenesis, and Dandy-Walker malformation (DWM) spectrum. Discussion of all anomalies is beyond the current scope, and this chapter will focus on the more common posterior fossa anomalies. A subset of these more common posterior fossa malformations results from abnormal development of the posterior membranous area during fourth ventricular development.[27,28] They exist along a continuum and include classic DWM, vermian hypoplasia, and Blake pouch cyst.

DWM is characterized radiologically by (1) enlargement of the posterior fossa with superior displacement of

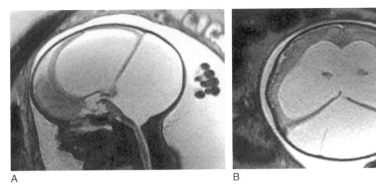

▲ **Figure 30–2.** Sagittal (**A**) and axial (**B**) T2 single-shot fast spin-echo image from fetal magnetic resonance imaging of a 32-week gestational age fetus with classic Dandy-Walker malformation with obstructive hydrocephalus.

both cerebellar tentorium and torcular, (2) a cystic dilatation of the fourth ventricle, and (3) a malformed vermis (Figure 30–2).[29,30] DWM is associated with a high rate of other CNS anomalies (61%) including ventriculomegaly (36%-76%) requiring ventriculoperitoneal shunt placement, agenesis of the corpus callosum (5%-50%), and extra-CNS structural anomalies and genetic syndromes (42.6%).[31,32] Neurodevelopmental outcome is better in children with no other CNS abnormalities with about 30% of this subgroup having normal development.[33]

Blake pouch is a normal embryologic structure that arises from the posterior membranous area from the roof of the primitive rhombencephalon.[28] This pouch fenestrates to varying degrees to create the foramina of Luschka and Magendie, allowing for normal outflow of the cerebrospinal fluid. Isolated persistence of Blake pouch with normal vermian size and morphology carries a favorable prognosis (Figure 30–3). Mild to moderate ventriculomegaly is the most common finding in prenatal imaging, which typically resolves or remains stable in about 84% of patients and progresses in about 16%.[34] Blake pouch remnant in isolation is typically an incidental finding, and greater than 90% of those affected have reportedly normal 5-year neurologic outcomes without intervention.[34] Given complications including hydrocephalus requiring shunt placement,[35] counseling should emphasize close follow-up with monitoring of head circumference postnatally.

▶ Vermian Hypoplasia

Vermian hypoplasia can occur in isolation or accompanied by other CNS and extra-CNS anomalies. Isolated inferior

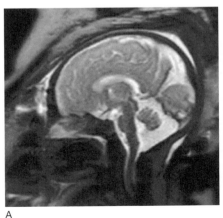
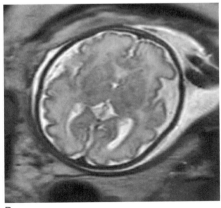

▲ **Figure 30–3.** **A.** Sagittal T2 single-shot fast spin-echo (SSFSE) image from fetal magnetic resonance imaging in a 32-week gestational age fetus with findings consistent with Blake pouch remnant. The vermis is rotated; however, it is normal in size and morphology. **B.** Axial T2 SSFSE image in the same fetus demonstrates no ventriculomegaly of the lateral ventricles.

vermian hypoplasia refers to the presence of this anomaly with no other associated abnormalities. When present as an isolated finding, studies report that greater than 70% of children have normal developmental outcome.[36,37] However, it can be difficult to determine prenatally whether vermian hypoplasia is present as an isolated condition or as part of a syndrome. One study found that in the presence of both additional intra- and extracranial anomalies, neurodevelopmental outcome was always abnormal.[36] Of note, Blake pouch remnant frequently coexists with vermian hypoplasia, marked by rotation of the vermis on imaging.

Compared to other CNS malformations, posterior fossa malformations are more likely to be associated with genetic conditions including CHARGE syndrome (coloboma of the eye, heart defects, atresia of the nasal choanae, retardation of growth and/or development, genital and/or urinary abnormalities, and ear abnormalities and deafness), trisomy 21, and Turner syndrome, as well as abnormalities of the limbs, kidneys, face, and heart.[7,32] Therefore, prenatal evaluation via MRI, echocardiogram, and genetic studies to identify additional abnormalities is encouraged to help provide accurate prognostic information. Counseling should emphasize delivery in centers with a level 3 or 4 neonatal intensive care unit, possible need for ventilatory and feeding support, and neurosurgical intervention. Long-term outcome is strongly dependent on presence of other syndromic, systemic, or genetic anomalies.

HOLOPROSENCEPHALY

Holoprosencephaly (HPE) is relatively common with incidence noted in 1 in 250 conceptions; however, only about 3% of fetuses with HPE survive to delivery. HPE occurs very early in gestation due to failure of cleavage of prosencephalon in the first 4 weeks of embryogenesis. There are 4 main types: alobar, semilobar, lobar, and middle hemispheric variant. Alobar HPE, the most frequently occurring form (40%-75% of cases), is characterized by a monoventricle with absent midline structures and thalamic fusion. Semilobar HPE is a fusion defect localized anteriorly with partial fusion of thalami, some degree of posterior interhemispheric fissure, and rudimentary lateral ventricles (Figure 30–4). Lobar HPE involves noncleavage of frontal lobes and separation of most of the cerebral hemisphere, rudimentary frontal horns, and absent anterior corpus callosum. Middle interhemispheric variant is the failure of separation of the posterior frontal and parietal lobes, with the poles of the frontal and occipital lobes well separated.[38-41] The etiology of HPE is complex and multifactorial. Chromosomal causes have been estimated to account for up to 25% to 50% of cases, with approximately half being trisomy 13 and the remainder largely trisomy 18 or triploidy.[42-44] HPE is also associated with recognized genetic syndromes including Smith-Lemli-Opitz, Meckel-Gruber, and other syndromes, which are estimated to account for 20% to 25% of cases.[45,46] Outcomes have been noted to be worse in those with chromosomal and syndromic causes of HPE.[47] A number of nonsyndromic monogenetic causes have also been identified and account for another 15% to 20% of cases.[48-50] The 4 most common genes, *SHH*, *ZIC2*, *SIX3*, and *TIGF*, make up 5% to 10% of all HPE cases but a much larger fraction of familial cases.[48-51] Multiple maternal or environmental factors, including maternal insulin-dependent diabetes and salicylate and alcohol exposure, have been proposed.[52] A subset of these mechanisms shares a role in cholesterol biosynthesis and/or downstream sonic hedgehog gene (*SHH*) signaling, which plays an important role in ventral neural tube patterning and, thus, forebrain development. Neurodevelopmental prognosis depends on the extent

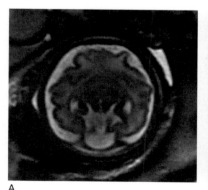
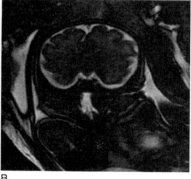
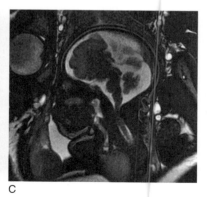

A   B   C

▲ **Figure 30–4.** Semilobar holoprosencephaly. **A.** Axial T2 single-shot fast spin-echo (SSFSE) image of a fetus at 34 weeks demonstrating lack of cleavage of the anterior hemisphere and normal separation of the posterior hemisphere. **B.** Coronal T2 steady-state free precession (SSFP) demonstrates lack of cleavage of the frontal lobes. **C.** Sagittal SSFP again showing nonseparation of the anterior hemisphere.

of brain malformation: Severe developmental delay is present in all cases of alobar holoprosencephaly, whereas 50% of lobar HPE patients achieve ambulation and verbal communication, and outcome in semilobar HPE is intermediate between alobar and lobar HPE.[53,54]

Fetal MRI continues to be the imaging modality with the best diagnostic accuracy.[54] A study by Riddle et al[55] found that of 63 patients identified by ultrasound to have concern for HPE, only 28 patients were confirmed on fetal MRI to meet diagnosis of HPE. This study found that mortality in the newborn period remained high, with most deaths occurring in the first month of life. Overall survival was 39%, and a variety of HPE subtypes including alobar were represented among survivors. Only one child achieved ambulation and speech, whereas the remainder had significant disability.[55] Olsen et al[56] identified several factors that correlated with mortality including syndromic features or chromosomal etiology and presence of congenital defects in organ systems not classically associated with HPE or a defined syndrome. Counseling needs to address survival after birth, complications, and expectations as babies may not die immediately after birth. Counseling should also engage pediatric palliative care services to guide families as they prepare to take home an infant with a limited life span.

AGENESIS/DYSGENESIS OF THE CORPUS CALLOSUM

Agenesis of the corpus callosum has a prevalence of about 1.8 per 10,000 live births (Figure 30–5). About 50% of patients have other CNS malformations; musculoskeletal (34%) and cardiac (28%) anomalies are the more common extra-CNS findings seen with this condition.[57] Callosal anomalies in the context of chromosomal abnormality have been found in about 17% of patients.[57] The majority of children with isolated agenesis of the corpus callosum do well, and studies find that over 75% of children have normal-range intelligence.[58-60] Gross motor and fine motor deficits are present in about 4% and 11% of patients, respectively, and epilepsy occurs in about 6% of patients.[58-60] No patients with isolated agenesis of the corpus callosum require long-term feeding or respiratory support.[7] Since callosal anomalies can occur with genetic or syndromic diagnoses, it is important to evaluate for these postnatally. In the presence of genetic syndromes, outcome is determined by these conditions and less defined by the intracranial anatomic abnormality.

ABSENT SEPTUM PELLUCIDUM

Cavum septum pellucidum is a marker of normal development of midline structures and detected via ultrasound during the 17th to 20th weeks of gestation. Absent septum pellucidum (ASP) can be associated with neurologic syndromes such as septo-optic dysplasia. It can also occur in isolation in the absence of accompanying CNS or systemic abnormalities. When ASP occurs in isolation, over 80% of patients have normal neurologic outcomes.[61,62] When detected prenatally, it is advisable for patients to undergo ophthalmologic and endocrine evaluation to evaluate for presence of anomalies suggestive of septo-optic dysplasia.

CONCLUSION

Improved diagnostic ability via fetal imaging has led to the emergence of the field of fetal neurology. Fetal MRI is fairly accurate, and postnatal imaging rarely changes an identified primary diagnosis. However, postnatal MRI is recommended in the immediate neonatal period when potential neurosurgical intervention is anticipated (eg, CAS, DWM, HPE, moderate or severe ventriculomegaly). Patients with prenatally

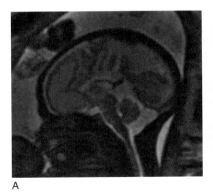 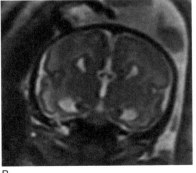 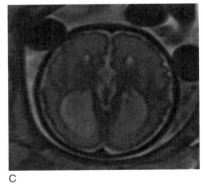

A   B   C

▲ **Figure 30–5.** Agenesis of the corpus callosum without associated anomaly at 31 weeks. **A.** Sagittal single-shot fast spin-echo (SSFSE) T2 imaging showing absence of corpus callosum and radial array of midline gyri. **B.** Axial SSFSE T2 with parallel configuration of lateral ventricles and colpocephaly. **C.** Coronal SSFSE T2 image with steer horn configuration of the frontal horns and third ventricle prominent extending interhemispheric due to absent corpus callosum.

detected mild ventriculomegaly should have close clinical follow-up, and head ultrasound may suffice initially. MRI can be performed more urgently if clinical concerns arise regarding head growth. In patients with identified or suspected cortical malformations or callosal agenesis/dysgenesis without intracranial cysts, imaging can be deferred until they are over 15 months of age when myelination is more optimal for better visualization of intracranial anatomy.

REFERENCES

1. Verburg B, Fink AM, Reidy K, Palma-Dias R. The Contribution of MRI after fetal anomalies have been diagnosed by ultrasound: correlation with postnatal outcomes. *Fetal Diagn Ther.* 2015;38:186-194.
2. Rossi AC, Prefumo F. Additional value of fetal magnetic resonance imaging in the prenatal diagnosis of central nervous system anomalies: a systematic review of the literature. *Ultrasound Obstet Gynecol.* 2014;44:388-393.
3. Kett JC, Woodrum DE, Diekema DS. A survey of fetal care centers in the United States. *J Neonatal Perinatal Med.* 2014;7: 131-135.
4. Kline-Fath BM, Bulas DI, Bahado-Singh R. *Fundamental and Advanced Fetal Imaging: Ultrasound and MRI.* Wolters Kluwer Health; 2015.
5. Levine D, Barnes PD, Robertson RR, Wong G, Mehta TS. Fast MR imaging of fetal central nervous system abnormalities. *Radiology.* 2003;229(1):51-61.
6. Sasaki-Adams D, Elbabaa SK, Jewells V, Carter L, Campbell JW, Ritter AM. The Dandy-Walker variant: a case series of 24 pediatric patients and evaluation of associated anomalies, incidence of hydrocephalus, and developmental outcomes. *J Neurosurg Pediatr.* 2008;2:194-199.
7. Arroyo MS, Hopkin RJ, Nagaraj UD, Kline-Fath B, Venkatesan C. Fetal brain MRI findings and neonatal outcome of common diagnosis at a tertiary care center. *J Perinatol.* 2019;39(8):1072-1077.
8. D'Addario V, Rossi AC. Neuroimaging of ventriculomegaly in the fetal period. *Semin Fetal Neonatal Med.* 2012;17(6):310-318.
9. Salomon LJ, Bernard JP, Ville Y. Reference ranges for fetal ventricular width: a non-normal approach. *Ultrasound Obstet Gynecol.* 2007;30(1):61-66.
10. Nagaraj UD, Kline-Fath BM. Imaging diagnosis of ventriculomegaly: fetal, neonatal, and pediatric. *Child Nerv Syst.* 2020; 36(8):1669-1679.
11. Parazzini C, Righini A, Doneda C, et al. Is fetal magnetic resonance imaging indicated when ultrasound isolated mild ventriculomegaly is present in pregnancies with no risk factors? *Prenat Diagn.* 2012;32(8):752-757.
12. Parilla BV, Endres LK, Dinsmoorm MJ, Curran L. In utero progression of mild fetal ventriculomegaly. *Int J Gynaecol Obstet.* 2006;93(2):106-109.
13. Griffiths PD, Reeves MJ, Morris JE, et al. A prospective study of fetuses with isolated ventriculomegaly investigated by antenatal sonography and in utero MR imaging. *AJNR Am J Neuroradiol.* 2010;31(1):106-111.
14. Gaglioti P, Oberto M, Todros T. The significance of fetal ventriculomegaly: etiology, short- and long-term outcomes. *Prenat Diagn.* 2009;29(4):381-388.
15. Scelsa B, Rustico M, Righini A, et al. Mild ventriculomegaly from fetal consultation to neurodevelopmental assessment:

16. Pagani G, Thilaganathan B, Prefumo F. Neurodevelopmental outcome in isolated mild fetal ventriculomegaly: systematic review and meta-analysis. *Ultrasound Obstet Gynecol.* 2014; 44(3):254-260.
17. Gaglioti P, Danelon D, Bontempo S, Mombrò M, Cardaropoli S, Todros T. Fetal cerebral ventriculomegaly: outcome in 176 cases. *Ultrasound Obstet Gynecol.* 2005;25(4):372-377.
18. Falip C, Blanc N, Maes E, et al. Postnatal clinical and imaging follow-up of infants with prenatal isolated mild ventriculomegaly: a series of 101 cases. *Pediatr Radiol.* 2007;37(10): 981-989.
19. Verhagen WI, Bartels RH, Fransen E, van Camp G, Renier WO, Grotenhuis JA. Familial congenital hydrocephalus and aqueduct stenosis with probably autosomal dominant inheritance and variable expression. *J Neurol Sci.* 1998;158(1):101-105.
20. Weller S, Gärtner J. Genetic and clinical aspects of X-linked hydrocephalus (L1 disease): mutations in the L1CAM gene. *Hum Mutat.* 2001;18(1):1-12.
21. Zhang J, Williams MA, Rigamonti D. Genetics of human hydrocephalus. *J Neurol.* 2006;253(10):1255-1266.
22. Jissendi-Tchofo P, Kara S, Barkovich AJ. Midbrain-hindbrain involvement in lissencephalies. *Neurology.* 2009;72(5):410-418.
23. Ishak GE, Dempsey JC, Shaw DW, et al. Rhombencephalosynapsis: a hindbrain malformation associated with incomplete separation of midbrain and forebrain, hydrocephalus and a broad spectrum of severity. *Brain.* 2012;135(Pt 5):1370-1386.
24. Kline-Fath BM, Arroyo MS, Calvo-Garcia MA, Horn PS, Thomas C. Prenatal aqueduct stenosis: association with rhombencephalosynapsis and neonatal outcome. *Prenat Diagn.* 2018; 38(13):1028-1034.
25. Levitsky DB, Mack LA, Nyberg DA, et al. Fetal aqueductal stenosis diagnosed sonographically: how grave is the prognosis? *AJR Am J Roentgenol.* 1995;164(3):725-730.
26. Adamsbaum C, Moutard ML, André C, et al. MRI of the fetal posterior fossa. *Pediatr Radiol.* 2005;35(2):124-140.
27. Barkovich AJ, Kjos BO, Norman D, Edwards MS. Revised classification of posterior fossa cysts and cystlike malformations based on the results of multiplanar MR imaging. *Am J Neuroradiol.* 1989;10(5):977-988. doi:10.1016/0899-7071(90)90031-6
28. Tortori-Donati P, Fondelli MP, Rossi A, Carini S. Cystic malformations of the posterior cranial fossa originating from a defect of the posterior membranous area. *Child's Nerv Syst.* 1996;12(6):303-308. doi:10.1007/bf00301017
29. Robinson AJ, Ederies MA. Diagnostic imaging of posterior fossa anomalies in the fetus. *Semin Fetal Neonatal Med.* 2016;21(5):312-320. doi:10.1016/j.siny.2016.04.007.
30. Massoud M, Guibaud L. Prenatal imaging of posterior fossa disorders. A review. *Eur J Paediatr Neurol.* 2018;22(6): 972-988.
31. D'Antonio F, Khalil A, Garel C, et al. Systematic review and meta-analysis of isolated posterior fossa malformations on prenatal ultrasound imaging (part 1): nomenclature, diagnostic accuracy and associated anomalies. *Ultrasound Obstet Gynecol.* 2016;47(6):690-697.
32. Ecker JL, Shipp TD, Bromley B, Benacerraf B. The sonographic diagnosis of Dandy-Walker and Dandy-Walker variant: associated findings and outcomes. *Prenat Diagn.* 2000;20(4):328-332.
33. Bolduc M-E, Limperopoulos C. Neurodevelopmental outcomes in children with cerebellar malformations: a systematic review. *Dev Med Child Neurol.* 2009;51(4):256-267.

a single center experience and review of the literature. *Eur J Paediatr Neurol.* 2018;22(6):919-928.

34. Gandolfi Colleoni G, Contro E, Carletti A, et al. Prenatal diagnosis and outcome of fetal posterior fossa fluid collections. *Ultrasound Obstet Gynecol.* 2012;39(6):625-631.

35. Cornips EMJ, Overvliet GM, Weber JW, et al. The clinical spectrum of Blake's pouch cyst: report of six illustrative cases. *Child's Nerv Syst.* 2010;26(8):1057-1064.

36. Patek KJ, Kline-Fath BM, Hopkin RJ, et al. Posterior fossa anomalies diagnosed with fetal MRI: associated anomalies and neurodevelopmental outcomes. *Prenat Diagn.* 2012;32(1):75-82.

37. Tarui T, Limperopoulos C, Sullivan NR, Robertson RL, du Plessis AJ. Long-term developmental outcome of children with a fetal diagnosis of isolated inferior vermian hypoplasia. *Arch Dis Child Fetal Neonatal Ed.* 2014;99(1):F54-F58.

38. DeMyer W, Zeman W, Palmer CG. The face predicts the brain: diagnostic significance of median facial anomalies for holoprosencephaly (arhinencephaly). *Pediatrics.* 1964;34:256-263.

39. Barkovich AJ, Quint DJ. Middle interhemispheric fusion: an unusual variant of holoprosencephaly. *AJNR Am J Neuroradiol.* 1993;14(2):431-440.

40. Hahn JS, Barnes PD, Clegg NJ, Stashinko EE. Septopreoptic holoprosencephaly: a mild subtype associated with midline craniofacial anomalies. *AJNR Am J Neuroradiol.* 2010;31(9):1596-1601.

41. Hahn JS, Barnes PD. Neuroimaging advances in holoprosencephaly: refining the spectrum of the midline malformation. *Am J Med Genet C Semin Med Genet.* 2010;154C(1):120-132.

42. Siebert JR, Kokich VG, Warkany J, Lemire RJ. Atelencephalic microcephaly: craniofacial anatomy and morphologic comparisons with holoprosencephaly and anencephaly. *Teratology.* 1987;36(3):279-285.

43. Dubourg C, Bendavid C, Pasquier L, Henry C, Odent S, David V. Holoprosencephaly. *Orphanet J Rare Dis.* 2007;2(1):8.

44. Tekendo-Ngongang C, Muenke M, Kruszka P. Holoprosencephaly overview. In: *GeneReviews.* December 27, 2000. University of Washington; 2020.

45. Bous SM, Solomon BD, Graul-Neumann L, Neitzel H, Hardisty EE, Muenke M. Holoprosencephaly-polydactyly/pseudotrisomy 13: a presentation of two new cases and a review of the literature. *Clin Dysmorphol.* 2012;21(4):183-190.

46. Kruszka P, Muenke M. Syndromes associated with holoprosencephaly. *Am J Med Genet C Semin Med Genet.* 2018;178(2):229-237.

47. Kauvar EF, Muenke M. Holoprosencephaly: recommendations for diagnosis and management. *Curr Opin Pediatr.* 2010;22(6):687-695.

48. Dubourg C, Kim A, Watrin E, et al. Recent advances in understanding inheritance of holoprosencephaly. *Am J Med Genet C Semin Med Genet.* 2018;178(2):258-269.

49. Solomon BD, Lacbawan F, Jain M, et al. A novel SIX3 mutation segregates with holoprosencephaly in a large family. *Am J Med Genet A.* 2009;149A(5):919-925.

50. Solomon BD, Mercier S, Velez JI, et al. Analysis of genotype-phenotype correlations in human holoprosencephaly. *Am J Med Genet C Semin Med Genet.* 2010;154C(1):133-141.

51. Roessler E, Velez JI, Zhou N, Muenke M. Utilizing prospective sequence analysis of SHH, ZIC2, SIX3 and TGIF in holoprosencephaly probands to describe the parameters limiting the observed frequency of mutant gene x gene interactions. *Mol Genet Metab.* 2012;105(4):658-664.

52. Johnson CY, Rasmussen SA. Non-genetic risk factors for holoprosencephaly. *Am J Med Genet C Semin Med Genet.* 2010;154C(1):73-85.

53. DeMyer W, Zeman W, Palmer CG. The face predicts the brain: diagnostic significance of median facial anomalies for holoprosencephaly (arhinencephaly). *Pediatrics.* 1964;34:256-263.

54. Kaliaperumal C, Ndoro S, Mandiwanza T, et al. Holoprosencephaly: antenatal and postnatal diagnosis and outcome. *Childs Nerv Syst.* 2016;32(5):801-809.

55. Riddle A, Nagaraj U, Hopkin RJ, Kline-Fath B, Venkatesan C. Fetal magnetic resonance imaging (MRI) in holoprosencephaly and associations with clinical outcome: implications for fetal counseling. *J Child Neurol.* 2021;36(5):357-364.

56. Olsen CL, Hughes JP, Youngblood LG, Sharpe Stimac M. Epidemiology of holoprosencephaly and phenotypic characteristics of affected children: New York State, 1984-1989. *Am J Med Genet.* 1997;73(2):217-226.

57. Glass HC, Shaw GM, Ma C, Sherr EH. Agenesis of the corpus callosum in California 1983-2003: a population-based study. *Am J Med Genet A.* 2008;146A(19):2495-2500. doi:10.1002/ajmg.a.32418

58. D'Antonio F, Pagani G, Familiari A, et al. Outcomes associated with isolated agenesis of the corpus callosum: a meta-analysis. *Pediatrics.* 2016;138:e20160445.

59. Siffredi V, Anderson V, Leventer RJ, Spencer-Smith MM. Neuropsychological profile of agenesis of the corpus callosum: a systematic review. *Dev Neuropsychol.* 2013;38:36-57.

60. Siffredi V, Anderson V, McIlroy A, Wood AG, Leventer RJ, Spencer-Smith MM. A neuropsychological profile for agenesis of the corpus callosum? Cognitive, academic, executive, social, and behavioral functioning in school-age children. *J Int Neuropsychol Soc.* 2018;24:445-455.

61. Vawter-Lee MM, Wasserman H, Thomas CW, et al. Outcome of isolated absent septum pellucidum diagnosed by fetal magnetic resonance imaging (MRI) scan. *J Child Neurol.* 2018;33(11):693-699. doi:10.1177/0883073818783460

62. Damaj L, Bruneau B, Ferry M, et al. Pediatric outcome of children with the prenatal diagnosis of isolated septal agenesis. *Prenat Diagn.* 2010;30(12-13):1143-1150.

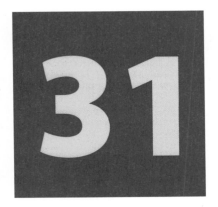

Neonatal Hypoxic Ischemic Encephalopathy

Krista Grande, MD

Charu Venkatesan, MD, PhD

 ESSENTIALS OF DIAGNOSIS AND TYPICAL FEATURES

▶ Neonatal encephalopathy is a clinical condition in the first days after birth manifested by alterations in consciousness, hypotonia, seizures, abnormal reflexes, and apnea.

▶ Hypoxic-ischemic injury in the peripartum period is the most common cause of neonatal encephalopathy and is referred to as hypoxic-ischemic encephalopathy (HIE).

▶ The diagnosis of neonatal HIE is based on multiple clinical and laboratory criteria, including Apgar scores, clinical appearance of the neonate, acidosis, multiorgan injury, and characteristic patterns of brain injury on magnetic resonance imaging (MRI).

▶ Moderate to severe neonatal HIE carries a high risk of death and disability.

▶ Therapeutic hypothermia is the standard of care for neonatal HIE in term infants and has been shown in multiple large trials to reduce risk of death and disability at 18 months and beyond.

▶ HIE is more common in preterm than in term infants, but there is no treatment with enough evidence to recommend as standard of care for preterm infants with HIE.

GENERAL CONSIDERATIONS

Neonatal encephalopathy is a term defined by the American College of Obstetricians and Gynecologists as "a clinically defined syndrome of disturbed neurologic function in the earliest days of life in an infant … manifested by a subnormal level of consciousness or seizures, and often accompanied by difficulty with initiating and maintaining respiration and depression of tone and reflexes."[1] Hypoxic-ischemic injury in the peripartum period is the most common cause of neonatal encephalopathy, and this chapter will focus on diagnosis and management of HIE. HIE is caused by failure of perfusion to the fetal brain due to uterine, placental, or umbilical cord compromise prior to or during delivery.

Hypoxic-ischemic injury as a cause of neonatal encephalopathy is often assumed, rather than certain, because few infants with encephalopathy have a known sentinel event such as placental abruption or cord prolapse.[2] Often, hypoxic-ischemic injury can be assumed without knowledge of a sentinel event in encephalopathic neonates in the presence of low Apgar scores, acidosis, and acute brain injury seen on MRI, or it may be diagnosed retrospectively in an older infant or child with cerebral palsy and MRI evidence of brain injury in a pattern typical of hypoxic-ischemic injury.

PATHOPHYSIOLOGY

The pathologic events of hypoxic-ischemic injury occur in 2 phases, primary energy failure and secondary energy failure, between which there is a latent phase that presents a window of opportunity for intervention.[3] Primary energy failure occurs as a result of the initial reduction of cerebral blood flow. Decreased cerebral blood flow leads to decreased availability of oxygen and glucose, which in turn leads to decreased production of adenosine triphosphate (ATP) and increased production of lactate.[4] Low ATP levels cause failure of many of the mechanisms that maintain cell integrity. Massive depolarization of neurons leads to release of excitotoxic neurotransmitters.[5] Eventually this pathway leads to necrosis and apoptosis of neurons. After cerebral blood flow is restored following resuscitation, there is a brief period of recovery characterized by normal cerebral metabolism.[6] Based on preclinical animal studies, the latent period is estimated to be approximately 6 hours.[6] The latent period is followed by secondary energy failure, which appears to be related to excitotoxicity, inflammation, and oxidative stress.[6]

PREVENTION

Unfortunately, despite advancements in obstetric care including the use of intrapartum markers of fetal distress such as fetal heart rate monitoring, the incidence of HIE has not declined.[7] Therefore, most of the research on treatment of HIE focuses on minimizing the extent of subsequent brain injury during the latent period.

CLINICAL FINDINGS

▶ Symptoms and Signs

Clinical signs of encephalopathy include changes in consciousness, alterations in tone and primitive reflexes, seizures, feeding difficulties, and apnea. The neonate may be hyperalert, irritable, lethargic, or comatose. Tone may be normal, increased, or decreased. The severity of symptoms depends on the timing and duration of the insult. Neonatal encephalopathy is progressive over the first days to week of life. Degree of encephalopathy is important in the evaluation for treatment and for later prognostication. Degree of encephalopathy is determined by serial neurologic examinations and is most commonly determined using the 3-stage scoring method first proposed by Sarnat and Sarnat,[8] which has since been modified for simplification. Severity can alter as the injury evolves, and the Sarnat score may change on repeat examinations. Each infant's initial score, obtained prior to 6 hours of life, is used to make initial treatment decisions. The infant's most severe score on serial examinations may be used to aid prognostication.[9]

▶ Laboratory Findings

Evaluation for HIE should include testing that supports the diagnosis as well as evaluation for sepsis and other organ damage. Multiorgan dysfunction is common in children with HIE.[10]

The following laboratory tests are typically obtained:

- Cord gas
- Infant blood gas within the first hour of life
- Glucose
- Electrolyte panel
- Creatinine and blood urea nitrogen
- Bilirubin
- Liver enzymes
- Partial thromboplastin time and prothrombin time
- Complete blood count and differential
- Blood cultures

If intracranial infection is suspected, lumbar puncture should be performed, and cerebrospinal fluid should be sent for cell counts, protein, glucose, culture and Gram stain, and viral studies. Empiric antimicrobials and antivirals are often started in encephalopathic neonates until culture results show no evidence of infection.

▶ Imaging Studies

Head Ultrasound

Head ultrasound is a simple bedside evaluation that should be completed early in all infants with suspected HIE. While abnormalities related to ischemia may be subtle and difficult to detect on head ultrasound, it is useful for evaluation of other causes of encephalopathy, including major brain malformations and hemorrhage.[11]

MRI

MRI is the preferred imaging technique for detecting the extent and pattern of hypoxic-ischemic injury in infants with HIE. MRI is a valuable prognostic tool in determining range and nature of expected disabilities. MRI should be performed within the first week of injury, as diffusion-weighted imaging changes peak 3 to 5 days after injury and become less apparent further out from injury.[12] Therefore, MRI performed within 7 to 10 days after injury may appear normal for a period of time even when injury is present, due to "pseudonormalization" of diffusion imaging values.[13,14]

There are 3 predominant patterns of hypoxic-ischemic injury in term neonates, which depend on the severity and duration of injury.[15]

- White matter and cortical injury in watershed zones: seen with prolonged partial asphyxia, such as prolonged difficult delivery, and with long-standing antenatal risk factors such as preeclampsia
- Basal ganglia and thalamus–predominant injury: seen with severe acute asphyxia, such as placental abruption, cord prolapse, or uterine rupture
- Global ischemia: the most severe pattern of injury; seen with severe prolonged asphyxia

In preterm infants, patterns of injury are different due to the relative immaturity of the brain.[12] Preterm infants who suffer severe acute ischemia are more likely to have injury to the brainstem and cerebellum.[16] In addition, the thalamus is usually more severely affected than the basal ganglia.[16] This may be because myelination occurs earlier in the thalamus than in the basal ganglia. Generally, the areas of most advanced myelination in the neonatal brain correspond to areas that are most metabolically active and therefore most vulnerable to hypoxia and ischemia.[16] In preterm infants who have milder ischemic events, the most common patterns of injury are germinal matrix hemorrhage and periventricular white matter injury. The germinal matrix is highly susceptible to oxygen deprivation due to its high vascularity and the high oxidative metabolic requirements of the capillary endothelium.[17] As the germinal matrix typically involutes by 34 weeks of gestation, germinal matrix hemorrhage is rare in term infants.

Magnetic Resonance Spectroscopy

Magnetic resonance spectroscopy (MRS) is not always obtained in infants with neonatal encephalopathy, but when available, it may be obtained concurrently with MRI to detect changes in cerebral metabolism after hypoxic-ischemic injury. Ratios of metabolites may be helpful in prognostication.[18] In addition, MRS is helpful in evaluating for metabolic disorders in neonates who present with encephalopathy and have clinical features suspicious for a metabolic disorder rather than, or in addition to, hypoxic-ischemic injury, because MRS features in common neurologic metabolic disease are well described.[19]

▶ Special Tests

All infants with HIE should undergo electroencephalogram (EEG) monitoring in order to monitor for seizures. HIE is the most common cause of neonatal seizures, and seizures occur in approximately 50% of neonates with HIE.[20] Seizures may compromise the infant's hemodynamic or respiratory status if frequent or prolonged. In addition, studies suggest that seizures during this critical period of brain development may exacerbate brain injury in children with HIE and may be independently associated with worse outcomes, including later risk for epilepsy.[21,22] Therefore, seizure detection and treatment are crucial. Most neonatal seizures are electrographic, or when there are clinical manifestations, they may be quite subtle,[23] underlining the importance of EEG monitoring. In addition, infants with HIE may have other paroxysmal movements that could be mistaken for seizures, such as tremor or jitteriness.

There are 2 main methods in common use for detection of neonatal seizures: conventional EEG and amplitude-integrated EEG (aEEG). aEEG displays filtered and compressed data derived from a single- or double-channel EEG recorded using fewer scalp electrodes than conventional EEG. aEEG is more easily applied and interpreted than conventional EEG, making it attractive for use in areas with fewer resources. However, sensitivity and specificity are better for conventional EEG.[24] Shorter seizures may be missed on aEEG due to time compression, and seizures further from the limited electrodes may also be missed.[25]

DIFFERENTIAL DIAGNOSIS

The etiology of neonatal encephalopathy is broad. Aside from hypoxic-ischemic injury, other causes of neonatal encephalopathy include sepsis, central nervous system infection, focal ischemic or hemorrhagic stroke, congenital brain malformations, neonatal epileptic encephalopathies, inborn errors of metabolism, and transient causes of encephalopathy including hypoglycemia and maternal anesthesia or analgesia.

COMPLICATIONS

Early complications of neonatal hypoxic-ischemic injury include respiratory failure, seizures, and feeding difficulties. Later complications include cerebral palsy, cognitive deficits, impairment in learning and attention, cortical vision impairment, hearing loss, and epilepsy, as well as persistent feeding difficulties.

TREATMENT

▶ Therapeutic Hypothermia

Therapeutic hypothermia is standard of care for treatment of moderate to severe HIE in term neonates. Preclinical trials of hypothermia showed marked reduction of secondary brain injury in developing rodents, fetal sheep, and neonatal monkeys.[26] Promising animal studies and early human trials led to the development of multiple major randomized controlled trials of therapeutic hypothermia in neonates with hypoxic-ischemic injury.[27-30] Current protocols are based on protocols established in these large trials. Typically, eligible infants who present before 6 hours of life are cooled to 33 to 34°C for 72 hours, followed by gradual rewarming. Other protocols have been studied, including using longer and deeper cooling, which does not provide additional benefits over current protocols.[31] There is insufficient evidence that cooling infants over 6 hours of age is beneficial.[32]

The major trials of hypothermia for neonatal HIE evaluated outcomes at 18 to 22 months. The National Institute of Child Health and Human Development (NICHD) found that whole-body hypothermia reduced the combined outcome of death and disability in neonates with HIE.[27] The Total Body Hypothermia (TOBY) trial found that moderate systemic hypothermia did not reduce the combined outcome of death or disability in neonates with HIE but that it did reduce risk of disability in survivors.[29] The CoolCap trial found that moderate head cooling with systemic hypothermia was not effective in a mixed group of neonates with HIE but did improve outcome in neonates with moderate, rather than severe, HIE.[28] The Infant Cooling Evaluation (ICE) trial found that whole-body hypothermia reduced the risk of death or major neurodevelopment disability in neonates with HIE.[30] The investigators in these trials continued to follow the enrolled children, and school-age outcomes have since been published.

NICHD, TOBY, and CoolCap have published outcomes in the enrolled children at 6 to 7 years old. NICHD found that the combined outcome of death or intelligence quotient

(IQ) less than 70 was not significantly reduced in school-aged children with neonatal HIE, but it did find that hypothermia resulted in lower death rates without increasing rates of severe disability among survivors.[33] Like NICHD, TOBY found that more children in the hypothermia group survived to school age.[34] Furthermore, surviving children in the hypothermia group were more likely to have normal IQ and less likely to have moderate to severe disability compared to children in the control group. In CoolCap, many children were lost to follow-up, and the study did not have significant power to detect whether treatment with hypothermia impacted long-term outcomes. However, CoolCap did show that outcomes in toddlers predicted school-age outcomes.[35]

Taken together, these follow-up studies show that benefits of hypothermia persist in childhood, hypothermia does not lead to increased survival of children with severe disabilities who would otherwise have passed away, and good outcomes at ages 18 to 21 months reliably predict good functional outcomes at school age.

Treatment of Seizures

There is no consensus on the ideal pharmacologic treatment of neonatal seizures. Phenobarbital is the most widely used first-line treatment for neonatal seizures. However, levetiracetam is now being widely used in clinical practice, as there is increasing evidence that it is an effective alternative to phenobarbital for neonatal seizures.[36,37] Given the association of seizures with worse outcomes in some studies and because some antiepileptic drugs (AEDs) may inhibit mediators of secondary energy failure (eg, topiramate), some have proposed prophylactic treatment with AEDs in an attempt to improve outcome. While there are ongoing trials examining the role of prophylactic AEDs in neonatal HIE, currently available evidence does not support this practice.[38]

Optimal duration of AED treatment remains unknown. There is no consensus on when to discontinue AEDs in neonates with acute symptomatic seizures secondary to AEDs, and practices vary greatly by institution. Most practitioners discontinue AEDs within a few months of the acute symptomatic seizures, provided that the infant remains seizure free. Recent evidence suggests that early discontinuation of AEDs, at the time of hospital discharge, does not impact risk of seizure recurrence.[39]

PROGNOSIS

Neurologic Examination

Both Sarnat scores and neurologic examination are correlated with outcomes. In general, the later an examination is performed, the better it correlates with outcome because examination evolves and typically improves over time, especially in infants who are cooled. The best predictive values

are therefore seen with neurologic examination at discharge (positive and negative predictive values of 86% and 72%, respectively).[40]

MRI

MRI patterns of neonatal brain injury are a marker of prognosis. The NICHD group used data from their neonatal hypothermia study to evaluate the prognostic ability of MRI obtained during the neonatal period to predict childhood neurodevelopment outcome. MRI patterns were divided into 6 categories: 0, normal MRI; 1A, minimal cerebral lesions with no injury to the basal ganglia, thalamus, or internal capsule, and no watershed infarcts; 1B, more extensive cerebral lesions with no injury to the basal ganglia, thalamus, or internal capsule, and no watershed infarcts; 2A, any basal ganglia, thalamus, internal capsule, or any watershed infarcts without other cerebral lesions; 2B, any basal ganglia, thalamus, internal capsule, or any watershed infarcts with other cerebral lesions; and 3, cerebral hemispheric devastation. The primary outcome of death or IQ less than 70 occurred in 8% of children with a normal MRI, 17% of children with pattern 1A injury, 25% of children with pattern 1B injury, 38% of children with pattern 2A injury, 65% of children with pattern 2B injury, and all children with pattern C injury.[33] No children with a normal neonatal MRI developed cerebral palsy. Numbers in this study were small, but the association between pattern of injury and primary outcome was significant. Importantly, hypothermia does not affect the prognostic value of MRI.[41]

MRI patterns of injury also predict risk of epilepsy, with injury to midbrain and brainstem regions associated with significantly higher risk of developing epilepsy.[42]

EEG Background and Presence of Seizures

EEG is an excellent bedside measure of cerebral function, and many studies have examined the significance of EEG features in predicting outcome of infants with HIE. A normal EEG is highly predictive of a normal outcome. Flat tracing, low voltage, and burst suppression predict poor outcome with good to excellent sensitivity and specificity.[43] In a large meta-analysis, flat tracing predicted a poor outcome with a pooled sensitivity of 0.78 and a pooled specificity of 0.99. Low voltage predicted poor outcome with a pooled sensitivity of 0.92 and a pooled specificity of 0.99. Burst suppression predicted poor outcome with a pooled sensitivity of 0.87 and a pooled specificity of 0.82.[43] Of note, poor outcome was defined differently in the studies comprising the meta-analysis, and outcome was evaluated using different means. The meta-analysis therefore pooled normal, minor abnormal, or mildly abnormal outcome into a "normal" category and moderate and severely abnormal outcomes or death into an "abnormal" category.

As EEG is routinely obtained during cooling and rewarming, it is reasonable to use the EEG data for both seizure detection and prognostication. Hypothermia can affect EEG continuity and needs to be interpreted cautiously for prognostication.[44] Severely abnormal background on early EEG is not always predictive of poor outcome in cooled infants.[44] EEG abnormalities that persist are more predictive of a poor outcome in cooled infants.[44]

REFERENCES

1. American College of Obstetricians and Gynecologists and the American Academy of Pediatrics. *Neonatal Encephalopathy and Neurologic Outcome.* 2nd ed. American College of Obstetricians and Gynecologists; 2014.

2. Nelson KB, Bingham P, Edwards EM, et al. Antecedents of neonatal encephalopathy in the Vermont Oxford Network Encephalopathy Registry. *Pediatrics.* 2012;130(5):878-86. doi: 10.1542/peds.2012-0714.

3. Cotten CM, Shankaran S. Hypothermia for hypoxic-ischemic encephalopathy. *Expert Rev Obstet Gynecol.* 2010;5(2)227-239. doi:10.1586/eog.10.7

4. Hanrahan JD, Sargentoni J, Azzopardi D, et al. Cerebral metabolism within 18 hours of birth asphyxia: a proton magnetic resonance spectroscopy study. *Pediatr Res.* 1996;39(4 Pt 1): 584-590. doi:10.1203/00006450-199604000-00004

5. Millar LJ, Shi L, Hoerder-Suabedissen A, Molnár Z. Neonatal hypoxia ischaemia: mechanisms, models, and therapeutic challenges. *Front Cell Neurosci.* 2017;11:78. doi:10.3389/fncel.2017.00078

6. Shalak L, Perlman JM. Hypoxic-ischemic brain injury in the term infant-current concepts. *Early Hum Dev.* 2004;80(2): 125-141. doi:10.1016/j.earlhumdev.2004.06.003

7. Alfirevic Z, Devane D, Gyte GM, Cuthbert A. Continuous cardiotocography (CTG) as a form of electronic fetal monitoring (EFM) for fetal assessment during labour. *Cochrane Database Syst Rev.* 2017;2(2):CD006066. doi:10.1002/14651858.CD006066.pub3

8. Sarnat HB, Sarnat MS. Neonatal encephalopathy following fetal distress. A clinical and electroencephalographic study. *Arch Neurol.* 1976;33(10):696-705. doi:10.1001/archneur.1976.00500100030012

9. Robertson C, Finer N. Term infants with hypoxic-ischemic encephalopathy: outcome at 3.5 years. *Dev Med Child Neurol.* 1985;27(4):473-484. doi:10.1111/j.1469-8749.1985.tb04571.x

10. Shah P, Riphagen S, Beyene J, Perlman M. Multiorgan dysfunction in infants with post-asphyxial hypoxic-ischaemic encephalopathy. *Arch Dis Child Fetal Neonatal Ed.* 2004; 89(2):F152-F155. doi:10.1136/adc.2002.023093

11. Rutherford MA, Pennock JM, Dubowitz LM. Cranial ultrasound and magnetic resonance imaging in hypoxic-ischaemic encephalopathy: a comparison with outcome. *Dev Med Child Neurol.* 1994;36(9):813-825. doi:10.1111/j.1469-8749.1994.tb08191.x

12. Huang BY, Castillo M. Hypoxic-ischemic brain injury: imaging findings from birth to adulthood. *Radiographics.* 2008;28(2):417-617. doi:10.1148/rg.282075066

13. McKinstry RC, Miller JH, Snyder AZ, et al. A prospective, longitudinal diffusion tensor imaging study of brain injury in newborns. *Neurology.* 2002;59(6):824-833. doi:10.1212/wnl.59.6.824

14. Bednarek N, Mathur A, Inder T, et al. Impact of therapeutic hypothermia on MRI diffusion changes in neonatal encephalopathy. *Neurology.* 2012;1;78(18):1420-7. doi: 10.1212/WNL.0b013e318253d589.

15. Okereafor A, Allsop J, Counsell SJ, et al. Patterns of brain injury in neonates exposed to perinatal sentinel events. *Pediatrics.* 2008;121(5):906-914.

16. Barkovich AJ, Sargent SK. Profound asphyxia in the premature infant: imaging findings. *AJNR Am J Neuroradiol.* 1995;16(9):1837-1846.

17. Volpe JJ. Intraventricular hemorrhage in the premature infant: current concepts. Part I. *Ann Neurol.* 1989;25(1):3-11. doi:10.1002/ana.410250103

18. Ancora G, Testa C, Grandi S, et al. Prognostic value of brain proton MR spectroscopy and diffusion tensor imaging in newborns with hypoxic-ischemic encephalopathy treated by brain cooling. *Neuroradiology.* 2013;55(8):1017-1025. doi:10.1007/s00234-013-1202-5

19. Cecil KM. MR spectroscopy of metabolic disorders. *Neuroimaging Clin N Am.* 2006;16(1):87-116. doi:10.1016/j.nic.2005.10.004

20. Yap V, Engel M, Takenouchi T, Perlman JM. Seizures are common in term infants undergoing head cooling. *Pediatr Neurol.* 2009;41(5):327-331. doi:10.1016/j.pediatrneurol.2009.05.004

21. Glass HC, Glidden D, Jeremy RJ, Barkovich AJ, Ferriero DM, Miller SP. Clinical neonatal seizures are independently associated with outcome in infants at risk for hypoxic-ischemic brain injury. *J Pediatr.* 2009;155:318-323.

22. De Haan TR, Langeslag J, van der Lee JH, et al. A systematic review comparing neurodevelopmental outcome in term infants with hypoxic and vascular brain injury with and without seizures. *BMC Pediatr.* 2018;18:147. doi:10.1186/s12887-018-1116-9

23. Nagarajan L, Palumbo L, Ghosh S. Classification of clinical semiology in epileptic seizures in neonates. *Eur J Paediatr Neurol.* 2012;16(2):118-125. doi:10.1016/j.ejpn.2011.11.005

24. Rakshasbhuvankar A, Paul S, Nagarajan L, Ghosh S, Rao S. Amplitude-integrated EEG for detection of neonatal seizures: a systematic review. *Seizure.* 2015;33:90-98. doi:10.1016/j.seizure.2015.09.014

25. Kadivar M, Moghadam EM, Shervin Badv R, Sangsari R, Saeedy M. A comparison of conventional electroencephalography with amplitude-integrated EEG in detection of neonatal seizures. *Med Devices (Auckl).* 2019;12:489-496. doi:10.2147/MDER.S214662

26. Shankaran S. Neonatal encephalopathy: treatment with hypothermia. *Neoreviews.* 2010;11(2):e85-e92.

27. Shankaran S, Laptook AR, Ehrenkranz RA, et al. Whole-body hypothermia for neonates with hypoxic-ischemic encephalopathy. *N Engl J Med.* 2005;353:1574-1584. doi:10.1056/NEJMcps050929.

28. Gluckman PD, Wyatt JS, Azzopardi D, et al; Cool Cap Study Group. Selective head cooling with mild systemic hypothermia after neonatal encephalopathy: multicentre randomized trial. *Lancet.* 2005;365:1319-1327.

29. Azzopardi DV, Strohm B, Edwards AD, et al. Moderate hypothermia to treat perinatal asphyxial encephalopathy. *N Engl J Med.* 2009;361:1349-1358.

30. Jacobs SE, Morley CJ, Inder TE, et al. Whole-body hypothermia for term and near-term newborns with hypoxic-ischemic encephalopathy: a randomized controlled trial. *Arch Pediatr Adolesc Med.* 2011;165(8):692-700. doi:10.1001/archpediatrics.2011.43

31. Shankaran S, Laptook AR, Pappas A, et al. Effect of depth and duration of cooling on death or disability at age 18 months

among neonates with hypoxic-ischemic encephalopathy: a randomized clinical trial. *JAMA*. 2017;318(1):57-67. doi:10.1001/jama.2017.7218

32. Laptook AR, Shankaran S, Tyson JE, et al. Effect of therapeutic hypothermia initiated after 6 hours of age on death or disability among newborns with hypoxic-ischemic encephalopathy: a randomized clinical trial. *JAMA*. 2017;318(16):1550-1560. doi:10.1001/jama.2017.14972

33. Shankaran S, McDonald SA, Laptoot AR, et al. Neonatal magnetic resonance imaging pattern of brain injury as a biomarker of childhood outcomes following a trial of hypothermia for neonatal hypoxic-ischemic encephalopathy. *J Pediatr*. 2015;167:987-993.

34. Azzopardi D, Strohm B, Marlow N, et al. Effects of hypothermia for perinatal asphyxia on childhood outcomes. *N Engl J Med*. 2014;371(2):140-149. doi:10.1056/NEJMoa1315788

35. Guillet R, Edwards AD, Thoresen M, et al. Seven- to eight-year follow-up of the CoolCap trial of head cooling for neonatal encephalopathy. *Pediatr Res*. 2012;71(2):205-209. doi:10.1038/pr.2011.30

36. Venkatesan C, Young S, Schapiro M, Thomas C. Levetiracetam for the treatment of seizures in neonatal hypoxic ischemic encephalopathy. *J Child Neurol*. 2017;32(2):210-214. doi:10.1177/0883073816678102

37. Sharpe C, Reiner GE, Davis SL, et al. Levetiracetam versus phenobarbital for neonatal seizures: a randomized controlled trial [published correction appears in Pediatrics. 2021 Jan;147(1):]. *Pediatrics*. 2020;145(6):e20193182. doi:10.1542/peds.2019-3182

38. Young L, Berg M, Soll R. Prophylactic barbiturate use for the prevention of morbidity and mortality following perinatal asphyxia. *Cochrane Database Syst Rev*. 2016;5:CD001240. doi:10.1002/14651858.CD001240.pub3

39. Fitzgerald MP, Kessler SK, Abend NS. Early discontinuation of antiseizure medications in neonates with hypoxic-ischemic encephalopathy. *Epilepsia*. 2017;58(6):1047-1053. doi:10.1111/epi.13745

40. Murray DM, Bala P, O'Connor CM, Ryan CA, Connolly S, Boylan GB. The predictive value of early neurological examination in neonatal hypoxic-ischaemic encephalopathy and neurodevelopmental outcome at 24 months. *Dev Med Child Neurol*. 2010;52(2):e55-e59.

41. Rutherford M, Ramenghi LA, Edwards AD, et al. Assessment of brain tissue injury after moderate hypothermia in neonates with hypoxic-ischaemic encephalopathy: a nested substudy of a randomised controlled trial. *Lancet Neurol*. 2010;9(1):39-45. doi:10.1016/S1474-4422(09)70295-9

42. Jung DE, Ritacco DG, Nordli DR, Koh S, Venkatesan C. Early Anatomical Injury Patterns Predict Epilepsy in Head Cooled Neonates With Hypoxic-Ischemic Encephalopathy. *Pediatr Neurol*. 2015;53(2):135-40. doi: 10.1016/j.pediatrneurol.2015.04.009.

43. Awal MA, Lai MM, Azemi G, Boashash B, Colditz PB. EEG background features that predict outcome in term neonates with hypoxic ischaemic encephalopathy: a structured review. *Clin Neurophysiol*. 2016;127(1):285-296. doi:10.1016/j.clinph.2015.05.018

44. Hamelin S, Delnard N, Cneude F, Debillon T, Vercueil L. Influence of hypothermia on the prognostic value of early EEG in full-term neonates with hypoxic ischemic encephalopathy. *Neurophysiol Clin*. 2011;41(1):19-27. doi:10.1016/j.neucli.2010.11.002

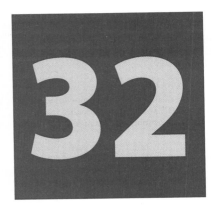

Childhood Stroke

J. Michael Taylor, MD

INTRODUCTION

Stroke is a rare cause of childhood morbidity and mortality. Vascular emergencies result from disruption of the arterial supply or venous return leading to energy failure and cell death. Acute development of a focal neurologic deficit is the hallmark of clinical presentation, although age and comorbid clinical findings may obscure the diagnosis. Children have higher rates of acute seizures and headaches complicating stroke presentation. The risk factors promoting ischemia and hemorrhage vary in the fetus, neonate, child, and adolescent, making the diagnostic workup challenging and broad in these diseases. Evidence supporting hyperacute treatment of vascular emergencies in children remains incomplete, with uncertainties about the safety and implementation of strategies used in adults with similar pathology. Throughout this disease, the affected child requires expertise from child neurologists familiar with stroke management and the resulting complications of developmental delay, cerebral palsy, epilepsy, cognitive difficulties, and neurobehavioral symptoms.

EPIDEMIOLOGY

While the overall rate of stroke in neonates and children is low, high-risk intervals and populations are well defined. Among infants born at term, the risk of ischemic stroke is estimated at 1 in 3500 live births, with an overall stroke rate, including hemorrhage, of 1 in 2700 live births.[1] Throughout life, the 2 highest single-week risks for stroke are at the time of delivery—for both the mother and child.[2] Older infants and children have a lower incidence of stroke, with estimates ranging from 1.3 to 5.4 per 100,000 children.[3] A population-based study indicates the rate of incident stroke has been stable over the past 2 decades.[3]

Unlike adults, in whom stroke is strongly skewed toward ischemic disease (~85%), pediatric cerebrovascular presentation is equally ischemic and hemorrhagic, the latter associated with congenital vascular malformations that are symptomatic in childhood.[4] Stroke is more common in males and is found in higher rates in Black and Asian children in the United States.[4] The highest-risk group is children with sickle cell disease—disproportionately affecting Black families—with a rate of 761 cases of stroke per 100,000 persons.[5] Fortunately, case rates for sickle cell disease–related stroke are falling in developed countries that have widespread screening and prevention strategies in place.[6] A similar finding has thus far not been observed in sub-Saharan Africa, where multiple studies have reported the problems of screening and treatment allocation.[7,8]

ETIOLOGIES OF CHILDHOOD STROKE

The causes of ischemic and hemorrhagic stroke are many. A comprehensive review of risk must consider the age, genetic predeterminants, exposures, comorbid diagnoses, and medical condition at the onset of stroke (Table 32–1).[9,10] Note significant overlap between risk factors for arterial, venous, and hemorrhagic stroke subtypes, suggesting a child may be at risk for multiple events. Arterial ischemic stroke is most highly associated with arteriopathy, which is also a predictor of stroke recurrence, and cardiac disease.[9,11] Hemorrhagic stroke is associated with arteriovenous malformation (14%-46%), coagulation disorders (10%-30%), and brain tumor.[10] Often, a multiplicity of risk factors converging on a single individual may precipitate stroke onset.[9] As an example, the fetus with a COL4A1 mutation and maternal alloimmune thrombocytopenia may suffer intraparenchymal hemorrhage in utero. An adolescent with vascular-type Ehlers-Danlos syndrome may be uniquely susceptible to traumatic dissection of the carotid artery in a motor vehicle collision. A comprehensive evaluation for stroke etiology is recommended to identify cases where further management is indicated, prevent stroke recurrence, and provide diagnostic certainty.

Table 32–1. Partial list of childhood stroke etiologies.

Etiology	Arterial Stroke	Venous Stroke	Hemorrhagic Stroke
Anemia	X	X – Iron deficiency anemia and CSVT	
Aneurysm • Congenital (sporadic or syndrome associated) • Acquired (mycotic aneurysm in endocarditis)	X	X	X
Arteriopathy • Congenital or acquired, iatrogenic, may be progressive, uni- or multifocal	X – Most common risk factor; highest risk for stroke recurrence		X – Moyamoya is hemorrhagic in adults
Arteriovenous (AV) shunt lesions • AV malformation (congenital, 20% familial) • AV fistula; may be congenital or acquired • Vein of Galen malformation	X – Steal and embolic	X – Venous hypertension causes chronic ischemia	X – Most common risk factor
Cardiac defects • Risk for embolic disease, arteriopathy • Antithrombotic often required in treatment	X	X – Increased thoracic pressure impairs venous return	X – Risk for hemorrhage with cardiac support devices, bypass, transplant
Cancer • Hyperviscosity in liquid tumors, thrombocytosis • Mechanical effects of CNS tumors • Multiple risk factors with treatments (chemotherapy, radiotherapy)	X	X – L-Asparaginase and CSVT	X – Brain tumors hemorrhage internally
Cavernous malformation (familial in 20% of cases)			X
Coagulopathy (congenital, acquired, iatrogenic)	X	X	X
Dehydration	X	X	
Fever	X	X	
Genetic disorders	X	X	X
Iatrogenic (ECMO, line-associated thrombus, postoperative)	X	X	X
Illicit drugs (amphetamines, cocaine)	X		X
Infection (intracranial or systemic—sepsis)	X	X	X
Ischemic stroke			X – Hemorrhagic transformation
Hemoglobinopathy • Sickle cell disease (SCD), SS is most important risk • Marked reduction in SCD stroke with targeted HbS fraction management	X	X	X
Hemorrhagic stroke	X – Vasospasm causes delayed ischemia	X – Compression, herniation	
Hypertension (hypertensive emergency and PRES)		X	X
Metabolic (eg, MELAS, Fabry disease)	X	X	X
Migraine	X	X	X
Obesity	X	X	X
Pregnancy (risk for mother and child, twin gestation)	X	X	X – Preterm infants at risk for germinal matrix hemorrhage

(Continued)

Table 32–1. Partial list of childhood stroke etiologies. (*Continued*)

Etiology	Arterial Stroke	Venous Stroke	Hemorrhagic Stroke
Steroids (OCP, implications in gender dysphoria)	X	X	
Thyroid disease		X	X
Trauma (blunt or penetrating, inflicted or accidental)	X	X	X
Venopathy (Sturge-Weber syndrome)		X	X

CNS, central nervous system; CSVT, cerebral sinovenous thrombosis; ECMO, extracorporeal membrane oxygenation; HbS, hemoglobin S; MELAS, mitochondrial encephalopathy, lactic acidosis, and stroke-like episodes; OCP, oral contraceptive pill; PRES, posterior reversible encephalopathy syndrome.

SYMPTOMS OF STROKE

The classic clinical finding of stroke is the immediate development of a focal neurologic symptom, typically in a defined arterial or venous distribution. The clinical examination can be localized to a specific territory corresponding to the finding on imaging. Monitoring the child after vascular injury relies critically on the physical examination to judge lesion stability, secondary injury from edema and medical support, and eventual stabilization of a fixed deficit. This task is made more difficult in young children with immature nervous systems who may not have full connectivity to regions undergoing injury. Consider the neonate who may present with focal status epilepticus after arterial ischemic stroke involving the left middle cerebral artery territory who does not have evidence of right hemiparesis on exam. Serial follow-up with that child may reveal right-sided disuse and hypertonia not previously detectable. Consider a different child with a mature motor system who experiences a right frontal hemorrhage from a cerebral cavernoma rupture at age 4. She may have brief motor symptoms related to edema after hemorrhage and surgical excision with apparent complete resolution. Years later, symptoms of behavioral disinhibition and obsessive thoughts may emerge that localize to the disrupted subcortical networks in the injured frontal lobe. This pattern of immediate and evolving delayed signs and symptoms is a hallmark of pediatric stroke.

In arterial ischemic stroke, toddlers and older children experience acute findings of hemiparesis, language abnormalities, visual field cut, and ataxia.[12] Seizures are more common in the acute interval (15%-25%) in pediatric patients, whereas this is a subacute finding in adults.[12] Nonspecific findings of acute encephalopathy and complaint of headache are also more common in the pediatric stroke population. In the fetus and neonate, stroke onset may be silent or associated with focal seizures, in both cases followed by delayed emergence of lateralizing signs.[13]

Venous stroke may have fewer discrete localizing signs and present more gradually. The infant born with periventricular venous infarction may show lateralizing signs at 6 to 18 months of life but is less frequently found to have seizure or cognitive disability due to relative sparing of overlying cortical tissue.[14] Cerebral sinus venous thrombosis occurs most commonly in the neonatal period but can begin at any time during the life span. Roughly half of venous thrombosis cases will have corresponding ischemia, although symptoms are largely nonspecific, with headache, encephalopathy, and seizures predominating over focal symptoms.[12] Venous stroke is unique among vascular lesions, in that regional hypoperfusion may be bilateral, extending the territory of at-risk tissue.

Hemorrhagic stroke is the least robustly studied and likely most heterogenous subtype in pediatrics. The symptom complexes are likely defined by the causative vascular lesion or associated comorbid condition. In one pediatric cohort, mental status change was present in over 50% of cases, with seizure, vomiting, respiratory distress, and weakness occurring at lower frequencies.[15] More data are needed from prospectively collected population-based studies to further delineate symptoms in pediatric hemorrhagic stroke.

DIAGNOSIS

The emergence of acute focal neurologic symptoms should prompt evaluation for stroke. Complicating this evaluation is the inherent instability of a child with a new vascular compromise with dynamic changes in intracranial pressure and threat for recurrent injury. Often, the evaluation begins in the trauma suite upon presentation to the hospital with an initial battery of laboratory studies and imaging. This targeted evaluation screens for mimics of stroke and begins the diagnostic process for etiology.[16] Several studies have demonstrated the value of acute stroke response teams in the pediatric hospital to speed time to diagnosis and treatment decisions with the goal of improving disease outcome.[17-19]

Selection of a first imaging modality is largely driven by the resources of the institution.[20] Computed tomography (CT) is widely available, fast, and cost effective. The sensitivity for acute hemorrhage is highest with CT, but ischemia will be undetectable for up to 6 hours. Magnetic resonance imaging (MRI) is free from ionizing radiation, immediately diagnostic for ischemic stroke (diffusion-weighted imaging), more sensitive to stroke mimics, and increasingly available for use in all hospital settings.[20] Drawbacks for MRI include limited access to available scanners and longer study times, which potentially limits utility in younger children who may have difficulty remaining still for the scan. Recent development of fast MRI protocols allows for a shorter study time and is increasingly used in the evaluation of trauma,[21] ventriculoperitoneal shunt malfunction,[22] and stroke[23,24] with promising results. Either imaging modality should be paired with appropriate vascular imaging of the arteries (magnetic resonance or CT angiography) or veins (magnetic resonance or CT venography) during the initial evaluation of stroke.

Stroke diagnosis is strongly influenced by the pattern of injury identified on the index scan, which prompts further targeted workup (Figure 32–1). One example is the child with focal cerebral arteriopathy who has a characteristic stroke in the basal ganglia, corresponding steno-occlusive changes on the ipsilateral middle cerebral artery, and small distal ischemic lesions from artery-to-artery embolism (Figure 32–1B). This pattern may prompt an evaluation for vascular inflammation or central nervous system infection. Ischemic lesions in multiple vascular territories with many appearing at the gray-white interface are strongly suspicious for proximal embolism, making the evaluation for a source lesion imperative. CT angiography may show a "spot sign" within an intracranial hemorrhage.[25] This centrally placed leak of contrast is predictive of hematoma expansion and rebleeding. Utilization of imaging biomarkers helps predict outcome and aids the diagnostic workup.[26,27]

The balance of the diagnostic phase screens for precipitating risk factors.[12] These include cardiac evaluation with echocardiogram and agitated saline bubble study to find valvular disease, intracardiac thrombus, heart failure, or thoracic level shunt; and electrocardiogram to screen for dysrhythmia. Inflammatory testing for infectious or rheumatologic disorders may reveal previously occult comorbid diagnoses. Coagulation testing may reveal aberrations in clotting cascade, selective factor deficiencies, genetic thrombophilia, or acquired dysfunction (eg, protein-losing enteropathy in intestinal failure). Special circumstances may trigger additional targeted workup, including lumbar puncture for spinal fluid analysis, screening for genetic disorders, vascular biopsy, or catheter angiography. Several controversies remain regarding optimal secondary prevention strategies after discovery of modifiable risk factors (eg, patent foramen ovale). Consultation between appropriate specialists and an experienced pediatric stroke provider is strongly advised to arrive at a consensus management strategy.

Neonates and infants identified with presumed perinatal stroke are again guided by different recommendations. Studies have demonstrated low diagnostic yield and high false-positive screening for infants evaluated for stroke that occurred at delivery.[28,29] Pathologic evaluation of the placenta may be informative for stroke etiology but is not routinely ordered if no concerns are raised for the infant at birth.[30] In most circumstances, imaging is the only evaluation for ischemic stroke in this population.[12]

In a minority of cases, no inciting cause of stroke is identified. This circumstance is termed idiopathic or cryptogenic in both ischemic and hemorrhagic cases. Fortunately, data

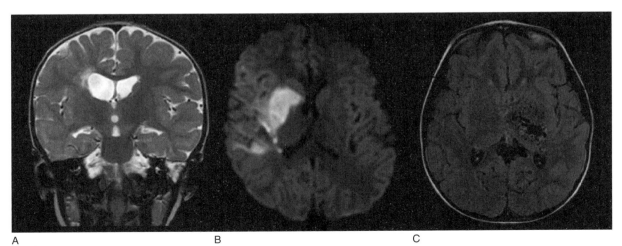

A   B   C

▲ **Figure 32–1.** Examples of pediatric cerebrovascular disorders. **A.** Right hemispheric venous infarction with asymmetric lateral ventricle, overlying gliosis and white matter volume loss. **B.** Acute arterial ischemic stroke in the right putamen and insular cortex secondary to focal cerebral arteriopathy. **C.** Left thalamic arteriovenous malformation with a complex network of dilated vascular structures.

suggest that the rate of recurrent stroke is low when a thorough evaluation fails to identify a cause of stroke.[11,31,32]

TREATMENT

Management of stroke occurs throughout the disease. Upon initial presentation, there is an opportunity in arterial ischemic stroke to clear a blockage and restore perfusion. Hemorrhagic lesions require targeted neurocritical care support and may warrant surgical intervention emergently. After immediate stabilization, the next management phase targets mitigation of secondary injury through careful physiologic manipulation. Deescalated from the intensive care unit, a subacute to chronic phase focuses on secondary prevention and chronic rehabilitation.

Pediatric stroke providers, having struggled to develop the highest-quality evidence-based treatment paradigms (in large part due to lower disease incidence), have adapted management of adults for their population. In hyperacute arterial ischemic stroke therapy in childhood, a multicenter randomized prospective trial of thrombolysis was closed early in 2013 due to failure of accrual, prompting a broad look at readiness for stroke intervention trials in pediatric patients.[33,34] Evidence supporting treatment with thrombolysis (tissue plasminogen activator) or endovascular approaches targeting reperfusion[35,36] has been published in multiple case series and meta-analyses, although widespread implementation of hyperacute therapies remains controversial. Literature supports development of networks and multidisciplinary teams with expertise in pediatric stroke to guide management of hyperacute stroke therapy on an individualized patient basis.[12] In the critical care setting, literature supports targeted management of cerebral perfusion, avoidance of hyperthermia and hyperglycemia, and management of intracranial pressure and seizures.[12] The selection of antithrombotic treatment in both arterial and venous stroke is a matter of controversy guided by inconsistent literature, consensus statements from professional societies, provider experience, and institutional practice.[37] As a general recommendation, antiplatelet agents (eg, aspirin) are used for arteriopathy, and anticoagulants (eg, warfarin, enoxaparin) are used for venous clots. The direct oral anticoagulants (eg, rivaroxaban) have an emerging role in clinical practice and have shown early safety and efficacy in pediatric stroke.[38] Evidence-based therapies for many specific etiologies of stroke remain under investigation, including the role of glucocorticoids in focal cerebral arteriopathy; optimal approaches, timing, and follow-up biomarkers in cerebral revascularization for moyamoya; and pharmacotherapies to reduce vascular complications of ionizing radiation for brain tumor. There are tremendous opportunities for advancement in the science of pediatric stroke management.

To advance this field, hospital systems are challenged to support the multidisciplinary care teams needed to provide best-quality care to stroke patients. These systems include cooperation between neurology, neurosurgery, hematology, diagnostic and interventional radiology, critical care medicine, rehabilitation, and other disciplines.[17,39] Care teams at large academic medical centers are well suited to support the financial costs and offer training opportunities to physicians to meet these care demands.[40]

OUTCOME

Childhood stroke has significant morbidity and mortality. These costs are seen in many forms. Among all pediatric age cohorts, stroke is among the top 10 leading causes of death.[41] Among survivors, children remain in recovery for many years, participating in therapies for physical, language, cognitive, behavioral, and emotional symptoms. In ischemic stroke, these outcomes can be quantified and tracked with the pediatric stroke outcome measure.[42] A corollary, validated measure has not been developed for hemorrhagic stroke in childhood. Symptomatic sequelae of stroke add to the morbidity, as epilepsy is known to predict higher severity scores on the referenced outcome measure.[43] Vascular brain injury results in lower overall intelligence, communication disorders, emotional dysregulation, executive dysfunction, and many other cognitive symptoms.[44-46] The impact these changes have on academic performance and occupational trajectory are assured but not robustly quantified.[47,48] Further investigation is needed to minimize stroke disability and maximize recovery outcome.

REFERENCES

1. Agrawal N, Johnston SC, Wu YW, Sidney S, Fullerton HJ. Imaging data reveal a higher pediatric stroke incidence than prior US estimates. *Stroke.* 2009;40(11):3415-3421. doi:10.1161/STROKEAHA.109.564633

2. Moatti Z, Gupta M, Yadava R, Thamban S. A review of stroke and pregnancy: incidence, management and prevention. *Eur J Obstet Gynecol Reprod Biol.* 2014;181:20-27. doi:10.1016/j.ejogrb.2014.07.024

3. Lehman LL, Khoury JC, Taylor JM, et al. Pediatric stroke rates over 17 years: report from a population-based study. *J Child Neurol.* 2018;33(7):463-467. doi:10.1177/0883073818767039

4. Fullerton HJ, Wu YW, Zhao S, Johnston SC. Risk of stroke in children: ethnic and gender disparities. *Neurology.* 2003; 61(2):189-194. doi:10.1212/01.wnl.0000078894.79866.95

5. Powars D, Wilson B, Imbus C, Pegelow C, Allen J. The natural history of stroke in sickle cell disease. *Am J Med.* 1978;65(3): 461-471. doi:10.1016/0002-9343(78)90772-6

6. Fullerton HJ, Adams RJ, Zhao S, Johnston SC. Declining stroke rates in Californian children with sickle cell disease. *Blood.* 2004;104(2):336-339. doi:10.1182/blood-2004-02-0636

7. Kirkham FJ, Lagunju IA. Epidemiology of stroke in sickle cell disease. *J Clin Med.* 2021;10(18):4232. doi:10.3390/jcm10184232

8. Abdullahi SU, Wudil BJ, Bello-Manga H, et al. Primary prevention of stroke in children with sickle cell anemia in sub-Saharan Africa: rationale and design of phase III randomized clinical trial. *Pediatr Hematol Oncol.* 2021;38(1):49-64. doi:10.1080/08880018.2020.1810183

9. Mackay MT, Wiznitzer M, Benedict SL, et al. Arterial ischemic stroke risk factors: the International Pediatric Stroke Study. *Ann Neurol*. 2011;69(1):130-140. doi:10.1002/ana.22224

10. Jordan LC, Hillis AE. Hemorrhagic stroke in children. *Pediatr Neurol*. 2007;36(2):73-80. doi:10.1016/j.pediatrneurol.2006.09.017

11. Fullerton HJ, Wintermark M, Hills NK, et al. Risk of recurrent arterial ischemic stroke in childhood: a prospective international study. *Stroke*. 2016;47(1):53-59. doi:10.1161/STROKEAHA.115.011173

12. Ferriero DM, Fullerton HJ, Bernard TJ, et al. Management of stroke in neonates and children: a scientific statement from the American Heart Association/American Stroke Association. *Stroke*. 2019;50(3):e51-e96. doi:10.1161/STR.0000000000000183

13. Kirton A, Deveber G. Stroke in the fetus and neonate. *Future Cardiol*. 2006;2(5):593-604. doi:10.2217/14796678.2.5.593

14. Dunbar M, Kirton A. Perinatal stroke. *Semin Pediatr Neurol*. 2019;32:100767. doi:10.1016/j.spen.2019.08.003

15. Lo WD. Childhood hemorrhagic stroke: an important but understudied problem. *J Child Neurol*. 2011;26(9):1174-1185. doi:10.1177/0883073811408424

16. Shellhaas RA, Smith SE, O'Tool E, Licht DJ, Ichord RN. Mimics of childhood stroke: characteristics of a prospective cohort. *Pediatrics*. 2006;118(2):704-709. doi:10.1542/peds.2005-2676

17. Catenaccio E, Riggs BJ, Sun LR, et al. Performance of a pediatric stroke alert team within a comprehensive stroke center. *J Child Neurol*. 2020;35(9):571-577. doi:10.1177/0883073820920111

18. Ladner TR, Mahdi J, Gindville MC, et al. Pediatric acute stroke protocol activation in a children's hospital emergency department. *Stroke*. 2015;46(8):2328-2331. doi:10.1161/STROKEAHA.115.009961

19. Bernard TJ, Friedman NR, Stence NV, et al. Preparing for a "pediatric stroke alert". *Pediatr Neurol*. 2016;56:18-24. doi:10.1016/j.pediatrneurol.2015.10.012

20. Khalaf A, Iv M, Fullerton H, Wintermark M. Pediatric stroke imaging. *Pediatr Neurol*. 2018;86:5-18. doi:10.1016/j.pediatrneurol.2018.05.008

21. Lindberg DM, Stence NV, Grubenhoff JA, et al. Feasibility and accuracy of fast MRI versus CT for traumatic brain injury in young children. *Pediatrics*. 2019;144(4):e20190419. doi:10.1542/peds.2019-0419

22. Boyle TP, Paldino MJ, Kimia AA, et al. Comparison of rapid cranial MRI to CT for ventricular shunt malfunction. *Pediatrics*. 2014;134(1):e47-e54. doi:10.1542/peds.2013-3739

23. Chung MS, Lee JY, Jung SC, et al. Reliability of fast magnetic resonance imaging for acute ischemic stroke patients using a 1.5-T scanner. *Eur Radiol*. 2019;29(5):2641-2650. doi:10.1007/s00330-018-5812-5

24. Christy A, Murchison C, Wilson JL. Quick brain magnetic resonance imaging with diffusion-weighted imaging as a first imaging modality in pediatric stroke. *Pediatr Neurol*. 2018;78:55-60. doi:10.1016/j.pediatrneurol.2017.09.020

25. Wada R, Aviv RI, Fox AJ, et al. CT Angiography "spot sign" predicts hematoma expansion in acute intracerebral hemorrhage. *Stroke*. 2007;38(4):1257-1262. doi:10.1161/01.str.0000259633.59404.f3

26. Domi T, deVeber G, Shroff M, Kouzmitcheva E, MacGregor DL, Kirton A. Corticospinal tract pre-wallerian degeneration: a novel outcome predictor for pediatric stroke on acute MRI. *Stroke*. 2009;40(3):780-787. doi:10.1161/STROKEAHA.108.529958

27. Devela G, Taylor JM, Zhang B, et al. Quantitative arterial tortuosity suggests arteriopathy in children with cryptogenic stroke. *Stroke*. 2018;49(4):1011-1014. doi:10.1161/strokeaha.117.020321

28. Lehman LL, Beaute J, Kapur K, et al. Workup for perinatal stroke does not predict recurrence. *Stroke*. 2017;48(8):2078-2083. doi:10.1161/STROKEAHA.117.017356

29. Curtis C, Mineyko A, Massicotte P, et al. Thrombophilia risk is not increased in children after perinatal stroke. *Blood*. 2017;129(20):2793-2800. doi:10.1182/blood-2016-11-750893

30. Bernson-Leung ME, Boyd TK, Meserve EE, et al. Placental pathology in neonatal stroke: a retrospective case-control study. *J Pediatr*. 2018;195:39-47 e5. doi:10.1016/j.jpeds.2017.11.061

31. Fullerton HJ, Wu YW, Sidney S, Johnston SC. Risk of recurrent childhood arterial ischemic stroke in a population-based cohort: the importance of cerebrovascular imaging. *Pediatrics*. 2007;119(3):495-501. doi:10.1542/peds.2006-2791

32. Fullerton HJ, Wu YW, Sidney S, Johnston SC. Recurrent hemorrhagic stroke in children: a population-based cohort study. *Stroke*. 2007;38(10):2658-2662. doi:10.1161/STROKEAHA.107.481895

33. Bernard TJ, Rivkin MJ, Scholz K, et al. Emergence of the primary pediatric stroke center: impact of the thrombolysis in pediatric stroke trial. *Stroke*. 2014;45(7):2018-2023. doi:10.1161/STROKEAHA.114.004919

34. Rivkin MJ, deVeber G, Ichord RN, et al. Thrombolysis in pediatric stroke study. *Stroke*. 2015;46(3):880-885. doi:10.1161/STROKEAHA.114.008210

35. Sporns PB, Sträter R, Minnerup J, et al. Feasibility, safety, and outcome of endovascular recanalization in childhood stroke. *JAMA Neurol*. 2020;77(1):25. doi:10.1001/jamaneurol.2019.3403

36. Cobb MI-PH, Laarakker AS, Gonzalez LF, Smith TP, Hauck EF, Zomorodi AR. Endovascular therapies for acute ischemic stroke in children. *Stroke*. 2017;48(7):2026-2030. doi:10.1161/strokeaha.117.016887

37. Boucher AA, Taylor JM, Luchtman-Jones L. Aspirin in childhood acute ischemic stroke: the evidence for treatment and efficacy testing. *Pediatr Blood Cancer*. 2019;66(6):e27665. doi:10.1002/pbc.27665

38. Connor P, Sánchez Van Kammen M, Lensing AWA, et al. Safety and efficacy of rivaroxaban in pediatric cerebral venous thrombosis (EINSTEIN-Jr CVT). *Blood Adv*. 2020;4(24):6250-6258. doi:10.1182/bloodadvances.2020003244

39. Barry M, Le TM, Gindville MC, Jordan LC. In-hospital pediatric stroke alert activation. *Pediatr Neurol*. 2018;88:31-35. doi:10.1016/j.pediatrneurol.2018.08.003

40. Wainwright MS, Grimason M, Goldstein J, et al. Building a pediatric neurocritical care program: a multidisciplinary approach to clinical practice and education from the intensive care unit to the outpatient clinic. *Semin Pediatr Neurol*. 2014;21(4):248-254. doi:10.1016/j.spen.2014.10.006

41. Lynch JK, Hirtz DG, DeVeber G, Nelson KB. Report of the National Institute of Neurological Disorders and Stroke workshop on perinatal and childhood stroke. *Pediatrics*. 2002;109(1):116-123. doi:10.1542/peds.109.1.116

42. Kitchen L, Westmacott R, Friefeld S, et al. The pediatric stroke outcome measure: a validation and reliability study. *Stroke*. 2012;43(6):1602-1608. doi:10.1161/STROKEAHA.111.639583

43. Fox CK, Jordan LC, Beslow LA, Armstrong J, Mackay MT, deVeber G. Children with post-stroke epilepsy have poorer outcomes one year after stroke. *Int J Stroke*. 2018;13(8):820-823. doi:10.1177/1747493018784434

44. Westmacott R, Askalan R, MacGregor D, Anderson P, Deveber G. Cognitive outcome following unilateral arterial ischaemic stroke in childhood: effects of age at stroke and

lesion location. *Dev Med Child Neurol.* 2010;52(4):386-393. doi:10.1111/j.1469-8749.2009.03403.x

45. Ballantyne AO, Spilkin AM, Trauner DA. Language outcome after perinatal stroke: does side matter? *Child Neuropsychol.* 2007;13(6):494-509. doi:10.1080/09297040601114878

46. O'Keeffe F, Stark D, Murphy O, Ganesan V, King J, Murphy T. Psychosocial outcome and quality of life following childhood stroke: a systematic review. *Dev Neurorehabil.* 2017;20(7): 428-442. doi:10.1080/17518423.2017.1282052

47. Deotto A, Westmacott R, Fuentes A, deVeber G, Desrocher M. Does stroke impair academic achievement in children? The role of metacognition in math and spelling outcomes following pediatric stroke. *J Clin Exp Neuropsychol.* 2019;41(3):257-269. doi:10.1080/13803395.2018.1533528

48. Hawks C, Jordan LC, Gindville M, Ichord RN, Licht DJ, Beslow LA. Educational placement after pediatric intracerebral hemorrhage. *Pediatr Neurol.* 2016;61:46-50. doi:10.1016/j.pediatrneurol.2016.05.004

Central Nervous System Tumors in Childhood

Heather M. Wied, MD, PhD

Peter de Blank, MD, MSCE

Central nervous system (CNS) tumors are the most common solid tumor of childhood and are the leading cause of death in children diagnosed with cancer. The number of children 0 to 19 years old in the United States diagnosed with a CNS tumor is approximately 6.21 per 100,000 per year as estimated by the Central Brain Tumor Registry of the United States.[1]

CNS tumors have variable treatments and prognoses based on their location, histology, immunohistochemistry, and molecular classification, which has been most recently updated in 2021 by the World Health Organization Classification of Tumors of the Central Nervous System (WHO CNS5).[2] The classification of tumors of the CNS is constantly being updated as new information is learned. Recently, WHO CNS5 updated the classifications of numerous pediatric CNS tumors, including pediatric diffuse low-grade gliomas and diffuse high-grade gliomas; circumscribed astrocytic gliomas; glioneuronal tumors and neuronal tumors, including dysembryoplastic neuroepithelial tumors; ependymal tumors; choroid plexus tumors; embryonal tumors such as medulloblastoma; pineal tumors; cranial and paraspinal nerve tumors; meningiomas; mesenchymal and nonmeningothelial tumors; melanocytic tumors; hematolymphoid tumors, including lymphomas and histiocytic tumors; germ cell tumors; tumors of the sellar region; and metastases to the CNS.

Pediatric low-grade gliomas are the most common brain tumor in childhood. They occur throughout the CNS and in a broad range of ages with multiple different tumor histologies. When low-grade gliomas can be completely surgically resected, they may not require further treatment. However, tumors that occur in critical or inaccessible regions of the brain are frequently unable to undergo complete surgical resection.

Medulloblastoma, a common pediatric embryonal tumor, is the most common malignant brain tumor of childhood. It is found in the cerebellum, although it may metastasize to other CNS locations, and is typically seen in children younger than 10 years old. Fortunately, it is associated with increased survival rates due to advances in risk stratification and combination therapies including radiation to the craniospinal axis and chemotherapy.

The second most common malignant brain tumor of childhood is ependymoma, which is found throughout the CNS. Ependymomas most frequently occur in children younger than 5 years old with variable prognosis. These are typically treated with surgery and radiation, with variable use of chemotherapy. Unlike other CNS tumors, the risk of relapse continues long into typical survivorship.

High-grade gliomas occur at all ages and anywhere in the CNS and lead to poor outcomes. Diffuse intrinsic pontine gliomas are a particularly aggressive type of glioma centered in the pons of the brainstem. Despite radiation or other treatments, these tumors almost always lead to devastating outcomes with a very poor survival rate. Overall median survival is 1 year, with a 2-year overall survival rate of less than 10%.[3]

Spinal tumors are rare and account for approximately 5% of all CNS tumors in children and adolescents.[1]

CLINICAL PRESENTATION

The clinical presentation of a CNS tumor can vary widely depending on many factors including the age of the patient, the area of the CNS affected, and rate of growth of the tumor.

The child may present with vague symptoms or more focal symptoms. The most common symptoms include headaches, nausea and vomiting, abnormal gait, and seizures. In addition, more specific focal neurologic deficits can be seen, such as cranial nerve palsies, difficulty swallowing, double vision, abnormal eye movements, and focal motor weakness. Other nonspecific changes may be noted such as behavior changes, increased fatigue, irritability, regression of skills, weight loss, or poor growth. In an infant, the clinical presentation can include macrocephaly, bulging fontanelle with splayed sutures, enlarging head circumference, or "setting sun" sign with downward deviation of the eyes and impaired upgaze.

For spinal tumors, the most common presenting symptom is back pain, but other symptoms may include motor weakness, paresthesias, torticollis, abnormal curvature of the spine, or sphincter dysfunction.

Headaches

Headaches are the most common symptom of children presenting with intracranial tumors, occurring in up to 30% of children. Severe headaches may present as irritability in younger children who are unable to communicate or may be associated with developmental delays. Headaches of particular concern include those in children younger than 5 years old, those that awaken a child at night, and those that occur first thing in the morning. Often, children will feel relief after they vomit. Headaches are likely due to increased intracranial pressure.

Nausea and Vomiting

Nausea and vomiting (often associated with headaches) can be common symptoms of brain tumors, particularly if associated with impaired cerebrospinal fluid drainage and increased intracranial pressure.

Seizures

Seizure may be the first presenting symptom of a child's brain tumor. Seizures are more typically seen in patients with low-grade supratentorial lesions.[4,5] Often these seizures will be focal seizures that may secondarily generalize based on the tumor location.

Abnormal Gait

In a child with a posterior fossa tumor, the gait may change, and the child may become clumsier or appear uncoordinated with increased difficulty walking or running. Changes in the way a child walks may also be concerning for possible spinal cord tumor.

DIAGNOSIS

Neuroimaging should be obtained when a child presents with concerning signs or symptoms such as headaches, seizures, or abnormal gait. A head computed tomography scan can quickly evaluate for larger masses or hydrocephalus that might be associated with increased intracranial pressure. However, the preferred modality for full evaluation in nonemergent cases is a brain and/or spine magnetic resonance imaging (MRI) scan with contrast for any symptoms of concern. If a concerning mass is found, imaging of the complete craniospinal axis should be considered, in addition to advanced imaging techniques such as magnetic resonance spectroscopy or positron emission tomography imaging to help determine potential targets for biopsy. If a mass is identified, referral to a pediatric neurosurgeon is critical for further evaluation, including management of intracranial hypertension and to obtain a tissue biopsy for histologic and molecular diagnosis. In tumors that have a potential for metastasis, obtaining an MRI of the spine with contrast and cerebrospinal fluid cytology is helpful to determine staging.

TREATMENTS

Brain and spinal tumors are treated using a combination of surgery (removal when feasible or debulking), radiation, and chemotherapy. The tumor type, growth pattern, and patient symptoms often determine the best treatment regimen.

Surgery

Tumors that are causing threatening symptoms often require maximum safe resection by a pediatric neurosurgeon. Depending on the tumor characteristics, this may involve anything from a biopsy to a complete resection. After surgery, a repeat brain MRI is often performed to determine the extent of the resection and any postsurgical complications. Dexamethasone is often used perioperatively to reduce surgical edema. During this perioperative period, it is important to closely monitor for complications of brain surgery such as syndrome of inappropriate antidiuretic hormone secretion or cerebral salt wasting. Depending on the tumor type, additional treatments with a combination of chemotherapy and/or radiation are typically required.

Children with seizures prior to their surgery should be continued on their antiseizure medications around the time of surgery. An increase in seizures can occur during the perioperative period. Neurosurgeons may prefer to place certain patients who have undergone tumor resection on antiseizure medication prophylaxis for 7 days postoperatively. However, it is not recommended to continue antiseizure medications past this time if the patient has never had a seizure previously.[6] Risk factors for perioperative seizures in children who have not had previous seizures include tumors located supratentorially, age less than 2 years, and hyponatremia due to syndrome of inappropriate antidiuretic hormone or cerebral salt wasting.[7]

After surgeries to the posterior fossa, a possible complication is posterior fossa syndrome. This syndrome is associated with mutism, ataxia, hypotonia, cranial nerve palsies, and emotional lability. Although the mutism typically improves, dysarthria and ataxia may persist due to the disruption of the dentato-thalamo-cortical pathway. Patients with posterior fossa syndrome should undergo intensive comprehensive rehabilitation to help with the numerous deficits of this condition.

Radiation

Radiation therapy is an important treatment of CNS tumors in children but is often avoided when possible due to the long-term consequences of radiation in children. For instance, neurocognitive impairment is a common effect of radiation in a developing brain and is related to the dose of radiation used, the age of the patient, and the volume and location of tissue irradiated. Younger children are more sensitive to the effects of radiation on cognition. Children who have undergone radiation therapy have been reported to have a decline in their overall global intelligence quotient.[8-10] Using proton beam radiation therapy has helped to minimize damage to surrounding brain tissue, as it targets only the areas of interest, and has been found to decrease the effects of radiation on cognitive development.[10] Radiation to the hypothalamic-pituitary axis can result in hormone deficiency, with growth hormone most commonly affected. Other side effects that can occur from radiation therapy include hearing loss, cerebrovascular disease resulting in moyamoya, cavernomas, strokes, and stroke-like migraine attacks after radiation therapy (SMART syndrome).[11,12] In addition, radiation therapy is known to cause secondary tumors, most commonly meningiomas and high-grade gliomas.

Chemotherapy

Chemotherapy is often used in conjunction with surgery and/or radiation for CNS tumors. Due to improved understanding of the molecular characteristics of tumors, many targeted therapies are now being developed.[13] However, challenges remain in pharmacologic therapies due to the poor permeability of the blood-brain barrier. Side effects of these treatments are generally specific to the agents used but can include peripheral neuropathy, leukoencephalopathy, or posterior reversible encephalopathy syndrome.

NEUROLOGIC COMPLICATIONS

Emergency Complications

Children with CNS tumors may present to the emergency department prior to their diagnosis or due to a complication from their tumor or treatment. Children who present with symptoms of increased intracranial pressure, seizures including nonconvulsive status epilepticus, cerebrovascular accidents, or concerns for spinal cord compression require immediate evaluation and treatment.

Long-Term Neurologic Complications

Seizures are one of the most common complications of pediatric brain tumors, occurring in up to 24% of children at initial presentation.[14] Seizures may be caused by the tumor or occur after treatment as a sequela of surgery, radiation, or chemotherapy. Children with tumors located supratentorially with gray matter involvement, such as dysembryoplastic neuroepithelial tumors and gangliogliomas, are at greater risk of having seizures that are difficult to control.[15] Seizures also have a long-term impact on childhood cancer survivors, affecting functional and psychological outcomes independent of cancer treatments.[16] Typically, non–enzyme-inducing antiseizure medications are preferred to avoid possible interactions with chemotherapy and corticosteroids. Thus, medications such as levetiracetam, lamotrigine, lacosamide, valproic acid, topiramate, and zonisamide are preferred over cytochrome P450 inducers such as phenytoin or carbamazepine. If a child with a brain tumor has not had seizures, it is not recommended to start antiseizure medications prophylactically.[6] After antiseizure medications have been started, it is appropriate to attempt to wean the patient off these medications after 2 years of seizure freedom, similar to other children with epilepsy.

It is important for neurologists to have a high index of suspicion for possible nonconvulsive status epilepticus in a child with a history of a brain tumor who presents with altered mental status. When this occurs, the child should have emergent imaging to rule out increased intracranial pressure or stroke. If these imaging studies are negative, an electroencephalogram may help evaluate for status epilepticus.

PROGNOSIS

The prognosis for children with CNS tumors varies widely depending on the age of the child and tumor characteristics. Overall, treatment advances and therapies have increased survival rates for many children with medulloblastomas and low-grade gliomas with a 5-year survival rate of greater than 75%. The prognosis for many other tumors, including high-grade gliomas and diffuse intrinsic pontine gliomas, unfortunately remains poor.

As survival improves among children with CNS tumors, it is important to continue to offer support needed for initial treatment as well as long-term care to optimize their outcomes. This is best addressed in a multidisciplinary center with integrated resources that include pediatric oncology, neurosurgery, neuroradiology, neuropathology, neurology, endocrinology, neuro-ophthalmology, rehabilitation, neuropsychology, genetics, and palliative care.

REFERENCES

1. Ostrom QT, Cioffi G, Waite K, Kruchko C, Barnholtz-Sloan JS. CBTRUS statistical report: primary brain and other central nervous system tumors diagnosed in the United States in 2014-2018. *Neuro Oncol.* 2021;23(12 suppl 2):iii1-iii105.
2. Louis DN, Perry A, Wesseling P, et al. The 2021 WHO classification of tumors of the central nervous system: a summary. *Neuro Oncol.* 2021;23(8):1231-1251.

3. Rashed WM, Maher E, Adel M, Saber O, Zaghloul MS. Pediatric diffuse intrinsic pontine glioma: where do we stand? *Cancer Metastasis Rev.* 2019;38(4):759-770.

4. Fattal-Valevski A, Nissan N, Kramer U, Constantini S. Seizures as the clinical presenting symptom in children with brain tumors. *J Child Neurol.* 2013;28(3):292-296.

5. Wells EM, Gaillard WD, Packer RJ. Pediatric brain tumors and epilepsy. *Semin Pediatr Neurol.* 2012;19(1):3-8.

6. Walbert T, Harrison RA, Schiff D, et al. SNO and EANO practice guideline update: anticonvulsant prophylaxis in patients with newly diagnosed brain tumors. *Neuro Oncol.* 2021;23(11):1835-1844.

7. Hardesty DA, Sanborn MR, Parker WE, Storm PB. Perioperative seizure incidence and risk factors in 223 pediatric brain tumor patients without prior seizures. *J Neurosurg Pediatr.* 2011;7(6):609-615.

8. Ellenberg L, McComb JG, Siegel SE, Stowe S. Factors affecting intellectual outcome in pediatric brain tumor patients. *Neurosurgery.* 1987;21(5):638-644.

9. Ris MD, Walsh K, Wallace D, et al. Intellectual and academic outcome following two chemotherapy regimens and radiotherapy for average-risk medulloblastoma: COG A9961. *Pediatr Blood Cancer.* 2013;60(8):1350-1357.

10. Kahalley LS, Peterson R, Ris MD, et al. Superior intellectual outcomes after proton radiotherapy compared with photon radiotherapy for pediatric medulloblastoma. *J Clin Oncol.* 2020;38(5):454-461.

11. DeNunzio NJ, Yock TI. Modern radiotherapy for pediatric brain tumors. *Cancers (Basel).* 2020;12(6):1533.

12. Partap S. Stroke and cerebrovascular complications in childhood cancer survivors. *Semin Pediatr Neurol.* 2012;19(1):18-24.

13. Pollack IF, Agnihotri S, Broniscer A. Childhood brain tumors: current management, biological insights, and future directions. *J Neurosurg Pediatr.* 2019;23(3):261-273.

14. Ullrich NJ, Pomeroy SL, Kapur K, Manley PE, Goumnerova LC, Loddenkemper T. Incidence, risk factors, and longitudinal outcome of seizures in long-term survivors of pediatric brain tumors. *Epilepsia.* 2015;56(10):1599-1604.

15. Sánchez Fernández I, Loddenkemper T. Seizures caused by brain tumors in children. *Seizure.* 2017;44:98-107.

16. Phillips NS, Khan RB, Li C, et al. Seizures' impact on cognition and quality of life in childhood cancer survivors. *Cancer.* 2022;128(1):180-191.

Infections of the Nervous System

Marissa Vawter-Lee, MD
Zachary Willis, MD, MPH

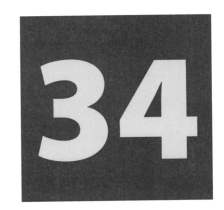

INTRODUCTION

Many pathogens of all classes—bacterial, viral, parasitic, and fungal—can affect the nervous system, both centrally and peripherally. The risks and short- and long-term outcomes from exposure to a pathogen vary significantly depending on a patient's age, with a fetus and an adolescent having very different responses to the same pathogen. This chapter begins with a brief introduction to different types of neurologic infections and then briefly covers the most common infectious pathogens in each pediatric age range (fetal, neonatal, and infant/childhood/adolescent). We then briefly discuss neurologic infections unique and common in the developing world, in immunocompromised children, and in children with neurologic hardware.

TYPES OF NERVOUS SYSTEM INFECTIONS

There are several mechanisms for pathogens to cause nervous system injury. Meningitis is defined as direct invasion and inflammation of the meninges itself. Common meningitis symptoms in children include fever, headache, nuchal rigidity (in those with a closed anterior fontanelle), vomiting, seizures, cranial neuropathies, and altered mental status. Brudzinski and Kernig signs are both used during neurologic exams to look for signs of meningitis but are not sensitive in those with an open anterior fontanelle.

Encephalitis, in contrast, is inflammation of the brain itself. Clinical symptoms of encephalitis are similar to meningitis, but typically, the altered mental status is more severe. Other neurologic symptoms, such as seizures, ataxia, and focal deficits, may occur. Meningitis and encephalitis often co-occur, and patients are referred to as having meningoencephalitis when symptoms of both are present.

At times, focal infections in the nervous system can become encapsulated, causing a purulent abscess, most commonly in fungal and bacterial infections, or an enclosed

cyst, as in neurocysticercosis. This can be seen after localized extension of infections from elsewhere (eg, sinusitis, ear infections, mastoiditis, dental infections). If the collection is in the subdural space, it is classified as a subdural empyema. Ventriculitis denotes significant involvement of the ventricles, most commonly in bacterial meningitis, which may cause hydrocephalus.

Even when there is no direct invasion of the central or peripheral nervous systems, some infections can have postinflammatory effects that lead to neurologic diseases, such as acute disseminated encephalomyelitis (ADEM), Bell's Palsy, focal cerebral arteriopathy and vasculitis, Guillain-Barré syndrome, plexitis, or Sydenham chorea.

FETAL INFECTIONS OF THE NERVOUS SYSTEM

Fetal life is one of the most dangerous times for the central nervous system (CNS) to be exposed to an infection, as the fetus's CNS is undergoing critical periods of neurodevelopment for the entire duration of pregnancy. Infections that cause minimal or no nervous system injury in postnatal life, such as rubella and cytomegalovirus (CMV), may be devastating during fetal development. The most common fetal infections are frequently remembered by the mnemonics TORCH (toxoplasmosis, other, rubella, CMV, and herpes simplex) and SCRATCHES (syphilis, CMV, rubella, AIDS, toxoplasmosis, chickenpox/varicella, herpes simplex, and *Enterovirus*) (Table 34–1).[1] Infections during fetal development can cause inflammatory or destructive effects or can interrupt normal neurodevelopment (ie, affect neuronal migration); some infections do both.[1]

The most common congenital CNS infection is CMV.[1] CMV exposure is relatively common during pregnancy; risk of fetal infection is significantly higher if the pregnant person is seronegative, but infection with a new strain or CMV reactivation in a seropositive individual may also result in fetal infection.[2] It is important to note that the vast majority

Table 34–1. Common fetal nervous system infections.

Infection	Key Clinical Features
Cytomegalovirus	Most common congenital infection in industrialized countries. Usually asymptomatic, but infants may have periventricular calcifications, hearing loss, rash, anemia, thrombocytopenia, hepatosplenomegaly, IUGR, microcephaly.
Enterovirus	Asymptomatic, IUFD, myocarditis, may have sepsis and fulminant liver failure.
Herpes simplex	Vesicular rash, hepatic dysfunction, lethargy, poor feeding, irritability, focal seizures.
HIV/AIDS	Usually asymptomatic until 1-2 months of age.
Lymphocytic choriomeningitis virus	Periventricular calcifications, chorioretinitis, microcephaly.
Parechovirus	Seizures, brain MRI pattern that is similar to hypoxic-ischemic encephalopathy, fever.
Parvovirus B19	Hydrops fetalis, intrauterine fetal demise.
Rubella	Heart disease, cataracts, IUGR, thrombocytopenia, and rash; may have severe cognitive deficits.
Syphilis	May cause stillbirth; lymphadenopathy, hepatosplenomegaly, sinusitis, bony abnormalities, abnormal teeth, hearing loss; neonates usually asymptomatic at birth.
Toxoplasmosis	Ventriculomegaly with multifocal cortex calcifications, meningoencephalitis, jaundice, rash, chorioretinitis.
Varicella-zoster virus	Rash, skin scarring, hypoplasia of bone/muscle.
Zika virus	Progressive microcephaly with "occipital shelf," cerebral calcifications, hydrocephalus.

IUFD, intrauterine fetal death; IUGR, intrauterine growth restriction; MRI, magnetic resonance imaging.

(~90%) of neonates with congenital CMV are asymptomatic.[3] The most common symptoms of CMV at birth are petechial rash, anemia, thrombocytopenia, intrauterine grown restriction, microcephaly, hearing loss, hepatosplenomegaly, hyperbilirubinemia, chorioretinitis, and pneumonia; on imaging, periventricular calcifications are the hallmark sign, although malformations of the brain are quite common.[3,4] Neonates who are symptomatic from congenital CMV are much more likely to have long-term complications.[3] The vast majority of infants with symptomatic congenital CMV will have progressive hearing loss. Infants with congenital CMV and neurologic involvement are at high risk for neurosequelae including intellectual disability, cerebral palsy, and seizures. Antiviral therapy substantially improves hearing and may also improve developmental outcomes.[5]

There are overlapping symptoms among congenital infections, but symptoms from viruses and parasites include microcephaly, irritability, meningoencephalitis, hydrocephalus, chorioretinitis, cerebral calcifications and cysts, and skin lesions. Many of the pathogens have one unique feature that lets clinicians hone in on that pathogen, such as a brain imaging pattern that mimics hypoxic-ischemic encephalopathy (*Parechovirus*), brain imaging with ventriculomegaly and multifocal cortex calcifications (toxoplasmosis), or the degree of microcephaly (Zika virus).[6-8] Other congenital infections, such as syphilis and HIV, are most often asymptomatic at birth and usually detected by prenatal screening.

Certain clinical findings, such as progressive microcephaly or irritability appearing at 3 to 6 months of life, may appear typical for congenital infection, distracting providers from a noninfectious diagnosis. Aicardi-Goutières syndrome, in particular, has been missed, and infants have been mislabeled as having a presumed unknown in utero infection.[9] In cases without confirmed evidence of in utero infection, clinicians should carefully consider the family history, physical exam, and whether genetic evaluation is warranted.

NEONATAL INFECTIONS OF THE NERVOUS SYSTEM

Neonates are the age group at highest risk for bacterial meningitis.[10] Symptoms of neonatal meningitis include temperature instability, poor feeding, vomiting, irritability, tachypnea and apnea, and lethargy; in older neonates, seizures may occur. A bulging fontanelle is a classic physical finding but is only seen in 25% to 50% of neonates with meningitis.[1,11]

The most common cause of meningitis in neonates is group B *Streptococcus* (GBS),[12] with *Escherichia coli* accounting for a growing proportion.[13] Table 34–2 lists other bacterial pathogens that frequently cause neonatal bacterial meningitis. Obstetricians now routinely screen pregnant mothers for GBS, as the treatment of GBS in these mothers lowers the rate of early-onset (within the first 6 days of life) GBS; however, screening of pregnant women has not affected the rate of late-onset (after the sixth day of life) GBS disease. Risk factors for neonatal meningitis include prematurity,

Table 34–2. Common neonatal pathogens of the nervous system.

Enteroviruses
Escherichia coli, Klebsiella, and other gram-negative enteric bacilli
Group B *Streptococcus*
Herpes simplex virus
Listeria monocytogenes

chorioamnionitis, prolonged rupture of membranes, intra-partum fever, and presence of indwelling catheters.[1] Of note, there is racial disparity in rates of neonatal GBS infections, with African-American infants at higher risk.[12] Infants with symptoms consistent with meningitis, including fever alone in the first few weeks of life, require careful evaluation, often including cerebrospinal fluid (CSF) examination and empiric antibiotics.[14]

Herpes simplex virus (HSV) is the most common viral cause of CNS infections in neonates. HSV is most commonly transmitted perinatally, although some cases are transmitted postnatally through direct skin contact (eg, from kissing the neonate or herpetic whitlow).[15] Primary HSV infection, in which the pregnant person has a new genital infection with HSV-1 or -2, poses very high risk to the neonate due to high viral burden and lack of transplacentally acquired type-specific antibodies. Neonates exposed to recurrent HSV lesions or asymptomatic shedding are also at risk, although it is significantly lower. Exposed neonates can be managed according to American Academy of Pediatrics guidelines.[16] Note that the mothers of many infants with neonatal HSV report no history of genital HSV infection; lack of maternal history does not rule out HSV. HSV in neonates can be localized to eyes, skin, or mouth; localized to the brain; or disseminated to multiple organs. Symptoms include vesicular rash (which is not universally present), conjunctivitis, jaundice, irritability, and seizures. HSV should be strongly suspected in infants under 6 weeks of age with these symptoms.[17] Mortality from neonatal HSV is quite high; most survivors have neurologic sequelae. Acyclovir is very effective in neonatal HSV and should be initiated whenever HSV is suspected.

Preterm infants are at unusually high risk of meningitis in the context of invasive infections that would not cause meningitis in other patient populations. In addition to GBS, gram-negative bacilli and even low-virulence pathogens such as coagulase-negative staphylococci and enterococci can cause meningitis; invasive candidiasis has a particular propensity to cause meningitis in this population.

Acute complications of neonatal meningitis and encephalitis include ventriculitis, hydrocephalus, abscess, subdural empyema, cerebral edema, increased intracranial pressure, stroke, and cerebral venous thrombosis.[1] Certain pathogens, such as gram-negative bacilli, are more likely to cause intracranial pyogenic complications. Long term, these infections can lead to cystic encephalomalacia and gliosis in the brain.[1] Hearing loss is the most common complication of infant and childhood meningitis.

INFANT, CHILDHOOD, AND ADOLESCENT INFECTIONS OF THE NERVOUS SYSTEM

As children grow older, the incidence of bacterial meningitis declines, falling from 81 per 100,000 in neonates, to 7 per 100,000 in children 2 to 24 months old, 0.6 per 100,000 in

Table 34–3. Common infant (>3 months old) and childhood infections of the nervous system.

Arboviruses (California-La Crosse, eastern equine, Japanese, St. Louis, West Nile)
Bartonella henselae
Borrelia burgdorferi
Enteroviruses
Haemophilus influenzae
Herpes simplex virus
Influenza
Mycoplasma pneumoniae
Neisseria meningitidis
Streptococcus pneumoniae
Tuberculosis

children 2 to 10 years old, and 0.4 per 100,000 in children 11 to 17 years old.[10] Vaccination against *Haemophilus influenzae* type b and *Streptococcus pneumoniae* has substantially decreased the overall incidence of bacterial meningitis in young children. Common pathogens in young infants are still GBS and *E coli*. But in infants over 3 months old and young children, the bacterial pathogens of meningitis are quite different (Table 34–3) and include *S pneumoniae*, *Neisseria meningitidis*, and *H influenzae*.[18] Clinical symptoms of meningitis at this age include bulging fontanelle, nuchal rigidity (after the fontanelle closes), irritability, fever, vomiting, headache, lethargy, and seizures.[19]

Similar to meningitis, the rate of encephalitis declines as children get older, with neonates and infants younger than 12 months old having an incidence of 18 per 100,000, but children 1 to 18 years old having an overall incidence of 10 per 100,000.[20] In most encephalitis epidemiology studies, the incidence continues to decline with increasing age, with rates decreasing down to 1 per 100,000 in children 15 to 18 years old.[20] In the vaccine era, the causes of encephalitis have also shifted dramatically, as vaccines have almost completely eliminated measles, mumps, and varicella-zoster virus (VZV) as causes of viral encephalitis in many parts of the world.[20] Enteroviruses are now the most common infectious encephalitis cause, and ADEM is the most common immune-mediated encephalitis cause.[21] Arboviruses can also cause pediatric encephalitis in the United States, with California encephalitis virus, La Crosse encephalitis virus, and St. Louis encephalitis virus each endemic in different regions of the United States. HSV, *Mycoplasma*, CMV, Epstein-Barr virus (EBV), and VZV are additional viral etiologies to consider for pediatric encephalitis.[22] The causative agent of encephalitis is often difficult to diagnose, and there is significant clinical overlap between infectious causes of encephalitis and noninfectious causes, such as autoimmune encephalitis.[23]

Careful exposure history, neurologic examination, and laboratory and radiologic testing are essential in building a differential diagnosis.[22]

Although generally more severe in adults, West Nile virus (WNV) can also cause pediatric neurologic complications, including encephalitis, meningitis, and acute flaccid paralysis. WNV causes extremity paralysis and weakness, with notable areflexia on exam, by injuring the motor neuron (anterior horn cell).[24]

Not all pathogens with neurologic consequences present with meningitis or encephalitis. Some present with focal neurologic findings such as weakness, paralysis, cranial nerve palsies, headaches, or seizures. Since 2014, acute flaccid myelitis (AFM) has occurred in biennial peaks in the United States. Affected patients, mostly children, present with acute onset of weakness and paralysis, usually following a prodromal illness. AFM is thought to cause symptoms by a similar mechanism of action to WNV, with injury to the anterior horn cell. A direct pathologic link between infection and AFM has not been definitively established, although Enterovirus D68 is strongly suspected.[25]

Many relatively common infections may rarely present with distinct neurologic symptoms. *Mycoplasma pneumoniae*, a relatively common cause of respiratory tract infections, can cause meningoencephalitis by an unknown mechanism in a small proportion of infected individuals.[26] Cat-scratch disease (CSD), caused by *Bartonella henselae*, is an infection to consider in patients presenting with altered mental status, seizures, and lymphadenopathy. CSD can also present with optic neuritis or retinitis.[27] Lyme disease, a tickborne infection caused by the spirochete *Borrelia burgdorferi*, can present weeks to months after initial infection with multiple neurologic findings in children, including headaches, aseptic meningitis, encephalitis, and facial nerve palsy.[28] Roseola, caused by human herpesvirus-6 (HHV-6), is characterized by high fever and rash and is the most common cause of febrile seizures in children.[29] *Rickettsia rickettsii* causes Rocky Mountain spotted fever, which typically presents with fever, myalgia, and rash; neurologic symptoms can include headaches (frequently present at time of presentation) and, if treatment is delayed, meningitis, meningoencephalitis, or seizures.[30]

NEUROLOGIC INFECTIONS IN THE IMMUNOCOMPROMISED CHILD

In children who are immunocompromised (eg, premature infants or children undergoing chronic steroid treatment, diagnosed with HIV/AIDS, with solid organ or hematopoietic stem cell transplantation, with autoimmune disease, or undergoing chemotherapy), development of new neurologic symptoms calls for an aggressive diagnostic evaluation. The differential should include typical bacterial and viral infections (including EBV and VZV) as well as fungal pathogens,

including *Candida*, *Cryptococcus neoformans*, *Coccidioides immitis*, and *Histoplasma capsulatum*. Symptoms of fungal infections include headaches, fever, vomiting, papilledema, and altered mental status (including personality changes). The type and degree of immunocompromise are important to understand when planning such an evaluation. For example, cryptococcal meningoencephalitis is classically associated with HIV/AIDS, whereas HHV-6 causes encephalitis primarily in hematopoietic stem cell transplant recipients. Children can have meningitis, focal abscesses, and increased intracranial pressure. *Nocardia* should also be considered if a brain abscess is present.

NEUROLOGIC INFECTIONS IN CHILDREN AND ADOLESCENTS IN THE DEVELOPING WORLD

Outside of developed countries, there are pathogens that must be considered as a source of nervous system infection in the developing world. Limitations on public sanitation, public health, and access to vaccines account for the persistent presence of these infections. Practitioners in developed nations must be aware of these infections, as they may occur in visitors, immigrants, or returning travelers. Cerebral malaria is still a significant source of neurologic problems throughout the world. One study estimated that 70% of status epilepticus in Africa was triggered by an infection, with malaria accounting for the majority.[31] Cerebral malaria presents with neurologic symptoms that include headaches, seizures, focal neurologic deficits, and altered mental status (including coma). The mortality and morbidity from cerebral malaria are still alarmingly high (15%-25% mortality and 25% morbidity in survivors).[32] Seizures associated with malaria are typically complex (multiple, longer than 15 minutes, and focal).[33]

Rabies, a zoonotic virus usually transmitted by the bite of an infected animal, remains endemic in much of the developing world and causes around 59,000 deaths per year.[34] Rabies has both an encephalitic form (presenting with muscle spasms, delirium, autonomic changes, seizures, hypersalivation, and meningismus) and a paralytic form (presenting with flaccid paralysis). Symptoms typically present 1 week to multiple months after the bite from the infected animal; once symptoms emerge, it is almost universally fatal. Combined active and passive immunization, with rabies immune globulin plus rabies vaccine, is highly effective when administered within days of suspected exposure; the vast majority of deaths occur in developing countries where treatment is not available.[35]

Tuberculosis (TB), due to *Mycobacterium tuberculosis* complex, frequently presents with meningoencephalitis in young children, which is far less common in older children and adults. Meningitis may progress to hydrocephalus, tuberculomas, and infarcts, particularly in the basal ganglia.[36] A high index of suspicion is required, as diagnosis is challenging and delayed treatment may result in mortality or significant permanent neurologic injury.[37] Because of the long incubation period, tuberculous meningitis may present in children who have immigrated from countries with a high incidence of TB or in children residing with people born in high-incidence countries. TB neurologic involvement in children can also include spinal TB (also known as Pott disease).[38]

Other pathogens with high neurologic disease burden include neurocysticercosis from *Taenia solium* (estimated to cause 30% of epilepsy cases in endemic countries), poliomyelitis from poliovirus (as of 2021, still endemic in 2 countries throughout the world), schistosomiasis, and tetanus from *Clostridium tetani*.[39,40] Neonatal tetanus alone is estimated to cause around 25,000 newborn deaths per year.[41]

NERVOUS SYSTEM INFECTIONS SECONDARY TO HARDWARE

CNS devices generally increase the risk of CNS infection with bacterial and fungal pathogens by providing passage through the blood-brain barrier and safe haven from the host's immune system. Ventricular drainage devices, including external ventricular drains and internalized ventricular shunts such as ventriculoperitoneal shunts, constitute a major risk factor for ventriculitis and meningitis. The timing is usually within weeks after device placement, but infection may occur at any time.[42] The most common causative organisms are skin colonizers such as coagulase-negative staphylococci and *Cutibacterium acnes*, but more virulent pathogens such as *Staphylococcus aureus*, gram-negative bacilli, and fungi may also be involved.[42] Treatment generally requires removal of the affected catheter with alternative CSF drainage until definitive CSF sterilization permits placement of a new indwelling catheter, if required.[43]

Placed for intractable epilepsy, vagal nerve stimulators (VNS) are an important antiseizure tool that child neurologists use. It is important for child neurologists to be aware that 2% to 8% of VNSs will become infected after insertion, typically with *S aureus*.[44,45]

Deep-brain stimulation can be done for pediatric-onset dystonia. This too has a significant risk of infection, with 8% to 10% of deep-brain stimulations becoming infected.[46] Cochlear implants also slightly increase the risk of bacterial meningitis; this risk can be mitigated with vaccinations and prompt management of acute otitis media.[47]

SEQUELAE OF CENTRAL NERVOUS SYSTEM INFECTIONS

Children of any age exposed to CNS infections can have long-term sequelae. The sequelae from fetal exposures are well known, but children exposed as infants and during childhood and adolescence can also have significant long-term complications. These vary significantly by specific type of infection and can include hearing loss, seizures, developmental delays and impairments, intellectual disability, motor disability (including cerebral palsy), and visual deficits, among others.[48]

REFERENCES

1. Volpe JJ. *Neurology of the Newborn*. 5th ed. Saunders Elsevier; 2008.
2. Mussi-Pinhata MM, Yamamoto AY, Aragon DC, et al. Seroconversion for cytomegalovirus infection during pregnancy and fetal infection in a highly seropositive population: "the BraCHS study." *J Infect Dis*. 2018;218(8):1200-1204. doi:10.1093/infdis/jiy321
3. Dreher AM, Arora N, Fowler KB, et al. Spectrum of disease and outcome in children with symptomatic congenital cytomegalovirus infection. *J Pediatr*. 2014;164(4):855-859. doi:10.1016/j.jpeds.2013.12.007
4. Fink KR, Thapa MM, Ishak GE, Pruthi S. Neuroimaging of pediatric central nervous system cytomegalovirus infection. *Radiographics*. 2010;30(7):1779-1796. doi:10.1148/rg.307105043
5. Kimberlin DW, Jester PM, Sánchez PJ, et al. Valganciclovir for symptomatic congenital cytomegalovirus disease. *N Engl J Med*. 2015;372(10):933-943. doi:10.1056/NEJMoa1404599
6. Amarnath C, Helen Mary T, Periakarupan A, Gopinathan K, Philson J. Neonatal parechovirus leucoencephalitis-radiological pattern mimicking hypoxic-ischemic encephalopathy. *Eur J Radiol*. 2016;85(2):428-434. doi:10.1016/j.ejrad.2015.11.038
7. Driggers RW, Ho CY, Korhonen EM, et al. Zika virus infection with prolonged maternal viremia and fetal brain abnormalities. *N Engl J Med*. 2016;374(22):2142-2151. doi:10.1056/NEJMoa1601824
8. Malinger G, Werner H, Rodriguez Leonel JC, et al. Prenatal brain imaging in congenital toxoplasmosis. *Prenat Diagn*. 2011;31(9):881-886. doi:10.1002/pd.2795
9. Rice G, Patrick T, Parmar R, et al. Clinical and molecular phenotype of Aicardi-Goutieres syndrome. *Am J Hum Genet*. 2007;81(4):713-725. doi:10.1086/521373
10. Thigpen MC, Whitney CG, Messonnier NE, et al. Bacterial meningitis in the United States, 1998-2007. *N Engl J Med*. 2011;364(21):2016-2025. doi:10.1056/NEJMoa1005384
11. Chotpitayasunondh T. Bacterial meningitis in children: etiology and clinical features, an 11-year review of 618 cases. *Southeast Asian J Trop Med Public Health*. 1994;25(1):107-115.
12. Nanduri SA, Petit S, Smelser C, et al. Epidemiology of invasive early-onset and late-onset group B streptococcal disease in the United States, 2006 to 2015: multistate laboratory and population-based surveillance. *JAMA Pediatr*. 2019;173(3):224-233. doi:10.1001/jamapediatrics.2018.4826
13. Stoll BJ, Puopolo KM, Hansen NI, et al. Early-onset neonatal sepsis 2015 to 2017, the rise of *Escherichia coli*, and the need for novel prevention strategies. *JAMA Pediatr*. 2020;174(7):e200593. doi:10.1001/jamapediatrics.2020.0593
14. Pantell RH, Roberts KB, Adams WG, et al. Evaluation and management of well-appearing febrile infants 8 to 60 days old. *Pediatrics*. 2021;148(2):e2021052228. doi:10.1542/peds.2021-052228
15. Kimberlin DW. Herpes simplex virus infections of the newborn. *Semin Perinatol*. 2007;31(1):19-25. doi:10.1053/j.semperi.2007.01.003

16. Kimberlin DW, Baley J; Committee on Infectious Diseases; Committee on Fetus and Newborn. Guidance on management of asymptomatic neonates born to women with active genital herpes lesions. *Pediatrics*. 2013;131(2):e635-e646. doi:10.1542/peds.2012-3216

17. Cruz AT, Nigrovic LE, Xie J, et al. Predictors of invasive herpes simplex virus infection in young infants. *Pediatrics*. 2021;148(3):e2021050052. doi:10.1542/peds.2021-050052

18. Nigrovic LE, Kuppermann N, Malley R; Bacterial Meningitis Study Group of the Pediatric Emergency Medicine Collaborative Research Committee of the American Academy of Pediatrics. Children with bacterial meningitis presenting to the emergency department during the pneumococcal conjugate vaccine era. *Acad Emerg Med*. 2008;15(6):522-528. Recomm Rep. doi:10.1111/j.1553-2712.2008.00117.x

19. Johansson Kostenniemi U, Norman D, Borgström M, Silfverdal SA. The clinical presentation of acute bacterial meningitis varies with age, sex and duration of illness. *Acta Paediatr*. 2015;104(11):1117-1124. doi:10.1111/apa.13149

20. Koskiniemi M, Korppi M, Mustonen K, et al. Epidemiology of encephalitis in children. A prospective multicentre study. *Eur J Pediatr*. 1997;156(7):541-545. doi:10.1007/s004310050658

21. Pillai SC, Hacohen Y, Tantsis E, et al. Infectious and autoantibody-associated encephalitis: clinical features and long-term outcome. *Pediatrics*. 2015;135(4):e974-e984. doi:10.1542/peds.2014-2702

22. Tunkel AR, Glaser CA, Bloch KC, et al. The management of encephalitis: clinical practice guidelines by the Infectious Diseases Society of America. *Clin Infect Dis*. 2008;47(3):303-327. doi:10.1086/589747

23. Bloch KC, Glaser CA. Encephalitis surveillance through the emerging infections program, 1997-2010. *Emerg Infect Dis*. 2015;21(9):1562-1567. doi:10.3201/eid2109.150295

24. Sejvar JJ, Bode AV, Marfin AA, et al. West Nile virus-associated flaccid paralysis. *Emerg Infect Dis*. 2005;11(7):1021-1027. doi:10.3201/eid1107.040991

25. Vawter-Lee M, Peariso K, Frey M, et al. Acute flaccid myelitis: a multidisciplinary protocol to optimize diagnosis and evaluation. *J Child Neurol*. 2021;36(6):421-431. doi:10.1177/0883073820975230

26. Yiş U, Kurul SH, Cakmakçi H, Dirik E. *Mycoplasma pneumoniae*: nervous system complications in childhood and review of the literature. *Eur J Pediatr*. 2008;167(9):973-978. doi:10.1007/s00431-008-0714-1

27. Canneti B, Cabo-López I, Puy-Núñez A, et al. Neurological presentations of *Bartonella henselae* infection. *Neurol Sci*. 2019;40(2):261-268. doi:10.1007/s10072-018-3618-5

28. Gerber MA, Shapiro ED, Burke GS, Parcells VJ, Bell GL. Lyme disease in children in southeastern Connecticut. Pediatric Lyme Disease Study Group. *N Engl J Med*. 1996;335(17):1270-1274. doi:10.1056/NEJM199610243351703

29. Suga S, Suzuki K, Ihira M, et al. Clinical characteristics of febrile convulsions during primary HHV-6 infection. *Arch Dis Child*. 2000;82(1):62-66. doi:10.1136/adc.82.1.62

30. Buckingham SC, Marshall GS, Schutze GE, et al. Clinical and laboratory features, hospital course, and outcome of Rocky Mountain spotted fever in children. *J Pediatr*. 2007;150(2):180-184, 184.e1. doi:10.1016/j.jpeds.2006.11.023

31. Newton CR, Kariuki SM. Status epilepticus in sub-Saharan Africa: new findings. *Epilepsia*. 2013;54(suppl 6):50-53. doi:10.1111/epi.12277

32. World Health Organization. Severe malaria. *Trop Med Int Health*. 2014;(19 suppl 1):7-131.

33. Kariuki SM, Rockett K, Clark TG, et al. The genetic risk of acute seizures in African children with falciparum malaria. *Epilepsia*. 2013;54(6):990-1001. doi:10.1111/epi.12173

34. Centers for Disease Control and Prevention. Rabies around the world. Accessed November 18, 2021. https://www.cdc.gov/rabies/location/world/index.html

35. Manning SE, Rupprecht CE, Fishbein D, et al. Human rabies prevention—United States, 2008: recommendations of the Advisory Committee on Immunization Practices. *MMWR Recomm Rep*. 2008;57(RR-3):1-28.

36. Principi N, Esposito S. Diagnosis and therapy of tuberculous meningitis in children. *Tuberculosis (Edinb)*. 2012;92(5):377-383. doi:10.1016/j.tube.2012.05.011

37. Chiang SS, Khan FA, Milstein MB, et al. Treatment outcomes of childhood tuberculous meningitis: a systematic review and meta-analysis. *Lancet Infect Dis*. 2014;14(10):947-957. doi:10.1016/S1473-3099(14)70852-7

38. Cruz AT, Starke JR. Pediatric tuberculosis. *Pediatr Rev*. 2010;31(1):13-25; quiz 25-26. doi:10.1542/pir.31-1-13

39. Reddy DS, Volkmer R. Neurocysticercosis as an infectious acquired epilepsy worldwide. *Seizure*. 2017;52:176-181. doi:10.1016/j.seizure.2017.10.004

40. Polio Eradication Initiative. Polio endemic countries. Accessed November 18, 2021. https://polioeradication.org/

41. World Health Organization. Tetanus. Accessed November 18, 2021. https://www.who.int/health-topics/tetanus

42. van de Beek D, Drake JM, Tunkel AR. Nosocomial bacterial meningitis. *N Engl J Med*. 2010;362(2):146-154. doi:10.1056/NEJMra0804573

43. Tunkel AR, Hasbun R, Bhimraj A, et al. 2017 Infectious Diseases Society of America's clinical practice guidelines for healthcare-associated ventriculitis and meningitis. *Clin Infect Dis*. 2017;64(6):e34-e65. doi:10.1093/cid/ciw861

44. Entezami P, German JW, Adamo MA. Does one week of postoperative antibiotic prophylaxis reduce the rate of infection after vagus nerve stimulator surgery? *World Neurosurg*. 2021;149:e546-e548. doi:10.1016/j.wneu.2021.01.140

45. Air EL, Ghomri YM, Tyagi R, Grande AW, Crone K, Mangano FT. Management of vagal nerve stimulator infections: do they need to be removed? *J Neurosurg Pediatr*. 2009;3(1):73-78. doi:10.3171/2008.10.PEDS08294

46. Kaminska M, Perides S, Lumsden DE, et al. Complications of deep brain stimulation (DBS) for dystonia in children: the challenges and 10 year experience in a large paediatric cohort. *Eur J Paediatr Neurol*. 2017;21(1):168-175. doi:10.1016/j.ejpn.2016.07.024

47. Wei BP, Clark GM, O'Leary SJ, Shepherd RK, Robins-Browne RM. Meningitis after cochlear implantation. *BMJ*. 2007;335(7629):1058. doi:10.1136/bmj.39380.598380.80

48. Ouchenir L, Renaud C, Khan S, et al. The epidemiology, management, and outcomes of bacterial meningitis in infants. *Pediatrics*. 2017;140(1):e20170476. doi:10.1542/peds.2017-0476

Demyelinating Diseases of the Central Nervous System

Helen Wu, MD, PhD
Kristen Fisher, DO

ACUTE DISSEMINATED ENCEPHALOMYELITIS

Acute disseminated encephalomyelitis (ADEM) is a central nervous system (CNS) inflammatory syndrome characterized by rapid-onset encephalopathy along with multifocal neurologic deficits. While ADEM is frequently thought to occur in the context of preceding illness, the specific microbial trigger is rarely identified, and the pathophysiology of the disorder is thought to be immune-mediated.[1] Magnetic resonance imaging (MRI) of the brain typically demonstrates large, diffuse, and poorly demarcated T2-hyperintense lesions predominantly affecting white matter. These lesions are apparent during the initial acute to subacute phase (typically 3 months, by definition) and can resolve in the weeks following. Further clinical workup includes lumbar puncture (LP), which is typically remarkable for cerebrospinal fluid (CSF) pleocytosis with lymphocytic predominance and elevated protein. Additional findings may include elevated immunoglobulin (Ig) G index, but oligoclonal bands are rarely positive in ADEM.

Although ADEM is typically monophasic, a smaller subset of children can experience multiphasic ADEM (MDEM) with another attack occurring 3 or more months following the initial attack.[2,3] In cases of MDEM, the diagnosis should be considered thoughtfully as ADEM may be the initial presentation of neuromyelitis optica spectrum disorder (NMO-SD), or rarely, ADEM is followed by a non-ADEM event and meeting criteria for a diagnosis of multiple sclerosis (MS). ADEM may also be followed by optic neuritis (ADEM-ON), which more recently has been seen to have high association with myelin oligodendrocyte glycoprotein (MOG) antibodies.

Initial treatment for ADEM is typically intravenous (IV) methylprednisolone. In severe cases, IV immunoglobulin (IVIG) or plasma exchange should be considered, especially in patients requiring intensive care.

The majority of patients have good recovery, but there can be long-standing neuropsychological and neurobehavioral symptoms.[4]

CLINICALLY ISOLATED SYNDROME

Clinically isolated syndrome (CIS) is defined as an isolated occurrence of acute CNS inflammatory demyelination without encephalopathy. Approximately 30% to 70% of patients with CIS can go on to develop MS, with increased risk of progression in female patients, patients over 10 years of age, and patients with multifocal symptoms at onset, presence and appearance of brain lesions on MRI, and presence of oligoclonal bands.[5]

The clinical presentation of CIS varies depending on location of demyelination in the CNS. Most commonly in CIS, demyelination involves the optic nerves and the spinal cord. If a diagnosis of CIS is being considered, then workup for underlying neuroimmune etiologies such as NMO-SD and MOG antibody-associated disease (MOGAD), in addition to MS, should be considered.

▶ Optic Neuritis

Inflammation of the optic nerves, or optic neuritis (ON), can lead to an acute presentation typically with acute, unilateral or bilateral vision loss and retro-orbital pain that worsens with eye movement. Visual field perimetry, optical coherence tomography, MRI, and serologic and CSF fluid will be helpful to make the correct diagnosis as well as to monitor disease progression and response to treatment.[6] ON may be the initial presentation of a relapsing condition such as MS or NMO-SD, so a thorough evaluation for these conditions should be performed on initial presentation, especially in patients with presence of brain or spinal cord demyelination.

Transverse Myelitis

Transverse myelitis (TM) is characterized by acute to subacute onset of sensory, motor, or autonomic dysfunction caused by inflammatory demyelination of the spinal cord. The lesion may be partial (part of the spinal cord below the lesion is affected), complete (bilateral spinal cord involvement), and longitudinally extensive (involves at least 3 vertebral segments). In addition to sensory and motor symptoms, other symptoms of spinal cord inflammation that will require intervention include bowel or bladder dysfunction and acute respiratory failure. TM on MRI is typically characterized by a T2 hyperintense signal involving the central cord and surrounding white matter that often enhances with gadolinium contrast (up to 74% of cases).[7]

Initial treatment for CIS, including ON and TM, should consist of an IV steroid. Depending on the clinical presentation, plasmapheresis may be used. Plasmapheresis especially should be used in patients with severe bilateral ON in consideration of possible NMO-SD diagnosis to aid in long-term visual outcomes. Recovery from ON is dependent on suspected underlying etiology, where isolated ON and MS-associated ON is typically expected to have better recovery compared to NMO-SD. Recovery from TM can be variable, and supportive measures such as rehabilitation and adaptive technologies are frequently needed to optimize recovery and quality of life. In some cases, use of disease-modifying therapy may be considered for CIS if there is believed to be high risk for progression to MS or NMO-SD diagnosis.

MYELIN OLIGODENDROCYTE GLYCOPROTEIN ANTIBODY–ASSOCIATED DISEASE

MOGAD is an antibody-mediated CNS inflammatory and demyelinating disorder. Numerous clinical syndromes have been described with MOGAD, including ADEM, MDEM, ADEM-ON, relapsing ON, NMO-SD, and autoimmune encephalitis. The presence of MOG antibodies has been reported in 18% to 35% of pediatric acute demyelinating syndromes.[8,9] Clinical presentation of patients with MOGAD can vary depending on clinical syndrome and areas of demyelination and neuroinflammation. In case series, approximately 50% of patients with MOGAD have been seen to have a relapsing course.[8]

Laboratory evaluation for patients with MOG antibodies typically reveals CSF pleocytosis with lymphocytic predominance and normal to elevated CSF protein. CSF oligoclonal bands are less commonly positive in MOGAD. Diagnosis of MOGAD is based on positive serum MOG-IgG by cell-based assay.

At acute presentation, patients with MOGAD are treated with IV steroids, IVIG, or plasmapheresis depending on severity of presentation. Although patients with MOGAD are at increased risk of relapsing course, patients are only placed on longer-term treatment if relapse were to occur or if the patient were to meet criteria for NMO-SD. Case series have reported treatment regimens of monthly IVIG, monthly IV steroids, rituximab, mycophenolate mofetil, and azathioprine. There are no standards for the duration of treatment, but most recommend ongoing treatment for up to 2 years if patients have a relapsing course.

MULTIPLE SCLEROSIS

MS is an immune-mediated disease of the CNS, leading to demyelination in the brain, spinal cord, and optic nerves. MS typically affects young adults in their 20s to 40s, but onset can occur prior to age 18 in up to 10% of these patients.[10] There are current guidelines for a diagnosis of MS in pediatrics, most using the 2017 McDonald criteria and the International Pediatric MS Study Group definition.[11,12] These definitions require presence of dissemination in space on MRI with demyelination in at least 2 defined regions (periventricular, juxtacortical/cortical, infratentorial, and spinal cord) and evidence of dissemination in time, which can be demonstrated by more than one clinical event, presence of both enhancing and nonenhancing lesions on MRI, or presence of oligoclonal bands on LP.[11]

Typical presenting symptoms include ON, TM, brainstem symptoms, and long-tract symptoms, which include motor or sensory changes. However, these symptoms are nonspecific to MS, so further workup to differentiate MS from NMO-SD and MOGAD is needed. In addition to symptoms from acute clinical attacks, pediatric MS patients report symptoms including anxiety, depression, and cognitive complaints affecting school and work performance.

Treatment for the initial acute phase of MS typically consists of IV steroids or plasmapheresis in more severe presentations. Following the acute phase, the mainstay of treatment is prevention of further relapses as ongoing relapses lead to accrual of disability over time. Although in the past, a step-up or escalation approach to treatment was employed, more evidence recently has supported early use of high-efficacy disease-modifying therapy.[13] Currently, the only US Food and Drug Administration–approved treatment for pediatric-onset MS is fingolimod, but clinical trials are ongoing for approval of further treatments.

NEUROMYELITIS OPTICA SPECTRUM DISORDER

NMO-SD is an autoimmune neurologic disorder that is associated with aquaporin-4 antibodies (AQP4-IgG). Aquaporin-4 is a water channel protein that has been demonstrated to be preferentially expressed in the retina, optic nerve, hypothalamus, cerebellum, periventricular and periaqueductal regions, and spinal cord. AQP4-IgG drives complement-dependent necrosis of astrocytes, subsequently leading to demyelination, preferentially in the areas where aquaporin-4 is more prevalent. This can lead to typical demyelinating syndromes, most commonly ON and TM. Additional syndromes associated with NMO-SD include area postrema syndrome, acute brainstem syndromes, symptomatic narcolepsy/acute diencephalic syndrome, and symptomatic cerebral syndrome. NMOSD typically affects young adults in their 30s to 40s, although an estimated 3% to 5% of cases have pediatric onset.[14]

Presence of at least one core clinical syndrome together with AQP4-IgG seropositivity is sufficient to make a diagnosis of NMO-SD in the absence of a better alternative diagnosis. NMO-SD diagnosis can still be made in the absence of AQP4-IgG but will rely on the presence of additional core clinical characteristics and other key MRI features, such as optic nerve involvement, longitudinally extensive TM, dorsal medulla/area postrema lesions, or periependymal brainstem lesions.[15]

In acute attacks, IV methylprednisolone is generally considered first-line therapy. In cases of ON, use of plasmapheresis has been shown to improve visual outcomes overall and should be considered in patients with ON that is believed to be related to NMO-SD.[16] Additionally, use of IVIG has been shown to be beneficial in acute relapses that do not fully respond to steroids. Depletion of B-lymphocytes using anti-CD20 monoclonal antibodies, such as rituximab, is particularly effective in prevention of NMO-SD relapses.[14] Additional long-term therapies shown to be effective in NMO-SD include eculizumab, satralizumab, inebilizumab, azathioprine, or mycophenolate mofetil.[17]

REFERENCES

1. Tenembaum S, Chitnis T, Ness J, Hahn JS. Acute disseminated encephalomyelitis. *Neurology.* 2007;68(16 suppl 2):S23-S26. doi: 10.1212/01.wnl.0000259404.51352.7f

2. Dale RC, de Sousa C, Chong WK, Cox TCS, Harding B, Neville BGR. Acute disseminated encephalomyelitis, multiphasic disseminated encephalomyelitis and multiple sclerosis in children. *Brain.* 2000;123(12):2407-2422. doi:10.1093/brain/123.12.2407

3. Krupp LB, Tardieu M, Amato MP, et al. International Pediatric Multiple Sclerosis Study Group criteria for pediatric multiple sclerosis and immune-mediated central nervous system demyelinating disorders: revisions to the 2007 definitions. *Mult Scler.* 2013;19(10):1261-1267. doi:10.1177/1352458513484547

4. Kuni BJ, Banwell BL, Till C. Cognitive and behavioral outcomes in individuals with a history of acute disseminated encephalomyelitis (ADEM). *Dev Neuropsychol.* 2012;37(8):682-696. doi: 10.1080/87565641.2012.690799

5. Miller D, Barkhof F, Montalban X, Thompson A, Filippi M. Clinically isolated syndromes suggestive of multiple sclerosis, part I: natural history, pathogenesis, diagnosis, and prognosis. *Lancet Neurol.* 2005;4(5):281-288. doi:10.1016/S1474-4422(05)70071-5

6. Bennett JL. Optic neuritis. *Continuum.* 2019;25(5):1236-1264. doi:10.1212/CON.0000000000000768

7. Pidcock FS, Krishnan C, Crawford TO, Salorio CF, Trovato M, Kerr DA. Acute transverse myelitis in childhood: center-based analysis of 47 cases. *Neurology.* 2007;68(18):1474-1480. doi:10.1212/01.wnl.0000260609.11357.6f

8. Chitnis T. Pediatric central nervous system demyelinating diseases. *Continuum.* 2019;25(3):793-814. doi:10.1212/CON.0000000000000730

9. Fernandez-Carbonell C, Vargas-Lowy D, Musallam A, et al. Clinical and MRI phenotype of children with MOG antibodies. *Mult Scler.* 2016;22:174-184. doi:10.1177/1352458515587751

10. Renoux C, Vukusic S, Confavreux C. The natural history of multiple sclerosis with childhood onset. *Clin Neurol Neurosurg.* 2008;110(9):897-904. doi:10.1016/j.clineuro.2008.04.009

11. Thompson AJ, Banwell BL, Barkhof F, et al. Diagnosis of multiple sclerosis: 2017 revisions of the McDonald criteria. *Lancet Neurol.* 2018;17(2):162-173. doi:10.1016/S1474-4422(17)30470-2

12. Tardieu M, Banwell B, Wolinsky JS, Pohl D, Krupp LB. Consensus definitions for pediatric MS and other demyelinating disorders in childhood. *Neurology.* 2016;87(9):S8-S11. doi:10.1212/WNL.0000000000002877

13. Gross RH, Corboy JR. Monitoring, switching, and stopping multiple sclerosis disease-modifying therapies. *Continuum.* 2019;25(3):715-735. doi:10.1212/CON.0000000000000738

14. Tenembaum S, Chitnis T, Nakashima I, et al. Neuromyelitis optica spectrum disorders in children and adolescents. *Neurology.* 2016;87(9):S59-S66. doi:10.1212/WNL.0000000000002824

15. Wingerchuk DM, Banwell B, Bennett JL, et al. International consensus diagnostic criteria for neuromyelitis optica spectrum disorders. *Neurology.* 2015;85(2):177-189. doi:10.1212/WNL.0000000000001729

16. Siritho S, Srisupa-Olan T, Sathukitchai C, Prayoonwiwat N. Beneficial effect of plasma exchange in acute attack of neuromyelitis optica spectrum disorder. *J Neurol Sci.* 2017;381:115-121. doi:10.1016/j.jns.2017.08.3002

17. Tenembaum S, Yeh EA. Pediatric NMOSD: a review and position statement on approach to work-up and diagnosis. *Front Pediatr.* 2020;8:339. doi:10.3389/fped.2020.00339

Inflammatory Diseases of the Central Nervous System

Kelsey Poisson, MD
Kristen Fisher, DO

IMMUNE-MEDIATED ENCEPHALOPATHIES

▶ Autoimmune Encephalitis

Autoimmune encephalitis (AE) involves an abnormal immune response of the central nervous system (CNS) to autoantibodies binding to extracellular antigens such as neuronal cell surface proteins, synaptic receptors, and ion channels.[1] Symptoms in children are typically subacute in onset, may involve an infectious prodrome, and include altered level of consciousness, seizures, movement disorders, cognitive/speech decline, psychiatric symptoms, sleep disturbance, focal deficits, and/or autonomic disturbances. Established diagnostic criteria for pediatric AE (summarized below) exist to guide treatment decisions.[2]

Possible AE: Acute or subacute (<3 months) onset of at least 2 of the following clinical criteria and reasonable exclusion of other etiologies:

1. Altered mental status or electroencephalogram (EEG) abnormalities (epileptiform or slowing)
2. Focal neurologic deficits
3. Cognitive difficulties
4. Acute developmental regression
5. Movement disorder (excludes tics)
6. Psychiatric symptoms
7. Seizures not explained by previously diagnosed condition

Probable antibody-negative AE: Fulfills all clinical criteria and at least one of the following paraclinical criteria:

1. Cerebrospinal fluid (CSF) white blood cell count greater than 5 or positive oligoclonal bands
2. Abnormal magnetic resonance imaging (MRI) suggestive of encephalitis
3. Brain biopsy with inflammatory infiltrates consistent with AE

Definite AE: Fulfills clinical criteria and has presence of antibody associated with AE

The most common autoantibodies in children are myelin oligodendrocyte glycoprotein (MOG; discussed separately), anti-N-methyl-D-aspartate receptor (NMDAR), GAD65, GABA$_A$, and glycine receptor.[2,3] Serum laboratory evaluation generally includes inflammatory markers, infectious evaluation, rheumatologic autoantibodies, thyroid autoantibodies, and encephalopathy autoantibody panel. MRI of the brain with and without contrast should be performed, which may demonstrate focal areas of enhancement or T2/fluid-attenuated inversion recovery (FLAIR) hyperintensity. CSF evaluation is required for autoantibody and infectious disease testing. Most common CSF findings include pleocytosis, protein elevation, presence of oligoclonal bands, or elevated immunoglobulin (Ig) G index. Malignancy screening should be pursued, although malignancy is less common in pediatric patients.

After reasonable exclusion of alternative etiologies, particularly infectious encephalitis, first-line immunomodulatory treatment with intravenous (IV) steroids and/or IV immunoglobulin (IVIG) should be initiated while awaiting workup. Assuming a diagnosis of probable or definite AE is made, rituximab is an appropriate next-line therapy. For treatment-refractory cases, other options include cyclophosphamide, tocilizumab, and bortezomib.

▶ NMDAR Encephalitis

NMDAR encephalitis typically presents with seizures, movement disorders, psychiatric symptoms, insomnia, reduced speech, cognitive decline, autonomic instability, and/or catatonia. The disease is more likely to present in children than adults with movement disorders (particularly orofacial dyskinesias and chorea) and seizures, with psychiatric symptoms often being less prominent at presentation.[4] In younger children and toddlers, NMDAR encephalitis can present with early symptoms of developmental regression. In young woman, there may be an association with ovarian teratoma, but this is less commonly seen in pediatric NMDAR encephalitis.

First-line immunotherapy involves IV methylprednisolone, as well as IVIG and/or plasmapheresis. Plasmapheresis should be initiated concurrently with steroids for severe presentations. Use of rituximab has increasingly become standard of care as second-line immunotherapy in NMDAR encephalitis, and retrospective studies have shown improved long-term outcomes and increased likelihood of monophasic disease course with use.[5] If symptoms are more refractory despite rituximab use, escalation to cyclophosphamide or tocilizumab should be considered. Maintenance immunosuppression may be pursued with IV steroids, IVIG, and/or rituximab. Evidence is lacking with regard to duration of immunotherapy, but consensus guidelines suggest 3 to 18 months are appropriate depending on the severity of presentation.[6] The relapse rate is estimated at 12% to 24% (and is lower for those with an excised ovarian teratoma) and has been shown to be lower with early and adequate treatment.[4] In pediatrics, mild cognitive problems in language and memory can persist beyond 1 year, but 85% of children have only minimal residual deficits or full recovery at 2 years.[7,8]

Steroid-Responsive Encephalopathy Associated With Autoimmune Thyroiditis

Steroid-responsive encephalopathy associated with autoimmune thyroiditis (SREAT), previously referred to as Hashimoto encephalopathy, presents with neuropsychiatric symptoms in association with antithyroglobulin or antithyroid peroxidase antibodies and often hypothyroidism. Clinical presentation can vary widely in severity and may include cognitive decline, coma, seizures, hallucinations, myoclonus, and/or stroke-like episodes. Proposed adult criteria require encephalopathy with any of the aforementioned symptoms, subclinical or mild thyroid disease, presence of antithyroid antibodies, and lack of other etiology.[9] However, children may not present with abnormal thyroid function and may still benefit from immunotherapy.[10] EEG is abnormal in 82%, and MRI is normal or shows nonspecific white matter changes.[11] The syndrome is characteristically steroid responsive in 91% of cases with overall good outcomes; however, occasionally second-line therapy with IVIG or plasmapheresis is required.[11] Treatment for dysthyroidism, if present, is also indicated. Reports of relapse rates vary widely in the literature and are as low as 16% in adults and about one-third in children.[11,12] Treatment/outcomes data are limited in children, and optimal duration of steroid treatment is unknown, ranging from weeks to years, although a steroid taper is advised.

Opsoclonus-Myoclonus Ataxia Syndrome

Opsoclonus-myoclonus ataxia syndrome (OMAS) is a rare syndrome with a mean age of onset of 18 to 22 months and an association with neuroblastoma in about half of cases.[13] Diagnostic criteria require 3 of the following: ataxia/myoclonus, opsoclonus, irritability or sleep disturbance, and presence of neuroblastoma. OMAS is thought to be a B-cell–mediated disease process, although no causative autoantibody has yet been identified. CSF may show evidence of neuroinflammation, with pleocytosis or presence of oligoclonal bands. Evaluation for neuroblastoma includes urine catecholamine metabolites, serum neuron-specific enolase, lactate dehydrogenase, and whole-body imaging including metaiodobenzylguanidine (MIBG). Tumor resection alone is insufficient in treatment and prevention of relapse. Aggressive initial treatment is generally pursued with steroids, IVIG, and cyclophosphamide or rituximab and then ongoing maintenance treatment with steroids and IVIG. In more severe cases, use of adrenocorticotrophic hormone is considered preferential over oral steroids for ongoing immunotherapy. A multimodal approach and reduction in relapse frequency are thought to improve the poor cognitive, behavioral, and motor outcomes.[14] Despite this, many patients have ongoing residual neurocognitive and neurobehavioral symptoms.

IMMUNE-MEDIATED EPILEPSY SYNDROMES

Febrile Infection-Related Epilepsy Syndrome

Febrile infection-related epilepsy syndrome (FIRES) is a rare neurologic disorder characterized by new onset of refractory status epilepticus following febrile illness. Children with FIRES typically have a standard febrile illness followed by new-onset seizures up to 2 weeks following illness. The seizures are typically abrupt in onset and quickly evolve into status epilepticus that is refractory in nature. Patients generally require an intensive care unit level of care in the acute phase as well as use of multiple antiepileptic medications and anesthetic agents for seizure control. In the chronic phase of the disease, there is ongoing refractory epilepsy and varying levels of neuropsychological impairments.[15] Children with FIRES have activation of the innate immune system and have been found to have elevated CSF proinflammatory cytokines that have been shown to be epileptogenic.[16-18] This activation of the innate immune system leads to neuroinflammation leading to epileptogenic potential.

FIRES is a diagnosis of exclusion. There is not one diagnostic study or specific marker leading to diagnosis. Clinical evaluation for patients with suspected FIRES should include workup for infectious, autoimmune, and genetic etiologies. CSF studies should be collected including CSF neopterin and cytokines to aid in diagnosis. MRI studies performed at the initial presentation of patients with FIRES are normal in the majority of patients, but over time, they can show varying degrees of atrophy and mesial temporal sclerosis.[19]

The initial treatment of FIRES is focused on antiepileptic medications and anesthetic agents to achieve seizure control and obtain burst suppression. Immune-modulating therapy including IV steroids, IVIG, and plasmapheresis is often used in patients in the early stages of FIRES due to possible AE but generally with minimal response. There have been data supporting the early use of a ketogenic diet showing improved neurocognitive outcomes. Thus, a ketogenic diet should be considered early in presentation.[20] Additionally, the use of anakinra, an interleukin (IL)-1 receptor antagonist, has been shown to be effective in retrospective cohort studies.[16,21]

Rasmussen Encephalitis

Rasmussen encephalitis (RE) is a chronic, progressive, unilateral hemispheric neuroinflammatory disease with refractory epilepsy and progressive unilateral motor and cognitive decline. Patients with RE typically present with focal-onset seizures. Some patients present with epilepsia partialis continua (EPC). Seizures are typically refractory in nature. Ongoing disease can lead to hemiparesis, hemianopia, and cognitive decline within 1 year of disease onset. RE is believed to be mediated by cytotoxic T cells, and pathology generally shows T-cell infiltration.[22,23]

Clinical workup for patients with suspected RE should exclude other potential etiologies of presentation including infectious, autoimmune, and genetic causes. MRI is the most sensitive tool in making a diagnosis of RE. Early findings may include unilateral atrophy or unilateral T2 FLAIR signal. Over time, there is evolution of these changes characterized by progressive atrophy and increased T2 FLAIR signal.[24]

Antiseizure medications (ASMs) can be of benefit, but seizures often persist. EPC tends to be more refractory to ASMs than other seizure types. Currently, functional hemispherectomy is the only highly effective treatment to achieve seizure freedom in RE. Small case studies have shown treatments such as IV steroids, IVIG, tacrolimus, natalizumab, rituximab, cyclophosphamide, alemtuzumab, and intrathecal methotrexate to be beneficial, but further studies are needed.[22,25] In general, these immunotherapy treatments do not appear to be effective in halting the disease process but may only slow progression.

OTHER INFLAMMATORY BRAIN DISEASES

Primary CNS Vasculitis

CNS vasculitis can be a primary or secondary (related to infection or systemic inflammation) inflammatory process in the cerebral blood vessels leading to focal neurologic deficits, cognitive dysfunction, or psychiatric presentation.

Primary CNS vasculitis in children, termed *childhood primary angiitis of the CNS* (cPACNS), occurs in a child without an underlying systemic illness or inflammatory condition. cPACNS can affect small, medium, and large vessels of the CNS. The clinical presentation varies depending on size and location of vasculature involved. MRI in patients with cPACNS may show nonspecific inflammatory lesions and leptomeningeal enhancement in small vessel involvement or ischemic findings in large and medium vessel involvement. Magnetic resonance angiography may show gadolinium enhancement of the vessel wall in large vessel involvement. Conventional angiography may aid in the diagnosis of medium and large vessel disease. Small vessel involvement of cPACNS may be more difficult to diagnose, and at times, brain biopsy with lymphocytic infiltration can support the diagnosis. Additional supporting diagnostic evaluation includes CSF pleocytosis, elevated opening pressure on lumbar puncture, and presence of oligoclonal bands isolated to CSF.[26] Treatment regimens vary depending on vessel size but include use of anticoagulation, corticosteroids, cyclophosphamide, mycophenolate mofetil, and azathioprine.[27]

Primary Rheumatologic Conditions With Neurologic Manifestations

Systemic Lupus Erythematosus

Systemic lupus erythematosus (SLE) is an autoimmune condition that causes widespread inflammation in the body, which can include the CNS and peripheral nervous system. CNS involvement in SLE occurs due to breakdown of the blood-brain barrier, inflammatory cytokines, autoantibodies, and immune complexes, leading to vascular disease and parenchymal damage.[28] Neurologic manifestations of SLE can include headache, seizures, psychosis, cerebrovascular disease, demyelination, movement disorder, cognitive dysfunction, and myelopathy. There is currently no biomarker specific for neuropsychiatric lupus (NPSLE); thus, thoughtful, multidisciplinary evaluation for possible NPSLE should be considered. Treatment regimens for pediatric SLE and NPSLE should be made in conjunction with pediatric rheumatology.

Sarcoidosis

Sarcoidosis is a systemic condition leading to granulomatous inflammation. Common presenting symptoms of sarcoidosis include pulmonary disease, hilar adenopathy, arthritis, and erythema nodosum, among others.[29] The most commonly seen neurologic presentation of sarcoidosis is cranial neuropathy, but it should be considered in patients with "typical" neurologic manifestations that have been associated with sarcoidosis, including aseptic meningitis, conus or cauda equina syndrome, encephalopathy, myelopathy, peripheral polyneuropathy, elevated intracranial pressure, seizures, uveoparotid fever, and vascular syndromes.[30] CSF studies may be helpful in the diagnosis of neurosarcoidosis, including but not limited to angiotensin-converting enzyme and soluble IL-2 receptor, although they are not always sensitive or specific for sarcoidosis.[31]

Behçet Disease

Behçet disease (BD) is a small and large vessel inflammatory vasculitis that can affect the CNS. Common presentations of BD are oral aphthae, genital ulcers, skin lesions, arthritis, uveitis, and thrombophlebitis. BD may show direct parenchymal involvement, more commonly affecting the brainstem and basal ganglia, but can also involve the spinal cord. Presenting symptoms vary depending on location and degree of involvement. CSF studies can aid in the diagnosis of neuro-BD, including elevated levels of IL-6, although it is not sensitive or specific to the diagnosis.[32]

There are numerous other rheumatologic conditions including autoimmune and autoinflammatory conditions such as those with genetic etiologies that may cause neurologic manifestations. These diagnoses are important considerations for children with neurologic symptoms but also with coexisting systemic manifestations.

REFERENCES

1. Dalmau J, Graus F. Antibody-mediated encephalitis. *N Engl J Med*. 2018;378(9):840-851. doi:10.1056/nejmra1708712
2. Cellucci T, van Mater H, Graus F, et al. Clinical approach to the diagnosis of autoimmune encephalitis in the pediatric patient. *Neurol Neuroimmunol Neuroinflamm*. 2020;7(2):e663. doi:10.1212/NXI.0000000000000663
3. Brenton JN, Goodkin HP. Antibody-mediated autoimmune encephalitis in childhood. *Pediatr Neurol*. 2016;60:13-23. doi:10.1016/j.pediatrneurol.2016.04.004
4. Titulaer MJ, McCracken L, Gabilondo I, et al. Treatment and prognostic factors for long-term outcome in patients with anti-NMDA receptor encephalitis: an observational cohort study. *Lancet Neurol*. 2013;12(2):157-165. doi:10.1016/S1474-4422(12)70310-1
5. Nosadini M, Eyre M, Molteni E, et al. Use and safety of immunotherapeutic management of N-methyl-D-aspartate antibody encephalitis: a meta-analysis. *JAMA Neurol*. 2021;78(11):1333-1344. doi:10.1001/jamaneurol.2021.3188
6. Nosadini M, Thomas T, Eyre M, et al. International consensus recommendations for the treatment of pediatric NMDAR antibody encephalitis. *Neurol Neuroimmunol Neuroinflamm*. 2021;8(5):e1052. doi:10.1212/NXI.0000000000001052
7. Armangue T, Titulaer MJ, Málaga I, et al. Pediatric anti-N-methyl-D-aspartate receptor encephalitis: clinical analysis and novel findings in a series of 20 patients. *J Pediatr*. 2013;162(4):850-856.e2. doi:10.1016/j.jpeds.2012.10.011
8. Shim YK, Kim SY, Kim H, et al. Clinical outcomes of pediatric Anti-NMDA receptor encephalitis. *Eur J Paediatr Neurol*. 2020;29:87-91. doi:10.1016/j.ejpn.2020.10.001
9. Graus F, Titulaer MJ, Balu R, et al. A clinical approach to diagnosis of autoimmune encephalitis. *Lancet Neurol*. 2016;15(4):391-404. doi:10.1016/S1474-4422(15)00401-9
10. Adams A, Mooneyham GLC, van Mater H, Gallentine W. Evaluation of diagnostic criteria for Hashimoto encephalopathy among children and adolescents. *Pediatr Neurol*. 2020;107:41-47. doi:10.1016/j.pediatrneurol.2019.12.011
11. Laurent C, Capron J, Quillerou B, et al. Steroid-responsive encephalopathy associated with autoimmune thyroiditis (SREAT): characteristics, treatment and outcome in 251 cases from the literature. *Autoimmun Rev*. 2016;15(12):1129-1133. doi:10.1016/j.autrev.2016.09.008
12. Hilberath JM, Schmidt H, Wolf GK. Steroid-responsive encephalopathy associated with autoimmune thyroiditis (SREAT): case report of reversible coma and status epilepticus in an adolescent patient and review of the literature. *Eur J Pediatr*. 2014;173(10):1263-1273. doi:10.1007/s00431-014-2391-6
13. Matthay KK, Blaes F, Hero B, et al. Opsoclonus myoclonus syndrome in neuroblastoma a report from a workshop on the dancing eyes syndrome at the advances in neuroblastoma meeting in Genoa, Italy, 2004. *Cancer Lett*. 2005;228(1-2):275-282. doi:10.1016/j.canlet.2005.01.051
14. Mitchell WG, Wooten AA, O'Neil SH, Rodriguez JG, Cruz RE, Wittern R. Effect of increased immunosuppression on developmental outcome of opsoclonus myoclonus syndrome (OMS). *J Child Neurol*. 2015;30(8):976-982. doi:10.1177/0883073814549581
15. Lam SK, Lu WY, Weng WC, Fan PC, Lee WT. The short-term and long-term outcome of febrile infection-related epilepsy syndrome in children. *Epilepsy Behav*. 2019;95:117-123. doi:10.1016/j.yebeh.2019.02.033
16. Kenney-Jung DL, Vezzani A, Kahoud RJ, et al. Febrile infection-related epilepsy syndrome treated with anakinra. *Ann Neurol*. 2016;80(6):939-945. doi:10.1002/ana.24806
17. Sakuma H, Tanuma N, Kuki I, Takahashi Y, Shiomi M, Hayashi M. Intrathecal overproduction of proinflammatory cytokines and chemokines in febrile infection-related refractory status epilepticus. *J Neurol Neurosurg Psychiatry*. 2015;86(7):820-822. doi:10.1136/jnnp-2014-309388
18. Kothur K, Bandodkar S, Wienholt L, et al. Etiology is the key determinant of neuroinflammation in epilepsy: elevation of cerebrospinal fluid cytokines and chemokines in febrile infection-related epilepsy syndrome and febrile status epilepticus. *Epilepsia*. 2019;60(8):1678-1688. doi:10.1111/epi.16275
19. Culleton S, Talenti G, Kaliakatsos M, Pujar S, D'Arco F. The spectrum of neuroimaging findings in febrile infection-related epilepsy syndrome (FIRES): a literature review. *Epilepsia*. 2019;60(4):585-592. doi:10.1111/epi.14684
20. Peng P, Peng J, Yin F, et al. Ketogenic diet as a treatment for super-refractory status epilepticus in febrile infection-related epilepsy syndrome. *Front Neurol*. 2019;10:423. doi:10.3389/fneur.2019.00423
21. Lai YC, Muscal E, Wells E, et al. Anakinra usage in febrile infection related epilepsy syndrome: an international cohort. *Ann Clin Transl Neurol*. 2020;7(12):2467-2474. doi:10.1002/acn3.51229
22. Orsini A, Foiadelli T, Carli N, et al. Rasmussen's encephalitis: from immune pathogenesis towards targeted-therapy. *Seizure*. 2020;81:76-83. doi:10.1016/j.seizure.2020.07.023
23. al Nimer F, Jelcic I, Kempf C, et al. Phenotypic and functional complexity of brain-infiltrating T cells in Rasmussen encephalitis. *Neurol Neuroimmunol Neuroinflamm*. 2017;5(1):e419. doi:10.1212/NXI.0000000000000419
24. Cay-Martinez KC, Hickman RA, McKhann GM, Provenzano FA, Sands TT. Rasmussen encephalitis: an update. *Semin Neurol*. 2020;40(2):201-210. doi:10.1055/s-0040-1708504

25. Liba Z, Vaskova M, Zamecnik J, et al. An immunotherapy effect analysis in Rasmussen encephalitis. *BMC Neurol.* 2020;20(1):359. doi:10.1186/s12883-020-01932-9

26. Gowdie P, Twilt M, Benseler SM. Primary and secondary central nervous system vasculitis. *J Child Neurol.* 2012;27(11):1448-1459. doi:10.1177/0883073812459352

27. Beelen J, Benseler SM, Dropol A, Ghali B, Twilt M. Strategies for treatment of childhood primary angiitis of the central nervous system. *Neurol Neuroimmunol Neuroinflamm.* 2019;6(4):e567. doi:10.1212/NXI.0000000000000567

28. Popescu A, Kao AH. Neuropsychiatric systemic lupus erythematosus. *Curr Neuropharmacol.* 2011;9(3):49-457.

29. Gaddam M, Ojinnaka U, Ahmed Z, et al. Sarcoidosis: various presentations, coexisting diseases and malignancies. *Cureus.* 2021;13(8):e16967. doi:10.7759/cureus.16967

30. Ibitoye RT, Wilkins A, Scolding NJ. Neurosarcoidosis: a clinical approach to diagnosis and management. *J Neurol.* 2017;264(5):1023-1028. doi:10.1007/s00415-016-8336-4

31. Otto C, Wengert O, Unterwalder N, Meisel C, Ruprecht K. Analysis of soluble interleukin-2 receptor as CSF biomarker for neurosarcoidosis. *Neurol Neuroimmunol Neuroinflamm.* 2020;7(4):e725. doi:10.1212/NXI.0000000000000725

32. Caruso P, Moretti R. Focus on neuro-Behcet's disease: a review. *Neurol India.* 2018;66(6):1619-1628. doi:10.4103/0028-3886.246252

Concussion and Post-traumatic Headache

Joanne Kacperski, MD, FAHS
Todd Arthur, MD

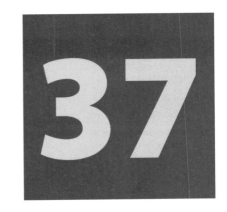

INTRODUCTION

Traumatic brain injury (TBI) is one of the most common injuries in the pediatric age group. It is estimated that as many as half a million children younger than 15 years sustain TBIs that require hospital-based care in the United States each year, with the majority of these injuries being mild in severity.[1] A national cross-sectional study in the United States estimated that 1 of every 220 pediatric patients seen in emergency departments receive a diagnosis of mild traumatic brain injury (mTBI).[2] Headaches are the most common symptom after mTBI or concussion and often occur with a constellation of physical, cognitive, emotional, and behavioral signs and symptoms. Headaches may affect a child's ability to function and participate in school and extracurricular activities, which can cause disability and impair their quality of life.[3]

CONCUSSION (MTBI DEFINITION)

The Consensus Statement on Concussion in Sport from the 5th International Conference on Concussion in Sport held in Berlin in October 2016[4] defines concussion using the following criteria:

Sport-related concussion (SRC) is a TBI induced by biomechanical forces. Several common features that may be utilized in clinically defining the nature of a concussive head injury include:

A. SRC may be caused either by a direct blow to the head, face, neck or elsewhere on the body with an impulsive force transmitted to the head.

B. SRC typically results in the rapid onset of short-lived impairment of neurological function that resolves spontaneously. However, in some cases, signs and symptoms evolve over a number of minutes to hours.

C. SRC may result in neuropathological changes, but the acute clinical signs and symptoms largely reflect a functional disturbance rather than a structural injury and, as such, no abnormality is seen on standard structural neuroimaging studies.

D. Results in a range of clinical signs and symptoms that may or may not involve loss of consciousness. Resolution of the clinical and cognitive features typically follows a sequential course. However, in some cases symptoms may be prolonged. The clinical signs and symptoms cannot be explained by drug, alcohol, or medication use, other injuries (such as cervical injuries, peripheral vestibular dysfunction, etc) or other comorbidities (eg, psychological factors or coexisting medical conditions).

INITIAL EVALUATION OF CONCUSSION

The initial evaluation of a suspected concussion involves a thorough history, including patient self-report and knowledge from others (eg, family, teacher, trainer), and a thorough exam.

The Centers for Disease Control and Prevention (CDC)[5] has summarized recommendations in the initial evaluation of concussions. It is highly recommended the reader study the original document. Below are the recommendations used most consistently in our practice. The focus of evaluation and treatment often falls on addressing some combination of headache, dizziness, sleep issues, attentional issues, cognitive issues, mood/personality changes, or visual issues (eg, accommodative issues).

1. Healthcare professionals should counsel patients and families that most (70%-80%) children with mTBI do not show significant difficulties that last more than 1 to 3 months after injury.

2. Healthcare professionals should counsel children and families completing preparticipation athletic examinations and children with mTBI, as well as their families,

that recovery from mTBI might be delayed in those with the following:

- Premorbid histories of mTBI
- Lower cognitive ability (for children with an intracranial lesion)
- Neurologic or psychiatric disorder
- Learning difficulties
- Increased preinjury symptoms (ie, similar to those commonly referred to as "postconcussive")
- Family and social stressors (moderate; level B).

3. Routine neuroimaging is not recommended.

   - However, healthcare professionals should use validated clinical decision rules to identify children with mTBI at low risk for intracranial injury (ICI) in whom head computed tomography (CT) is not indicated, as well as children who may be at higher risk for clinically important ICI and thus may warrant head CT. **Our practice uses the Pediatric Emergency Care Applied Research Network (PECARN) decision rules.**[6]

4. Healthcare professionals should use an age-appropriate, validated symptom rating scale as a component of the diagnostic evaluation in children seen with acute mTBI.

5. Healthcare professionals may use validated, age-appropriate computerized cognitive testing in the acute period of injury as a component of the diagnosis of mTBI.

6. The Standardized Assessment of Concussion should not be exclusively used to diagnose mTBI in children aged 6 to 18 years.

7. Healthcare professionals should not use biomarkers outside of a research setting for the diagnosis of children with mTBI.

8. In providing education and reassurance to the family, the healthcare professional should include the following information:

   - Warning signs of more serious injury
   - Description of injury and expected course of symptoms and recovery
   - Instructions on how to monitor postconcussive symptoms
   - Prevention of further injury
   - Management of cognitive and physical activity/rest
   - Instructions regarding return to play/recreation and school
   - Clear clinician follow-up instructions

9. Rest and return-to-activity counseling are cornerstones of treatment (covered in the following section, Return to School/Play).

An example of a validated symptom rating scale is the Post-Concussion Symptom Scale from Lovell and Collins.[7] Symptom scales are very useful for objectively following recovery. They also can focus the clinical visit to improve time management during a busy clinic.

RETURN TO SCHOOL/PLAY

It is generally accepted that complete rest for the first 24 to 48 hours is standard care following a concussion. Our practice is to minimize physical and cognitive efforts (eg, take care of activities of daily living only, limit screen or phone time to 1 hour per day, no schoolwork) for the first 2 days and then start a program of gradual return to school and activity (pacing). Pacing has one rule: Don't do anything that will get you knocked down or hit in the head. The patient then attempts their normal routine (school/cognitive and physical activity) as described in the diagram below (Figure 37–1). Symptom control during the first 14 days relies heavily on activity pacing, good sleep hygiene, and headache care (covered in a separate section later).

Other symptoms that may arise less frequently but can have an equally disabling effect include dizziness, visual issues, emotional lability, and cognitive or concentration issues. If orthostatic symptoms arise, check orthostatic blood pressures to diagnose and treat orthostatic intolerance. If visual symptoms arise (eg, losing place on page, poor focusing of vision at close distance), be sure to test accommodation and introduce corrective exercises if necessary

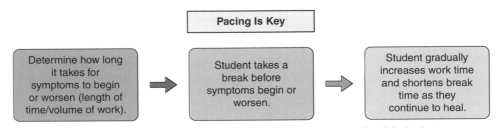

Pacing Is Key

Determine how long it takes for symptoms to begin or worsen (length of time/volume of work). → Student takes a break before symptoms begin or worsen. → Student gradually increases work time and shortens break time as they continue to heal.

Example: If symptoms begin after 20 minutes of work, take a break after 15 minutes of work for 5 minutes.

▲ **Figure 37–1.** Return to activity.

(eg, a pen or pencil pushup [hold a pen or pencil at arm's length and pull toward face until tip of pen/pencil gets blurry, then stop and push pen away until clear again, and then pull toward face until blurry; perform 20 repetitions 3 times a day until pen/pencil can be held at reading/screen distance and remains clear]).

We advise the school and patient on return to learn using a standardized letter with the overriding principles of slowing down the pace of school and controlling symptom-exacerbating environmental factors (Figure 37–2).

Once a patient is (1) not reliably triggering or worsening symptoms of their concussion with activities of daily living and with full school days and (2) has a reasonably low Post-Concussion Symptom Scale score (often adjusted if patient had preinjury headaches), they may attempt a return-to-play progression. The CDC (Figure 37–3) provides guidelines to return to sports in a general sense that we then modify to each sport.[8] Once a patient clears all stages of recovery, the concussion is resolved. Progressing from step 4 to step 5 involves reevaluation by the treating clinician. Finishing the steps means the concussion is fully resolved.

POSTTRAUMATIC HEADACHES

Headache after concussion, referred to as posttraumatic headache (PTH), is one of the most common and disabling symptoms after a head injury. Headache has been reported in as many as 86% of high school and college athletes who have suffered from head trauma.[9] Eisenberg et al[10] reported that 85% of pediatric patients presented to a pediatric emergency department with headache following an mTBI. Kuczynski et al[11] reported that 11% of pediatric patients who presented to a university hospital emergency department with mTBI continued to report headache 2 weeks after injury.

▶ Definition

The International Classification of Headache Disorders, Third Edition (ICHD-3) classifies PTHs as acute if lasting less than 3 months and persistent if lasting more than 3 months. The classification for acute and persistent PTH is summarized in Tables 37–1 and 37–2. Although the ICHD-3 criteria state that PTHs begin within 7 days after injury to the head or after regaining consciousness, this 7-day cutoff is arbitrary, and some experts believe that headaches may develop after a longer interval.[12]

▶ Risk Factors

Predictive factors for the development of PTH in the pediatric population may include age, sex, prior history of headaches, and family history.[13] Some studies suggest that females are more likely to endorse both preinjury and postinjury headaches consistent with migraine.[14] In a study of 400 patients from a pediatric concussion clinic, although 90% of females versus 79% of males reported PTH, females also demonstrated a longer duration of symptoms compared to males (median recovery time of 80 days vs 34 days),[15] indicating that the role of sex remains uncertain. Prior headache history may also play a role in the development of PTH. In a pediatric study, 51% of children with persistent PTH at 3 months after mTBI had a preexisting history of headaches, and 31% had headaches fulfilling the ICHD-3 criteria for migraine or probable migraine prior to the injury. Fifty-six percent of the children with persistent PTH also had a positive family history of migraine.[11] Chronic pain, nonsteroidal anti-inflammatory drug (NSAID) use prior to injury, and a family history of headache have also been associated with increased risk of developing PTH.[13] Patients with prior mTBI, preexisting anxiety and/or depression, and/or with maladaptive coping styles seem to be at higher risk for PTH.[16] A 2019 trial found that the only risk factor for the development of PTH was a past history of primary headache and that, in 90% of cases, the PTH phenotyped to migraine.[17]

▶ Phenotypes

Despite being classified as a secondary headache type, headache attributed to mTBI often presents with clinical features seen in other primary headache disorders. Like other secondary headache types, PTH has no defining or identifying features. Prospective studies of PTH have found that migraine is the most common phenotype in adults and children. In one study of 378 participants older than 16 years admitted for acute inpatient rehabilitation following mTBI, migraine was the most frequent headache phenotype after injury in 38%. Probable migraine was suspected in up to 25%, tension-type headache in 21%, and cervicogenic headache in 10%.[14]

▶ Evaluation

Assessment of pediatric PTH is similar to the assessment of a primary headache disorder. Evaluation should exclude secondary causes of headache, including the possibility of a structural cause such as intracranial hemorrhage, cerebral edema, stroke, traumatic dissection (carotid or vertebral), or acute cervical/thoracic neck injury.[13] The history should include evaluation of prior head injuries, preinjury symptoms (eg, preexisting headaches or migraines, anxiety, depression, sleep disturbance), risk factors (eg, family history, learning disabilities), details regarding the injury, current symptoms (eg, location, quality, associated symptoms), and the progression of symptoms after the injury. It is important to ask about other postconcussion symptoms such as dizziness, nausea, sleep disturbances, mood changes, and cognitive changes and to assess for medication overuse.[18] A thorough general and neurologic examination should be completed, including fundoscopy to rule out papilledema and head and neck exam to evaluate for neuralgias.[19]

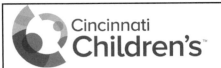

Brain Health and Wellness Center
{DIVISION:26715}

Return to Learning Following Brain Injury: School Recommendations

Patient Name: @NAME@   Date of Appointment/Medical Evaluation: @TD@
Duration of Recommendations: ☒ {DURATION:26809}
Follow up appointment: @FOLLOWUP@ **These recommendations will be reassessed at that time.**

@FNAME@ has been diagnosed with a brain injury and is currently under the care of the Brain Health & Wellness Center at Cincinnati Children's Hospital Medical Center. Proper treatment of concussion/traumatic brain injury in the first days and weeks after injury is vital to optimize recovery. It is important for @FNAME@'s school team to recognize signs and symptoms of brain injury. We request flexibility and supports during this recovery period. The following are our recommendations for academic adjustments needed to address the student's medical condition and should be individualized for the student as deemed appropriate in the school setting. **If there is consensus between the patient, their family, and school, these recommendations may be applied/removed as needed as the student's symptoms improve/worsen.**

Pacing Is Key

Determine how long it takes for symptoms to begin or worsen (length of time/volume of work)	⟹	Student takes a break before symptoms begin or worsen.	⟹	Student gradually increases work time and shortens break time as they continue to heal.

Example: If symptoms begin after 20 minutes of work, take a break after 15 minutes of work for 5 minutes.

Attendance
- ☐ No school: Please excuse the above-mentioned absences.
- ☐ Partial school days gradually increasing as tolerated:
- ☐ Full school days as tolerated by the student
- ☒ Please excuse school absence for today's appointment.

Visual Stimulus
- ☒ Change classroom seating as necessary (i.e. move closer to board or farther away from bright projector screen)
- ☒ Allow student to wear sunglasses/hat/hood in school
- ☒ Pre-printed notes, presentation slides, and/or note taker
- ☒ Limited computer, bright electronic screen/device use (allow student to request items be printed on paper/provide pre-printed curriculum materials)
- ☒ Reduce brightness on monitors and screens
- ☐ Please help student read assignments on electronics, have another student help, or allow access to audio or text-to-speech

Workload/Multi-Tasking
- ☒ Reduce amount of make-up class work and homework
- ☒ Consider exemption from non-essential assignments and a reduction of essential assignments for current work (ex. prioritize assignments to display mastery of content)
- ☒ Extra time/flexible deadlines for work as needed/requested
- ☒ Allow student to 're-do' assignments/tests completed when performance may have been impacted by injury symptoms
- ☐ Allow for an extra set of books to be provided for home

Physical Exertion
- ☒ No contact sports
- ☒ No physical exertion/athletics/Physical Education class/recess
- ☐ Walking/light-aerobic activity in Physical Education class/on recess only

Additional Recommendations
- ☒ Permission to use a water bottle (filled with any non-caffeinated drink) and lenient restroom privileges. If helpful for headache pain, allow student to have access to a snack.
- ☒ Access to a "point person" who can work with the student to develop a plan to complete any assignments that he/she will need to complete to compensate for his or her missed class time during his or her initial recovery period. Regular meetings or "check ins" are recommended.
- ☒ Increased opportunities for repetition and review of material. This could be with a tutor, during guided study hall, or through after-school help (if available).
- ☐ Consider supplemental home-based instruction, to help the student to complete make-up assignments and "catch-up" on their missed work. We recommend one hour of instruction for every full school day missed.
- ☐ Consider student for a functional behavioral assessment or behavior plan
- ☐ Consider referral for school-based counseling/therapy
- ☐ Consider consultation with school speech pathologist or occupational therapist to support executive-functioning deficits
- ☐ Consider discussing a formal support plan (504 or IEP) with school officials
- ☐ This patient is being recommended for a full neuropsychological evaluation through our hospital.
- ☐
- ☐

Breaks
- ☒ Access to breaks in a quiet area as needed/allow student to lay head on desk
- ☒ Access to nurse as needed
- ☒ Allow student to go home if symptoms do not subside
- ☐ Scheduled rest break (see pacing guide above):

Audible Stimulus
- ☒ Allow student to wear earplugs, earbuds, or noise blocking headphones
- ☒ Lunch in a quiet area if requested/needed
- ☐ Allow extra time for class transitions (i.e. before or after peers)
- ☐ No choir, band, music, or shop classes

Testing
- ☒ Excuse from all tests until material is fully learned and make-up work is complete
- ☒ Provide additional time and breaks for tests/quizzes/assessments
- ☐ Allow for scribe, oral response, and oral delivery of questions if needed/available
- ☐ Modify test requirements/format as needed (i.e. paper test rather than digital to reduce screen time; provide word bank, etc.)
- ☐ Limit amount of test/quizzes per day

- ☐ Access to school elevator
- ☐ Student needs peer or adult assistance due to symptoms
- ☐ Begin return to play protocol as outlined by return to activity guidelines

@SIGNATURE@

▲ **Figure 37–2.** Return to learn/school recommendations used by the Cincinnati Children's Hospital Medical Center Brain Health Wellness Collaborative (Reproduced with permission from Brain Health and Wellness Center, v. 2. Revised 2-24-22).

Step 1: Back to regular activities (such as school)

Athlete is back to their regular activities (such as school) and has the green light from their healthcare provider to begin the return to play process. An athlete's return to regular activities involves a stepwise process. It starts with a few days of rest (2-3 days) and is followed by light activity (such as short walks) and moderate activity (such as riding a stationary bike) that do not worsen symptoms.

Step 2: Light aerobic activity

Begin with light aerobic exercise only to increase an athlete's heart rate. This means about 5 to 10 minutes on an exercise bike, walking, or light jogging. No weight lifting at this point.

Step 3: Moderate activity

Continue with activities to increase an athlete's heart rate with body or head movement. This includes moderate jogging, brief running, moderate-intensity stationary biking, moderate-intensity weightlifting (less time and/or less weight from their typical routine).

Step 4: Heavy, non-contact activity

Add heavy non-contact physical activity, such as sprinting/running, high-intensity stationary biking, regular weightlifting routine, non-contact sport-specific drills (in 3 planes of movement).

Step 5: Practice & full contact

Young athlete may return to practice and full contact (if appropriate for the sport) in controlled practice.

Step 6: Competition

Young athlete may return to competition.

▲ **Figure 37–3.** Returning to sports and activities per Centers for Disease Control and Prevention Heads Up. (Reproduced with permission from Centers for Disease Control and Prevention. Heads up. Brain injury basics. Returning to sports and activities. https://www.cdc.gov/headsup/basics/return_to_sports.Html).

CT and magnetic resonance imaging (MRI) are not necessary to establish the diagnosis of mTBI and PTH in children and are not recommended during the acute evaluation unless there are risk factors for ICI or clinical concern for significant injuries that could result in intracranial hemorrhage or a cervical spine injury.[18,20]

▶ **Treatment**

Acute Therapies

The goal of acute treatment in children with PTH should be a consistent response with minimum side effects and a rapid return to normal function. The treatments should be properly dosed and used as quickly as possible, while minimizing the potential for medication overuse. Acute treatment

Table 37–1. International Classification of Headache Disorders, Third Edition (ICHD-3) definition of acute headache attributed to traumatic injury to the head.

5.1 Acute headache attributed to traumatic injury to the head
  A. Any headache fulfilling criteria C and D
  B. Traumatic injury to the head[a] has occurred
  C. Headache is reported to have developed within 7 days after one of the following:
    1. The injury to the head
    2. Regaining consciousness following the injury to the head
    3. Discontinuation of medication(s) that impair ability to sense or report headache following the injury to the head
  D. Either of the following:
    1. Headache has resolved within 3 months after the injury to the head
    2. Headache has not yet resolved, but 3 months have not yet passed since the injury to the head
  E. Not better accounted for by another ICHD-3 diagnosis

5.1.2 Acute posttraumatic headache attributed to mild traumatic injury to the head
  A. Headache fulfilling criteria for 5.1
  B. Injury to the head fulfilling none of the following:
    1. Associated with none of the following:
      a) Loss of consciousness for >30 minutes
      b) Glasgow Coma Scale (GCS) score <13
      c) Posttraumatic amnesia[b] lasting >24 hours
      d) Altered level of awareness for >24 hours
      e) Imaging evidence of traumatic head injury, eg, intracranial hemorrhage and/or brain contusion
    2. Associated immediately following the head injury, with one or more of the following symptoms and/or signs:
      a) Transient confusion, disorientation, or impaired consciousness
      b) Loss of memory for events immediately before or after the head injury
      c) Two or more other symptoms suggestive of mild traumatic brain injury: nausea, vomiting, visual disturbances, dizziness and/or vertigo, impaired memory, and/or concentration

[a]Traumatic injury to the head is defined as a structural or functional injury resulting from the action of external forces on the head. These include striking the head with or the head striking an object, penetration of the head by a foreign body, forces generated from blasts or explosions, and other forces yet to be defined.
[b]The duration of posttraumatic amnesia is defined as the time between head injury and recovery of memory of current events and those occurring in the last 24 hours.
Data from Headache Classification Committee of the International Headache Society (IHS). The International Classification of Headache Disorders, 3rd ed. (Beta version) *Cephalalgia*. 2013;33(9):629–808.

Table 37–2. International Classification of Headache Disorders, Third Edition (ICHD-3) definition of persistent posttraumatic headaches.

5.2 Persistent headache attributed to traumatic injury to the head
  A. Any headache fulfilling criteria C and D
  B. Traumatic injury to the head[a] has occurred
  C. Headache is reported to have developed within 7 days after one of the following:
    1. The injury to the head
    2. Regaining consciousness following the injury to the head
    3. Discontinuation of medication(s) that impair ability to sense or report headache following the injury to the head
  D. Headache persists for >3 months after the injury to the head
  E. Not better accounted for by another ICHD-3 diagnosis

5.2.2 Persistent headache attributed to mild traumatic injury to the head
  A. Headache fulfilling criteria for 5.2
  B. Head injury fulfilling both of the following:
    1. Associated with none of the following:
      a) Loss of consciousness for >30 minutes
      b) Glasgow Coma Scale (GCS) score <13
      c) Posttraumatic amnesia[b] lasting >24 hours
      d) Altered level of awareness for >24 hours
      e) Imaging evidence of traumatic head injury, eg, intracranial hemorrhage and/or brain contusion
    2. Associated immediately following the head injury, with one or more of the following symptoms and/or signs:
      a) Transient confusion, disorientation, or impaired consciousness
      b) Loss of memory for events immediately before or after the head injury
      c) Two or more other symptoms suggestive of mild traumatic brain injury: nausea, vomiting, visual disturbances, dizziness and/or vertigo, impaired memory, and/or concentration

[a]Traumatic injury to the head is defined as a structural or functional injury resulting from the action of external forces on the head. These include striking the head with or the head striking an object, penetration of the head by a foreign body, forces generated from blasts or explosions, and other forces yet to be defined.
[b]The duration of posttraumatic amnesia is defined as the time between head injury and recovery of memory of current events and those occurring in the last 24 hours.
Data from Headache Classification Committee of the International Headache Society (IHS). The International Classification of Headache Disorders, 3rd ed. (Beta version) Cephalalgia. 2013;33(9):629–808.

should be incorporated into the child's life with the ability to receive these treatments in the school or at home, without missing school or social activities. To avoid the development of medication overuse headache (MOH), abortive medications should be used for no more than 3 days per week. When prescribed, migraine-specific drugs, particularly the triptans,

should be used fewer than 9 times per month.[20] Thus, the clinician should make every effort to classify the headache type because this may have treatment implications.[21]

The initial outpatient treatment strategy should include over-the-counter medications, including ibuprofen and acetaminophen. Ibuprofen (10 mg/kg) is considered safe and effective, and acetaminophen (15 mg/kg) is probably as effective. Naproxen sodium (10 mg/kg) has been effective and routinely recommended in adults as a reasonable option for acute migraine with good response to a similar previously used NSAID and is often tried in children with acute migraine, often when ibuprofen is ineffective. Aspirin (10 mg/kg) can be considered in adolescents 16 years and older due to concerns for Reye syndrome in younger children.[15] Consistent with migraine management in pediatrics, opioids should be avoided due to lack of evidence for efficacy and concern for abuse and MOH or chronification.[20,21]

Triptans may be administered to patients whose headaches phenotype to migraine. Caution should be used in the very acute setting of mTBI because of the theoretical risk of vasospasm, which may exacerbate hypoperfusion in children who may have an underlying vascular injury to the brain. Imaging should be done prior to triptan administration in any child with headache and persistent altered mental status or focal neurologic findings.[21] Once ruled out, triptans should be taken at the onset of headache and can be repeated 2 hours later if needed. The dosage maximum per day and per week differs for each of the seven triptan medications, but all should be limited to no more than 9 days per month to avoid MOH. An adverse effect of triptan use includes tightness of the chest, throat, or head, which is often brief and transient.[11]

Preventive Treatments

There are no accepted guidelines to aid the clinician on the timing of initiation of preventive therapy. Some have argued that earlier initiation of such agents could potentially decrease the likelihood of developing persistent PTH.[22] Prophylaxis should be limited to children whose headaches occur with sufficient frequency and/or severity to warrant a daily preventive medication and should be considered if acute treatments are ineffective, poorly tolerated, contraindicated, or overused. The goals of treatment should be outlined at onset. Medications should be titrated to goal dose slowly. Delayed onset of preventive medication effect, often up to 6 to 8 weeks after initiation, must be highlighted to families. A treatment goal of having less than 3 to 4 headaches per month for a sustained period of 4 to 6 months is recommended prior to discontinuing therapy.[20,22] Few medications have been studied for PTH in a systematic way, and most are extrapolated from the migraine literature. There are no placebo-controlled randomized trials of how children with PTH respond to pharmacologic treatment strategies used for primary headache.

Nonpharmacologic Treatments

Nonpharmacologic treatments have established good evidence in children and adolescents with chronic headaches.[23] The US Headache Consortium found that cognitive behavioral therapy was supported by Grade A evidence for the prevention of migraine.[24] Lifestyle modifications are often discussed with patients, including hydration, sleep hygiene, and a well-balanced diet.

REFERENCES

1. Bazarian JJ, McClung J, Shah MN, Cheng YT, Flesher W, Kraus J. Mild traumatic brain injury in the United States, 1998–2000. *Brain Inj.* 2005;19(2):85-91.

2. Meehan WP 3rd, Mannix R. Pediatric concussions in United States emergency departments in the years 2002 to 2006. *J Pediatr.* 2010;157(6):889-893.

3. Powers SW, Andrasik F. Biobehavioral treatment, disability, and psychological effects of pediatric headache. *Pediatr Ann.* 2005;34(6):461-465.

4. McCrory P, Meeuwisse W, Dvorak J, et al. Consensus statement on concussion in sport—the 5th international conference on concussion in sport held in Berlin, October 2016. *Br J Sports Med.* 2017;51:838-847.

5. Lumba-Brown A, Yeates KO, Sarmiento K, et al. Centers for Disease Control and Prevention guideline on the diagnosis and management of mild traumatic brain injury among children [published correction appears in JAMA Pediatr. 2018 Nov 1; 172(11):1104]. *JAMA Pediatr.* 2018;172(11):e182853.

6. Kuppermann N, Holmes JF, Dayan PS, et al; Pediatric Emergency Care Applied Research Network (PECARN). Identification of children at very low risk of clinically-important brain injuries after head trauma: a prospective cohort study. *Lancet.* 2009;374(9696):1160-1170.

7. Lovell MR, Collins MW. Neuropsychological assessment of the college football player. *Head Trauma Rehabil.* 1998;13(2):9-26.

8. Centers for Disease Control and Prevention. Heads up. Brain injury basics. Returning to sports and activities. Accessed July 13, 2022. https://www.cdc.gov/headsup/basics/return_to_sports.html

9. Guskiewicz KM, Weaver NL, Padua DA, Garrett WE. Epidemiology of concussion in collegiate and high school football players. *Am J Sports Med.* 2000;28:643-650.

10. Eisenberg MA, Meehan WP, Mannix R. Duration and course of post-concussive symptoms. *Pediatrics.* 2014;133(6):999-1006.

11. Kuczynski A, Crawford S, Bodell L, Dewey D, Barlow K. Characteristics of post-traumatic headaches in children following mild traumatic brain injury and their response to treatment: a prospective cohort. *Dev Med Child Neurol.* 2013;55:636-641.

12. Headache Classification Committee of the International Headache Society (IHS). The International Classification of Headache Disorders, 3rd edition (beta version). *Cephalalgia.* 2013; 33(9):629-808.

13. Blume HK. Headaches after concussion in pediatrics: a review. *Curr Pain Headache Rep.* 2015;19(9):1-11.

14. Lucas S, Hoffman JM, Bell KR, Walker W, Dikmen S. Characterization of headache after traumatic brain injury. *Cephalalgia.* 2012;32(8):600-606.

15. Bramley H, Heverley S, Lewis MM, Kong L, Rivera R, Silvis M. Demographics and treatment of adolescent posttraumatic headache in a regional concussion clinic. *Pediatr Neurol.* 2015;52(5):493-498.

16. Morgan CD, Zuckerman SL, Lee YM, et al. Predictors of post-concussion syndrome after sports-related concussion in young athletes: a matched case-control study. *J Neurosurg Pediatr.* 2015;15(6):589-598.

17. Lane R, Davies P. Post traumatic headache (PTH) in a cohort of UK compensation claimants. *Cephalalgia.* 2019;39(5):641-647.

18. Pinchefsky E, Dubrovsky AS, Friedman D, Shevell M. Part I: evaluation of pediatric post-traumatic headaches. *Pediatr Neurol.* 2015;52(3):263-269.

19. Blume HK. Posttraumatic headache in pediatrics: an update and review. *Curr Opin Pediatr.* 2018;30(6):755-763.

20. Kacperski J, Arthur T. Management of post-traumatic headaches in children and adolescents. *Headache.* 2016;56(1):36-48.

21. Wilson MB, Krolczyk SJ. Pediatric post-traumatic headache. *Curr Pain Headache Rep.* 2006;10(5):387-390.

22. Pinchefsky E, Dubrovsky AS, Friedman D, Shevell M. Part II: management of pediatric post-traumatic headaches. *Pediatr Neurol.* 2015;52(3):270-280.

23. Blume HK, Brockman LN, Breuner CC. Biofeedback therapy for pediatric headache: factors associated with response. *Headache.* 2012;52(9):1377-1386.

24. Campbell JK, Penzien DB, Wall EM. Evidenced-based guidelines for migraine headache: behavioral and physical treatments. US Headache Consortium, American Academy of Neurology. 2000. Accessed July 13, 2022. http://www.aan.com/professionals/practice/pdfs/gl0089.pdf

38

Neurologic Complications of Systemic Disease

Kris Wesselkamper, MD

The nervous system is undoubtedly complex and susceptible to a wide range of ailments and diseases. What is equally true, and perhaps even more impressive, is the effect that all the other systems of the body, their diseases, and the treatments of those diseases can have on the nervous system. Delving into the neurologic complications of systemic disease is a book in itself, and in fact, there are several available. This chapter is going to provide a framework (and a few examples) of how to think about whether a systemic process, including the treatments, can affect the nervous system.

One way to think about neurologic complications of systemic disease is to think of the different systems in the body that get diseased. Those systems include, but are not limited to, the cardiac, vascular, pulmonary/respiratory, gastrointestinal, renal, urologic, skeletal, hematologic, endocrine, dermatologic, and reproductive systems. Now think about the diseases of those systems. That gets overwhelming very quickly. To add to that burden, think of the treatments for those diseases. That is a bit more than the mind can handle. Now try to list and prioritize which systems and diseases are the most important in causing neurologic complications. Are those the only ones that need to be learned about? Of course not! An alternate, and maybe simplified, way to think about how the nervous system is affected by systemic disease is to think about the ways the nervous system can be affected. By thinking this way, one can give anticipatory guidance about systemic diseases and treatments. It also allows for quicker identification of the cause of symptoms and the resolution of symptoms.

The acronym VITAMINS, which has variations, is used to think of the differential diagnoses of the nervous system. It can also be used to think of the different ways the nervous system can be affected by systemic disease. Admittedly,

thinking this way can lead to much overlap of categories; however, that is preferred to missing a complication.

V	Vascular – intracranial and extracranial
I	Infectious/inflammatory
T	Trauma/toxin
A	Autoimmune/allergic
M	Metabolic
I	Inflammatory/ingestion/iatrogenic
N	Neoplasm
S	Structural

VASCULAR

It is important to remember that vascular system causes of neurologic symptoms can come from the heart, intracranial vessels, extracranial vessels, large vessels, small vessels, arteries, and veins. The most obvious primary vascular nervous system disease is related to the larger intracranial vessels and results in ischemia or hemorrhagic strokes. When discussing pediatric complications of systemic disease, it is typically not the larger intracranial vessels that are the problem. Common conditions that lead to nervous system complications from systemic disease arise from the heart (congenital defects of valves; abnormal chambers; abnormal or defective septae; pulmonary vasculature anomalies; and smaller vascular anomalies as seen in moyamoya, cavernomas, arteriovenous malformations, and angiomas). Those can be conditions in of themselves or part of other conditions or syndromes. For example, moyamoya is more common in patients with Down syndrome, patients who have had intracranial radiation, patients who have neurofibromatosis type 1, patients who are of Asian descent, patients who have sickle cell disease, and patients who have a family history of moyamoya.

The large arteries are not the cause of strokes in pediatric patients. The venous system must also be considered. Patients can have cerebral sinovenous thrombosis (CSVT) from oral contraceptive pills, clotting disorders, infections, dehydration, cancer and its treatments, autoimmune disorders, inflammatory bowel disease, kidney disease, head or neck trauma, and cortical venous thrombosis.

The small intracranial arterioles can also be involved in complications. Posterior reversible encephalopathy syndrome is suspected to be the result of the small intracranial arterioles dilating and "leaking." This condition is frequently seen in pediatric patients with high blood pressure from kidney disease, patients who take immune-suppressing medications, patients who have lupus, patients who use illicit drugs, and patients with autonomic dysfunction.

Vasculitis is another complication of systemic disease that is seen on brain vessel imaging or angiography and that can affect the large, medium, and small intracranial vessels. Central nervous system (CNS) vasculitis can be the primary presenting symptom of many types of viral, bacterial, fungal, and other infections. It can also be a result of complications of autoimmune disorders, metabolic disorders, collagen disorders, genetic conditions, channelopathies, rheumatologic conditions, and other diseases associated with high inflammatory states (inflammatory bowel disease or Kawasaki disease). CNS vasculitis in children is known as childhood primary angiitis of the CNS.

Lastly, extracranial vein and artery disease can lead to neurologic complications. Sometimes the conditions need to be just right for symptoms to develop. Think about a patient with a deep vein thrombosis that causes a stroke through a patent foramen ovale. With that in mind, the extracranial vascular system should always be considered as a source of complications in managing patients with trauma, immobility, prolonged hospital stays, hypercoagulable states, and autoimmune conditions.

INFECTIONS

Primary infections in the CNS clearly cause neurologic symptoms, but it is important to remember that systemic infection can cause neurologic complications. Secondary abscesses or even direct infiltration of the infection is always possible. Conditions that exemplify this point are Pott puffy tumor from frontal sinusitis and acute otitis media or mastoiditis disseminating and causing meningitis. Lemierre syndrome, which also could be listed as a vascular cause, can lead to CSVT and even meningitis in a small percentage of patients. Other infection-related conditions that can cause infectious complications of the nervous system

include immunosuppression, indwelling lines or catheters, prolonged hospitalization for any reason, and postoperative states.

TRAUMA

Trauma to the head is a common cause of CNS symptoms in the pediatric population. It is important to remember that trauma to other systems of the body can lead to CNS complications. Trauma itself can lead to hypocoagulable states early after the injury and then to hypercoagulable states as more time passes after the injury. The CNS is susceptible to injury in both of those states. Pelvic bone and long bone fractures can result in fat embolism. The fat embolism can go to the lung and cause hypoxia, which can lead to CNS complications, or the emboli can go to the brain and cause cerebral fat embolism syndrome. In the same manner that a fat embolism can cause secondary hypoxia, a pericardial injury can also lead to anoxia or hypoxia depending on the extent cardiac output is affected. A third potential way the CNS can be affected by trauma is through hypoxia or anoxia in pulmonary contusion or pneumothorax. After the acute phase of the trauma, the recovery phase of the traumatic injury can lead to complications. Prolonged bed rest and immobility can lead to the formation of a deep vein thrombosis. Prolonged bed rest can also lead to skin breakdown and infections.

AUTOIMMUNE DISEASE AND NEOPLASM

Autoimmune disease has been mentioned several times already as having the potential to cause neurologic complications. Unfortunately, systemic autoimmune conditions are frequently identified based on their neurologic symptom presentations. Although that is true, the neurologic symptoms can also be the result of a complication. Those CNS symptoms can include vascular complications, encephalitis, seizures, mental status changes, and balance problems.

As mentioned, systemic autoimmune conditions can be diagnosed based on their neurologic symptoms. This is true of myasthenia gravis and its variants, neuromyelitis optic spectrum disorders, myelin oligodendrocyte glycoprotein antibody disorder, GAD65 limbic encephalitis, Guillain-Barré syndrome and its variants, neuromyotonia, and faciobrachial dystonic seizures. Therefore, if a patient has these conditions, then it is important to be aware of how complications may present.

A group within the autoimmune category where the neurologic symptoms lead to the systemic disease diagnoses is the paraneoplastic conditions. Sometimes it is hard to separate the 2 terms. As such, I added the "N" of VITAMINS in the autoimmune group. The most frequently associated neoplasms in children leading to autoimmune disease are neuroblastoma, thymoma, ovarian teratoma, and Hodgkin lymphoma.

METABOLIC

The metabolism of glucose, protein, and carbohydrates is affected in many systemic diseases. The conditions that first come to mind should include endocrinologic disorders and infections. Gastrointestinal diseases that affect intake or absorption, such as inflammatory bowel disease, eosinophilic esophagitis, or celiac disease, can cause nutrient deficiencies, as well as more systemic inflammation that can be seen as nervous system symptoms. Gastrointestinal processes such as bariatric surgery, bowel resection, trauma, and pancreatic islet cell transplantation can also lead to neurologic symptoms.

Oxygen is not often thought of as a nutrient, but it is essential to the proper functioning of the body and neurologic system. Diseases that cause hypoxia directly affect the nervous system, but they can also lead to neurologic complications by affecting other organs that then cause neurologic complications.

INFLAMMATORY

Organ dysfunction from injury, disease, or neoplasms can lead to inflammation. The reverse is also true, in that inflammation can lead to organ dysfunction. Sometimes, it is hard to tell which comes first. Regardless of which order the inflammation happens, neurologic complications are possible. The inflammation can be rapid in onset or be the result of a long-standing problem. The complications can be from the organ that is not performing its intended task, as is seen in hyperammonemia with liver dysfunction, or it can be the inflammation itself that is causing secondary neurologic symptoms, as is seen with coagulopathies from liver disease. The liver is not the only organ to be concerned about. The kidneys, heart, lungs, and thyroid are some of the other organs that cause neurologic symptoms.

STRUCTURAL

There are no systemic structural problems that lead to neurologic conditions that have not been discussed in another section.

BIBLIOGRAPHY

Alavi S. Paraneoplastic neurologic syndromes in children: a review article. *Iran J Child Neurol*. 2013;7(3):6-14.

Eilbert W, Singla N. Lemierre's syndrome. *Int J Emerg Med*. 2013;6(1):40.

Herard K, Khanni JL, Alusma-Hibbert K, et al. Neurological disorders associated with glutamic acid decarboxylase antibodies. *Cureus*. 2019;11(5):e4738.

Moore EE, Moore HB, Kornblith LZ, et al. Trauma-induced coagulopathy. *Nat Rev Dis Primers*. 2021;7(1):30.

Ndu IK, Ayuk AC, Onukwuli VO. Challenges of diagnosing pediatric posterior reversible encephalopathy syndrome in resource poor settings: a narrative review. *Glob Pediatr Health*. 2020;7:2333794X20947924.

Punnett A, Betcherman L. Paraneoplastic syndromes in children with Hodgkin lymphoma. *Oncol Hematol Rev*. 2017;13(1):41-44.

Twilt M, Benseler S. Childhood primary angiitis of the central nervous system. UpToDate. Last updated: March 4, 2021. Accessed July 13, 2022. https://www.uptodate.com/contents/childhood-primary-angiitis-of-the-central-nervous-system

Disorders of the Spinal Cord

S. Katie Ihnen, MD, PhD

ESSENTIALS OF DIAGNOSIS

► Spinal cord disorders can be organized into categories based on chronicity and etiology, keeping in mind that the categories are not rigid (eg, some entities can present either acutely or subacutely):

- Nontraumatic
  - Chronic
  - Subacute
  - Acute
- Traumatic
  - Acute

► Pathophysiology and epidemiology vary significantly by etiology.

► Certain anatomic variants (eg, spinal canal stenosis, disk herniation, osteophytes, abnormal ligamentous structures), chromosomal anomalies (eg, trisomy 21), connective tissue disorders (eg, Ehlers-Danlos), and bleeding diatheses (eg, hemophilia) can predispose to or worsen the impact of spinal cord injury.

► Some of the following sections are treated separately for nontraumatic and traumatic etiologies.

GENERAL CONSIDERATIONS, EPIDEMIOLOGY, AND PREVENTION

Nontraumatic

Epidemiology varies by etiology.

Traumatic

Spinal cord injuries affect many young people under age 30 years, with a male predominance.[1] Spinal cord injuries often result in significant medical, psychological, and economic sequelae, with lifetime expenses among patients with high cervical cord injury, for example, topping several million dollars.[1] Preventative strategies include the consistent use of safety devices such as seat belts and helmets.

PATHOGENESIS

Nontraumatic

Pathophysiology varies by etiology.

Traumatic

Pathophysiology includes primary injury (transient or persistent compression, cord laceration, or cord transection) as well as secondary injury (early hypoxia and hypoperfusion, followed by reperfusion, inflammation, and blood–spinal cord barrier disruption). Cord swelling peaks at 3 to 6 days and then subsides over weeks.[2]

CLINICAL FINDINGS

History

Nontraumatic

Chronicity and progression of symptoms are key historical details. Motor, sensory (including pain), and higher-order (cortical) symptoms should be queried, and their precise anatomic patterns discerned, keeping in mind that sensory *symptoms* can be more reliable than sensory *signs*. Sensory complaints can be elicited by asking, "Does water temperature feel the same everywhere when you shower or bathe?" When symptom onset is acute, the patient should be asked about urine and stool output over the past 24 hours. Vague abdominal discomfort and delay or loss of lower extremity motor function may suggest a thoracic lesion in a child. Clumsy gait may suggest a slowly progressive disorder. Another helpful clinical pearl is that transverse myelitis can evolve quite dramatically over a time course of hours.

Traumatic

Relevant medical history questions include the presence of genetic disorders or bleeding disorders since these diagnoses make a patient more vulnerable to spinal cord injury. Spinal shock may complicate the initial evaluation, manifesting as flaccid paralysis, areflexia, sensory loss, loss of bladder tone, and autonomic dysregulation. Traumatic brain injury co-occurs in 25% to 50% of spinal cord injury cases, and its evaluation should be considered.[2]

▶ Physical Exam

Physical exam should be comprehensive and timely, including close monitoring of vital signs for the presence of dysautonomia. The entire spine should be palpated for tenderness or deformity, and the skin overlying the base of the spine should be examined carefully for hair tufts, pits, masses, or abnormal pigmentation. For the neurologic exam, specific attention should be paid to the motor, deep tendon reflex, and sensory examinations. An ice-filled glove is more effective than the handle of a tool such as a reflex hammer for assessing temperature sensitivity. The sensory examination should include an attempt to establish a sensory level, which is the most caudal dermatomal level at which both light touch and sharp/dull discrimination are intact. If possible, sensory level should be assessed systematically on both sides of the body (left and right) and both on the back as well as the front of the body. Useful anatomic landmarks for remembering the dermatomes include the position of the nipples (at T4) and the umbilicus (at T10).[3] In some cases, the subjective sensory level may be higher than the objective sensory level. A positive Romberg sign suggests sensory ataxia and may help localize to the dorsal columns. An anorectal examination is mandatory, in part because sacral sparing helps distinguish an incomplete from a complete lesion. There are additional examination maneuvers that can be helpful in the evaluation of myelopathy, for example, the bulbocavernous, abdominal cutaneous, cremasteric, and anal wink reflexes. See Box 39–1 for additional useful exam manuevers.

The American Spinal Injury Association (ASIA) and International Medical Society of Paraplegia (IMSOP) have produced a document titled "International Standards for Neurological Classification of Spinal Cord Injury" that is useful for establishing an objective physical assessment that can be shared between providers.[3]

Box 39–1

- **Wheel-and-flare reaction:** The skin is scratched longitudinally in the paraspinal region, and the absence of a skin response indicates presence of an autonomic level
- **Upgoing toe:** Extension of great toe with or without splaying of toes in response to scratching the dorsum of the foot along the lateral side to the middle metatarsophalangeal joint; specific (but not sensitive) sign of corticospinal tract dysfunction
- **Hoffman sign:** Thumb and/or index finger flexes when middle fingernail is flicked down; specific (but not sensitive) sign of corticospinal tract dysfunction
- **Beevor sign:** Upward displacement of the umbilicus when a patient sits up or flexes the neck; suggests thoracic cord lesion
- **Lhermitte sign:** Electric sensation running down the back elicited by neck flexion; suggestive of a dorsal column lesion in the cervical spine

▶ Laboratory Findings

For acute myelopathies, unless there is a clearly compressive etiology, a lumbar puncture with cerebrospinal fluid (CSF) analysis should be obtained. Tests should include cell count, protein, glucose, culture, oligoclonal bands, immunoglobulin (Ig) G index, and other studies as appropriate. Serum studies may be indicated (eg, anti–aquaporin-4 and anti–myelin oligodendrocyte glycoprotein in patients with longitudinally extensive myelitis).

▶ Imaging Studies

Stabilize the cervical spine and obtain immediate imaging if the onset is acute.[2] Computed tomography (CT) is best to evaluate for bony involvement, although 3-view plain films can be substituted. In children, the cervical spine is more flexible than it is in adults, so bony injury may not be evident, despite cord injury. Magnetic resonance imaging (MRI) is more sensitive than CT to ligamentous injury.

For evaluating the cord itself, whole-spine MRI is appropriate for screening for neoplastic lesions or cord compression; otherwise, image segments of the cord is based on clinical localization. Gadolinium should be used when there is concern for inflammation or neoplasm.[4] T2 short tau inversion recovery is useful for lesions containing lipids. T2 is better than T1 for parenchymal lesions. It is crucial to review images in multiple planes. Also, spine MRI is highly susceptible to artifacts (related to motion, respiration, CSF pulsation, arterial pulsation, and swallowing); these can be especially problematic in children and may lead to falsely negative imaging.[5] Alternatively, the clinical pattern may not match the observed MRI abnormality. For this reason, one should not be overly reliant on imaging; myelopathy is a clinical diagnosis! Consider adding brain MRI when there is myelitis of unclear etiology.

Special Tests: Bowel and bladder

Early in an acute spinal cord disorder, bowel and bladder dysfunction can be problematic (and are sometimes overlooked and undertreated). Have a low threshold to perform a bladder scan and perform urinary catheterization if necessary. Beware that recurrent "constipation" can herald myelopathy. Ongoing bowel and bladder monitoring should be considered.

Special Tests: Respiratory

High cervical spine lesions may cause respiratory failure, which is typically not subtle. However, lower cervical and some upper thoracic lesions can also cause respiratory weakness and even failure. Keep in mind that "asthma" and weakness might not be asthma at all. If respiratory symptoms are suspected, obtain objective measures of neuromuscular function, and do not rely on oxygen saturation monitoring. In our center, we ask the respiratory therapists to record and trend parameters including negative inspiratory force and forced vital capacity.

Special Tests: Electromyography and Nerve Conduction Studies

In cases with unclear localization between spinal cord and peripheral nerves, electromyography and nerve conduction studies may be useful. If necessary, children can be sedated for these studies.

DIFFERENTIAL DIAGNOSIS AND COMMON ETIOLOGIES

For anatomic localization, a lesion must be at or above the established sensory level (since the spinothalamic tracts ascend as they decussate, the lesion will actually be *2 to 3* vertebral segments above the level with normal pain and temperature sensation).[6] A motor level can be determined by deciding whether the muscles innervated by a single spinal nerve are affected. Patterns of symptoms can be helpful; Table 39–1 lists the spinal cord syndromes with their associated symptoms,[7] as well as the common traumatic and nontraumatic etiologies.

Nontraumatic

These designations by typical chronicity are not fixed; some entities can present at more than one time scale.

Chronic

- Spinal dysraphism (eg, tethered cord in association with a fatty filum terminale, a dermal sinus, or a lipoma)
- Genetic/metabolic (eg, hereditary spastic paraplegia, adrenomyeloneuropathy, spinal muscular atrophy, Friedrich ataxia, spinocerebellar ataxia)

- Neoplastic (in children, most likely ependymoma or astrocytoma)
- Nutritional (eg, vitamin B_{12}, copper, and vitamin E deficiencies)
- Multiple sclerosis (MS)
- Toxic (eg, chemotherapy-related, nitrous oxide poisoning)
- Others (more common in adults) (eg, spinal dural arteriovenous fistula, amyotrophic lateral sclerosis)

Subacute

- Spinal epidural abscess (back pain and fever are useful clues)
- Spinal epidural hematoma (more likely in children with underlying bleeding diatheses)
- Neuromyelitis optica spectrum disorders (NMOSD), MS, and other inflammatory conditions (note that the number of involved vertebral segments in myelopathy due to NMOSD will be 3 or more, as compared to MS, in which lesions spanning fewer than 3 vertebral segments are seen[8])
- Infectious (eg, HIV and syphilis)
- Infectious (eg, acute flaccid myelitis associated with enterovirus D68, Lyme disease, West Nile disease; of note, an infectious etiology for spinal cord dysfunction was first described by Hippocrates, probably in reference to tuberculosis[9])
- Toxic (eg, nitrous oxide exposure)

Acute

- Spinal cord infarction/postoperative hypoperfusion (may present with pure motor signs; can be seen in neonates following umbilical artery catheterization; other etiologies in pediatric patients include fibrocartilaginous embolism and vertebral dissection[10])
- Acute transverse myelitis (primary or secondary; represents important category in pediatrics; defined by the onset of bilateral signs and symptoms with a clearly defined sensory level progressing over the course of several hours to 3 weeks; CSF should demonstrate pleocytosis and/or elevated IgG index; lesion on spinal MRI should enhance)
- Acute disseminated encephalomyelitis (encephalopathy is a key clue)

Traumatic

Important causes of acute spinal cord injuries in children include motor vehicle accidents (52%), sports-related injuries (27%), falls (15%), and child abuse (3%), as well as gunshot

Table 39–1. Spinal cord syndromes.

Syndrome	Symptoms	Nontraumatic Etiologies	Traumatic Mechanisms	Notes
Complete cord	Complete sensory, motor, and autonomic dysfunction below level of lesion	Severe tumor suppression, transverse myelitis, epidural abscess	Transection in the setting of high-impact trauma	
Central cord	Paresis of arms > legs, distal > proximal; variable sensory change (often, cape-like distribution of pain and temperature loss with relative preservation of lower limb sensation)	Syringomyelia, intramedullary tumor (the latter of which is usually associated with cord expansion)	Neck hyperextension	White matter more affected than gray matter
Anterior (ventral) cord	Motor function +/− pain and temperature lost distal to injury	Anterior spinal artery infarction	Flexion injury of retropulsed disk or bone	Posterior columns spared; poor prognosis for recovery
Posterior (dorsal) column	Vibration and proprioception (+/− some motor) lost distal to injury	Infectious, toxic/metabolic, inflammatory, compression	Neck hyperextension	Subacute combined degeneration defines the condition when due to vitamin B_{12} deficiency (in which case, lateral columns are also involved)
Brown-Séquard	Ipsilateral motor, vibration, and proprioception lost at level of injury, contralateral pain and temperature lost 1-2 dermatomes below level of injury	Multiple sclerosis affecting lateral half of the cord	Penetrating injury (less commonly, blunt trauma)	Bladder spared
Cervicomedullary	Respiratory compromise, hypotension, tetraparesis (arms worse than legs), hyperesthesia, onion-skin sensory loss over the face		Injuries to atlantoaxial complex, burst fractures	Risk factors include trisomy 21, rheumatoid arthritis, ankylosing spondylitis
Conus medullaris	Early and prominent sphincter dysfunction (bowel and bladder); symmetric motor impairment that may be distal > proximal; diminished ankle DTRs with brisk patella DTRs; saddle anesthesia/hypesthesia; sexual dysfunction	Disk herniation, neoplastic	Burst fracture or fracture-dislocation in thoracolumbar region (above L2)	Upper *and* lower motor neuron involvement
Cauda equina	Saddle anesthesia/hypesthesia; radicular pain in lower back and/or legs; diminished lower extremity reflexes; sexual dysfunction; +/− asymmetric lower extremity weakness	Disk herniation, neoplastic, inflammatory, infiltrative	Burst fracture or fracture-dislocation in lumbar region (usually L4/L5, L5/S1)	Lower motor neuron involvement only; lower extremity involvement only

DTR, deep tendon reflexes.

wounds and other less frequent injuries.[11] The vast majority of spinal cord injuries in children involve the cervical spine. Of the various spinal cord syndromes listed in Table 39–1, central cord injuries are the most common.

TREATMENT

▶ Nontraumatic

Treat respiratory, bowel, and bladder dysfunction. Identify and treat the underlying etiology, involving other medical specialists as necessary. Some entities require a high index of suspicion due to the need for prompt treatment (eg, spinal epidural abscess).

▶ Traumatic

Traumatic myelopathy should be treated as a neurologic emergency. Initial management is likely to occur in the intensive care unit with the assistance of the critical care, neurosurgery, rehabilitation, and palliative care teams. Stabilize the cervical spine. Manage immediate complications including spinal shock (oxygenate and perfuse), neurogenic shock (administer fluids and vasopressors), and respiratory failure (ventilate). Place nasogastric tube and Foley catheter. Determine candidacy for decompressive surgery, with some data showing improved outcomes if surgery is performed within 24 hours.[12] Current guidelines from the American Association of Neurological Surgeons and Congress of Neurological Surgeons do not advocate for the use of steroids, with National Acute Spinal Cord Injury Study trials[13,14] showing higher morbidity and mortality associated with steroid use. Another randomized controlled trial found no improvement in neurologic outcomes at 1 year for patients with spinal cord injury who were treated with methylprednisolone acutely.[15] Ongoing studies are examining a potential role for therapeutic hypothermia for acute spinal cord injury.[16] Some data suggest roles for riluzole, minocycline, and fibroblast growth factor, but treatment with these agents is not standardized. Research into the potential utility of stem cell therapy for those with spinal cord injury is ongoing.[17]

PROGNOSIS

Overall, factors that modulate prognosis include age, spinal cord level, neurologic grade, and medical comorbidities.

▶ Nontraumatic

Prognosis varies by etiology.

▶ Traumatic

Acute in-hospital mortality rates range from 4% to 17%.[1] The ASIA/IMSOP Spinal Cord Impairment Scale is a 5-level scale indicating level of impairment, ranging from A, denoting complete impairment, through E, indicating normal motor and sensory function (B, C, and D describe increasingly milder degrees of incomplete impairment).[3]

COMPLICATIONS

Short-term complications relevant during the acute admission include refractory shock, respiratory failure, dysphagia, infections, venous thromboembolism, and stress gastroduodenal ulcers. Long-term sequelae of acute spinal cord injury are also important and include urinary retention, constipation, neuropathic pain, spasticity, autonomic dysreflexia (especially for injuries at T6 or higher), decubitus ulcers, syringomyelia, sexual dysfunction, venous thromboembolism, obesity, heterotopic ossification, depression, and other mental health disorders.[1] Preparing the home for optimal supportive care should be a priority at the time of discharge from the hospital. Psychological care for easing the transition to a new level of function should be sought proactively. Physical therapy, gait training, and adaptive technology should be pursued as appropriate. The involvement of social work, the utilization of available community resources, and

a supportive friend/family network are all extremely helpful for best long-term outcomes.

REFERENCES

1. Ahuja CS, Wilson JR, Nori S, et al. Traumatic spinal cord injury. *Nat Rev Dis Primers.* 2017;3:17018. doi:10.1038/nrdp.2017.18
2. Rabinstein AA. Traumatic spinal cord injury. *Continuum (Minneap Minn).* 2018;24(2):551-566. doi:10.1212/CON.0000000000000581
3. Kirshblum SC, Burns SP, Biering-Sorensen F, et al. International standards for neurological classification of spinal cord injury (revised 2011). *J Spinal Cord Med.* 2011;34(6):535-546. doi:10.1179/204577211X13207446293695
4. Diehn FE, Krecke KN. Neuroimaging of spinal cord and cauda equina disorders. *Continuum (Minneap Minn).*2021;27(1):225-263. doi:10.1212/CON.0000000000000926
5. Hamilton MG, Myles ST. Pediatric spinal injury: review of 174 hospital admissions. *J Neurosurg.* 1992;77(5):700-704. doi:10.3171/jns.1992.77.5.0700
6. Diaz E, Morales H. Spinal cord anatomy and clinical syndromes. *Semin Ultrasound CT MR.* 2016;37(5):360-371. doi:10.1053/j.sult.2016.05.002
7. Hardy TA. Spinal cord anatomy and localization. *Continuum (Minneap Minn).* 2021;27(1):12-29. doi:10.1212/CON.0000000000000899
8. Lopez Chiriboga S, Flanagan EP. Myelitis and other autoimmune myelopathies. *Continuum (Minneap Minn).* 2021;27(1):62-92. doi:10.1212/CON.0000000000000900
9. New PW. A narrative review of pediatric nontraumatic spinal cord dysfunction. *Top Spinal Cord Inj Rehabil.* 2019;25(2):112-120. doi:10.1310/sci2502-112
10. Zalewski NL. Vascular myelopathies. *Continuum (Minneap Minn).* 2021;27(1):30-61. doi:10.1212/CON.0000000000000905
11. Huisman TA, Wagner MW, Bosemani T, Tekes A, Poretti A. Pediatric spinal trauma. *J Neuroimaging.* 2015;25(3):337-353. doi:10.1111/jon.12201
12. Badhiwala JH, Wilson JR, Witiw CD, et al. The influence of timing of surgical decompression for acute spinal cord injury: a pooled analysis of individual patient data. *Lancet Neurol.* 2021;20(2):117-126. doi:10.1016/S1474-4422(20)30406-3
13. Bracken MB, Shepard MJ, Collins WF, et al. A randomized, controlled trial of methylprednisolone or naloxone in the treatment of acute spinal-cord injury. Results of the Second National Acute Spinal Cord Injury Study. *N Engl J Med.* 1990;322(20):1405-1411. doi:10.1056/NEJM199005173222001
14. Bracken MB, Shepard MJ, Holford TR, et al. Administration of methylprednisolone for 24 or 48 hours or tirilazad mesylate for 48 hours in the treatment of acute spinal cord injury. Results of the Third National Acute Spinal Cord Injury Randomized Controlled Trial. National Acute Spinal Cord Injury Study. *JAMA.* 1997;277(20):1597-1604.
15. Pointillart V, Petitjean ME, Wiart L, et al. Pharmacological therapy of spinal cord injury during the acute phase. *Spinal Cord.* 2000;38(2):71-76. doi:10.1038/sj.sc.3100962
16. Alkabie S, Boileau AJ. The role of therapeutic hypothermia after traumatic spinal cord injury: a systematic review. *World Neurosurg.* 2016;86:432-449. doi:10.1016/j.wneu.2015.09.079
17. Shende P, Subedi M. Pathophysiology, mechanisms and applications of mesenchymal stem cells for the treatment of spinal cord injury. *Biomed Pharmacother.* 2017;91:693-706. doi:10.1016/j.biopha.2017.04.126

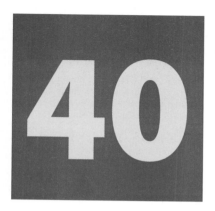

Deafness, Dizziness, and Disorders of Equilibrium

Kris Wesselkamper, MD

The eighth cranial nerve (vestibulocochlear nerve) has the dual function of sending input about noise and position to the brain.

DEAFNESS

INTRODUCTION

Hearing is one of the 5 major senses. It is crucial for the ability to learn and interact with the environment we live in. The loss of hearing, whether partial or complete, can be devastating for development at any time. The loss of hearing in early development can be even more detrimental. Without the ability to hear a parent's voice, one's own cry, or one's own babbling, the future ability to produce language and, ultimately, the ability to verbally communicate will be impaired. The many reasons for hearing loss vary across the neonate, infant, toddler, child, and adolescent. Hearing loss can be caused by a congenital defect from an infection, a toxic exposure, or a genetic cause. Hearing loss can be acquired from frequent ear infections or fluid behind the tympanic membrane (TM). Metabolic, traumatic, and compressive nerve injuries can also cause hearing loss.

Whether a child is brought in for concerns about hearing or being seen for a well-child check, screening for hearing function at every opportunity is crucial. The family will provide clues to help determine if there are concerns about hearing function. Knowledge of normal development is a necessity to be able to identify when development is abnormal. The exam is used to give additional clues to help determine the onset of the deafness and the severity.

PRESENTATION

▶ Hearing Loss in Neonates and Infants

Expectations of normal development must be used to determine whether hearing is abnormal. The history should be used to screen if the baby has an intact Moro reflex. Since most parents may not know what that is, ask if the patient reacts to a dog barking, doors slamming, a car horn beeping, or sirens. Did the infant ever respond to any of those things? Does the baby turn to sound both ways? This will help determine if the hearing loss is unilateral or bilateral. It is possible for the hearing loss to be asymmetrical, so asking about response to different levels of noise is also important. Ask about the noises the baby makes. The age of the patient will guide the level of sound they should be making. Does the patient coo or babble? Does the baby have different cries? Are any consonant sounds being made? Do they say "dada," "mama," or any other consonant words? How many words do they have? Do they use 2-word sentences?

▶ Hearing Loss in Toddlers and Older Children

Indicators that are suspicious of hearing loss in older children are similar to those in neonates and infants. Such clues include not turning to the source of a sound without a visual clue, not following commands, ignoring people frequently, or not paying attention frequently. Other clues can include if they sing the wrong words to songs or if the volume of their music or television is higher than seems necessary. One important question to ask families that will help guide a differential is whether these clues are acute in onset or have progressed over time.

TESTING

Screening for hearing function ideally begins in neonates in the nursery before discharge. Getting the report is always beneficial to know if hearing was ever normal. The Centers for Disease Control and Prevention, American Academy of Pediatrics, American Academy of Audiology, Joint Committee on Infant Hearing, American

Speech-Language-Hearing Association, and National Center for Hearing Assessment and Management all have guidelines for some components of screening, rescreening (if needed), testing (when suspected/identified), development of an intervention plan, and implementation of a treatment plan. The key to a successful outcome in hearing loss and deafness is early detection.

Regardless of the degree of concern about hearing loss, a child not screened before discharge from the nursery should be screened before 1 month of age. A baby who failed the screen should have the test repeated before 3 months of age.

PATHOPHYSIOLOGY

The prevalence of hearing loss varies throughout life. The prevalence of permanent sensorineural hearing loss (SNHL) is reported as 1 to 3 in 1000. Newborn nursery hearing loss is reported at 1 in 1000. Babies in the newborn intensive care unit have a 10-fold increased incidence compared with the newborn nursery, with a hearing loss rate of 10 in 1000. The rate at the time of school is reported to be 6 in 1000. By the age of 65 years, 1 in 3 people have enough irreversible hair cell damage to have hearing loss.

There are several forms of hearing loss and varying degrees of each type. Conductive hearing loss is the dysfunction in hearing caused by the restriction of sound waves from reaching the inner ear where they are turned into sounds. This happens when there is an obstruction in the outer or middle ear. SNHL refers to the dysfunction of the nerve that carries the signal to the brain. Both types of loss can occur at the same time. There is also an auditory neuropathy spectrum disorder in which sound is not organized in a way that the brain can understand.

When discussing hearing loss, the degree of loss is also important to know. With mild loss, a person may hear some speech sounds but it is hard to hear soft sounds. Moderate loss results in almost no speech being heard when another person is talking at a normal level. Severe loss causes a person to hear no speech when a person is talking at a normal level, and they hear only some loud sounds. In profound hearing loss, a person hears no speech and only very loud sounds.

EXAM

An easy way to test hearing, and the Moro reflex, during an exam is to watch the patient's response to hands clapped close to their ear. It is best performed if the patient does not see that the clap is going to happen. Otherwise, observation will give you an idea of the patient's degree of language.

In an office setting with a cooperative patient, you can use a 512-Hz tuning fork to help determine the patient's type of hearing loss. In normal hearing, air conduction is better than bone conduction. The Rinne test is used to compare unilateral bone conduction versus air conduction. The tuning fork is placed on the mastoid and then moved adjacent to the ear, with tuning fork tines perpendicular to the ear canal. When air conduction hearing is perceived longer than bone conduction hearing, the test is positive and indicates normal hearing or SNHL. If the sound is heard longer with bone conduction than air conduction, then the test is negative, and a conductive hearing loss is present.

The Weber test uses a 512-Hz tuning fork placed on the midline vertex, forehead, or teeth of the patient. The sound should be heard equally in both ears. With unilateral conductive loss, the sound lateralizes to the affected ear. With SNHL, the sounds localize to the normal-hearing ear.

DIFFERENTIAL DIAGNOSIS OF HEARING LOSS

- Vascular: cortical deafness
- Infectious: intrauterine cytomegalovirus, toxoplasmosis, herpes simplex virus, measles, mumps, rubella, syphilis, Zika; meningitis; recurrent/chronic otitis media (external and acute otitis media, serous otitis media)
- Traumatic: external ear and canal injuries, ruptured TM, temporal bone fractures, ossicle or cochlear fracture
- Autoimmune/inflammatory: neuronitis
- Metabolic/toxin: hyperbilirubinemia, asphyxia, teratogen exposure, medication exposure; mitochondrial; heavy metal exposure
- Inherited: microtia, genetic causes with or without a known syndrome
- Neoplastic: schwannoma
- Structural: cerumen or foreign body, TM cholesteatoma, exostoses or osteomas, otosclerosis, perilymph fistula, excessive nerve damage

EVALUATION

The first step in identifying hearing loss is having the awareness to screen for it. The second step is identifying what specialists the child should see for further evaluation.

Confirming the diagnosis of hearing loss, regardless of age, is best accomplished by having a formal hearing screen performed by an audiologist. There are several testing options available. The most common are the auditory brainstem response, the otoacoustic emissions test, and the behavior auditory evaluation. The audiologist will determine which test to perform based on the patient's age and ability to cooperate.

If hearing loss is confirmed, then a referral to an otolaryngologist (ie, ear-nose-throat [ENT]) is warranted. They will be able to evaluate the hearing loss and treat cerumen impaction, persistent fluid behind the TM, frequent or recurrent otitis media, and other potential causes of conductive hearing loss. The otolaryngologist will then determine what type of additional testing is needed. The most common additional testing will consist of imaging with magnetic resonance imaging (MRI) or computed tomography.

Other specialists who may be of value to the patient and family are geneticists. They can help determine if there is a heritable cause for the hearing loss, even if there is no family history.

TREATMENT

The treatment for hearing loss depends on the age of the patient at the time of diagnosis, the developmental level of the patient, and, of course, the cause. Some interventions may focus on restoring hearing (hearing aids), some may focus on preventing further loss (tumor debulking), and some may focus on improving communication, whether it be verbal or another type (speech-language therapy and communication devices).

Surgical interventions are quite variable. They include the common pressure equalization (PE) tubes, more formally known as tympanostomy tubes or ventilating tubes; cochlear or brainstem implants; and bone-anchored hearing aids.

▼ EQUILIBRIUM AND BALANCE

INTRODUCTION

The sense of balance is determined by the vestibular system, which is composed of the peripheral (inner ear) and central nervous system structures. The peripheral structures include the 3 semicircular canals, cochlea, and otolith organs. The central nervous system structures include the vestibulocochlear nerve, cerebellum, and vestibular nuclei. The vestibulocochlear nerve receives input from the peripheral vestibular system and sends the message to the cerebellum. The semicircular canals detect rotational head movement, and the otolith organs detect linear acceleration and gravitational forces. Any disruption to the system can present with ataxia (dizziness, lightheadedness) and vertigo (the sensation of movement when there is none).

PRESENTATION

Children with problems with the vestibular system can present with trouble walking, episodes of clinging to their parents, or frequent falls. The terms *lightheaded* and *ataxia* are frequently used, often incorrectly. The episodes can be acute in onset, subacute, or even chronic in some cases. Determining if falls happen in the same direction can be valuable. It is sometimes difficult to get some of the details about what a child is experiencing. Other symptoms of vestibular dysfunction can include tinnitus, nausea, and hearing loss.

PATHOPHYSIOLOGY

Any disruption of normal function along the system can result in symptoms. Inflammation, infection, compression, trauma, toxins, and tumors can all affect the way position and balance are detected. It is important to remember that the cerebellar hemispheres control the ipsilateral body.

EXAM

The exam is crucial in determining the level of concern for the complaints of vertigo. There is an advantage to seeing more children who complain of balance problems because determining a real balance problem from a functional problem can be difficult. Watching for nystagmus is beneficial, but its absence does not rule out a pathologic cause, especially if symptoms are intermittent. The Dix-Hallpike maneuver can be beneficial to help induce symptoms in patients who have an otolith that has been dislodged. Gait and tandem gait are also beneficial. The side of the unsteadiness or the direction of falling can be useful. Identifying whether there are coordination problems in the upper and lower extremities can also be of benefit.

DIFFERENTIAL DIAGNOSES

- Central causes
  - Constant
  - Hearing intact
  - Other cranial nerve findings
  - Single direction
- Peripheral causes
  - Episodic, acute onset
  - Hearing loss
  - Tinnitus
  - No other cranial nerve findings
  - Ataxia with eyes closed
  - Can have nystagmus
  - Variable direction
- Vascular: transient ischemic attack, stroke, migraine
- Infectious: meningitis, labyrinthitis, neuronitis, cerebellitis, encephalitis, otitis
- Traumatic
- Autoimmune: multiple sclerosis
- Metabolic/toxin: drugs, medications

- Inherited: epilepsy
- Neoplastic: neuromas, schwannomas, cerebellar tumors
- Structural: Ménière, trauma

EVALUATION

Evaluation includes MRI of the brain, vestibular testing, and lumbar puncture.

TREATMENT

Treatment varies greatly based on the identified cause but can include steroids, antibiotics, antivirals, vestibular physical therapy, antiepileptic medications, clot removal and antiplatelets, migraine medications, stopping medications, surgical interventions for neoplasms, and diuretics for Ménière disease.

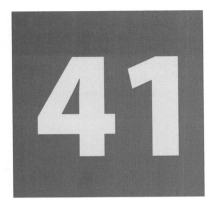

Approach to Pediatric Vision Disorders

Kevin X. Zhang, PhD

Veeral S. Shah, MD, PhD

INTRODUCTION

At their core, human beings are visual beings, and this is evidenced by the fact that most of the human brain is devoted to the visual system. The visual sensory or afferent pathways not only include the retina, optic nerve, chiasm, optic tract, lateral geniculate nucleus, optic radiations, and primary visual cortex, but also the parietal and temporal lobes, which are involved in processing visual information to produce a rich and vibrant sensory experience. The motor or efferent visual system, which directs eye movement to optimize target-specific viewing of the object of interest and capture visual information, requires extraocular muscles, cranial nerves, and their nuclei, which are found in the midbrain, pons, and brainstem. However, they also require the supranuclear network found in the frontal eye fields, parietal lobe, supplementary eye fields, superior colliculus, basal ganglia, and reticular formation.

In human development, there is a dynamic interplay between the sensory and motor visual pathways, which depend on each other at critical periods to establish normal vision. Moreover, abnormalities in development and/or childhood-acquired dysfunction in either motor or sensory domains can ultimately disrupt development of both areas. Disorders of vision and ocular motility in pediatric patients can impede other areas of normal development and later affect a child's independence, education, social interactions, and daily function.

In this chapter, we focus on disorders of subnormal vision and ocular dysmotility by reviewing pediatric neuro-ophthalmic history and examination. Furthermore, this chapter is intended to serve as a framework to approach the child with abnormal visual behavior and abnormal eye movements.

PEDIATRIC NEURO-OPHTHALMIC HISTORY

History in our complex neurologic patients can be quite time consuming. To expedite data collection during the interview, patients and their families are often requested to bring neuroimaging, prior ocular or neurologic exams, and any testing (eg, laboratory workup, ocular imaging) to the office visit.

▶ History of Present Illness

History taking ought to be open-ended and general so as not to bias responses from the child or the parents. Below is a framework for organizing questions to cover the principal aspects of functional vision in a new pediatric patient:

1. **Introductory questions:** "Do you have any concerns about your child's vision?" and "What do you think your child can and cannot see?" are some examples of introductory questions. The answers to these general questions can help direct the interview to focus on specific domains of vision and ocular motility.

2. **Peripheral vision:** Asking how the child navigates their environment can reveal localizable visual field deficits such as hemianopsias. Example questions include "How does your child get around the room or house?" and "Does your child bump into things?" It should be noted that unusual head movements or postures might not always implicate visual field defects but may rather suggest ocular motility disorders such as nystagmus or diplopia.

3. **Central vision (visual acuity):** This can best be ascertained by asking the parents to bring books or pictures to which they know the child responds. The smaller and more detailed an object or text that garners a response from the child, the better is the functional acuity.

4. **Near and distance vision:** Asking how close the child holds objects (books or toys) to their eyes or how far they sit from the television can provide information on the likelihood of certain conditions over others.

5. **Color vision:** Direct questioning on whether the child sees certain colors better than others can help guide

decision making toward conditions that affect color vision and contrast sensitivity. For example, good contrast sensitivity is required to be able to make out people's facial features.

Past Medical History

In children with abnormal visual behavior and/or eye movements, it is important to determine if there were any signs of central nervous system (CNS) damage in early development. It is very important to obtain prenatal, birth, and postnatal history for these children.

Prenatal history can include maternal infections (eg, cytomegalovirus, HIV, *Toxoplasma*), preeclampsia/eclampsia, gestational diabetes, in utero drug exposure, and trauma. Also important are any abnormalities noted on neuroimaging or in utero ultrasound (eg, enlarged ventricles). Birth history can include prematurity, intrauterine growth restriction, forceps trauma, perinatal infections, or abnormal Apgar scores. Postnatal history can include any systemic developmental abnormalities (eg, hypotonia, cleft lip, midface hypoplasia, craniofacial/craniosynostosis), immunodeficiencies, and metabolic/neurodegenerative/genetic disorders.

Family History

It is crucial to inquire about ocular history with regard to primary and extended family, as many visual conditions contain genetic or hereditary components. Example conditions with evidence of familial etiology are listed in Table 41–1.

Surgical History

Taking a comprehensive surgical history is crucial to augment understanding of previous ocular and neurologic problems. With respect to a child's vision, both prior eye surgeries and intracranial surgeries are especially important. Notable intra- and extraocular pediatric surgeries can include cataract extraction, glaucoma, orbital surgery, orbital fracture repair, eyelid surgery, and extraocular muscle surgery for strabismus. In reference to intracranial surgical history, procedures such as craniosynostosis repair, hydrocephalus or elevated intracranial pressure surgery (eg, ventriculostomy, ventriculoperitoneal shunting), tumor resection, and intracranial hemorrhage evacuation are important to ask about.

Medication and Allergies

It is important to ask the child or parents about present and past medications for both ocular and medical conditions. Typical ocular medications include artificial tears, antiallergy eyedrops, and antiglaucoma eyedrops. Many medications are important in the etiology of many neuro-ophthalmic conditions. It is also helpful to assess compliance by asking whether the family has been able to use their medication as prescribed. In instances where medication is found to be ineffective, understanding patient compliance and potential barriers can guide decision making.

It is also important to review allergies to medications or other substances.

PEDIATRIC NEURO-OPHTHALMIC EXAMINATION

The goals of the pediatric neuro-ophthalmic examination are to properly assess the refractive, binocular, accommodative, sensory, and motor functions of the visual system, while taking into account special vision demands and needs of the patient. Although there are many components of a comprehensive ophthalmic examination, this section focuses specifically on those that relate to neuro-ophthalmology and can be

Table 41–1. Pediatric disorders of the visual system with genetic components organized by anatomy.

Anterior segment	• Congenital abnormalities of the cornea
	  • Axenfeld-Rieger syndrome
	  • Sclerocornea
	  • Peter anomaly
	• Keratoconus
	• Corneal dystrophies
	• Congenital cataract
	• Metabolic diseases
	  • Hunter syndrome
	  • Hurler syndrome
	  • Galactosemia
	• Childhood glaucoma
	• Aniridia
	• Albinism

Posterior segment	• Retinoblastoma
	• Retinitis pigmentosa
	• High refractive errors
	• Leber congenital amaurosis
	• Choroideremia
	• Achromatopsias
	• Retinal and macular dystrophies
	  • Cone-rod dystrophy
	  • Stargardt disease
	• Other rare inherited diseases
	  • Norrie disease
	  • Batten disease

Optic nerve and tract	• Optic nerve hypoplasia • Optic nerve atrophy • Leber hereditary optic neuropathy • Kjer optic neuropathy
Central nervous system	• Seizure disorders • Cerebral visual impairment • Williams-Beuren syndrome • Arnold-Chiari malformation

evaluated by a pediatric neurologist without the need for specialized ophthalmic equipment and instruments. It should be noted that different exam techniques may be suitable for patients of a specific age group. An overall framework for organizing the exam is as follows:

- General appearance and external exam
- Base vision exam (including acuity, refraction, and stereopsis)
- Ocular motility and alignment
- Pupils
- Visual fields
- Color vision
- Anterior examination
- Posterior examination
- Miscellaneous adjuncts

▶ General Appearance and External Exam

The external exam of the eye should follow a systematic approach (ie, from front to back or from external to internal). Begin with the lids by observing the position with regard to the fellow eye to look for signs of ptosis. Redness or swelling of the lids can be a clue indicating an infectious process such as orbital cellulitis or an inflammatory process such as angioedema. Look for signs of lacerations (trauma), lumps/bumps (chalazion, stye, sebaceous cysts), rashes, ulcerations, thickening, or discolorations. Check the eyelashes and look for signs of redness, discharge, or crusting (blepharitis, ectropion, entropion). Examine the lacrimal system and the puncta for possible redness, blockage, swelling, discharge, or pain. Next, observe the conjunctiva for color, injection, pallor, cysts, ulcerations, or discharge. Everting the lids may be necessary to look for the presence of foreign bodies, follicles, or papillae. Finally, examine the ocular surface or cornea for clarity. Take note regarding whether the child is wearing contact lenses. Examining the anterior chamber is limited without a slit lamp, but observe for presence of pus (hypopyon) or blood (hyphema).

▶ Base Vision Exam

A patient's base vision exam provides the first and often most important objective set of metrics for visual function. In pediatric patients, it primarily consists of visual acuity, refraction, and stereopsis. Visual acuity in infants and toddlers can be qualitatively assessed by using preferential looking methods, such as assessing a child's ability to show steady fixation of a target and to follow the target using smooth pursuit movements. Visual acuity in preschool-age children can begin leveraging the child's verbal responses through symbol or letter optotype matching/testing. Visual acuity in school-age children can be assessed with adult methods such as Snellen

visual acuity, at distance and near vision, with or without the child's spectacle or contact lens correction, if applicable.

Refraction should be performed in infants and toddlers using retinoscopy with loose lenses primarily because of their short attention span and poor fixation ability. Cycloplegic retinoscopy with an appropriate agent (0.5% cyclopentolate hydrochloride) will provide the most reliable quantification of refractive error in the presence of visual conditions such as strabismus, amblyopia, and anisometropia. Preschool-age children and school-age children may be more amenable to either static (distance) retinoscopy or subjective refraction if cooperative. Autorefraction with a tabletop instrument may be a useful alternative but should not totally substitute a manual method.

Testing of stereopsis for infants becomes viable after 6 months of age, where it can provide a sensitive measure of visual development. A variety of validated methods exist for assessing stereopsis in infants and toddlers and include the Lang, Frisby, stereo fly, Toegepast Natuurwetenschappelijk Onderzoek (TNO), and dynamic random dot tests. The sensitivity and reliability of these tests increase when used on preschool-age and school-age children.

▶ Ocular Motility and Alignment

Proper testing of ocular motility and alignment is the primary means of evaluating visual efferent function. Any fixation target can be used to test ocular motility in practically any age group. These include lighted toys, soft noises or music, or even the examiner's face for infants. Help can be enlisted from a parent or an assistant to maintain the child's head position during motility testing if necessary. For ocular alignment, the cover-uncover test at distance and near is still the mainstay. However, infants and toddlers may resist the test due to their dislike or fear of occluders. The Hirschberg test examining the corneal light reflex is a useful alternative in young patients who are less cooperative. For horizontal alignment testing, if the corneal light reflex lands temporal to the pupil, the tested eye is exotropic. If the light reflex lands nasal to the pupil, the tested eye is esotropic. Prisms can then be used (Krimsky test) to align the corneal reflex and provide an estimate of the magnitude of the deviation.

▶ Pupils

Pupils should be checked for size, symmetry, red reflex, and reactivity to light under bright and dim conditions. Many aspects of pupillary testing will be similar between pediatric and adult patients, with some specific considerations. Evaluating the patient's pupils should be done while the child is fixating on a distant target. Children have profound pupillary constriction in response to accommodation for near targets compared to adults. The retinoscope provides an excellent means to check for the presence of anisocoria from a distance. Set the light bar at 180 degrees, position yourself far enough from the child to have the light hover over both pupils, and look into the retinoscope to obtain a quick and accurate comparison of pupillary size. To check for an afferent pupillary defect, perform the swinging flashlight test, while keeping in mind that pupillary hippus (rhythmic <1 mm fluctuation of pupillary size) is also more pronounced in younger patients.

▶ Visual Fields

Confrontation visual field testing can be used to detect peripheral defects and areas of constricted vision in children. Older children can be tested in a similar manner as adults. For infants and toddlers, a "2-toy" method can be used. First, have the child fixate on a toy directly in front of them and then slowly bring a second toy into the child's visual field. If the child either saccades or turns their head toward the second object, it indicates that their peripheral field is intact in that direction. Repeat for all 4 quadrants.

▶ Color Vision

Most children can be reliably evaluated for color vision deficiency after 5 years of age. Having an undiagnosed color vision deficiency, whether congenital or acquired, may create profound learning barriers for a child's development, including the risk of misidentifying the child as learning disabled. Hence, identification of possible color vision deficiency prior to school age is important. In addition, a deficiency in color discrimination could also be a manifest sign of a separate ocular health problem.

Most Ishihara pseudoisochromatic plate tests can only detect protanopia and deuteranopia deficits in color vision. More recent electronic color vision tests have the robustness to characterize the specific deficiency and grade it as mild, moderate, or severe. The advent of genetic testing has also improved our understanding and diagnosis of inherited color vision deficiency, and genetic testing has continued to become cheaper and more accessible.

▶ Anterior and Posterior Exam

In young children or infants, the anterior exam can be completed with a direct ophthalmoscope, a hand-held slit lamp, or a 20-diopter lens. Indirect ophthalmoscopy remains the primary means of examining the fundus. Infants and young children may require distractions to evoke gaze in a particular direction in order to enable examination. In children with concerns for pathology that may require a more detailed exam that is not possible in clinic, an exam under anesthesia may be necessary.

▶ Miscellaneous Adjunct Testing

The interpretation of subjective and objective data gathered during the routine eye and vision exam may indicate the need for additional testing. These tests can assist in confirming or ruling out differential diagnoses, enable a more in-depth assessment of a particular domain of visual function, or act as an alternative means of evaluation in an uncooperative patient. These additional tests for infants and children may include:

- Electroretinogram (ERG)
- Visual evoked potentials (VEP)
- Ultrasonography
- Optical coherence tomography
- Fundus photography
- Corneal topography
- Neuroimaging (computed tomography or magnetic resonance imaging [MRI])

APPROACH TO DECREASED VISION

Visual impairment in infants and children, regardless of congenital or acquired causes, is always a concerning finding. Depending on the underlying cause, visual prognosis may range from normal vision to complete blindness. Early detection and accurate diagnosis must be initiated as early as possible to protect and maximize sight. In the case of newborns, the neurologist and ophthalmologist are confronted with the challenge of having to fathom a wide array of prenatal, perinatal, and postnatal pathologies that can be intraocular and extraocular. In the following sections, several neuro-ophthalmic clues are discussed that can help guide the differential diagnosis and the approach to decreased vision in a pediatric patient.

▶ Pupillary Responses

This relatively easy-to-perform test on noncooperative infants and newborns can provide valuable clues toward the diagnosis of impaired vision. Congenital retinal disorders causing blindness in infants will often show sluggishly reactive pupils, indicating a primary disorder in the visual afferent pathway. Conversely, infants with cerebral visual impairment (CVI) often have normal pupillary light reactions, along with a normal eye examination. Paradoxical pupillary responses (initial constriction in dark settings) may be indicative of specific rod or cone dystrophies such as congenital stationary night blindness (CSNB) or congenital achromatopsia.

▶ Nystagmus

The presence of nystagmus is a strong indication that the primary problem lies in the anterior visual pathway (pregeniculate structures). Accordingly, nystagmus is often absent in children with CVI. It is important to characterize the nystagmus by describing the direction and intensity of its movement "phases." Other attributes such as binocularity, conjugacy, frequency, waveform, null points, temporal profile, and age at first appearance are also crucial for classification. Beware of confusing nystagmus with other oscillatory eye movements, such as saccadic intrusions or oscillations.

Vestibulo-ocular Reflex

Presence of the vestibulo-ocular reflex (VOR) requires an intact vestibular system and saccadic and pursuit pathways. It is important to emphasize that even complete blindness does not impair VOR, as the reflex does not depend on visually generated information. In situations where VOR is impaired, motor conditions such as congenital ocular motor apraxia ought to be considered, whereby the initiation of ocular movements are impeded, falsely simulating blindness in an infant without head control.

Photophobia

Light aversion is an important finding that can share strong associations with both intraocular (retinal dystrophies, optic nerve hypoplasia) and extraocular (meningitis, migraine, head trauma, thalamic infarct) insults. Retinal disorders can cause varying degrees of photophobia, with congenital achromatopsia causing extreme aversion to light and dominant optic atrophy causing milder photophobia. Not all photophobia is of retinal origin, however, as glare from lenticular or corneal opacities has also been implicated, as well as iritis, aniridia, and media opacities. Photophobia has also been demonstrated in patients with CVI, presumably as a result of damage to thalamic or cortical areas. The photophobia is mostly mild but does not seem to share any relationship with the severity of visual loss from CVI. A child with congenital glaucoma can present with photophobia accompanied by epiphora (tearing), buphthalmos, and elevated intraocular pressure.

Retina Findings

The retina exam remains the primary means of diagnosing retinopathy of prematurity (ROP) in preterm infants because ROP does not initially present with any signs or symptoms when it first develops. If untreated, patients eventually develop nystagmus, white pupils (leukocoria), and ultimately vision loss. A consensus diagnostic classification for ROP has been developed and refined to characterize the disease by location (zones), severity (stage), and vascular characteristics in the posterior pole (normal, pre-plus, or plus disease).

Retinal dystrophies can also cause changes in retinal vasculature, often causing diffuse narrowing of the arterioles, and retinal pigmentary changes centrally or peripherally. Some of the more common dystrophies (eg, Leber congenital amaurosis) do not possess overt signs of retinal abnormalities, despite the retina being functionally impaired. Functional testing (VEP/ERG) may be required to confirm the diagnosis in high-suspicion cases.

SELECTED PEDIATRIC NEURO-OPHTHALMIC DISORDERS

The following section provides a brief overview of select categories of neuro-ophthalmic disorders that can be encountered in the pediatric patient with subnormal vision. The overall framework will include brief discussions of the underlying causes, clinical presentation, differential diagnoses, evaluation, and management.

Childhood Retinal Dystrophies

Hereditary diseases of the retina are a broad group of genetic disorders that result in progressive visual dysfunction that begins early in life. They should be suspected in children who present with a bilateral decrease in vision, color deficiency, time of day–specific visual impairment, or photophobia not easily explained by media opacities, refractive error, or anatomic defects on ophthalmic examination. Positive family history is a very specific finding for retinal dystrophies because many disorders in this category are recessively inherited. Some dystrophies present with characteristic features that are either highly suggestive or even diagnostic of a specific disorder. The clinical profiles of a few such disorders are reviewed in the following sections.

Leber Congenital Amaurosis

Leber congenital amaurosis (LCA) is a heterogeneous genetic disorder of the retina that often results in blindness at birth. At least 27 different gene mutations have been associated with causing LCA, and most involve elements of the photo-transduction pathway. Affected patients often present with nystagmus, sluggish or near-absent pupillary responses, photophobia, and high hyperopia. On exam, visual acuity is often 20/400 or worse, with a third of patients having no light perception. The retina on fundus exam initially appears normal but often develops pigmentary changes (salt-and-pepper pattern), foveal chorioretinal degeneration, subretinal flecks, macular colobomas, and pseudopapilledema over time. Electrophysiologic evaluation with ERG is especially specific for LCA, where it will often reveal an extinguished or remarkably attenuated response. A normal ERG essentially rules out LCA. LCA should be differentiated from nonocular causes of blindness such as CVI or delayed visual maturation. Other conditions that mimic LCA include achromatopsia, CSNB, retinitis pigmentosa, Joubert syndrome, and peroxisomal disorders. Treatment for LCA has recently made significant progress with US Food and Drug Administration approval of precision gene therapy (voretigene neparvovec-rzyl [Luxturna]) for a subset of LCA patients with biallelic mutations in RPE65.

Stargardt Disease

Also known as Stargardt macular degeneration, this disease is caused by mutations in the *ABCA4* gene, which encodes a rod photoreceptor-specific transport protein. The age of onset is often between childhood and early adolescence, with rare cases arising in adulthood. Earlier onset typically prognosticates worse vision outcomes. Patients with Stargardt disease are often asymptomatic in the early course of the disease but will later develop bilateral central visual loss, mild dyschromatopsia, photophobia, and central scotomas. Visual acuity often deteriorates rapidly from around 20/40 to the 20/200 to 20/400 range, where it remains stable. The retina usually appears normal during early disease but will begin to show atrophic macular degeneration, peripheral pigmentary clumping, bull's eye maculopathy, and fundus flecks as vision deteriorates. Fluorescein angiography typically shows the characteristic absence of signal in the choroid (termed *silent choroid*) in the majority of cases. Fundus autofluorescence often highlights the fundus flecks as small, irregular, hyperfluorescent lesions. ERG is typically unhelpful in the workup for Stargardt disease as it usually yields normal results early in the disease. There are currently no targeted treatment options for Stargardt disease, but it remains an attractive future candidate for gene replacement therapy given its single-gene etiology.

Achromatopsia

Achromatopsia is caused by a congenital defect in cone photoreceptors that results in decreased visual acuity, nystagmus, profound photophobia, day blindness (hemeralopia), severe dyschromatopsia, and paradoxical pupillary reactions (initial constriction to dim light). Multiple causative genes have been implicated in achromatopsia, with the most common mutation affecting cone-specific cyclic nucleotide–gated cation channel subunits encoded by *CNGA3* and *CNGB3*. Visual acuity can range from 20/40 to 20/400, depending on the extent of cone photoreceptor involvement. Fundus exam reveals a normal-looking retina. ERG is the gold standard for diagnosis, showing a diminished or absent cone response and a normal rod response. There is currently no approved treatment for achromatopsia. Associated high hyperopia can be managed with refractive error correction, and referral to a low vision specialist can help manage the debilitating photophobia.

▶ Cerebral Visual Impairment

Also called cortical visual impairment, CVI is the leading cause of visual impairment in children in developed countries. CVI results from damage to postgeniculate structures of the visual pathway, while the anterior pathway and the eye are normal. Damage can occur at the cortical or subcortical level, resulting in a heterogeneous spectrum of disease.

Perinatal injury to the developing visual system and brain remains the most common cause of CVI, with the most common etiologies listed below:

- Neonatal hypoxic-ischemic encephalopathy (HIE)
- Cerebral malformations (holoprosencephaly, lissencephaly)
- Hydrocephalus
- Meningitis/encephalitis
- Head trauma
- Intraventricular hemorrhage of the newborn
- Seizures, epilepsy, and other ictal phenomena
- Metabolic and neurodegenerative disorders (hypoglycemia, Fabry disease, Leigh disease)

The degree of visual impairment is highly dependent on the extent of damage to cerebral visual structures and can range from near-perfect vision to complete blindness. In most cases, the inability to properly assess visual function in CVI patients presents a unique challenge to the clinician, as traditional methods have little to no utility. Assessments of broader visual function (eg, light perception, fixate-follow behavior, optokinetic drum response, grating/vernier acuity) may prove more useful than attempting to measure visual acuity.

The most common neuro-ophthalmic signs in CVI patients are infantile exotropia, horizontal conjugate gaze deviation, absence of nystagmus, and mild atrophy of the optic discs. Other ophthalmic signs include refractive error (hyperopia > myopia) and bilateral inferior visual field defects. Nonocular features often reflect sequelae of systemic comorbidities such as cerebral palsy, developmental delay, neural tube defects, progressive degenerative disorders, and hypotonia.

CVI is a diagnosis of exclusion and may be isolated or co-present with associated disorders that are often the sequelae of the inciting insult that caused the CVI (eg, HIE, encephalitis, trauma). From a vision standpoint, it is important to distinguish whether an infant or child is unable to see, unable to interpret visual input (visual agnosia), or unable to move their eyes, prior to considering CVI as a diagnosis. Visual inattention and gaze avoidance are other behaviors that can be seen in certain disorders (autism) that can lead to CVI being frequently misdiagnosed.

Neuroimaging with MRI is typically first pursued to survey the extent of cortical damage. While the spectrum of results ranges from normal to extensive damage of the posterior pathway, frequent findings include areas of cerebral atrophy, watershed infarctions, periventricular leukomalacia, and cerebral dysgenesis. Interestingly, multiple studies have shown that visual outcomes poorly correlate with the severity of findings on neuroimaging.

While there is no specific treatment for CVI, multimodal visual rehabilitation is often pursued to help patients make the most of their vision. Children benefit the most from early intervention with vision therapy and educational support. Visual development occurs to varying degrees in children diagnosed with CVI, with over half demonstrating some form of improvement on follow-up. Without consideration of etiology, a broad prognostic factor is the degree of visual impairment at initial diagnosis, where patients with better visual acuity eventually demonstrate the greatest improvement over time.

▶ Optic Nerve Hypoplasia

Optic nerve hypoplasia (ONH) is the most common congenital optic disc anomaly, with an estimated prevalence of 1 in 10,000 children. Defined as an underdevelopment of the optic nerve, it can present either unilaterally or bilaterally and can occur by itself or in conjunction with maldevelopment of midline cerebral structures such as the septum pellucidum, corpus callosum, or pituitary gland. Visual acuity can range from 20/20 to no light perception and usually remains stable throughout life. However, ONH in children is amblyogenic, which can further deteriorate visual acuity over time. On exam, the optic nerve appears abnormally small and gray or pale in color, often surrounded by a peripapillary halo (double-ring sign). MRI is often first recommended in patients suspected to have ONH and achieves 2 goals: (1) to assess and measure the dimensions of the intracranial optic nerve and optic chiasm, and (2) to screen for the presence of midline CNS malformations. In ONH, T1-weighted MRI scans will typically show thinning and attenuation of the intracranial optic nerve. If the ONH presents bilaterally, coronal T1-weighted images will show symmetric thinning of the optic chiasm.

Septo-optic Dysplasia

ONH has been associated with a wide variety of CNS abnormalities, and among them, septo-optic dysplasia (SOD) represents a triad of ONH, absence of the septum pellucidum, and thinning or agenesis of the corpus callosum. This often leads to hypophyseal malformation and hormonal deficiencies, the most common being growth hormone (70%), followed by thyrotropin (43%), corticotropin (27%), and antidiuretic hormone (5%). Endocrinologic sequelae include hypothyroidism, panhypopituitarism, diabetes insipidus, and hyperprolactinemia. Among these, neonatal hypothyroidism is a significant risk factor for developmental delay. For these reasons, it is highly recommended to pursue a comprehensive endocrine evaluation if SOD is suspected, with the caveat that normal pituitary function does not preclude the development of endocrinopathy in the future. On MRI, the absence of the neurohypophysis (which often appears as a bright spot on T1-weighted sequences), along with attenuation or absence of the pituitary infundibulum, is often confirmatory of SOD.

Approach to Anisocoria in Children

Kevin X. Zhang, PhD
Veeral S. Shah, MD, PhD

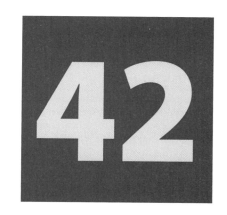

INTRODUCTION

Anisocoria in a young child is a frequent cause of concern among parents and is a common reason for referral to pediatric neurology/ophthalmology clinics. Many of these patients are eventually diagnosed with physiologic anisocoria, requiring no further evaluation. However, the differential diagnosis of anisocoria in a child contains more life-threatening conditions that should not be missed. These can include an acquired Horner syndrome secondary to a neuroblastoma of the paravertebral sympathetic chain or a third nerve palsy from a compressive intracranial process. Often, patients are referred to both a neurologist and a neuro-ophthalmologist to undergo an appropriate investigation for potential underlying problems that require further attention. The focus of this chapter is to guide the general pediatrician and pediatric neurologist through the clinical approach to a child presenting with anisocoria and to help inform decision making.

PHYSIOLOGY

Because anisocoria represents either impaired dilation or constriction of one pupil, it is important to review the sympathetic and parasympathetic pathways that control pupil size:

- Constriction of the pupil is achieved by the pupillary sphincter muscles, which are under parasympathetic control. The cholinergic fibers that innervate the pupillary sphincter muscle travel along the third cranial nerve.
- Dilation of the pupil occurs through the action of the iris dilator muscle, which is under sympathetic control. These fibers originate in the hypothalamus, descend to the sympathetic trunk, and reascend to the superior cervical ganglion before arriving in the orbit. Besides the iris dilator muscle, these oculosympathetic fibers also innervate Müller's muscle (also known as the superior tarsal muscle), which is a smooth muscle that assists with upper eyelid elevation.

COMMON CAUSES

Physiologic Anisocoria

The prevalence of physiologic anisocoria in the general population has been estimated to be approximately 20%, or around 1 in 5 clinic patients.[1] The anisocoria is usually more pronounced under dim light.[2] The major features that distinguish physiologic from pathologic anisocoria are as follows:

- Both pupils react briskly to light.
- There is no dilation lag.
- The degree of anisocoria is 1 mm or less.

Reviewing past photographs can help provide reassuring evidence that the child's anisocoria is potentially a chronic, likely benign condition. Photographs of parents and siblings may also help, as the anisocoria can be familial. Overall, physiologic anisocoria is asymptomatic, does not cause any problems with the development of vision in the child, and requires no further workup.

Horner Syndrome

Horner syndrome occurs from the disruption of the oculosympathetic chain, resulting in loss of pupillary dilation on the affected side (the affected pupil will be smaller). In children, Horner syndrome is classified as congenital or acquired, with acquired causes warranting higher concern for life-threatening etiologies. The degree of anisocoria is more pronounced, with studies in children showing an average pupillary difference of 1.37 mm in room light and 2 mm in dim light.[3] There is a prominent dilation lag of over 10 to 15 seconds in the affected eye.

Besides anisocoria and dilation lag, the other signs of Horner syndrome include unilateral ptosis and anhidrosis. In children, the anhidrosis can also be appreciated as a lack of redness (flushing) that would normally appear from heat, exertion, or emotional reactions. Although Horner syndrome does not typically cause vision problems, it is important because of its association with other systemic conditions.

Structural Causes

Certain ocular conditions may result in mechanical or physical barriers to pupillary constriction and dilation, resulting in anisocoria and sometimes abnormal pupillary shapes. Congenital defects in the anterior segment of the eye, including aniridia, polycoria, Axenfeld-Rieger syndrome, Peter anomaly, and persistent pupillary membrane, can all produce anisocoria and will have other notable ocular features on examination to aid in diagnosis.

Acquired ocular conditions can also produce anisocoria secondary to damage and compromise of the iris and surrounding structures. For instance, trauma can immediately distort the iris architecture and also predispose the patient to iris sphincter atrophy in the long term, leading to impaired constriction that is more pronounced in bright light. Intraocular inflammatory processes (eg, iritis, iridocyclitis, uveitis) can result in reactive fibrosis and adhesion formation between the iris and adjacent structures such as the lens. These conditions are often diagnosed through a comprehensive slit lamp examination by an ophthalmologist.

Pharmacologic

Exposure to various pharmacologic agents can produce anisocoria by modulating the sympathetic and/or parasympathetic pathways that control pupil size. This is generally due to exposure in only one eye, as systemic exposure would constrict or dilate both pupils equally. Accidental instillation of eye drops is the most common route of exposure, but other documented mechanisms include nebulized medications,[4] aerosol exposure,[5] and contact with certain plants.[6] Examples of medications or exposures that can cause either pharmacologic miosis or mydriasis are listed in Table 42–1. The diagnosis of pharmacologic mydriasis can be verified by confirmatory drop testing with 1% pilocarpine eye drops, an agonist of the M_3 muscarinic receptor. Pilocarpine acts on the neuromuscular junction of the pupillary constrictor muscle to cause profound and sustained miosis. If pilocarpine instillation does not constrict the pupil, then the pupil is pharmacologically dilated. It should be noted, however, that pilocarpine ophthalmic drops should be used sparingly in pediatric patients, particularly infants and young children, and only as a diagnostic exigent.

Third Nerve Palsy

Children presenting with third cranial nerve palsies can present with an enlarged pupil on the affected side, along with ptosis and extraocular movement deficits. The anisocoria

Table 42–1. Examples of pharmacologic agents that can cause anisocoria.

Type of Anisocoria	Examples of Causes
Affected pupil larger (mydriasis)	Adrenergic agonists • Phenylephrine • Epinephrine • Hydroxyamphetamine Sympatholytics • Ipratropium • Scopolamine • Atropine • Tropicamide • Cyclopentolate
Affected pupil smaller (miosis)	Systemic miotics (parasympathomimetics) • Carbachol • Methacholine • Organophosphates • Physostigmine Topical miotic • Pilocarpine

is often helpful in establishing the diagnosis when it copresents with these findings.

Tonic Pupil

Patients with a tonic pupil (also called Adie pupil) will present with a dilated pupil on the affected side that constricts poorly to light but better to accommodation. Most cases of tonic pupil are idiopathic and result from damage to the parasympathetic ciliary ganglion, followed by subsequent aberrant regeneration.[7] Patients who present with a tonic pupil may experience photophobia and difficulty adapting to the dark, owing to their pupillary sphincter dysfunction. The diagnostic approach shares many similarities to that of pharmacologic mydriasis, where low-concentration pilocarpine (0.05%-0.15%) will result in a larger degree of pupillary constriction in a tonic pupil but not a normal pupil.

DIAGNOSTIC APPROACH

History

The pediatric patient's anisocoria may have been first noticed by the child's parents or by the pediatrician during a well-child exam. Questions about when and how the anisocoria was first noticed, which pupil seems bigger (or smaller), whether the anisocoria is variable or constant, and differences under dim versus bright light are important. Besides the anisocoria itself, the history should also include general questions about the child's health and development, including if there was a history of birth trauma, particularly when Horner syndrome may be suspected. Complications during a difficult birth delivery may include Erb palsy or shoulder dystocia, which may damage the cervical portion of the oculosympathetic chain. Asking the parents for old photographs of their child may also help establish the chronicity of the anisocoria, especially when it is not clear whether it has been present since birth. Asking about the possibility of ocular trauma, neck manipulations or trauma (central line placement), and exposure to medications or plants should also be prioritized if traumatic or pharmacologic anisocoria is suspected. The history should end with a comprehensive neurologic review of systems.

Exam

The evaluation of the child with anisocoria should start with a general ocular examination, which includes measuring visual acuity using age-appropriate methods. The pupils should be checked for size, color, symmetry, and shape in both eyes prior to any light stimulation. Some congenital anomalies may present with irregular pupil shapes and colors (eg, coloboma, heterochromia, persistent pupillary membranes). Most children with physiologic anisocoria have only a mild difference in pupillary sizes (<0.4 mm), and the anisocoria is more noticeable in dim light.

A bright light source and a pupillary size gauge are the only tools needed to examine the pupillary reaction to light. The child should be relaxed, with their attention fixated on a distant object. Pupils should be examined in light and dark conditions, and a comparison of size, shape, and position of each pupil should be noted. Pupillary reactions are then assessed to light and near stimuli.

When a light source is shined into either eye, both pupils should constrict, and once the light is moved down and away from the eye, both pupils should dilate. The degree of the pupillary response should be equal and symmetric in both eyes, and the speed should be brisk. Any differences in magnitude, speed, and symmetry of the direct and consensual pupillary responses should be noted. If there is dilation lag, it is usually observed when the light source is moved away from the eye and the pupillary re-dilation between the 2 eyes is asymmetric in speed. This usually indicates a sympathetic innervation abnormality on the side of the affected pupil and may suggest underlying Horner syndrome or tonic pupil.

If there is no pupillary reaction, the etiology may be pharmacologic or structural/mechanical. If trauma is suspected, the child should be examined for other ocular or periocular injuries.

In general, the first step in a child with anisocoria is to determine whether the abnormal pupil is the large pupil or the small pupil. If the anisocoria is greater in the dark than in the light, the small pupil is abnormal, as it is not dilating

well in the dark. Poor pupillary constriction reflects an abnormality of the parasympathetic nervous system. However, if the anisocoria is the same in both light and dark conditions and the degree of pupillary constriction is symmetric to light stimuli, then the diagnosis is likely physiologic anisocoria. Poor pupillary dilation reflects an abnormality of the sympathetic nervous system. If the anisocoria is greater in the light than in the dark, the large pupil is abnormal because it is not reacting well to light and constricting appropriately.

Horner syndrome is a constellation of clinical findings that include: anisocoria (miotic pupil), ptosis, and anhidrosis (lack of sweating from the skin glands) as a result of disruption of sympathetic pupillary pathways that take a circuitous path from the hypothalamospinal tract down to the cervical spine and then ascend to the superior cervical ganglion, carotid artery, cavernous sinus, and ipsilateral orbit and terminate at the iris dilator muscles. Patients with Horner syndrome most commonly present with anisocoria and subtle ptosis and rarely present with the entire triad of clinical findings. Confirmatory diagnosis can be obtained by administering 10% cocaine eyes drops, which are administered twice in each eye, and observing 45 to 60 minutes later. Upon cocaine eye drop administration, the normal pupillary response is to dilate; however, a constricted pupil confirms Horner syndrome.

Other important aspects of the examination should include evaluation for ptosis and strabismus. In doing so, eyelid height (upper and lower eyelids), levator muscle function, and extraocular movements should be assessed. The presence of ptosis is strong evidence for an underlying third cranial nerve palsy or Horner syndrome; however, in the latter, the ptosis is milder since it affects the sympathetic innervation of the smaller Mueller muscle in both upper and lower eyelids. A swinging flashlight test should also be performed to assess for a relative afferent pupillary defect, which may indicate an abnormality of the afferent visual pathway (eg, optic neuropathy). A full cranial nerve exam should also be performed because deficits in specific nerves may help localize a specific lesion. For cooperative patients, a slit lamp examination can uncover the underlying etiology of the anisocoria.

DIFFERENTIAL DIAGNOSES

- Anisocoria greater in dim light (poor dilation)
  - Horner syndrome
  - Exposure to parasympathomimetics (cholinergic medications)
  - Posterior synechiae
- Anisocoria greater in bright light (poor constriction)
  - Third cranial nerve palsy
  - Exposure to cycloplegic medications

- Exposure to sympathomimetics
- Adie tonic pupil
- Traumatic mydriasis
- Migraine headache
- Intraocular inflammation (iritis, iridocyclitis, uveitis)
- Anisocoria equal in bright and dim light
  - Physiologic anisocoria

MANAGEMENT

In a child with mild anisocoria (difference in pupillary size <1 mm) and an otherwise normal ocular examination, no further evaluation is necessary. Reassurance of the benign nature of physiologic anisocoria should be provided. The management of other patients with anisocoria is dependent on the underlying etiology, which is often narrowed down by determining which pupil is abnormal. Treatment of the underlying condition will often resolve the anisocoria. Important diagnoses that should not be missed include Horner syndrome (which has a large variety of causes and management strategies) and third nerve palsy, particularly if the onset is acute, which may suggest a life-threatening cranial compressive process. These patients should receive emergent neuroimaging for further evaluation.

Similar to physiologic anisocoria, a tonic pupil also warrants no further evaluation and only requires observation and documentation (to prevent unnecessary workup in the future). Anisocoria due to pharmacologic exposure will resolve over time.

REFERENCES

1. Lam BL, Thompson HS, Corbett JJ. The prevalence of simple anisocoria. *Am J Ophthalmol.* 1987;104(1):69-73. doi:10.1016/0002-9394(87)90296-0
2. Lam BL, Thompson HS, Walls RC. Effect of light on the prevalence of simple anisocoria. *Ophthalmology.* 1996;103(5):790-793. doi:10.1016/s0161-6420(96)30614-3
3. Suh SH, Suh DW, Benson C. The degree of anisocoria in pediatric patients with Horner syndrome when compared to children without disease. *J Pediatr Ophthalmol Strabismus.* 2016;53(3):186-189. doi:10.3928/01913913-20160405-07
4. Royce L, Schulz C, Brown N. Case of a fixed and dilated pupil: acute anisocoria secondary to aerosol ipratropium bromide. *Arch Dis Child.* 2018;103(11):1090. doi:10.1136/archdischild-2017-314054
5. Gunderson CA. Unilateral mydriasis associated with exposure to flea spray. *Arch Ophthalmol.* 2002;120(5):665.
6. Serin HM, Ozen B, Yilmaz S. A rare cause of acute anisocoria in a child: the angel's trumpet plant. *J Pediatr Ophthalmol Strabismus.* 2018;55:e33-e35. doi:10.3928/01913913-20181009-01
7. McGee S. The pupils. In: *Evidence-Based Physical Diagnosis.* New York, NY: Elsevier; 2012:161-179.

The Congenital Neuromuscular Disorders

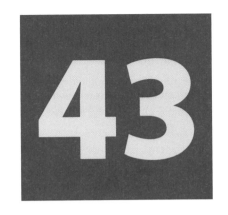

Cuixia Tian, MD

Congenital neuromuscular disorders are a group of genetic diseases affecting nerves, muscles, and neuromuscular junctions (eg, congenital myopathies, congenital muscular dystrophies, congenital myasthenic syndromes, and congenital myotonic dystrophy).

CONGENITAL MYOPATHIES

ESSENTIALS OF DIAGNOSIS AND TYPICAL FEATURES

▶ A heterogeneous group of early-onset muscle diseases

▶ Characteristic myopathic findings on muscle biopsy

▶ Clinically present with hypotonia and muscle weakness at birth or in infancy

▶ Mutations in a heterogeneous group of genes have been identified

The congenital myopathies are a rare, heterogeneous group of hereditary genetic muscle diseases that are defined by architectural abnormalities in the muscle fibers. Besides the clinical features, muscle biopsy and genetic analyses are essential in the diagnosis. Based on the findings on muscle biopsy, congenital myopathies can be further classified into core myopathies, nemaline myopathies, centronuclear myopathies, congenital fiber-type disproportion myopathies, and myosin storage myopathies. Management is provided by a multidisciplinary neuromuscular team. To date, only supportive treatment is available.

▶ Clinical Findings

Symptoms and Signs

Patients present with similar symptoms, with either a floppy infant at birth or later with muscle weakness. Polyhydramnios due to decreased swallowing function and reduced fetal movements in utero can be seen in patients with prenatal onset. Other clinical presentations include muscle weakness, delayed motor development milestones, respiratory insufficiency, feeding difficulties, and arthrogryposis. Severe infantile presentations are associated with marked weakness and may lead to death from respiratory failure in early life, whereas other affected children mostly have a relatively benign course with static weakness and hypotonia. Deep tendon reflexes are usually depressed or absent.

Laboratory Findings

Serum creatine kinase (CK) levels may be normal or mildly elevated. Electromyography (EMG) is usually normal but may show mild and nonspecific myopathic features. Nerve conduction studies (NCSs) are normal. Histologically, muscle biopsy findings in most congenital myopathies demonstrate type 1 myofiber predominance and atrophy with superimposed characteristic morphologic features most commonly including nemaline body, central core, central nucleation, and multiple minicores. In addition to muscle biopsy, genetic testing that demonstrates mutations in causative genes will further aid in establishing the diagnosis.

▶ Differential Diagnosis

Differential diagnoses include broad categories such as congenital muscular dystrophy, congenital myotonic dystrophy, congenital myasthenic syndrome, infantile-onset motor neuron diseases, and metabolic myopathy.

Complications

Feeding intolerance, respiratory deficiency, neuromuscular scoliosis, hip joint subluxations, and arthrogryposis are common complications. Cardiomyopathies can also be complications in some patients.

Treatment

Supportive treatment managed through several medical disciplines is provided typically through a multidisciplinary pediatric neuromuscular care center. The management is typically orchestrated by a pediatric neurologist, in collaboration with other specialties, including cardiology, pulmonary, dietary, gastroenterology, orthopedics, genetics, rehabilitation medicine, physical therapy, occupational therapy, and speech therapy.

CONGENITAL MUSCULAR DYSTROPHIES

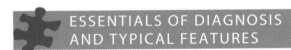

ESSENTIALS OF DIAGNOSIS AND TYPICAL FEATURES

▶ A heterogeneous group of early-onset muscle diseases
▶ Characteristic dystrophic findings on muscle biopsy
▶ Clinically present with hypotonia and muscle weakness at birth or in infancy
▶ Mutations in a heterogeneous group of genes have been identified

The congenital muscular dystrophies are a rare, heterogeneous group of hereditary genetic muscle diseases that are defined by early onset and progressive muscle weakness with dystrophic abnormalities in the muscle fibers. Besides the clinical features, muscle biopsy and genetic analyses are essential in the diagnosis. Dystrophic findings on muscle biopsy demonstrate muscle fiber atrophy, degeneration, and fibrofatty tissue infiltration. Management is provided by a multidisciplinary neuromuscular team. To date, only supportive treatment is available.

Clinical Findings

Symptoms and Signs

Polyhydramnios due to decreased swallowing function and reduced fetal movements in utero can be seen in patients with prenatal onset. At birth, patients present as floppy infants with a weak cry and minimal spontaneous movements of the extremities. Other clinical presentations include muscle weakness, delayed motor development milestones, respiratory insufficiency, feeding difficulties, and arthrogryposis. Severe infantile presentations are associated with marked weakness and may lead to death from respiratory failure in early life, while other affected children have significant motor delay and impaired mobility, with initial limited improvement of motor function during early childhood followed by a course of gradual progressive worsening of muscle weakness. Deep tendon reflexes are usually depressed or absent.

Laboratory Findings

Serum CK levels may vary from normal to significantly elevated. EMG may show myopathy features. NCSs are normal. Histologically, muscle biopsy findings in most congenital muscular dystrophies demonstrate muscle fiber atrophy with dystrophic features including myofibril degeneration and regeneration, and fibrofatty infiltrations. Immunohistochemistry and electron microscopy may help to identify specific diseases based on staining patterns. In addition to muscle biopsy, genetic testing that demonstrates mutations in causative genes will further aid in establishing the diagnosis.

Imaging and Other Findings

Imaging of the brain with magnetic resonance imaging is indicated because specific brain abnormalities are associated with certain types of congenital muscular dystrophy, especially muscle-eye-brain disease. Echocardiography and electrocardiography are recommended to look for cardiomyopathy and abnormal cardiac conduction. Eye abnormalities such as myopia, strabismus, cataract, and glaucoma can be seen in a subset of patients, such as those with Fukuyama dystrophy and muscle-eye-brain disease.

Differential Diagnosis

Differential diagnoses include broad categories such as congenital myopathy, congenital myotonic dystrophy, congenital myasthenic syndrome, infantile-onset motor neuron diseases, and metabolic myopathy.

Complications

Feeding intolerance, respiratory deficiency, neuromuscular scoliosis, hip joint subluxations, and arthrogryposis are common complications. Cardiomyopathies and cardiac conduction delay can also be complications in some patients.

Treatment

Supportive treatment managed through several medical disciplines is provided typically through a multidisciplinary pediatric neuromuscular care center. The management is typically orchestrated by a pediatric neurologist, in collaboration with other specialties, including cardiology, pulmonary, dietary, gastroenterology, orthopedics, genetics, rehabilitation medicine, physical therapy, occupational therapy, and speech therapy.

CONGENITAL MYASTHENIC SYNDROMES

 ESSENTIALS OF DIAGNOSIS AND TYPICAL FEATURES

▶ A heterogeneous group of early-onset neuromuscular junction diseases

▶ Genetic mutations in genes coding for proteins residing in the nerve terminal, the synaptic basal lamina, and the postsynaptic region of the motor endplate

▶ Normal or nonspecific findings on muscle biopsy

▶ Clinically present with fatigable muscle weakness affecting especially the ocular muscles at birth to early childhood

▶ EMG/NCS showing decremental response with repetitive stimulations

▶ Medical treatment is available, and a genetic diagnosis helps in selecting the appropriate treatment drug

The congenital myasthenic syndromes are a rare, heterogeneous group of hereditary genetic muscle diseases that are defined by early-onset muscle weakness with fatigability of voluntary muscles. Most commonly, the eyelids and extraocular muscles are involved. Bulbar involvement can be seen with swallowing and chewing difficulties. Muscle biopsy is normal or with nonspecific abnormalities in the muscle fibers. Besides the clinical features, EMG and NCS with repetitive stimulation testing and genetic analyses are essential in the diagnosis. Management is provided by a multidisciplinary neuromuscular team. Medical and supportive treatments are available.

▶ Clinical Findings

Symptoms and Signs

Prenatally, polyhydramnios and reduced fetal movements can be seen. Most patients present with onset at or shortly after birth or in early childhood. Fatigable muscle weakness affecting ocular, bulbar, and limb muscles and ptosis are seen commonly. At birth, patients present as floppy infants with a weak cry and minimal spontaneous movements of the extremities. Delayed motor development milestones, respiratory insufficiency, feeding difficulties, and arthrogryposis are also common findings. Severe infantile presentations

are associated with marked weakness and may lead to death from respiratory failure in early life, whereas other affected children have significant motor delay and impaired mobility. Rarely, symptoms may not manifest until later in childhood. Deep tendon reflexes are usually depressed or absent.

Laboratory Findings

Serum CK levels are normal or mildly elevated in rare cases. EMG and NCS show a decremental EMG response of the compound muscle action potential on low-frequency (2-3 Hz) repetitive stimulations; if available, a single-fiber EMG is preferred. However, some patients with symptoms present later in life, the weakness can affect proximal and torso rather than cranial muscles, and the decremental EMG response may be detected only after prolonged subtetanic stimulation. Tests for anti–acetylcholine receptor (AChR) and anti–muscle-specific kinase (MuSK) antibodies are indicated in sporadic patients after the age of 1 year and in arthrogrypotic infants even if the mother has no myasthenic symptoms. Genetic testing that demonstrates mutations in causative genes will further aid in establishing the diagnosis and determining medical treatment. Congenital myasthenic syndromes can also occur in combination with centronuclear myopathies and with plectin-related myopathies or muscular dystrophies.

▶ Differential Diagnosis

Differential diagnoses include broad categories such as congenital myopathy, congenital muscular dystrophy, congenital myotonic dystrophy, infantile-onset motor neuron diseases, passively transferred or autoimmune myasthenia gravis, and metabolic myopathy.

▶ Complications

Feeding intolerance, respiratory deficiency, neuromuscular scoliosis, hip joint subluxations, and arthrogryposis are common complications. Cardiac and smooth muscles are typically not affected.

▶ Treatment

Current medical therapies for congenital myasthenic syndromes include cholinergic agonists, including pyridostigmine and 3,4-diaminopyridine (3,4-DAP); long-lived open channel blockers of the AChR ion channel (fluoxetine and quinidine); and adrenergic agonists (albuterol and ephedrine). It is important to note that agents that benefit one type of congenital myasthenic syndrome can be ineffective or harmful in another type (eg, patients harboring a low-expressor or fast-channel mutation in AChR benefit from cholinergic agonists, whereas patients with slow-channel mutations in AChR are worsened by these medications). It is essential that a genetic or molecular diagnosis inform the choice of therapy. It is also important to note that the cholinergic agonists pyridostigmine and 3,4-DAP exert their effect as soon as the medication is absorbed, whereas the adrenergic agonists and the AChR channel blockers act more slowly over days, weeks, or months.

In addition, supportive treatment managed through several medical disciplines is provided typically through a multidisciplinary pediatric neuromuscular care center. The management is typically orchestrated by a pediatric neurologist, in collaboration with other specialties, including cardiology, pulmonary, dietary, gastroenterology, orthopedics, genetics, rehabilitation medicine, physical therapy, occupational therapy, and speech therapy.

CONGENITAL MYOTONIC DYSTROPHY

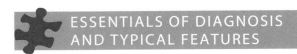

ESSENTIALS OF DIAGNOSIS AND TYPICAL FEATURES

▶ An autosomal dominant genetic disorder caused by expansion of trinucleotide CTG repeats in the 3′ untranslated, noncoding region of the DMPK gene

▶ Transcription of mutated DNA results in a mutant RNA that causes sequestration of splicing factors, leading to disturbance of cellular signaling and toxic effects on muscle metabolism and RNA processing

▶ Clinically presents with significant hypotonia, muscle weakness, myopathic facies, and contractures at birth

▶ Respiratory insufficiency and feeding intolerance are common complications during neonatal period

▶ Increased internalized nuclei and type 1 fiber atrophy are common findings on muscle biopsy; however, these findings are nonspecific

Myotonic dystrophy type 1 is an autosomal dominant, multisystem disorder with the primary manifestation being progressive distal and facial muscle weakness associated with myotonia. Congenital myotonic dystrophy is a severe form of myotonic dystrophy type 1 with symptoms present at birth, with its mildest form being hypotonia in the newborn but more severe phenotypes involving mechanical respiratory failure and oropharyngeal and gastrointestinal motility dysfunction. Its genetic cause is the expansion of trinucleotide CTG repeats in the 3′ untranslated, noncoding region of the DMPK gene. Muscle biopsy typically shows nonspecific abnormalities of increased internalized nuclei in the muscle fibers. Besides the clinical features, genetic testing is essential in establishing the diagnosis. Management is provided by a multidisciplinary neuromuscular team with primarily supportive treatment.

▶ Clinical Findings

Symptoms and Signs

Prenatally, polyhydramnios and reduced fetal movements can be seen. Most patients present with onset at or shortly after birth or in early childhood, with muscle weakness affecting facial, bulbar, and limb muscles. At birth, patients present as floppy infants with a weak cry and decreased spontaneous movements of the extremities. Congenital club feet are commonly seen. Delayed motor development milestones, respiratory insufficiency, and feeding difficulties are common findings. With advanced respiratory and feeding support, most infants survive and achieve motor development milestones, with about 70% achieving independent ambulation. Past infancy, the child often experiences cognitive impairment, gastrointestinal dysfunction, cardiac conduction delay and arrhythmias, insulin resistance, thyroid dysfunction, cataracts, and psychiatric issues.

Laboratory Findings

Serum CK levels are normal or mildly elevated. Genetic testing that demonstrates mutations in causative genes aids in establishing the diagnosis and determining medical treatment.

▶ Differential Diagnosis

Differential diagnoses include broad categories such as congenital myopathy, congenital muscular dystrophy, congenital myasthenic syndrome, infantile-onset motor neuron diseases, and metabolic myopathy.

▶ Complications

Feeding intolerance, respiratory deficiency, neuromuscular scoliosis, cardiac conduction delay and arrhythmias, hip joint subluxations, and arthrogryposis are common complications.

▶ Treatment

Medical treatment is largely supportive in nature, is managed through several medical disciplines, and is provided typically through a multidisciplinary pediatric neuromuscular care center. The management is typically orchestrated by a pediatric neurologist, in collaboration with other specialties, including cardiology, pulmonary, endocrinology, ophthalmology, dietary, gastroenterology, orthopedics, genetics, rehabilitation medicine, physical therapy, occupational therapy, and speech therapy.

BIBLIOGRAPHY

Engel A, Shen XM, Selcen D, Sine SM. Congenital myasthenic syndrome: pathogenesis, diagnosis, and treatment. *Lancet Neurol.* 2015;14(4):420-434.

Finsterer J. Congenital myasthenic syndromes. *Orphanet J Rare Dis.* 2019;14(1):57.

Ho G, Carey KA, Cardamone M, Farrar MA. Myotonic dystrophy type 1: clinical manifestations in children and adolescents. *Arch Dis Child.* 2019;104(1):48-52.

Kang P, Morrison L, Iannaccone ST, et al. Evidence-based guideline summary: evaluation, diagnosis, and management of congenital muscular dystrophy: report of the guideline development subcommittee of the American Academy of Neurology and the practice issues review panel of the American Association of Neuromuscular & Electrodiagnostic Medicine. *Neurology.* 2015;84(13):1369-1378.

Schorling D, Kirschner J, Bönnemann CG. Congenital muscular dystrophies and myopathies: an overview and update. *Neuropediatrics.* 2017;48(4):247-261.

Thornton C. Myotonic dystrophy. *Neurol Clin.* 2014;32(3):705-719.

Zapata-Aldana E, Ceballos-Sáenz D, Hicks R, Campbell C. Prenatal, neonatal, and early childhood features in congenital myotonic dystrophy. *J Neuromuscul Dis.* 2018;5(3):331-340.

The Muscular Dystrophies

Cuixia Tian, MD

The muscular dystrophies are a group of genetic diseases that affect muscle and cause myofibril degeneration and regeneration and are characterized by progressive muscle wasting and weakness. They are subdivided into several groups, including congenital forms (congenital muscular dystrophy [CMD]); Duchenne muscular dystrophy (DMD) and Becker muscular dystrophy (BMD); limb-girdle muscular dystrophy (LGMD); Emery-Dreifuss muscular dystrophy (EDMD); oculopharyngeal; distal; and facioscapulohumeral. Here we are focusing on the muscular dystrophies primarily or commonly affecting children: DMD, BMD, LGMD, and EDMD. CMD is discussed in Chapter 43.

DUCHENNE AND BECKER MUSCULAR DYSTROPHIES

ESSENTIALS OF DIAGNOSIS AND TYPICAL FEATURES

► X-linked recessive muscle dystrophies primarily affecting boys

► Duchenne mutations are typically out of frame, whereas Becker mutations are in frame in *DMD* gene

► Characteristic dystrophic findings with myofiber degeneration and regeneration on muscle biopsy, with primarily absent dystrophin protein expression in DMD and decreased dystrophin protein expression in BMD

► Clinically present with motor difficulty, calf pseudohypertrophy, and pelvic girdle muscle weakness; onset of symptoms for DMD is before age 5, whereas that for BMD is typically around age 12 or later

► Multisystem involvement, including progressive weakening of respiratory and cardiac muscles, leads to respiratory insufficiency and dilated cardiomyopathy

DMD and BMD are X-linked recessive degenerative muscle diseases caused by genetic mutations in the *DMD* gene that primarily affect boys. In addition, DMD is the most common childhood-onset muscle disease. Besides the clinical features, genetic analyses and/or muscle biopsy are essential to establish the diagnosis. Management is provided by a multidisciplinary neuromuscular team. Glucocorticoid steroids are standard treatment for DMD in addition to supportive care, and various genetic modification therapies are now available for DMD patients with specific genetic mutations (eg, exon-skipping medications). Cardiac medications are routinely prescribed to slow down the progression of cardiomyopathy and to optimize cardiac function.

► Clinical Findings

Symptoms and Signs

Symptom onset varies from early childhood before age 5 for DMD to around age 12 or later for BMD. Delayed motor development milestones are common in DMD. Patients present with symptoms of motor difficulty, calf pseudohypertrophy, and progressive pelvic girdle muscle weakness. Muscle weakness is more proximal and affects the lower extremities initially. Patients have difficulty with running and getting up from the floor with a positive Gowers sign due to weak knee and hip extensors. Subsequently, weakness worsens and spreads to the upper extremities as well. Deep tendon reflexes are usually depressed or absent. Patients have increased difficulty with step climbing, walking, and ambulation, eventually becomes impaired with ambulation. DMD patients lose independent ambulation around age 12 in most cases, whereas BMD patients lose independent ambulation in adolescence or later in adult life. In addition to skeletal muscle involvement, cardiac and respiratory muscles are affected. Patients have progressively decline in pulmonary function and cardiac systolic function. Chewing and swallowing functions are affected later. Cognitive function impairment and behavioral disturbances, such as anxiety and obsessive features, are common. About 5% to 10% of female carriers for DMD and BMD have symptoms of muscle weakness, and some have enlarged calves. Their muscle weakness can be static or slowly progressive, varies in onset from childhood to later, and is often asymmetric. Female carriers may develop dilated cardiomyopathy even without apparent skeletal muscle weakness.

Laboratory Findings

Serum creatine phosphokinase (CPK) levels are significantly elevated, ranging from 50 to 200 times the upper limit of normal in DMD and 20 to 200 times in BMD. Serum aminotransferases (aspartate aminotransferase [AST] and alanine aminotransferase [ALT]), blood aldolase, and lactate dehydrogenase are also elevated in DMD and BMD, which are not indicative of liver disease. CPK levels are elevated in about 50% of female carriers to about 2 to 10 times the upper limit of normal. Genetic testing demonstrating mutation in the DMD gene will aid in establishing the diagnosis in most cases. Muscle biopsy may be necessary when genetic testing is unable to identify a pathogenic DMD genetic mutation or there is discrepancy between a clinical phenotype and an identified DMD mutation (eg, a patient with an in-frame DMD mutation with muscle weakness consistent with a DMD phenotype clinically). Histologically, muscle biopsy findings demonstrate dystrophic changes with myofibril degeneration and regeneration, inflammatory infiltrates seen in the perimysium, and progressive replacement of degenerative fibers with connective tissue and fat. Absent or markedly reduced immunostaining of dystrophin protein is seen in DMD, whereas reduced dystrophin staining is seen in BMD.

▶ Differential Diagnosis

Differential diagnoses include LGMD, especially the sarcoglycanopathies; CMD; metabolic myopathies; spinal muscular atrophy type 3; and Pompe disease.

▶ Complications

DMD patients are at high risk for development of malignant hyperthermia, and specific anesthesia precautions to avoid causative medications are recommended. In advanced stages, cardiomyopathy, respiratory deficiency, neuromuscular scoliosis, feeding difficulty, and constipation are common complications. In steroid-treated patients, steroid-induced osteoporosis, growth suppression, obesity, puberty delay, and adrenal insufficiency are common side effects. Cardiopulmonary complications are the most common cause of death. Fat embolism affecting the brain and lungs is increasingly recognized as a leading cause of death in DMD patients after incidental falls or fractures.

▶ Treatment

Oral glucocorticoid steroid treatment is recommended as standard care. Daily prednisone and deflazacort are most commonly used. Compared with prednisone treatment, deflazacort treatment has relatively fewer behavioral and weight gain concerns and studies have shown more favorable outcome in preserving ambulation. Alternative dosing regimens (eg, intermittent 10 days on and 10 days off or high-dose weekend dosing) are also used with oral prednisone in DMD patients, especially when there are concerns for significant side effects with daily use of steroids.

Several disease-modifying medications have recently become available, including weekly intravenous infusions of exon-skipping medications that are available now in the United States for patients with exon 51, 53, and 45 skippable DMD mutations. Ataluren is a nonsense suppression medication that has been approved in Europe for DMD patients with nonsense mutations.

Cardiac medications to prevent and treat heart failure are recommended as standard care. First-line therapy is angiotensin-converting enzyme inhibitors (ACEis). In addition, the mineralocorticoid receptor antagonist eplerenone combined with an ACEi may offer additional benefit to lessen the decline in ventricular function. With continued ventricular dysfunction or elevated heart rate, β-adrenergic blockers are added.

Anticipatory management of respiratory weakness, prophylactic immunizations, and prompt treatment of respiratory infections are essential pulmonary treatments. Supportive treatment is provided typically through a multidisciplinary pediatric neuromuscular care center and managed through several medical disciplines, including neurology, cardiology, pulmonary, endocrinology, dietary, gastroenterology, orthopedics, rehabilitation medicine, physical therapy, and occupational therapy.

LIMB GIRDLE MUSCULAR DYSTROPHIES

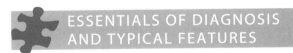

ESSENTIALS OF DIAGNOSIS AND TYPICAL FEATURES

- ▶ A heterogeneous group of muscular dystrophies with weakness that affects primarily the proximal limb girdle musculature
- ▶ Heterogeneous genetic mutations that can be autosomal dominant or recessive inheritance
- ▶ Associated with cardiomyopathies in some cases
- ▶ Dystrophic muscle findings on muscle biopsy include variations in fiber size, muscle fiber degeneration, inflammation, and replacement of muscle fiber by fat and connective tissue
- ▶ Treatment is supportive and multidisciplinary

The LGMDs are a group of heterogeneous, genetic degenerative muscle diseases primarily affecting proximal musculature. They clinically present with progressive proximal muscle weakness and elevated CPK. Muscle imaging over the course of disease demonstrates degenerative changes, and muscle biopsy demonstrates dystrophic findings. Besides the clinical features, genetic analyses and/or muscle biopsy are essential to establish the diagnosis. Management is supportive care provided by a multidisciplinary neuromuscular team. Cardiac medications and monitoring are routinely prescribed in patients with associated cardiac involvement to optimize cardiac function.

Clinical Findings

Symptoms and Signs

Symptom onset varies from early childhood after an individual has achieved independent ambulation to adulthood. Patients present with symptoms of motor difficulty and progressive pelvis and shoulder girdle muscle weakness and wasting. In addition to skeletal muscle involvement, cardiac and respiratory muscles can be affected in some types of LGMD. Chewing and swallowing function can also be affected in more advanced stages.

Laboratory Findings

Serum CPK levels vary from mildly to markedly elevated. Serum aminotransferases (AST and ALT), blood aldolase, and lactate dehydrogenase can be elevated if CPK levels are high and are not indicative of liver disease. Genetic testing demonstrating a mutation in a corresponding gene will aid in establishing the diagnosis in most cases. More than 30 genes have been identified to be associated with LGMD. Muscle biopsy may be necessary when genetic testing is unable to identify a pathogenic mutation. Histologically, muscle biopsy findings can vary from nonspecific myopathic changes to dystrophic features with myofibril degeneration and regeneration, inflammatory infiltrates, and progressive replacement of degenerative fibers with connective tissue and fat. Because muscle biopsy findings can vary depending on the severity of the weakness of the muscle biopsied, normal muscle histopathologic findings do not necessarily exclude a muscular dystrophy. Immunostaining for a specific protein in muscle tissue can aid in the diagnosis of some of the LGMD types (eg, sarcoglycanopathy, calpainopathy, dysferlinopathy, and dystroglycanopathy).

Imaging Findings

Fatty infiltration, replacement, and inflammation in affected musculature are typical degenerative findings demonstrated on muscle magnetic resonance imaging (MRI) that progressively increase over the course of disease development. Unique MRI findings have been found to be associated with specific types of LGMD (eg, studies have shown that thigh adductors, glutei, and posterior thigh muscles are the earliest and most severely affected muscles in sarcoglycanopathies). Normal or relatively preserved MRI findings of distal leg muscles and sparing of distal quadriceps are characteristics of all the sarcoglycanopathies.

Differential Diagnosis

Differential diagnoses include DMD, BMD, CMD, metabolic myopathies, congenital myasthenic syndrome, distal myopathies, myotonic dystrophy, and EDMD.

Complications

Specific anesthesia precautions to avoid malignant hyperthermia are recommended in patients with LGMD. Cardiomyopathy and symptoms related to central nerve system involvement can be seen in some LGMD types. Respiratory deficiency, neuromuscular scoliosis, feeding difficulty, and constipation are common complications in patients with advanced disease.

Treatment

Supportive treatment is typically managed through a multidisciplinary pediatric neuromuscular care center by several medical disciplines, including neurology, cardiology, pulmonary, dietary, gastroenterology, orthopedics, rehabilitation medicine, physical therapy, and occupational therapy.

EMERY-DREIFUSS MUSCULAR DYSTROPHY

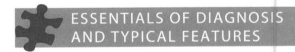

ESSENTIALS OF DIAGNOSIS AND TYPICAL FEATURES

► A heterogeneous group of muscular dystrophies with heterogeneous genetic mutations
► Presents with muscle weakness, early contractures, cardiac conduction abnormalities, cardiomyopathy, and life-threatening cardiac complications
► Dystrophic muscle findings on muscle biopsy
► Genetic diagnosis is essential
► Treatment is supportive and multidisciplinary

EDMD is a rare muscular dystrophy. EDMD clinically presents with joint contractures that begin in early childhood, slow progressive limb muscle weakness, and wasting. Symptoms related to cardiac conduction abnormalities and cardiomyopathy may manifest as palpitations, presyncope and syncope, poor exercise tolerance, and congestive heart failure, along with variable cardiac rhythm disturbances. The onset and severity of symptoms vary by subtype and individual, ranging from early onset and severe presentation in childhood to later onset with slow progression in adulthood. Besides the clinical features and dystrophic findings on muscle biopsy, genetic analyses are essential to establish the diagnosis. To date, at least 9 genes have been found to be associated with EDMD. Management is supportive care provided by a multidisciplinary neuromuscular team. Close cardiac monitoring is essential. Cardiac medications are routinely prescribed for patients who develop cardiac complications.

Clinical Findings

Symptoms and Signs

Symptom onset varies from early onset in childhood to late onset in adulthood. Patients present with early contractures affecting the elbow, neck, or spine, followed by symptoms of motor difficulty and progressive muscle weakness and wasting that begins in a humeroperoneal distribution and subsequently affects the scapular and pelvic girdle muscles. In addition to skeletal muscle involvement, cardiac complications are common and include both cardiac conduction abnormalities and cardiomyopathy. In advanced disease, respiratory function and chewing and swallowing function can also be affected.

Laboratory Findings

Serum CPK levels can be normal or mildly to markedly elevated (up to 15 times the upper limit of normal). Serum aminotransferases (AST and ALT), blood aldolase, and lactate dehydrogenase can be elevated if CPK levels are high and are not indicative of liver disease. Genetic testing demonstrating mutations in corresponding genes can help establish the diagnosis in most cases. Muscle biopsy may be necessary when genetic testing is unable to identify a pathogenic mutation. Histologically, muscle biopsy findings can vary from nonspecific myopathic changes to dystrophic features. Protein-specific immunostaining of muscle tissue can aid in the diagnosis of specific subtypes.

Imaging Findings

Fatty infiltration, replacement, and inflammation in affected musculature are typical degenerative findings demonstrated on muscle MRI that progressively increase over the course of disease development. Unique MRI findings have been found to be associated with specific types of EDMD (eg, studies have shown that in patients with laminopathies, muscle MRI demonstrates fatty infiltration of the semimembranosus, long and short heads of the biceps femoris, adductor magnus, and vasti muscles, with relative sparing of the rectus femoris).

Differential Diagnosis

Differential diagnoses include LGMD, BMD, CMD, metabolic myopathies, and distal myopathies.

Complications

Specific anesthesia precautions to avoid malignant hyperthermia are recommended in patients with EDMD. Cardiac involvement, including conduction abnormalities and cardiomyopathy, is common. Respiratory deficiency, neuromuscular scoliosis, and feeding difficulty are common complications in patients with advanced disease.

Treatment

Supportive treatment is typically managed through a multidisciplinary pediatric neuromuscular care center and provided by several medical disciplines, including neurology, cardiology, pulmonary, dietary, gastroenterology, orthopedics, rehabilitation medicine, physical therapy, and occupational therapy.

BIBLIOGRAPHY

Bockhorst J, Wicklund M. Limb girdle muscular dystrophies. *Neurol Clin.* 2020;38(3):493-504.

Domingos J, Sarkozy A, Scoto M, Muntoni F. Dystrophinopathies and limb-girdle muscular dystrophies. *Neuropediatrics.* 2017; 48(4):262-272.

Heller S, et al. Emery-Dreifuss muscular dystrophy. *Muscle Nerve.* 2020;61(4):436-448.

Liewluck T, Shih R, Kalra R, Kang PB. Untangling the complexity of limb-girdle muscular dystrophies. *Muscle Nerve.* 2018;58(2): 167-177.

Mercuri E, Bönnemann CG, Muntoni F. Muscular dystrophies. *Lancet.* 2019;394(10213):2025-2038.

Waldrop M, Flanigan KM. Update in Duchenne and Becker muscular dystrophies. *Curr Opin Neurol.* 2019;32(5):722-727.

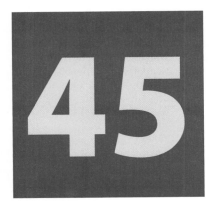

Motor Neuron Disease

Cuixia Tian, MD

Motor neuron diseases are a group of rare diseases affecting spinal motor neurons. They clinically present with progressive degenerative muscle weakness and wasting and lead to impairment in mobility, speech, swallowing, and breathing functions. Spinal muscular atrophy (SMA) is the leading cause for motor neuron disease in children. Here, we focus on SMAs, including the most common SMA, also known as proximal or 5q-SMA, as well as atypical SMA, also known as SMA plus, especially riboflavin-responsive motor neuron disease, which is a treatable childhood-onset motor neuron disease.

SPINAL MUSCULAR ATROPHY

ESSENTIALS OF DIAGNOSIS AND TYPICAL FEATURES

► A diverse group of genetic disorders associated with spinal motor neuron loss

► The most common form of SMA is 5q-SMA (also called proximal SMA), which is caused by homozygous deletion or mutation of the survival motor neuron 1 (*SMN1*) gene

► Clinically presents with muscle weakness, with onset of symptoms ranging from the prenatal period to adulthood

► Multisystem involvement; progressive weakening of respiratory and swallow muscles leads to respiratory insufficiency and feeding intolerance

► Genetic testing is essential for establishing diagnosis

► Genetic modification treatments are now available for 5q-SMA

SMAs are a group of degenerative neurologic diseases affecting spinal motor neurons caused by genetic mutations in a group of genes. The most common form of SMA is 5q-SMA (also called proximal SMA), which is caused by homozygous deletion or mutation of the *SMN1* gene. It accounts for up to 95% of SMA cases. Besides the clinical features, genetic analyses are essential to establish the diagnosis. Management is provided by a multidisciplinary neuromuscular team. Various genetic modification medications are now available for patients with 5q-SMA (eg, nusinersen and risdiplam for gene transcription modification treatment and onasemnogene abeparvovec-xioi for gene delivery therapy).

► Clinical Findings

Symptoms and Signs

For 5q-SMA, symptom onset varies from the prenatal period to adulthood. Patients present with symptoms of progressive proximal muscle weakness. Traditionally, 5q-SMA has been classified into types 1 to 3. Type 1 patients clinically present with symptoms beginning after birth and before age 6 months; affected patients have generalized hypotonia and are unable to sit independently. Breathing and swallowing functions are affected, and patients need breathing and feeding support to survive. Type 1 patients typically die before 2 years of age. Type 2 patients have symptoms that begin between 6 and 18 months. They achieve the ability to sit usually by 9 months but are never able to stand or walk. Type 3 patients present with symptom onset between 18 months and adulthood. Standing or walking without support is achieved, although many lose these abilities later in life with disease progression. Muscle weakness is more proximal and affects the lower extremities more than the upper extremities. Deep tendon reflexes are usually depressed or absent. Hand tremor can be seen in type 2 and 3 patients.

Tongue atrophy with fasciculation is a characteristic finding on exam. Facial and eye muscles are typically spared. Impairment of swallowing and breathing functions is common in advanced stages of disease. Scoliosis is common and contributes to restrictive ventilation defects. The majority of type 2 patients survive to age 25, and many patients live much longer with advanced support. Type 3 patients have a normal life span.

Atypical SMAs, also known as SMA plus syndromes, are disorders in which lower motor neuron dysfunction is the primary but not the sole feature of the disease. It is associated with genetic mutations in a diverse group of genes and a wide spectrum of clinical presentations. The clinical symptoms vary with regard to onset of symptoms, disease severity, weakness pattern, and multisystem involvement. Weakness can be proximal (SMA with progressive myoclonic epilepsy, congenital SMA with arthrogryposis and fractures, and SMA caused by mitochondrial disorders) or distal with predominantly lower extremity involvement (SMA with lower extremity predominance) or scapuloperoneal (scapuloperoneal SMA). Respiratory insufficiency is common, especially in SMA with respiratory distress, acute respiratory failure due to diaphragm paralysis is typically the initial presenting symptom.

Laboratory Findings

Molecular genetic testing is the standard tool for diagnosis of 5q-SMA and atypical SMA. Muscle biopsy and electrodiagnostic testing are no longer necessary due to the wide availability of genetic testing. Electromyogram and muscle biopsy showing features of denervation can be helpful for diagnosis if genetic testing is unrevealing.

▶ Differential Diagnosis

The differential diagnosis is broad. For type 1 5q-SMA, all other causes of hypotonic weakness in the infant should be considered, including central nervous system causes, congenital myopathy, congenital muscular dystrophy, and metabolic disorders, among others. For type 2 or 3 5q-SMA, Duchenne and Becker muscular dystrophies, limb-girdle muscular dystrophies, metabolic myopathies, inflammatory myopathies, neuropathy, neuromuscular junction disorders, and other motor neuron disorders should be considered.

▶ Complications

SMA patients are at high risk for the development of respiratory deficiency, neuromuscular scoliosis, and feeding difficulty. Pulmonary complications are the most common cause of death.

▶ Treatment

Several disease-modifying medications for 5q-SMA have recently become available. The antisense oligonucleotide medications nusinersen and risdiplam are gene modification therapies targeting *SMN2* gene transcription; they were approved for treatment of all types of 5q-SMA patients. The gene delivery medication onasemnogene abeparvovecxioi, which targets the *SMN1* gene, was approved for treating 5q-SMA patients younger than 2 years. Motor function improvement or stabilization was observed in symptomatic patients treated with these medications. In presymptomatic patients, treatment with these medications demonstrated stabilization and improvement of motor function and, in some cases, prevention of disease development, with type 1 patients achieving age-appropriate motor milestones. Because of the encouraging outcomes with these disease-modifying treatments, neonatal screening for SMA has become mandatory in many states in the United States.

Anticipatory management of respiratory weakness, prophylactic immunizations, and prompt treatment of respiratory infections are essential treatments. Supportive treatment is typically managed through a multidisciplinary pediatric neuromuscular care center by several medical disciplines, including neurology, pulmonary, dietary, gastroenterology, orthopedics, rehabilitation medicine, physical therapy, and occupational therapy.

RIBOFLAVIN-RESPONSIVE MOTOR NEURON DISEASE

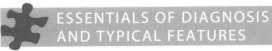

ESSENTIALS OF DIAGNOSIS AND TYPICAL FEATURES

- ▶ A subtype of atypical SMA
- ▶ A rare autosomal recessive neurologic disorder of pontobulbar motor neurons
- ▶ Presents with progressive facial and bulbar weakness, optic atrophy, arm and hand weakness, and ataxia, with or without hearing loss preceding neurologic symptoms
- ▶ High-dose riboflavin treatment is standard treatment, along with supportive and multidisciplinary management

Riboflavin-responsive motor neuron disease is also known as Brown-Vialetto-Van Laere (BVVL) syndrome and Fazio-Londe syndrome. It clinically presents with progressive facial and bulbar weakness, optic atrophy, arm and hand weakness, and ataxia. Sensorineural hearing loss typically presents before neurologic symptoms in BVVL syndrome, whereas

Fazio-Londe syndrome has no hearing loss. Besides the clinical features, genetic analyses are essential to establish the diagnosis. Management includes disease-modifying treatment with high-dose riboflavin, in addition to supportive care provided by a multidisciplinary neuromuscular team.

Clinical Findings

Symptoms and Signs

Symptom onset varies from early childhood to adulthood. BVVL syndrome clinically presents with progressive facial and bulbar weakness, dysphagia, tongue amyotrophy and fasciculations, sensorineural deafness, optic atrophy, weakness primarily affecting arms and hands, and sensory ataxia that leads to impaired ambulation. Hearing loss typically presents before the onset of neurologic symptoms. Fazio-Londe syndrome presents similar to BVVL syndrome except no hearing loss is present. The disease course is progressive and variable. Respiratory failure may develop over 6 to 18 months in early-onset cases, leading to recurrent chest infections and death. However, with optimal care, survival to the sixth decade has been reported. In addition to skeletal muscle involvement, vision and hearing impairments are common, and breathing, chewing, and swallowing functions are usually affected in advanced stages.

Laboratory Findings

Elevation of serum medium-chain acylcarnitines and deficient flavin levels are seen in some patients. Electrophysiology testing demonstrates absent brainstem auditory responses and a sensorimotor neuropathy. Molecular genetic testing is essential to aid diagnosis. BVVL syndrome is caused by homozygous or compound heterozygous mutations in *SLC52A2* or *SLC52A3* or heterozygous mutations in *UBQLN1*. Fazio-Londe syndrome is genetically related to *SLC52A3* pathogenic variants.

Differential Diagnosis

Differential diagnoses include other atypical SMAs, toxic myopathy, metabolic myopathy, inflammatory myopathy, and toxic or inflammatory neuropathies.

Complications

Hearing and vision impairments are common. Respiratory deficiency, neuromuscular scoliosis, and chewing and feeding difficulty are common complications in patients with advanced disease.

Treatment

Treatment is high-dose oral riboflavin supplementation at a dose ranging from 10 to 80 mg/kg/d. Clinical response varies; there can be rapid improvement in motor function, strength, hearing, and vision, with weaning of respiratory support and normalization of neurophysiologic parameters over days; gradual improvement over 12 months; stabilization; or in rare cases, no response.

Generally, the most positive responses are reported in patients who receive riboflavin supplementation shortly after disease onset. There have been reports of genetically diagnosed asymptomatic patients with positive family history who remained free of symptoms with high-dose riboflavin treatment. Abnormal acylcarnitine profiles and flavin levels normalize after riboflavin supplementation.

Supportive treatment is typically managed through a multidisciplinary pediatric neuromuscular care center by several medical disciplines, including neurology, pulmonary, ENT, audiology, ophthalmology, dietician, gastroenterologist, orthopedics, rehab medicine, physical therapy, and occupational therapy.

BIBLIOGRAPHY

Arnold WD, Kassar D, Kissel JT. Spinal muscular atrophy: diagnosis and management in a new therapeutic era. *Muscle Nerve.* 2015;51(2):157-67.

Mercuri E, Pera MC, Scoto M, et al. Spinal muscular atrophy: insights and challenges in the treatment era. *Nat Rev Neurol.* 2020;16:707-715.

O'Callaghan B, Bosch AM, Houlden H. An update on the genetics, clinical presentation, and pathomechanisms of human riboflavin transporter deficiency. *J Inherit Metab Dis.* 2019;42(4):598-607.

Teoh HL, Carey K, Sampaio H, et al. Inherited paediatric motor neuron disorders: beyond spinal muscular atrophy. *Neural Plast.* 2017;2017:6509493.

Wirth B. Spinal muscular atrophy: in the challenge lies a solution. *Trends Neurosci.* 2021;44(4):306-322.

The Inflammatory, Metabolic, and Toxic Myopathies

46

Cuixia Tian, MD

Alexander M. Zygmunt, MD

Myopathies are a heterogeneous group of disorders that affect the structure, function, or both structure and function of muscle fibers manifested most commonly by weakness in the patient. They may also present with either positive myopathic symptoms, such as cramps, contracture, hypertrophy, myalgia, or myoglobinuria, or negative myopathic symptoms, such as exercise intolerance, fatigue, muscle atrophy, or weakness.

There are a wide range of potential etiologies. This chapter will address inflammatory, metabolic, and toxic myopathies.

INFLAMMATORY MYOPATHIES

ESSENTIALS OF DIAGNOSIS AND TYPICAL FEATURES

▶ Juvenile idiopathic inflammatory myopathies are a rare and heterogeneous group of disorders, the most common clinical phenotype of which is juvenile dermatomyositis.

▶ Clinically, these myopathies are characterized by weakness, chronic inflammation of skeletal muscles, and typical skin rashes (Gottron papules or heliotrope rash) with onset during childhood,

▶ Serum autoantibody classification and clinicopathologic phenotype are essential for prognosis and treatment of these diseases.

Although classically diagnosed via clinicopathologic criteria first established in 1975 by Bohan and Peters, the juvenile idiopathic inflammatory myopathies (JIIMs) have recently undergone a paradigm shift in classification with the rise of antibody testing. In 2017, the European League Against Rheumatism (EULAR) and the American College of Rheumatology (ACR) introduced a new methodology to classify JIIMs based on physical examination signs and ancillary testing, specifically antibody testing. In contrast, the clinicopathologic criteria subdivided inflammatory myopathies into several discrete phenotypic groups, including juvenile dermatomyositis (JDM), juvenile polymyositis (JPM), overlap myositis, immune-mediated necrotizing myositis (IMNM), and hypomyopathic dermatomyositis (HD) (Table 46–1).

For patients with symptom onset beginning at age less than 18 years, EULAR/ACR criteria subclassify JIIMs into JDM and juvenile myositis other than JDM because the sample size was too small in the other subgroups to further subclassify. As more information arises via antibody testing, clinicopathologic phenotypes are becoming less relevant than underlying disease mechanism for prognosis and treatment.

▶ Clinical Findings

Symptoms and Signs

Clinically, the presence of a characteristic rash, Gottron papules or heliotropic rash, differentiates JDM from juvenile myositis other than JDM (JPM, overlap myositis, IMNM, or HD).

Typically, patients with JIIMs develop weakness that is symmetric, proximal (effecting proximal shoulder or hip limb girdle), and progressive. Historical details that may point to proximal weakness include difficulty rising from chair or with squatting, difficulty climbing stairs, worsening exercise tolerance, difficulty performing activities that require lifting arms above the head such as brushing hair or lifting objects onto a shelf, and difficulty keeping up with peers in physical activities. In JIIMs, neck flexor weakness is more pronounced than neck extensor weakness. Pharyngeal muscles may also be involved, resulting in dysphagia, nasal speech, or hoarseness. Diffuse myalgias may be reported, but severe muscle pain is usually not present.

Table 46–1. Classic clinicopathologic phenotypes of juvenile idiopathic inflammatory myopathies (JIIMs).

Clinicopathologic Phenotype	Historical, Epidemiologic, and Physical Examination Notes	Muscle Biopsy	Outcomes and Potential Complications
Juvenile dermatomyositis (JDM)	• ~85% of JIIM • Youngest age of onset (median, 7.5 years) • Clinical features include symmetric proximal muscle weakness, Gottron papules or heliotrope rash, small vessel vasculopathy (periungual), and other photosensitive rash	• Perifascicular muscle atrophy • Inflammatory infiltrate in perimysium and pericapillary • Reduction in capillaries	• 2%-3% mortality • 24%-40% monocyclic course • 50%-60% chronic course • 20%-40% calcinosis • ~10% lipodystrophy • Rare GI ulcerations and pulmonary or GI air leaks
Overlap myositis	• 6%-11% of JIIM • Meet criteria for JIIM plus another autoimmune disease • Systemic lupus erythematosus, juvenile idiopathic arthritis, systemic sclerosis, scleroderma • Clinical features include Raynaud phenomenon, interstitial lung disease, Malar rash, and arthritis	• More commonly has findings of JDM but can have histopathologic appearance of JPM	• Higher mortality than JDM • Interstitial lung disease is often associated with overlap myositis
Juvenile polymyositis (JPM)	• 4%-8% of JIIM • Older age of onset (median, 11 years old) • Clinical features include proximal and distal muscle weakness in absence of typical rash, weight loss, rapid and severe onset, myalgias • Often misdiagnosed in patients who have noninflammatory myopathies	• Endomysial inflammation • CD8$^+$ T cells	• Mortality intermediate between JDM and overlap myositis • Cardiac involvement in 35% of patients
Hypomyopathic dermatomyositis	• Rare • Presence of Gottron papules and/or heliotrope rash for 6 months with no discernable weakness on exam	• Same findings as JDM	• Good prognosis, with many patients recovering without any therapy • Can still progress to JDM • Complications seen in adults (interstitial lung disease, malignancy, ulcerations) are rare in children • Cancer screening is not routinely recommended in pediatric population
Immune-mediated necrotizing myositis	• Rare • Proximal muscle weakness • Rare extramuscular involvement (<10%) • Can progress very slowly in pediatric population (over the course of years); sometimes misdiagnosed as limb girdle muscular dystrophy	• Necrosis of muscle fibers • Paucity of lymphocytes • Absent perivascular inflammation and perifascicular atrophy	• If common autoantibodies are found, then likelihood of cancer is very low • If no autoantibody can be identified, raises suspicion for underlying neoplasm

GI, gastrointestinal.

Skin manifestations also can aid in the diagnosis of JIIMs, specifically JDM. In other forms of juvenile myositis other than JDM, rash is not typically present. Two rashes that are pathognomonic for JDM are Gottron sign or Gottron papules and heliotrope rash. Gottron papules are raised erythematous papules or plaques that are distributed over extensor surfaces of bony prominences, typically located over the metacarpophalangeal joints and the proximal and distal interphalangeal joints of the fingers. Gottron sign is an erythematous rash in the same distribution but without the raised papules. Heliotrope rash is a violaceous rash involving the upper eyelids that may be accompanied by periorbital edema.

In addition to these pathognomonic rashes, patients with JDM may develop erythematous and occasionally pruritic rashes in distribution over photosensitive areas of the skin such as extensor surfaces, in a V shape in the anterior chest, over the back and shoulders (shawl sign), and in a malar distribution on the face. Resolving rashes can later become poikiloderma, hyper- or hypopigmented lesions on the upper back and extensor surfaces.

JIIMs may also feature calcinosis and vasculopathy, which are discussed later in the Complications section of this chapter.

Laboratory Findings

Most children with JIIMs will have elevation in at least one of several serum enzymes that are released when skeletal muscle is damaged. These enzymes include creatine phosphokinase, alanine aminotransferase (ALT), aspartate aminotransferase (AST), aldolase, and lactate dehydrogenase, although there is no consensus on which of these elevations is most useful diagnostically. In approximately 10% of children, all of these enzymes will be within normal limits. Serum γ-glutamyltransferase, which is liver specific, can be used in situations of elevated AST and ALT to help differentiate liver disease from muscle disease.

Antibody testing can help aid in diagnosis, classification, and prognosis for JIIM. Two major subdivisions of antibodies may be identified: myositis-specific antibodies, which are autoantibodies found exclusively in idiopathic inflammatory myopathies (IIMs), and myositis-associated antibodies, which are autoantibodies found in IIMs and other autoimmune conditions. Although the same autoantibodies found in adult IIMs are found in JIIMs, the most common autoantibodies found in JIIMs differ from those most commonly seen in adults. In children, the most common antibodies found in IIMs are anti-p155/140 and anti-MJ antibodies. A full list of antibodies and clinical associations can be found in Table 46–2.

Anti-p155/140 antibodies are seen in 23% to 30% of JIIMs and are most commonly associated with JDM phenotype or overlap myositis with JDM. Individuals who test positive for anti-p155/140 antibodies tend to have extensive photosensitive skin rashes, generalized lipodystrophy, and a more chronic disease course. Anti-MJ antibodies are seen in 12% to 23% of JIIMs and are most commonly associated with JDM clinicopathologic phenotype but are also seen in overlap myositis and JPM phenotype. They are associated with earlier onset and a more severe disease course. Individuals who test positive for anti-MJ antibodies tend to have frequent muscle cramps, muscle atrophy, joint contractures, dysphonia, and an absence of truncal rashes. Gastrointestinal (GI) ulcers are rarely seen in patients with anti-MJ antibodies, but they are seen at a more frequent rate than in patients with JIIM who lack this antibody.

Other testing modalities that have aided diagnoses in the past are nerve conduction studies (NCSs), electromyography (EMG), and muscle biopsy. These tests are less frequently performed currently due to concerns involving their invasive nature (concern for NCS/EMG and biopsy), the patchy distribution of JIIM (biopsy), and the need for cooperation (NCS/EMG). However, these tests can still shed light on the diagnosis and prognosis for JIIM.

On NCS/EMG, sensory and motor nerve conduction studies are typically normal. Sometimes, low-amplitude motor nerve responses can be seen when weakness is severe and diffuse. EMG will show signs of a myopathic process with membrane irritability with abnormal spontaneous activity, such as fibrillation potentials and positive sharp waves, and short-duration, low-amplitude motor unit potentials with an early recruitment pattern. Compared to patients with the other JIIMs, patients with IMNM tend to demonstrate more abnormal spontaneous activity while at rest.

Muscle biopsy features seen in cases of JIIMs are endomysial infiltration of mononuclear cells that surround, but do not invade, the myofibers; perimysial infiltration of mononuclear cells; perivascular infiltration of mononuclear cells; perifascicular atrophy; and rimmed vacuoles.

Imaging Studies

Muscle magnetic resonance imaging (MRI) can be useful in the diagnosis and to follow response to treatment of JIIM. T1-weighted and short tau inversion recovery (STIR) sequences of the hip girdle or shoulder girdle can be particularly helpful. T1-weighted sequences are best to demonstrate fatty atrophy. STIR sequences can detect muscle or fascial edema, which will appear as hyperintensity. The pattern of visualization of inflammatory changes in imaging is similar to the clinical picture in JIIMs, preferentially involving proximal muscles.

▶ Differential Diagnosis

There are several other diagnoses to be considered when suspecting JIIM, listed in Table 46–3. Some of the most common and important considerations should be given to other rheumatologic disorders. Given the presence of overlap myositis, other rheumatologic conditions such as lupus, scleroderma, and mixed connective tissue disease must be considered. For nonrheumatologic diseases, congenital myopathies and muscular dystrophy, infectious and postinfectious etiologies (especially postinfluenza myositis, coxsackie B virus, and HIV), and endocrinopathies (eg, adrenal and thyroid disease) should be investigated in the proper circumstances.

▶ Complications

An important complication to consider in JIIM is calcinosis, deposits of calcium under the skin and subcutaneous tissues. Calcinosis can present in multiple forms. Calcinosis

Table 46–2. Clinicopathologic phenotypes and association with autoantibodies.

| Clinicopathologic Phenotype | Myositis-Specific Autoantibodies | | Myositis-Associated Autoantibodies | |
	Commonly Associated Autoantibodies (frequency)	Findings Specific to Autoantibody	Commonly Associated Autoantibodies (frequency)	Findings Specific to Autoantibody
Juvenile dermatomyositis (JDM)	Anti-p155/140 (35%)	Classical JDM rashes and capillary changes, lipodystrophy risk, chronic disease course	Anti-Ro (5%)	Sometimes associated with anti-Jo autoantibodies
	Anti-MJ (22%)	More severe onset, cramps, calcinosis, monocyclic course		
	Anti-synthetase (3%)	Among JIIM, highest mortality due to interstitial lung disease	Anti-U1RNP (2%)	Raynaud phenomenon, arthritis, sclerodactyly
	Anti-Mi-2 (3%)	Classic JDM rashes, milder disease course		
Juvenile polymyositis	Anti-SRP (18%)	Severe weakness, frequent falls, very high CK levels, cardiac involvement, chronic course	Anti-U1RNP (12%)	Raynaud phenomenon, arthritis, sclerodactyly
	Anti-MJ (9%)	More severe onset, cramps, calcinosis, monocyclic course	Anti-PM/SCl (6%)	Arthritis, interstitial lung disease, Raynaud phenomenon, esophageal dysmotility
	Anti-synthetase (9%)	Among JIIM, highest mortality due to interstitial lung disease	Anti-Ro (6%)	Sometimes associated with anti-Jo autoantibodies
			Anti-Sm (3%)	None
Overlap myositis	Anti-p155/140 (17%)	Classical JDM rashes and capillary changes, lipodystrophy risk, chronic disease course	Anti-U1RNP (27%)	Raynaud phenomenon, arthritis, sclerodactyly
	Anti-MJ (15%)	More severe onset, cramps, calcinosis, monocyclic course	Anti-Ro (15%)	Sometimes associated with anti-Jo autoantibodies
	Anti-synthetase (12%)	Among JIIM, highest mortality due to interstitial lung disease	Anti-PM/Sci (10%)	Arthritis, interstitial lung disease, Raynaud phenomenon, esophageal dysmotility
	Anti-Mi-2 (2%)	Classic JDM rashes, milder disease course	Anti-Sm (10%)	None

CK, creatine kinase; JIIM, juvenile idiopathic inflammatory myopathy.

circumscripta forms superficial nodules or plaques. Tumoral calcinosis presents as calcium tumors that can extend into deeper tissues. Collections of calcium can form along fascial planes or along ligaments or tendons. Finally, calcium can form plates that can result in joint contractures known as exoskeletal calcinosis.

Other potential complications include vasculopathy, which is particularly apparent in the periungual capillaries. When affected with vasculopathy, the periungual capillaries become tortuous, dilated, and decreased in density, and cuticles appear irregularly thickened and distorted.

In late stages of disease and in some severe phenotypes, interstitial lung disease may develop. This complication is associated with poor outcome and higher mortality. The GI system may also be involved with vasculopathy, potentially leading to GI bleeding that can become dangerous. Finally, although rare, cardiac muscle can be involved, leading to cardiac arrhythmia or ejection fraction deficits.

▶ Treatment

Goals of treatment focus on normalizing muscle strength to promote function, controlling extramuscular manifestations, and minimizing medication adverse effects. Initial treatment usually encompasses combination therapy with prednisone (2 mg/kg/d) and methotrexate (15 mg/m² or 1 mg/kg/dose). In moderate to severe cases, intravenous (IV) methylprednisolone (30 mg/kg to maximum of 1 g) burst may be warranted because vasculopathy may limit absorption of oral medication.

Table 46–3. Differential diagnosis in suspected juvenile idiopathic inflammatory myopathy.

When Rash Is Present
Systemic lupus erythematosus
Scleroderma
Mixed connective tissue disease
Psoriasis
Eczema
Fungal infections
When Rash Is Absent
Muscular dystrophies
Congenital myopathies
Metabolic myopathies
Endocrinopathies (thyroid, parathyroid, adrenal insufficiency)
Viral or other infectious myositis (influenza, parainfluenza, coxsackie B virus, HIV, *Borrelia burgdorferi, Toxoplasmosis gondii,* trichinae, cysticercosis)
Toxic myopathies (steroids, statins, alcohol)

In severe or refractory cases, other medication options may be warranted. There is evidence to support IV immunoglobulin (IVIG; 2 g/kg every 2 weeks for 3 doses, then monthly) and mycophenolate mofetil (800-1350 mg/m²/d) in cases of JIIMs. Oral tacrolimus and IV pulse cyclophosphamide have been used with some success in very small cohorts with particularly refractory JIIMs.

Biologic agents may be helpful in refractory cases. There is evidence that patients with refractory IIMs who have received rituximab have shown clinical improvement. Infliximab, etanercept, anakinra, tocilizumab, and alemtuzumab have very sparse data to indicate effectiveness at this time.

Nonpharmacologic treatment can include protection from sun to help rashes to heal and vitamin D and calcium supplementation to promote bone health while on steroids.

▶ Prognosis

Generally, the prognosis of JIIMs is good. Mortality is estimated at less than 2%, and factors associated with higher mortality are inclusion in the subgroup of JIIM other than JDM, presence of pulmonary disease, and presence of anti-tRNA synthetase antibody.

At 2 years after disease onset, about 25% of patients will have had a single course, 25% of patients will have established a polycyclic course with periods of complete remission and recurrence, and the final 50% will demonstrate a chronic course requiring immunosuppressive medications continually during that time. Long-term complications of JIIMs can include persistent skin manifestations, morbidity secondary to calcinosis, and persistent weakness.

METABOLIC MYOPATHIES

ESSENTIALS OF DIAGNOSIS AND TYPICAL FEATURES

▶ Metabolic myopathies are a rare class of genetic disorders that occur due to inability to transform carbohydrates, fats, and proteins into adenosine triphosphate (ATP) at the cellular level.

▶ Clinically, these myopathies are very heterogenous and vary greatly in timing of onset, severity, and prognosis, but typical presentation includes muscle weakness, exercise intolerance, cramping, and intermittent rhabdomyolysis with other organ systems often also involved. External ophthalmoplegia may be a clue to mitochondrial myopathy.

▶ With the rise of targeted and rapid genetic testing, the clinical utility of muscle biopsy is decreasing in the field of metabolic myopathies.

Metabolic myopathies encompass a broad and heterogenous group of genetic diseases that are, as individual diseases, very rare. The uniting feature of these myopathies is that they result from the body's inability to transform carbohydrates, fats, and proteins into ATP, resulting in deficient energy production. These deficiencies can arise from mitochondrial disorders, glycogen storage disorders, or disorders of lipid metabolism. These myopathies should especially be suspected when myopathy is concurrent with other organ system involvement. When evaluating for primary mitochondrial myopathy, it is important to remember that nuclear DNA and mitochondrial DNA can be the underlying cause of respiratory chain dysfunction and that the concept of heteroplasmy can affect severity of disease.

▶ Clinical Findings

Symptoms and Signs

Metabolic myopathies refer to myopathies caused by deficient energy production at the cellular level due to a broad spectrum of genetic entities. These defects can occur because of primary mitochondrial disorders, which involve a failure of oxidative phosphorylation due to respiratory chain dysfunction; glycogen storage disorders, which involve the inability to transform stored carbohydrates into energy; or disorders of fatty acid oxidation, which involve the inability to transform stored fats into energy. There are some classically described phenotypic presentations for these hereditary diseases. The most common of these are summarized individually in Table 46–4.

Table 46–4. Common types of metabolic myopathies.

Disease	Key Clinical Features	Testing (nongenetic)	Genetic Considerations
Primary Mitochondrial Disorders With Myopathy as Key Symptom			
Myoclonic epilepsy with ragged red fibers (MERRF)	Progressive epilepsy, myoclonus, myopathy, sensorineural hearing loss, ataxia	Elevated lactate in serum and CSF, elevated CSF protein, muscle biopsy will show ragged red fibers on Gomori trichrome staining	Maternally inherited related to pathogenic variant in mitochondrial DNA most commonly in gene *MT-TK* encoding tRNA^{Lys}.
Mitochondrial encephalo-myopathy, lactic acidosis, and stroke-like syndrome (MELAS)	Strokes and stroke-like events in nonvascular territories, epilepsy, myopathy, cognitive impairment, sensorineural hearing loss	Elevated lactate in serum and CSF, MRI may demonstrate stroke-like lesions in nonvascular territories (most commonly parieto-occipital), ragged red fibers on muscle biopsy	Maternally inherited related to pathogenic variant in mitochondrial DNA most commonly in gene *MT-TL1* encoding tRNA^{Leu}.
Kearns-Sayre syndrome (KSS)	Onset <20 years, external ophthalmoplegia, myopathy, retinitis pigmentosa, sensorineural hearing loss, cardiac conduction block; more severe version of CPEO	Elevated lactate in serum and CSF, elevated CSF protein, ECG with conduction block, ragged red fibers on muscle biopsy	Large mitochondrial DNA deletion syndrome: most commonly sporadic mutation of mitochondrial DNA, can be maternally inherited. Typically, a deletion of 1.1-10 kb of mtDNA. KSS and CPEO considered a spectrum.
Chronic progressive external ophthalmoplegia (CPEO)	Bilateral ophthalmoparesis, myopathy, ptosis, oropharyngeal weakness; milder version of KSS	Clinical diagnosis, lactate may be elevated in serum and CSF	See above.
Mitochondrial myopathy due to thymidine kinase 2 (TK2) deficiency	Variable onset: if infantile onset, will typically have profound myopathy with encephalopathy; if juvenile onset, will typically have proximal muscle involvement; if older age onset, more commonly with facial weakness	Elevated creatinine kinase (CK)	Nuclear DNA pathogenic variant in TK2. Autosomal recessive inheritance pattern.
POLG-spectrum disorders	Multiple described disorders with varying onset and severity: explosive-onset epilepsy, lactic acidosis, liver dysfunction, myopathy, valproate toxicity, sensory ataxia, neuropathy, external ophthalmoplegia	Elevated serum and CSF lactate, elevated CSF protein	Multiple nuclear DNA genes implicated, most commonly *POLG*. Most commonly inherited in autosomal recessive fashion.
Glycogen Storage Disorders			
Glycogen storage disease type II (Pompe disease); deficient acid maltase	Infantile: <12 months onset, hypotonia, myopathy, hypertrophic cardiomyopathy. Last onset: <12 months without cardiac involvement or >12 months of age, proximal muscle weakness and respiratory insufficiency	Elevated CK serum levels, elevation of urine glucose, tetrasaccharide; abnormal analysis of acid α-glucosidase activity on dried blood spots	*GAA* gene on chromosome 17q25.3. Autosomal recessive inheritance.
Glycogen storage disease (GSD) type IIIa (Cori disease); deficient amylo-1,6-glucosidase	Infantile to early childhood onset of hepatomegaly that improves with age, myopathy with distal predominance mild in childhood but slowly worsens into adulthood with extremely variable course, cardiac hypertrophy sometimes seen	Neonatal hypoglycemia with normal lactate, normal uric acid, elevated ketone bodies; biochemical testing of liver biopsy specimen will show abnormal amylo-1,6-glucosidase activity	*AGL* gene on chromosome 1p21. If mutation is in exon 3 of gene, will have GSD type IIIb (liver involvement without muscle). If downstream of exon 3, will have type IIIa (muscle and liver). Autosomal recessive inheritance.

(Continued)

Table 46–4. Common types of metabolic myopathies. (*Continued*)

Disease	Key Clinical Features	Testing (nongenetic)	Genetic Considerations
GSD type V (McArdle disease); deficient myophosphorylase	Adult onset, muscle cramps, pain, and potentially rhabdomyolysis in first minutes of exercise, but "second wind" with improvement in symptoms as exercise continues	Elevated CK, uric acid increased, lactate does not increase with exercise	*PYGM* gene on chromosome 11q13. Poor genotype-phenotype correlation. Autosomal recessive inheritance.
GSD type VII (Tarui disease); deficient muscle phospho-fructokinase (PFK)	Similar to McArdle but with earlier onset, more severe weakness, no second-wind phenomenon, and worsening of symptoms if exercising after carbohydrate-rich meal	Lactate does not increase with exercise PFK deficiency by immunohistochemistry	*PFKM* gene on chromosome 12q13.11. Autosomal recessive inheritance.
Fatty Oxidation Disorders			
Carnitine palmitoyltransferase 2 (CPT2) deficiency	Nonketotic hypoglycemia, cardiomyopathy, myopathy, renal dysgenesis, seizures	Low free carnitine in plasma, long-chain acylcarnitine high in plasma	*CPT2* on chromosome 1p32.3. Multiple phenotypes with different inheritance patterns, either autosomal recessive or autosomal dominant.
Very-long-chain acyl-CoA dehydrogenase (VLCAD) deficiency	Three major phenotypes: Infantile: hypertrophic cardiomyopathy and liver failure; childhood: hypoketotic hypoglycemia; juvenile: recurrent rhabdomyolysis triggered by prolonged exercise or fasting	Increased serum long-chain acylcarnitine, nonketotic hypoglycemia	*ACADVL* gene on chromosome 17p13.1. Autosomal recessive inheritance.
Mitochondrial trifunctional protein (MTP) deficiency	Hepatopathy, hypoketotic hypoglycemia, rhabdomyolysis, myopathy, cardiomyopathy, capillary leak syndrome; if milder phenotype, will develop neuropathy over time	Elevated long-chain 3-hydroxyacylcarnitine and free fatty acids in serum, elevated dicarboxylic acid in urine	Encoded by 2 different genes: *HADHA* and *HADHB*, both on chromosome 2p23. Autosomal recessive inheritance.
Glutaric aciduria type II or multiple acyl-CoA dehydrogenase deficiency (MADD)	Hypoglycemia, encephalopathy, myopathy, cardiomyopathy; milder forms with isolated persistent weakness; some patients respond to riboflavin	Elevated urine glutaric acid, lactic acid, ethylmalonic acid, butyric acid, isobutyric acid, 2-methyl-butyric acid, and isovaleric acid	*ETFDH* gene on chromosome 4p32.1, *ETFA* gene on chromosome 15q24.2-q24.3, or *ETFB* gene on chromosome 19q13.41. All autosomal recessive inheritance.

CoA, coenzyme A; CSF, cerebrospinal fluid; ECG, electrocardiogram; MRI, magnetic resonance imaging; mtDNA, mitochondrial DNA.

Although clinically, these myopathies are diverse with variable onset, severity, and myopathic symptomatology, there may be some clues to point to the underlying metabolic etiology. The most common myopathic symptom in primary mitochondrial disease is painless exercise intolerance. External ophthalmoplegia or ptosis on examination should raise suspicion for mitochondrial myopathy. Mitochondrial diseases can be secondary to mutations in either nuclear DNA or mitochondrial DNA. Diseases affecting mitochondrial DNA are subject to extreme variability due to heteroplasmy (ie, variability in percentage and location of cells that contain mutations in mitochondrial DNA).

The most common myopathic symptoms in glycogen storage disorders are episodic exercise intolerance, myoglobinuria, and cramping, especially at the initiation of anaerobic exercise. Some glycogen storage disorders, such as glycogen storage disorder type V (McArdle disease), have the phenomenon of a "second wind," that is, as more time passes (approximately 10 minutes of exercising) and fatty acid oxidation metabolically begins, the symptoms improve.

A common myopathic clue to an underlying fatty acid oxidation disorder is the presence of episodic exercise intolerance or weakness in the setting of prolonged exercise such as hiking or in periods of illness.

An important clue to the presence of a metabolic myopathy is the involvement of other organ systems in addition to the above myopathic symptoms. Brain, eyes, heart, liver, kidney, pancreas, and GI system may all be involved concomitantly in cases of metabolic myopathy (Table 46–5).

Table 46–5. Organ systems concomitantly involved in metabolic myopathies.

Organ/Organ System	Symptoms
Central nervous system	Seizure, tremor, developmental delays, sensorineural hearing loss, stroke/stroke-like episodes, ataxia
Liver	Liver failure, hepatic steatosis
Ophthalmologic	Ptosis, external ophthalmoplegia, optic atrophy
Cardiac	Cardiomyopathy, conduction block
Renal	Fanconi syndrome, nephrotic syndrome, kidney failure
Pancreas	Diabetes
Gastrointestinal	Gut dysmotility, intestinal pseudo-obstruction, chronic diarrhea

Laboratory Studies

There are several laboratory tests that can help to screen for underlying metabolic myopathies. Creatinine kinase (CK) is elevated in some, but not all, metabolic myopathies. Serum lactic acid will often be elevated in metabolic myopathies, usually mitochondrial myopathies, although results should be interpreted carefully. If lab was drawn after tourniquet placement or after a significant amount of exercise, values may be spuriously elevated. Concurrent pyruvate level can help to establish a lactate/pyruvate ratio. An elevated lactate/pyruvate ratio (>30) indicates compromised aerobic energy metabolism (disorders of respiratory chain complex or tricarboxylic acid cycle). In some mitochondrial myopathies, serum amino acids may be abnormal, demonstrating elevated alanine (if fasting) with an alanine-to-lysine ratio greater than 4:1; low taurine, arginine, or citrulline; or elevated proline or sarcosine. In mitochondrial diseases and lipid myopathies, free carnitine levels may be low. Urine organic acids may demonstrate elevated lactic acid, pyruvic acid, dicarboxylic acids, and 3-methylglutaconic acid in mitochondrial myopathies and lipid myopathies.

As detailed in Table 46–4, specific enzyme assays may help to detect certain glycogen storage disorders and certain fatty acid oxidation disorders. Enzymatic analysis of the oxidative phosphorylation complex may aid in the diagnosis of mitochondrial myopathy. Muscle biopsy may also aid in diagnosis, with appearance of ragged red fibers on Gomori trichrome stain for certain mitochondrial myopathies. However, given the rise of less invasive molecular testing, utility of muscle biopsy is lessening.

Genetic studies have come to the forefront of the diagnostic approach to metabolic myopathies. In terms of mitochondrial myopathies, genes that affect the support and function of mitochondria are found in both nuclear DNA, inherited in Mendelian fashion, or in mitochondrial DNA. Mitochondrial DNA is inherited maternally; that is, any mitochondrial DNA variance in a mother will be passed on to all of her children and no mitochondrial DNA variance would be passed on by the father. Mitochondrial DNA is subject to heteroplasmy, which is a variability in percentage and location of affected cells. The higher the percent heteroplasmy, the more cells are affected by the mutation and the more severe the phenotype is likely to be. Inheritance pattern and clinical phenotype should be considered when considering genetic testing for suspected mitochondrial myopathy. Targeted gene panel or whole-exome or whole-genome sequencing could be helpful if pathogenic variance is suspected in nuclear DNA. However, if the underlying etiology is thought to be from mitochondrial DNA, then testing should be targeted to that (see Table 46–4 for some descriptions of presentations of mitochondrial disease).

Similarly, many single genes have been found as underlying etiologies to glycogen storage disorders and fatty acid oxidation disorders (see Table 46–4). If these metabolic processes are thought to be underlying a patient's symptomatology, gene panels targeting these genetic anomalies should be sent.

Imaging Studies

Imaging studies should be ordered based on suspicion of other systems involved. Brain MRI may be useful in cases of myopathy that have components of central nervous system (CNS) involvement. Like all features of metabolic diseases, the findings are variable in nature. The most common finding that suggests a metabolic disorder is symmetric signal abnormality involving the deep gray matter that appears hyperintense on T2 and FLAIR images and hypointense on T1 images. However, some patients with metabolic myopathy can have normal imaging findings or imaging with nonspecific findings. For instance, the most common imaging abnormality in patients with mitochondrial disease is nonspecific global delay in myelination with a "catch-up" period at an older age.

▶ Differential Diagnosis

The differential diagnosis for metabolic diseases will differ based on the primary symptom present and severity of the symptomatology. When myopathy is the primary symptom, the differential diagnosis should remain broad. If ptosis is present, myasthenia gravis should be considered. In hypotonic infants, systemic illness such as sepsis should be excluded. Endocrinopathies such as hypothyroidism, adrenal insufficiency, diabetes mellitus, and hypoparathyroidism can present with fatigue and exercise intolerance. Other potential etiologies for fatigue and exercise intolerance include inflammatory disorders such as systemic lupus erythematosus, congenital muscular dystrophies, anemia, vitamin deficiencies (eg, vitamin B_{12} deficiency, vitamin E deficiency, and other cobalamin disorders), fibromyalgia, and chronic fatigue syndrome.

▶ Complications

Potential complications are wide ranging and variable based on disease severity. Specific organ system involvement should be considered when assessing the patient. For metabolic myopathies that present with episodic rhabdomyolysis and myoglobinuria, kidney failure can occur if the rhabdomyolysis is severe. There is concomitant liver involvement with many of the metabolic myopathies, and liver failure is a potential complication. In metabolic myopathies with CNS involvement, progressive encephalopathy and progressive epilepsy are potential complications. Cardiomyopathy and heart failure are seen in many metabolic disorders. In mitochondrial disorders involving the eye, optic nerve atrophy and blindness can occur. Sensorineural hearing loss is a complication seen in many mitochondrial disorders. In the fatty acid oxidation disorder carnitine palmitoyltransferase 2 deficiency, malignant hyperthermia can occur with the use of inhaled anesthetics or with depolarizing muscle relaxants.

▶ Treatment

For mitochondrial disorders, care should be directed at symptomatic management and surveillance for potential complications based on organ systems involved. In cases of myopathy, an evaluation for sleep apnea can be beneficial, and noninvasive or invasive ventilation may be warranted.

There is no evidence to date of any pharmacologic agents that are effective in treating mitochondrial disease. Several vitamins and cofactors have traditionally been used in clinical practice, most commonly coenzyme Q10, riboflavin, and α-lipoic acid, and some patients anecdotally report improvement.

For glycogen storage disorders, therapy is typically targeted at changes in the diet to avoid hypoglycemia. Frequent high-protein meals during the daytime and uncooked cornstarch have shown benefit in patients with glycogen storage diseases. Pompe disease (glycogen storage disease type II) is an exception. Enzyme replacement therapy with alglucosidase alfa is now available for Pompe disease.

For fatty acid oxidation disorders, dietary modifications are also the mainstay of treatment. Fasting should be avoided. Long-chain fatty acids should be avoided and replaced with medium-chain fatty acids in the diet.

▶ Prognosis

Prognosis is also extremely variable. Generally, for primary mitochondrial disorders, the earlier the onset, the more severe and diffuse is the symptomatology. Most tend to progress at variable rates rather than stay static or improve.

Prognosis follows a similar rule of thumb for glycogen storage disorders, with more severe phenotypes presenting earlier in life, although these do not always progress and often improve with therapies. In glycogen storage disease type IIIa (Cori disease), liver dysfunction tends to improve with time.

Fatty acid oxidation disorders also have highly variable prognosis with a wide range of phenotypes in the same disease category. Some are progressive in nature, and earlier disease onset typically indicates a poor prognosis. Like glycogen storage disorders, milder fatty acid oxidation disorders tend to respond well to dietary therapies.

TOXIC MYOPATHIES

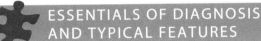

ESSENTIALS OF DIAGNOSIS AND TYPICAL FEATURES

▶ There are a wide range of toxins and medications that can cause myopathy via a variety of mechanisms, the most common of which are necrotizing myopathy via HMG-CoA reductase inhibitor (statin) use and amphiphilic myopathy via amiodarone or hydroxychloroquine and corticosteroid use, the mechanism of which is unclear.

▶ These myopathies are clinically diverse and usually occur soon after initiation of the new medication; however, in some cases, myopathies can occur months to years after starting medications.

▶ Although these myopathies will usually resolve within weeks of stopping the causative medication, recognition of agents that may trigger immune-mediated response is vital, and more medical management may be necessary in these cases.

▶ Clinical Findings

Toxic myopathies are a clinically and pathologically diverse group of myopathies that closely resemble many other causes of weakness. They typically occur soon after starting a new causative medication but can occur months or years after starting the causative agent. There are many pathologic mechanisms by which toxins can cause myopathy, including necrotizing, amphiphilic, inflammatory, mitochondrial, antimicrotubular, hypokalemic, and in some cases, unknown. Stopping the offending agent is the first line of treatment, and in cases of inflammatory myopathies, immunomodulatory therapy may be needed.

Symptoms and Signs

A detailed medication history and index of suspicion for toxic myopathy are crucial to diagnosis. The most commonly reported pathologic mechanism of toxic myopathy is necrotizing myopathy via HMG-CoA reductase inhibitors (statins). In cases of statin use that involve muscle, patients will typically experience myalgias in proximal muscle groups and cramping in small muscles of the hands that starts typically 1 to 6 months after starting the statin. Less commonly, patients have proximal muscle weakness and rhabdomyolysis. Symptoms can present more severely if statins are combined with other agents that can cause myopathy (Table 46–6) or with cytochrome P450 inhibitors. Other agents that can cause necrotizing myopathy are other cholesterol-lowering medications (eg, gemfibrozil, niacin,

Table 46–6. Pathologic mechanisms for toxic myopathies and common causative agents.

Pathologic Mechanism	Implicated Agents	Clinical Notes	Ancillary Testing	Comments
Necrotizing	HMG-CoA reductase inhibitors (statins), immunophilins, other lipid-lowering agents, labetalol, propofol	Proximal muscle myalgia, cramping of small muscles of hands, proximal muscle weakness, and rhabdomyolysis when severe	Level of CK elevation reflects clinical severity EMG with low-amplitude MUAP Necrosis on biopsy	In statin myopathy, may progress to inflammatory myopathy: HMG-CoA reductase Ab may help differentiate Propofol toxicity onset severity worse than other forms
Amphiphilic	Chloroquine, hydroxychloroquine, amiodarone	Proximal muscle weakness with distal neuropathy and sensory loss	CK normal to slightly elevated NCS with reduced-amplitude SNAP and CMAP, EMG with neuropathic motor units Autophagic vacuoles on biopsy	Similar presentation to antimicrotubular toxic myopathies
Inflammatory	HMG-CoA reductase inhibitors, D-penicillamine, cimetidine, TNF-α inhibitors, immune checkpoint inhibitors, imatinib, phenytoin, procainamide	Proximal muscle weakness, difficult to distinguish from inflammatory myopathies	CK elevated EMG with low-amplitude MUAP Biopsy with endomysial inflammation, perivascular inflammation	Must be considered in cases of statin myopathy Will require immunomodulatory therapy
Mitochondrial	Zidovudine, lamivudine, zalcitabine, didanosine, entecavir, telbivudine	Proximal muscle weakness, difficult to distinguish from HIV-associated myopathy	CK mildly elevated EMG with small-amplitude MUAP Biopsy with ragged red fibers	Zidovudine with higher likelihood of causing than other agents
Antimicrotubular	Colchicine and vincristine	Proximal muscle weakness with distal neuropathy and sensory loss	CK normal to slightly elevated NCS with reduced-amplitude SNAP and CMAP, EMG with neuropathic motor units Autophagic vacuoles on biopsy	Similar presentation to amphiphilic toxic myopathies
Hypokalemic	Laxatives, diuretics, toluene, excessive licorice, amphotericin, alcohol, corticosteroids	Proximal or generalized weakness	Hypokalemia on serum testing	Severe cases can cause rhabdomyolysis and renal failure
Other	Corticosteroids, alcohol, critical illness	Steroid: proximal weakness with Cushingoid features CIM: proximal weakness with spared bulbar muscles	CK may be normal in corticosteroid toxic myopathies. In CIM, CK may be initially high but can normalize	None

Ab, antibody; CIM, critical illness myopathy; CK, creatinine kinase; CMAP, compound muscle action potential; EMG, electromyography; MUAP, motor unit action potential; NCS, nerve conduction study; SNAP, sensory nerve action potential; TNF-α, tumor necrosis factor α.

fenofibrate, colesevelam), immunophilins (eg, cyclosporine, tacrolimus), labetalol, propofol, and some snake venoms.

Another pathologic mechanism for toxic myopathy is via amphiphilic medications that cause a drug-induced autophagic lysosomal myopathy. Chloroquine, hydroxychloroquine, and amiodarone have both hydrophilic and hydrophobic components that can disrupt the lysosomal membrane and cause autophagic vacuoles. Clinically, these entities tend to present as neuromyopathies with concomitant proximal weakness and distal neuropathy with sensory loss and loss of distal reflexes on examination.

Exposure to high-dose corticosteroids either via endogenous Cushing syndrome or via iatrogenic means can cause a myopathy with unclear pathologic mechanism. This clinically presents with cushingoid features in addition to proximal weakness more prominent in lower extremities than upper extremities that seems to spare distal, facial, and oculomotor musculature.

Some medications may cause an inflammatory myopathy. These are important to recognize early because immunomodulatory treatment may be indicated in addition to stopping the offending agent. The symptomatology may closely resemble that of inflammatory myopathies (see earlier section of this chapter for clinical signs and symptoms). Statins, in addition to causing necrotizing myopathy, can also rarely induce immune-mediated myopathy. The main differentiating factor between necrotizing myopathy caused by statin and inflammatory myopathy caused by statin is failure of symptom resolution for 2 months after cessation of statin. Other implicated medications include D-penicillamine; cimetidine; tumor necrosis factor α inhibitors such as adalimumab; the immune checkpoint inhibitors ipilimumab, nivolumab, durvalumab, and atezolizumab; the tyrosine kinase inhibitor imatinib; phenytoin; and rarely procainamide.

Mitochondrial toxicity due to use of antivirals is a known mechanism of toxic myopathy. The most commonly known medication to cause this pathology is the nucleoside analogue reverse transcriptase inhibitor zidovudine (azidothymidine). Clinical features of this toxicity are typically proximal muscle weakness that is difficult to distinguish clinically from other myopathies associated with HIV. Other antiviral agents implicated in this mechanism of myopathy are lamivudine, zalcitabine, didanosine, entecavir, and telbivudine.

The antimicrotubular agents colchicine and vincristine can cause myopathy via prevention of formation of microtubular structures. Clinically, patients present with progressive proximal muscle weakness and distal neuropathy.

Medications that cause hypokalemia may induce a myopathy that clinically presents with proximal or generalized weakness. If the hypokalemia is severe, myopathy may clinically appear as an acute necrotizing myopathy with rhabdomyolysis and renal failure. Alcohol misuse can cause a hypokalemic myopathy. Certain diuretics, laxatives,

amphotericin, excessive licorice, and corticosteroids have been implicated in causing hypokalemia-induced myopathy.

Two distinct entities that warrant discussion are critical illness myopathy and malignant hyperthermia. The mechanism of critical illness myopathy remains unclear. Patients with prolonged intensive care unit stays, multiorgan failure, mechanical ventilation, systemic inflammation, hyperglycemia, systemic corticosteroid use, or use of nondepolarizing neuromuscular agents are most at risk. Clinically, weakness is seen proximally more than distally with sparing of bulbar muscles. Concomitant polyneuropathy may be present.

Malignant hyperthermia is characterized clinically by severe muscle rigidity, fever, tachycardia, myoglobinuria, and arrhythmia in the acute setting of inhaled anesthetic or depolarizing muscle relaxant use. This is a rare occurrence that happens in patients with particular susceptibilities, including mutations of the ryanodine receptor, specific calcium and sodium channels, certain proteins, or carnitine palmitoyl transferase 2 (CPT2) deficiency (see earlier section titled Metabolic Myopathies).

Laboratory Studies

CK is typically markedly elevated in inflammatory and antimicrotubular myopathy caused by toxins. CK is mildly elevated in mitochondrial toxic myopathy. CK values tend to be normal to only slightly elevated in amphiphilic myopathies and normal in steroid toxic myopathies. In necrotizing toxic myopathies, CK levels are variable, and degree of elevation is reflective of severity of symptomatology with a higher degree of elevation seen in patients with more severe symptoms. In critical illness myopathy, CK can be elevated in the early stages but can normalize prior to detection of weakness. The presence or absence of HMG-CoA reductase antibodies can be helpful to distinguish necrotizing statin myopathy from inflammatory statin myopathy.

EMG/NCS is very similar in the majority of toxic myopathies. NCS is usually unremarkable with the exception of amphiphilic and antimicrotubular myopathies, which may demonstrate reduction in amplitudes, mildly prolonged latencies, and mildly reduced velocities in motor and sensory nerves if there is a superimposed neuropathy. EMG typically demonstrates increased insertional activity and can demonstrate fibrillations, positive sharp waves, complex repetitive discharges, or myotonic discharges. Motor unit action potentials (MUAPs) are typically small and of short duration with early recruitment. The exception to this rule is in amphiphilic and antimicrotubular neuromyopathies where distally, high-amplitude neurogenic MUAPs can be seen. EMG/NCS can be normal in steroid myopathy.

The hallmark histopathologic finding in necrotizing myopathy is muscle fiber necrosis. In amphiphilic toxic myopathy, biopsy shows acid phosphatase–positive autophagic vacuoles preferentially affecting type I fibers. The biopsy findings of inflammatory and mitochondrial myopathies are described earlier. Autophagic vacuoles are also seen on muscle biopsy specimens in cases of antimicrotubular toxic myopathies. In steroid myopathy, biopsy shows primarily type II fiber atrophy, which is also seen commonly in biopsies for critical illness myopathy.

Imaging Studies

Imaging is not typically indicated when toxic myopathy is suspected. If a toxin is thought to be contributing to inflammatory myopathy, then findings may be similar to those described in the earlier section of this chapter detailing inflammatory myopathies.

▶ Differential Diagnosis

When there is suspicion of toxic myopathy, the differential diagnosis is broad (Table 46–7). Other causes for myopathy should be considered, as well as endocrinopathies, infectious disease, and metabolic etiologies. If there is concern for immune-mediated toxic myopathy, JIIMs (see Inflammatory Myopathies section) must be considered. In cases of antiretroviral use, other HIV-associated myopathic processes could cause a similar picture. If corticosteroids are being used to treat a neuromuscular disorder, then the differential diagnosis for steroid toxic myopathy should include progression of underlying neuromuscular disease.

▶ Complications

In cases of toxic myopathies that can cause rhabdomyolysis with myoglobinuria, acute kidney failure can be a potential complication. In the case of statin myopathies, these can sometimes lead to inflammatory myopathy, as discussed earlier, which has a more prolonged course. Stopping a medication vital to a patient's treatment plan can come with complications of its own.

Table 46–7. Differential diagnosis for toxic myopathies.

Differential Diagnosis
Myopathy due to primary underlying disease (eg, HIV-related myopathy in cases of using zidovudine)
Inflammatory myopathies
Endocrinopathies (thyroid, parathyroid, adrenal insufficiency)
Muscular dystrophies
Congenital myopathies
Metabolic myopathies
Viral or other infectious myositis (influenza, parainfluenza, coxsackie B virus, HIV, *Borrelia burgdorferi*, *Toxoplasmosis gondii*, trichinae, cysticercosis)

▶ Treatment

Removal of the toxic agent is the most important step in treatment of toxic myopathies. The medication causing a patient's myopathy must be stopped. In cases of inflammatory toxic myopathies, immune-modulating therapies such as corticosteroids or IVIG, as described earlier in this chapter in the Inflammatory Myopathies section, are warranted.

▶ Prognosis

The prognosis is heterogenous for the various toxic myopathies but is generally good after the offending toxin is removed with partial to complete recovery usually occurring in a matter of months. Inflammatory myopathies require more treatment and may have a more chronic course. Critical illness myopathy has a much more protracted course, and patients may have mortality based on the nature of their critical illness.

BIBLIOGRAPHY

Ahmed ST, Craven L, Russell OM, Turnbull DM, Vincent AE. Diagnosis and treatment of mitochondrial myopathies. *Neurotherapeutics*. 2018;15(4):943-953. doi:10.1007/s13311-018-00674-4

American Association of Neuromuscular and Electrodiagnostic Medicine. AANEM glossary of terms in neuromuscular & electrodiagnostic medicine. *Muscle Nerve*. 2015;52:145-203. doi:10.1002/mus.24955

Berardo A, DiMauro S, Hirano M. A diagnostic algorithm for metabolic myopathies. *Curr Neruol Neurosci Rep*. 2010;10(2):118-126. doi:10.1007/s11910-010-0096-4

Bottai M, Tjärnlund A, Santoni G, et al. EULAR/ACR classification criteria for adult and juvenile idiopathic inflammatory myopathies and their major subgroups: a methodology report. *RMD Open*. 2017;3(2):1-10. doi:10.1136/rmdopen-2017-000507

Chawla J. Stepwise approach to myopathy in systemic disease. *Front Neurol*. 2011;2:49. doi:10.3389/fneur.2011.00049

Cohen BH. Mitochondrial and metabolic myopathies. *Contin Lifelong Learn Neurol*. 2019;25(6):1732-1766. doi:10.1212/CON.0000000000000805

Das AM, Steuerwald U, Illsinger S. Inborn errors of energy metabolism associated with myopathies. *J Biomed Biotechnol*. 2010;2010:340849. doi:10.1155/2010/340849

Doughty CT, Amato AA. Toxic myopathies. *Contin Lifelong Learn Neurol*. 2019;25(6):1712-1731. doi:10.1212/CON.0000000000000806

Goyal BNA. Immune-mediated myopathies. *Contin Lifelong Learn Neurol*. 2019;25(6):1564-1585. doi:10.1212/CON.0000000000000789

Huber AM. Juvenile idiopathic inflammatory myopathies. *Pediatr Clin North Am*. 2018;65(4):739-756. doi:10.1016/j.pcl.2018.04.006

Pasnoor M, Barohn RJ, Dimachkie MM. Toxic myopathies. *Neurol Clin*. 2014;32(3):647. doi:10.1016/j.ncl.2014.04.009

Pasnoor M, Dimachkie MM. Approach to muscle and neuromuscular junction disorders. *Contin Lifelong Learn Neurol*. 2019;25(6):1536-1563. doi:10.1212/CON.0000000000000799

Rider LG, Dankó K, Miller FW. Myositis registries and biorepositories: powerful tools to advance clinical, epidemiologic and pathogenic research. *Curr Opin Rheumatol*. 2014;26(6):724-741. doi:10.1097/BOR.0000000000000119

Rider LG, Katz JD, Olcay YJ. Developments in the classification and treatments of the juvenile idiopathic inflammatory myopathies. *Rheumatol Dis Clin North Am.* 2013;39(4):877-904. doi:10.1016/j.rdc.2013.06.001

Saneto RP, Friedman SD, Shaw DWW. Neuroimaging of mitochondrial disease. *Mitochondrion.* 2008;8(5-6):396-413. doi:10.1016/j.mito.2008.05.003

Shah M, Mamyrova G, Targoff IN, et al. The clinical phenotypes of the juvenile idiopathic inflammatory myopathies. *Medicine (United States).* 2013;92(1):25-41. doi:10.1097/MD.0b013e31827f264d

Valiyil R, Christopher-Stine L. Drug-related myopathies of which the clinician should be aware. *Curr Rheumatol Rep.* 2010;12(3):213-220. doi:10.1007/s11926-010-0104-3

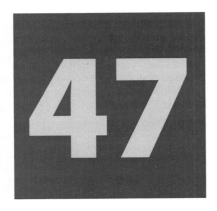

Myasthenia Gravis and Related Disorders of the Neuromuscular Junction

Alexander M. Zygmunt, MD

Cuixia Tian, MD

Pediatric disorders of the neuromuscular junction (NMJ), a group of disorders that affect the structure, function, or both the structure and function of the NMJ, can be acquired or congenital. Patients with NMJ disorders typically present with weakness that fluctuates throughout the day and is fatigable in nature. Classically, fluctuating weakness affects extraocular musculature early in the disease course, causing symptoms such as fluctuating ptosis or diplopia. Bulbar weakness is also commonly described in NMJ disorders, which can present as difficulty swallowing, choking, gagging, weak crying, nasal-sounding voice, or neck flexion or extension weakness.

This chapter discusses juvenile myasthenia gravis, other acquired NMJ disorders, and congenital myasthenic syndromes.

JUVENILE MYASTHENIA GRAVIS AND OTHER ACQUIRED NEUROMUSCULAR JUNCTION DISORDERS

 ESSENTIALS OF DIAGNOSIS AND TYPICAL FEATURES

- ▶ Juvenile myasthenia gravis is an autoimmune disease in which neuromuscular transmission is affected by antibodies that bind to the acetylcholine receptor or to related proteins on the NMJ's postsynaptic membrane.

- ▶ Clinically, juvenile myasthenia gravis is characterized by either isolated extraocular muscle weakness presenting with ptosis or diplopia or more generalized bulbar and limb weakness that is classically fluctuating and fatigable in nature.

- ▶ In the setting of relevant signs and symptoms, serum autoantibody testing can be diagnostic. In seronegative

patients with a clinical picture consistent with myasthenia gravis, electrodiagnostic studies including repetitive stimulation can help make the diagnosis.

- ▶ Other less common acquired disorders of the NMJ include neonatal myasthenia gravis, botulism, and pediatric Lambert-Eaton syndrome.

Juvenile myasthenia gravis (JMG), in which antibodies to components of the postsynaptic NMJ cause impaired synaptic transmission in patients under the age of 18, is a rare condition that more commonly occurs in children over the age of 10 years. The clinician must recognize JMG as a potential cause of fatigable weakness and institute proper antibody testing and immunosuppressive treatment as warranted by the clinical severity of the case. In the case of JMG, a high suspicion for progression to myasthenic crisis must be maintained.

▶ Clinical Findings

Symptoms and Signs

Clinically, patients with JMG will classically present with fluctuating, fatigable weakness. It is more commonly seen in adolescents than in young children, although it can occur at any age. This weakness can either exclusively affect the extraocular muscles (pure ocular myasthenia gravis) or have more generalized skeletal muscle involvement. All symptoms should be least noticeable after periods of rest and worsen with prolonged activity. Patients most commonly present first with ocular symptoms of asymmetric ptosis and binocular diplopia. Patients with bulbar involvement may report nasal speech that worsens with prolonged speaking. They may also report difficulty drinking through a straw, escape of liquids through the nose when drinking, difficulty chewing, or the sensation of food getting stuck when swallowing, all of which may cause meals to take a long time to eat. In the case of generalized skeletal muscle involvement, patients may note difficulty rising from a chair, climbing stairs, and reaching above their heads.

On examination, asymmetric ptosis or extraocular muscle weakness may be noticeable immediately, but severity can be variable depending on time of day. Asking the patient to sustain prolonged upward gaze can help to make ocular signs more apparent to the examiner. Other signs of extraocular muscle weakness include the "curtain sign," in which ptosis appears to worsen in the lesser affected eye when the opposite eyelid is lifted, and Cogan's lid twitch, in which the eyelid twitches as it overshoots when the eyes return to primary position after prolonged downgaze. Ptosis that improves with ocular cooling by placing an ice pack over the affected eye is suggestive of JMG as the cause of the ptosis rather than other potential causes.

Exam signs of bulbar weakness include neck weakness (flexion > extension); thus, neck flexion and extension should be examined routinely in patients with suspected JMG. Other signs of bulbar weakness are difficulty swallowing (which can appear as excessive oral secretions), nasal voice, and difficulty speaking for long periods of time. A single-breath count, during which the patient is asked to count to as high of a number as they can in one single breath, can serve as a quick assessment of vital capacity.

The examiner should pay close attention to examination of bulbar strength because diminishing neck flexor/extensor weakness, difficulty swallowing, and decreasing single-breath count could be signs of impending myasthenic crisis, which is a neurologic emergency.

During manual muscle testing, muscles can be fatigued by repeating testing in succession. Proximal musculature tends to be most prominently affected, although predominant weakness of triceps has been described. Diminishing strength after brief fatiguing exercises, such as repetitively activating deltoids against resistance or repeated deep knee bends, is suggestive. If possible, examining the patient multiple times at different times of the day can reveal the fluctuating weakness typical of myasthenia.

Laboratory Findings

Serum testing for autoantibodies is very useful in the diagnosis of JMG, although seronegative cases do occur at a higher rate in pediatric cases compared to adult cases. Positive autoantibodies are more commonly seen in generalized myasthenia compared to ocular myasthenia, and seroconversion can happen up to 5 years after onset of clinical symptoms; thus, periodic antibody testing is warranted in seronegative cases. The most common antibodies detected are those against the acetylcholine receptor (AChR). AChR-binding antibodies are most common, followed by AChR-blocking and AChR-modulating antibodies. In total, antibodies against AChR are found in an estimated 70% to 80% of cases. Less common are muscle-specific kinase (MuSK) antibodies, which account for 5% to 8% of cases. There are rare cases in which antibodies to low-density lipoprotein receptor-related protein 4 (LRP4) have been detected.

Electrophysiology

In the case of seronegative patients, electrophysiology may help to make the diagnosis of JMG. Two electrophysiologic tests that specifically target the NMJ are repetitive nerve stimulation (RNS) and single-fiber electromyography (EMG). RNS is the most specific electrophysiologic test for JMG, whereas single-fiber EMG is the most sensitive.

In RNS, slow (2-5 Hz), repetitive nerve supramaximal stimulation is applied and the patient is assessed for electrodecrement on weak muscles (most commonly tested are adductor digiti minimi, trapezius, and nasalis). Electrodecrement of greater than 10% on slow RNS from first supramaximal stimulation is highly specific for myasthenia. Although single-fiber EMG of a weak muscle is highly sensitive, it requires specific volitional movements from the patient and can be extremely difficult to perform accurately in pediatric patients.

Imaging Studies

Computed tomography (CT) scan of chest should be performed on patients with diagnosed myasthenia gravis to assess for thymoma or thymic hyperplasia.

▶ Differential Diagnosis

JMG must be differentiated from other disorders of the NMJ including congenital myasthenic syndrome, botulism, and the extremely rare pediatric Lambert-Eaton syndrome (all discussed later in this chapter). Other considerations include acute demyelinating inflammatory polyneuropathy (especially Miller Fisher variant, which can present with cranial neuropathies), mitochondrial disease (which often presents as extraocular weakness), Lyme disease, or brainstem ischemia.

▶ Complications

The most important complication of JMG is myasthenic crisis, which is a neurologic emergency. In myasthenic crisis, severe neuromuscular weakness causes respiratory failure and patients require respiratory support. The rate of myasthenic crisis in the pediatric population is unknown. It occurs in 15% to 20% of adult patients with myasthenia gravis, and up to 20% of adult patients have their first presentation with myasthenia gravis as myasthenic crisis.

Triggers for myasthenic crisis in JMG include infections, surgery, stress, heat, pregnancy, and many medications

Table 47-1. Potential triggers for myasthenic crisis.

Antibiotics: aminoglycosides, tetracyclines, fluoroquinolones, sulfonamides, penicillin, nitrofurantoin

Cardiac medications: β-blockers, calcium-channel blockers, quinidine

Magnesium (beware of laxatives and antacids)

Initiation of corticosteroids (must be cautious for first 2 weeks of induction of steroids)

Botulinum toxin

Depolarizing neuromuscular blockade or volatile anesthetics

Physiologic stress or infection

Surgery

Pregnancy or postpartum period

Bone marrow transplantation

including induction of high-dose steroids, magnesium-containing medications, neuromuscular blockade (eg, succinylcholine), and certain antibiotics, notably aminoglycosides, fluoroquinolones, and tetracyclines (Table 47–1).

Difficulty swallowing, trouble speaking in full sentences, worsening generalized weakness, and neck flexion and extension weakness are signs of developing myasthenic crisis. Patients who have suspected myasthenic crisis should be urgently evaluated at a healthcare facility that can provide respiratory support. Upon arrival, respiratory parameters such as forced vital capacity and negative inspiratory force should be evaluated to help determine the need for potential intubation.

Plasmapheresis (or plasma exchange [PLEX]) and intravenous immunoglobulin (IVIG) have been shown to speed recovery from myasthenic crisis, with equal effectiveness in studies performed to date. However, most important is supportive care, especially respiratory support, which is the hallmark of treatment. Low potassium, magnesium, phosphorus, and hematocrit should be repleted if needed, because low values can exacerbate weakness.

▶ **Treatment**

Symptomatic Therapy

First-line treatment for symptomatic management of myasthenia gravis is to treat with the cholinesterase inhibitor pyridostigmine. By inhibiting the action of acetylcholinesterase, this medication causes an increase in available acetylcholine in the NMJ, which can bind the available postsynaptic receptors and improve strength. Typical dosing ranges from 0.5 to 1.5 mg/kg, 4 to 5 times daily. Typically described adverse effects are diarrhea, abdominal pain/cramping, bronchoconstriction, hypersalivation, blurred vision, sweating, hypotension, and bradycardia. In the setting of high doses of pyridostigmine and worsening weakness, some of these symptoms can be erroneously confused with symptoms of impending myasthenic crisis. Of note, patients with MuSK antibodies often do not respond well to pyridostigmine.

Immunosuppressive Therapy

In the case of continued symptoms despite symptomatic treatment, immunosuppressive therapy can be considered. First-line immunosuppressive therapy is the corticosteroid prednisolone. It is important to note that children have a higher rate of remission than adults with myasthenia gravis and are more susceptible to the adverse effects of steroids, including growth suppression, infection, and osteopenia. Thus, steroid use should be limited to the lowest effective dose. When starting prednisolone, it is important to use a very low dose (0.25 mg/kg daily) because higher doses may induce myasthenic crisis. The dose can be slowly titrated to 1 mg/kg daily over the course of several weeks.

If the patient does not improve on dosing of corticosteroids, cannot be weaned to a reasonable dose of steroids, or has intolerable adverse effects from corticosteroid treatment, there are several other steroid-sparing regimens that can be considered, all with limited evidence in JMG. These include the purine analog azathioprine or the inosine-5′-monophosphate dehydrogenase inhibitor mycophenolate mofetil; these drugs are often used as first-line steroid-sparing agents in the adult population. In the case of refractory JMG or MuSK antibody–positive JMG, the anti-CD20 monoclonal antibody rituximab, which has shown the most benefit for MuSK antibody–positive adult patients, may be used. Maintenance dosing of IVIG or PLEX can be used in JMG as well, although IVIG and PLEX are typically reserved for exacerbations or crises, as described earlier, or used prior to surgery to prevent complications. In severe, refractory cases, methotrexate, cyclosporine, and cyclophosphamide can be considered. Eculizumab is a humanized monoclonal antibody that targets complement protein C5, thus inhibiting terminal complement-mediated damage at the postsynaptic membrane. It has been approved for use in AChR antibody–positive cases of myasthenia gravis in adults. Trials for approval of this medication in the pediatric population are currently ongoing.

Thymectomy

If the diagnosis of myasthenia gravis is made, chest CT should be obtained to assess for the presence of a thymoma or thymic hyperplasia. The presence of thymoma should prompt thymectomy. Even if thymoma is absent, thymectomy may be warranted. Thymectomy has demonstrated benefit in a large prospective cohort of adult nonthymomatous patients with AChR antibody positivity, and several retrospective studies have shown benefit for antibody-positive patients with generalized and purely ocular JMG.

Prognosis

Although hard to quantify with limited available data, generally, the prognosis of JMG is good. JMG has better remission rates than in adult patients with myasthenia gravis. Mortality is estimated at less than 5%. Myasthenic crisis represents the highest risk for mortality and is most common in the first several months after onset. Factors associated with higher remission rates that have been reported in the literature include seronegative status and normal RNS on initial examination.

Other Acquired Disorders of the Neuromuscular Junction

Transient Neonatal Myasthenia Gravis

Among neonates whose mothers have myasthenia gravis, between 10% and 20% develop transient neonatal myasthenia gravis shortly after birth because of transplacental passage of maternal antibodies. It more commonly occurs in mothers with positive AChR or anti-MuSK antibodies but can rarely occur in seronegative myasthenic mothers as well. Symptoms commonly appear in the first 12 to 48 hours after delivery and characteristically resolve within 18 to 21 days. However, there are cases in which symptoms can last up to 4 months. Ventilatory support and pyridostigmine should be administered as necessary until the symptoms have resolved.

Rarely, babies of myasthenic mothers can develop arthrogryposis multiplex congenita from reduced fetal movements in utero secondary to placental transfer of maternal antibodies.

Infantile Botulism

Infantile botulism occurs very rarely in children under the age of 1 year and is due to colonization of *Clostridium botulinum* in the gastrointestinal tract. Typical presentation begins with constipation and progresses to descending flaccid paralysis that includes difficulty feeding and managing oral secretions. On examination, patients will have diminished or absent reflexes, flaccid weakness, weak cry, and sluggish pupillary light reaction.

Diagnosis is made via stool testing for botulinum toxin. It is important to note that stool can be collected with the assistance of an enema, but glycerin suppositories should be avoided because they can invalidate the test.

The mainstays of treatment are supportive care and intubation if respiratory compromise is impending. Administration of intravenous human botulism immune globulin (BabyBIG) has been shown to speed the rate of recovery in patients with botulism.

Pediatric Lambert-Eaton Syndrome

Pediatric Lambert-Eaton myasthenic syndrome (LEMS), in which paraneoplastic or autoimmune antibodies disrupt the presynaptic membrane of the NMJ, is exceedingly rare. The typical presenting symptom of this acquired NMJ disorder is proximal lower extremity weakness that may improve with repeated use, although diurnal variations are far more subtle than in JMG. Patients may also present with ocular or bulbar symptoms, areflexia, and dysautonomia.

If this diagnosis is suspected, electrophysiologic testing should include repetitive stimulation before and after maximal voluntary contraction of muscles being tested. Electrophysiology that shows initially reduced compound muscle action potential with increment of greater than 100% after either maximal voluntary effort or high-frequency (10-50 Hz) repetitive stimulation is diagnostic. Antibodies to voltage-gated calcium channels are usually positive. Pediatric LEMS is more commonly a purely autoimmune rather than paraneoplastic syndrome in children, with neoplasms present in less than one-third of the reported cases, although tumor surveillance should be performed in cases of diagnosed pediatric LEMS.

Treatment of neoplasms, if present, and immunosuppressive therapies similar to those used in JMG are the mainstays of treatment. 3,4-Diaminopyridine (3,4-DAP) blocks presynaptic voltage-gated potassium channels, leading to increased acetylcholine release and can be useful for symptomatic treatment. Adverse effects of 3,4-DAP include paresthesia, nausea, headache, elevated transaminases, and seizure.

CONGENITAL MYASTHENIC SYNDROME

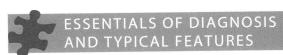

ESSENTIALS OF DIAGNOSIS AND TYPICAL FEATURES

▶ Congenital myasthenic syndromes (CMSs) are a spectrum of inherited disorders that cause disruption of NMJ signal transmission.

▶ Clinically, most CMSs share the element of fatigable weakness. However, there is great phenotypic diversity for other presenting symptoms and musculature affected by this fluctuating weakness.

▶ In the setting of relevant signs and symptoms, genetic testing for known causes of CMS may yield diagnosis. There is also a role for electrophysiology with RNS for suspected cases in which the genetic cause is unclear.

This topic is also discussed in the chapter on congenital neuromuscular disorders. Congenital myasthenic syndrome (CMS) represents a rare spectrum of disorders in which components of the presynaptic, synapse, postsynaptic, or both pre- and postsynaptic membranes of the NMJ are disrupted by genetic variants. Similar to JMG, the hallmark of CMS is fluctuating diurnal variation and fatigue in primarily extraocular muscles with variable bulbar musculature or generalized skeletal muscle involvement. However, CMS has a wide phenotypic variability, and different muscle groups may be initially involved depending on which component of the NMJ is affected by genetic variance. Genetic testing can confirm suspected diagnoses, and in cases in which genetic testing yields uncertain results, electrophysiology including RNS may help clinch the diagnosis. Some classifications focus on inheritance pattern, with the so-called "fast-channel" CMS typically representing autosomal recessive inheritance and the "slow-channel" CMS typically autosomal dominant inheritance. Another classification scheme focuses on location on NMJ of involved structure (pre-/postsynaptic or synapse).

Severity of disease is variable, and until genetic diagnosis is confirmed, acetylcholinesterase inhibitors should be used with caution because these medications can exacerbate symptoms in certain cases, most notably cases due to docking protein 7 (DOK7), collagen-like tail subunit of asymmetric acetylcholinesterase (COLQ), or slow-channel syndromes due to autosomal dominant forms of cholinergic receptor nicotinic subunit (CHRNA1, B1, D, or E) variants.

▶ Clinical Findings

Symptoms and Signs

Clinically, patients with CMS will classically present with fatigable weakness that demonstrates diurnal variation. However, clinically, the initial presenting phenotype is very diverse. Unlike JMG, CMS spectrum diseases are inherited and, thus, present most commonly in infancy or early childhood, although CMS can first manifest in later childhood, adolescence, or even adulthood in some cases. Similar to JMG (described earlier in this chapter), ptosis, weakness of extraocular musculature, and bulbar weakness are the most common presentations. Some patients may present with arthrogryposis multiplex congenita from reduced prenatal movement. Some presynaptic subtypes can present with sudden severe respiratory insufficiency with apnea and cyanosis, the most common of which is CMS due to variant in choline acetyltransferase (ChAT).

On examination, fluctuating, asymmetric ptosis or extraocular muscle weakness can be variable depending on the level of the patient's fatigue. The examiner can induce extraocular fatigue or fatigable ptosis by asking the patient to sustain prolonged upward gaze.

Neck flexion and extension should be examined routinely in patients with suspected CMS because weakness in that distribution can approximate bulbar weakness. Other signs of bulbar weakness include difficulty swallowing (which can appear as excessive oral secretions or poor feeding in a very young infant), nasal voice, weak cry, and difficulty speaking for long periods of time. A single-breath count, during which the patient is asked to count to as high of a number as they can in one single breath, can serve as a quick assessment of vital capacity. A fatiguing maneuver that may help draw out weakness in a very young infant would be to have the patient's parents feed the baby. In fatigable weakness, one would expect that the infant would have little difficulty at the initiation of feeding but would tire quickly as feeding continued for several minutes.

During manual muscle testing, muscles can be fatigued by repeating testing in succession. Diminishing strength after brief fatiguing exercises, such as repetitively activating deltoids against resistance or repeated deep knee bends, is suggestive. If possible, examining the patient multiple times at different times in the day can be revealing of fluctuating weakness typical of CMS.

Laboratory Findings

Genetic testing with a disease-specific panel is the most useful laboratory test in the setting of suspected CMS. There are greater than 30 genes implicated in CMS, and the 5 most commonly detected variants are in *CHRNE* (50%), receptor associated protein of the synapse (*RAPSN*; 10%-20%), *DOK7* (10%-15%), *COLQ* (10%-15%), and *ChAT* (4%-5%). Serum testing for autoantibodies may be useful to rule out JMG (discussed earlier in this chapter) if there is clinical concern, although seronegative cases of JMG are not uncommon and occur at a higher rate in pediatric cases compared to adult cases.

Electrophysiology

Electrophysiology may help to make the diagnosis of CMS. Two electrophysiologic tests that specifically target the NMJ are RNS and single-fiber EMG. RNS is the most specific electrophysiologic test for JMG, whereas single-fiber EMG is the most sensitive.

In RNS, slow (2-5 Hz), repetitive nerve supramaximal stimulation is applied and the patient is assessed for electrodecrement on weak muscles (most commonly tested are adductor digiti minimi, trapezius, and nasalis). Electrodecrement of greater than 10% on slow RNS from first supramaximal stimulation is highly specific for myasthenia. Although single-fiber EMG of a weak muscle is highly sensitive, it requires specific volitional movements from the patient and can be extremely difficult to perform accurately in pediatric patients.

Imaging Studies

Imaging is not typically indicated in the setting of CMS.

▶ Differential Diagnosis

CMS must be differentiated from other disorders of the NMJ including JMG, botulism, and the extremely rare pediatric LEMS (all discussed earlier in this chapter). Other considerations include congenital, metabolic, or mitochondrial myopathy depending on clinical presentation. Other causes of fatigue can include hypothyroidism, anemia, or connective tissue disorders such as Ehlers-Danlos syndrome.

Treatment

First-line treatment for symptomatic management of CMS is difficult to enact without clear genetic diagnosis. In most cases, the acetylcholinesterase inhibitor pyridostigmine is the best first choice of medication. Pyridostigmine causes an increase in available acetylcholine in the NMJ, which can bind the available postsynaptic receptors and improve strength. However, pyridostigmine can exacerbate symptoms in certain CMS subtypes, most notably CMS due to variants in *DOK7*, *COLQ*, or slow-channel syndromes, usually due to an autosomal dominant variant involving *CHRNA1* or *CHRNE*.

Typical dosing of pyridostigmine ranges from 0.5 to 1.5 mg/kg, 4 to 5 times daily. Typically described adverse effects are diarrhea, abdominal pain/cramping, bronchoconstriction, hypersalivation, blurred vision, sweating, hypotension, and bradycardia.

For cases in which there is inadequate symptomatic improvement with pyridostigmine, 3,4-DAP can be used to provide additional benefit. 3,4-DAP blocks the presynaptic potassium channels and increases acetylcholine release by prolonging action potential duration. While it may provide additional benefit to CMS that has responded to pyridostigmine, it should be avoided in the variants that are worsened by acetylcholinesterase inhibitors. Adverse effects include paresthesia, nausea, headache, elevated transaminases, and seizure.

In cases in which pyridostigmine should be avoided, oral administration of the β_2-adrenergic agonist albuterol has been used with success. It is specifically helpful in *DOK7*- and *COLQ*-related CMS. Time to effect is gradual and takes several weeks, with continuing improvement until plateau at approximately 6 months after treatment initiation. Side effects of adrenergic stimulation from albuterol include tachycardia, tremor, headache, and muscle aches.

Finally, in slow-channel syndromes, the selective serotonin reuptake inhibitor fluoxetine has been shown to be effective. Fluoxetine blocks the open slow channel, thus minimizing symptoms. The most common adverse effects of fluoxetine include nausea, diarrhea, insomnia, tremors, and dry mouth. Although the antiarrhythmic quinidine works similarly to fluoxetine, fluoxetine is generally preferred due to better side effect profile.

Prognosis

The prognosis of CMS is variable depending on the genetic variant involved and clinical phenotype. In cases of presynaptic CMS, especially *ChAT*-related, special care must be taken to avoid apneic episodes, which are frequently fatal.

BIBLIOGRAPHY

Balaraju S, Töpf A, McMacken G, et al. Congenital myasthenic syndrome with mild intellectual disability caused by a recurrent SLC25A1 variant. *Eur J Hum Genet.* 2020;28(3):373-377. doi:10.1038/s41431-019-0506-2

Barth D, Nabavi Nouri M, Ng E, Nwe P, Bril V. Comparison of IVIg and PLEX in patients with myasthenia gravis. *Neurology.* 2011;76(23):2017-2023. doi:10.1212/WNL.0b013e31821e5505

Beeson D. Congenital myasthenic syndromes. *Curr Clin Neurol.* 2018;0:251-274. doi:10.1007/978-3-319-73585-6_16

Ciafaloni E. Myasthenia gravis and congenital myasthenic syndromes. *Contin Lifelong Learn Neurol.* 2019;25(6):1767-1784. doi:10.1212/CON.0000000000000800

Elia N, Palmio J, Castañeda MS, et al. Myasthenic congenital myopathy from recessive mutations at a single residue in NaV1.4. *Neurology.* 2019;92(13):E1405-E1415. doi:10.1212/WNL.0000000000007185

Engel A, Xin-Ming S, Duygu S, Sine S. Congenital myasthenic syndromes: pathogenesis, diagnosis, and treatment. *Lancet Neurol.* 2015;4(14):420-434. doi:10.1038/nrendo.2014.139

Farmakidis C, Pasnoor M, Dimachkie M, Barohn R. Treatment of myasthenia gravis. *Clin Neurol.* 2018;36(2):311-337. doi:10.1016/j.physbeh.2017.03.040

Gamez J, Salvado M, Carmona F, et al. Intravenous immunoglobulin to prevent myasthenic crisis after thymectomy and other procedures can be omitted in patients with well-controlled myasthenia gravis. *Ther Adv Neurol Disord.* 2019;12(June):1-13. doi:10.1177/1756286419864497

Gilhus NE. Myasthenia gravis. *N Engl J Med.* 2016;375(26):2570-2581. doi:10.1056/NEJMra1602678

Hajjar M, Markowitz J, Darras BT, Kissel JT, Srinivasan J, Jones HR. Lambert-eaton syndrome, an unrecognized treatable pediatric neuromuscular disorder: three patients and literature review. *Pediatr Neurol.* 2014;50(1):11-17. doi:10.1016/j.pediatrneurol.213.08.009

Hassan A, Yasawy ZM. Myasthaenia gravis: clinical management issues before, during and after pregnancy. *Sultan Qaboos Univ Med J.* 2017;17(3):e259-e267. doi:10.18295/squmj.2017.17.03.002

Howard JF, Utsugisawa K, Benatar M, et al. Safety and efficacy of eculizumab in anti-acetylcholine receptor antibody-positive refractory generalised myasthenia gravis (REGAIN): a phase 3, randomised, double-blind, placebo-controlled, multicentre study. *Lancet Neurol.* 2017;16(12):976-986. doi:10.1016/S1474-4422(17)30369-1

Krueger J. Prognosis in pediatric myasthenia gravis. *Pediatr Neurol Briefs.* 2020;34(0):27358333. doi:10.15844/pedneurbriefs-34-24

Liew WKM, Powell CA, Sloan SR, et al. Comparison of plasmapheresis and intravenous immunoglobulin as maintenance therapies for juvenile myasthenia gravis. *JAMA Neurol.* 2014;71(5):575-580. doi:10.1001/jamaneurol.2014.17

Narayanaswami P, Sanders DB, Wolfe G, et al. International consensus guidance for management of myasthenia gravis: 2020 update. *Neurology.* 2021;96(3):114-122. doi:10.1212/WNL.0000000000011124

O'Connell K, Ramdas S, Palace J. Management of juvenile myasthenia gravis. *Front Neurol.* 2020;11(July):1-12. doi:10.3389/fneur.2020.00743

O'Connor E, Töpf A, Müller JS, et al. Identification of mutations in the MYO9A gene in patients with congenital myasthenic syndrome. *Brain.* 2016;139(8):2143-2153. doi:10.1093/brain/aww130

Rodríguez Cruz PM, Palace J, Beeson D. The neuromuscular junction and wide heterogeneity of congenital myasthenic syndromes. *Int J Mol Sci.* 2018;19(6):1-23. doi:10.3390/ijms19061677

Sanders DB, Wolfe GI, Benatar M, et al. International consensus guidance for management of myasthenia gravis: executive summary. *Neurology.* 2016;87(4):419-425. doi:10.1212/WNL.0000000000002790

Saxena A, Stevens J, Cetin H, et al. Characterization of an anti-fetal AChR monoclonal antibody isolated from a myasthenia gravis patient. *Sci Rep.* 2017;7(1):1-12. doi:10.1038/s41598-017-14350-8

Schorling DC, Rost S, Lefeber DiJ, et al. Early and lethal neurodegeneration with myasthenic and myopathic features: a new

ALG14-CDG. *Neurology.* 2017;89(7):657-664. doi:10.1212/WNL.0000000000004234

Vanhaesebrouck AE, Beeson D. The congenital myasthenic syndromes: expanding genetic and phenotypic spectrums and refining treatment strategies. *Curr Opin Neurol.* 2019;32(5):696-703. doi:10.1097/WCO.0000000000000736

Wendell LC, Levine JM. Myasthenic crisis. *Neurohospitalist.* 2011;1(1):16-22. doi:10.1177/1941875210382918

Zrelski MM, Kustermann M, Winter L. Muscle-related plectinopathies. *Cells.* 2021;10(2480):1-21. doi:10.3390/cells10092480

Neuromuscular Ionic Channelopathies

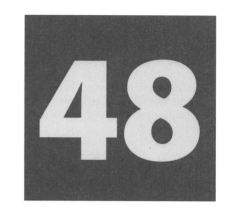

Cuixia Tian, MD

Ion channelopathies are a group of genetic disorders affecting functions of the ionic channels. The ionic channels are complex glycoprotein structures crossing the lipid cellular membrane, allowing the passage of electronically charged ions through the membrane. Neuromuscular ionic channelopathies include nondystrophic myotonias and primary periodic paralysis.

NONDYSTROPHIC MYOTONIAS

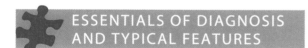

ESSENTIALS OF DIAGNOSIS AND TYPICAL FEATURES

- ▶ A heterogeneous group of skeletal muscle channelopathies
- ▶ Characteristic electrophysiologic findings of altered membrane excitability
- ▶ Clinically present with myotonia of varied severity and onset
- ▶ Mutations in a heterogeneous group of genes have been identified

The nondystrophic myotonias are a rare, heterogeneous group of hereditary genetic skeletal muscle ionic channelopathies including myotonia congenita, paramyotonia congenita, and sodium channel myotonia, defined by distinct clinical phenotypes ranging from severe neonatal myotonia to milder late-onset myotonia. Besides the clinical features, electromyogram (EMG) and genetic analyses are essential in the diagnosis. Causative genes include the skeletal muscle voltage-gated chloride channel gene (*CLCN1*) and the voltage-gated sodium channel gene (*SCN4A*). Management is provided by a multidisciplinary neuromuscular team. In

addition to supportive treatment, medical treatments primarily target reducing persistent muscle sodium currents or enhancing the conductance of mutant chloride channels.

▶ Clinical Findings

Symptoms and Signs

Patients present with muscle stiffness as a consequence of myotonia. The most severe type is a neonatal life-threatening presentation, with onset of myotonia symptoms at birth with respiratory deficiency. Others present with muscle stiffness or myotonia later in life, some may or may not have slow progression of disease, and some may have muscle weakness. Severe infantile presentations are associated with marked muscle stiffness and may lead to death from respiratory failure in early life. Other affected children may mostly have a relatively static course with muscle stiffness and myotonia, and some children may have slow disease progression with development of muscle weakness. Cardiac complications with primarily conductive abnormalities can be seen. Painful myotonia is commonly recognized in patients with nondystrophic myotonia, and some patients had severe and prolonged attacks.

Myotonia congenita is the most common form, with muscle stiffness and myotonia most pronounced during rapid voluntary movements following a period of rest and improvement with repeated activity, called the "warm-up" phenomenon. The causative genetic mutation is related to *CLCN1*. Compared to the autosomal dominant form, the recessive form tends to be more severe and more associated with transient muscle weakness, muscle hypertrophy, and depressed tendon reflexes.

Paramyotonia congenita is related to *SCN4A* mutations. The inheritance is autosomal dominant, and symptoms usually present in the first decade of life. Facial, tongue, and hand muscles are predominantly involved, and lower extremities are generally mildly affected. Myotonia typically lasts from seconds to minutes, but the weakness can persist up to hours and sometimes days. Episodic muscle cramps and paralysis are profoundly exacerbated by cold and exercise.

Sodium channel myotonia is autosomal dominant and related to *SCN4A* mutations, also known as potassium-aggravated myotonias. Symptoms present with cold-insensitive painful myotonia that was markedly exacerbated by potassium ingestion, typically with no attack of weakness. Some patients have marked improvement with acetazolamide treatment. In some patients, myotonia symptoms fluctuate dramatically and tend to occur with a more delayed onset, about 10 to 30 minutes after exercise, compared to the more immediate onset seen in myotonia congenita. Some patients have very severe persistent myotonia that significantly impairs respiration.

Laboratory Findings

Serum creatinine kinase (CK) levels may be normal or mildly elevated. EMG with specialized neurophysiologic protocols can reveal channel-specific patterns to help direct genetic testing (eg, early decrement in the compound muscle action potential [CMAP] with rapid recovery in short exercise test without cooling is specific for autosomal recessive myotonia congenita). Genetic testing demonstrating mutations in causative genes will further aid in establishing the diagnosis.

▶ Differential Diagnosis

Differential diagnoses include broad categories such as congenital muscular dystrophy, congenital myotonic dystrophy, congenital myasthenic syndrome, infantile-onset motor neuron diseases, and metabolic myopathy for the early-onset types and juvenile myotonic dystrophy, limb girdle muscular dystrophy, metabolic myopathy, and motor neuron disease for the later-onset types.

▶ Complications

Feeding intolerance and respiratory deficiency are complications in the neonatal severe types. Cardiac conduction abnormalities are complications in some patients, and although rare, they could lead to severe arrhythmia and death.

▶ Treatment

Medical advice regarding the avoidance of precipitating factors, such as cold exposure or strenuous exercise, is recommended. In patients with significant symptoms and disability from myotonia, a variety of medications have been used. Agents blocking sodium channels including anticonvulsants, local anesthetics, and antiarrhythmic drugs are most commonly used in the treatment of myotonia, although they lack evidence from large randomized studies. The class 1b antiarrhythmic mexiletine is considered to be a first-line treatment by many mycologists and is well tolerated and with minor side effects; however, it has proarrhythmic potential, requiring careful baseline cardiac evaluation

and close electrocardiogram monitoring. Acetazolamide use was reported to be beneficial in some studies but is generally not considered a first-line treatment of myotonia due to concerns for side effects (eg, one patient with paramyotonia developed quadriparesis 12 hours after the ingestion of acetazolamide). Supportive treatment is managed through several medical disciplines provided typically through a multidisciplinary pediatric neuromuscular care center. The management is typically orchestrated by a pediatric neurologist, in collaboration with other specialties.

PRIMARY PERIODIC PARALYSIS

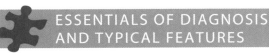

ESSENTIALS OF DIAGNOSIS AND TYPICAL FEATURES

▶ A heterogeneous group of rare neuromuscular channelopathies

▶ Caused by mutations in skeletal muscle sodium, calcium, and potassium channel genes

▶ Typically presents with attacks of flaccid weakness triggered by diet or rest after exercise in the first or second decades of life

▶ Genetic testing aids in confirming the diagnosis

▶ Medical treatment includes avoidance of triggers, diuretics, carbonic anhydrase inhibitors, and management of potassium levels

Primary periodic paralyses are a rare heterogeneous group of hereditary genetic neuromuscular channelopathies that are autosomal dominant inherited and associated with mutations in the skeletal muscle sodium, calcium, and potassium channels. Clinical symptoms are attacks of muscle paralysis, lasting from minutes to hours or days, that can cause morbidity. These attacks are often triggered by diet or behavior and often associated with alterations in serum potassium levels. Primary periodic paralyses include hypokalemic periodic paralysis (HypoPP), hyperkalemic periodic paralysis (HyperPP), and Anderson-Tawil syndrome. Sodium channel mutations are associated with most cases. In addition to clinical symptoms, genetic analyses are essential to establish the diagnosis. Management is provided by a multidisciplinary neuromuscular team. Medical treatment and supportive treatment are available.

▶ Clinical Findings

Symptoms and Signs

Most patients present with onset in the first or second decade of life, with episodic attacks of flaccid muscle paresis.

Symptoms are often triggered by diet or rest after exercise. Severe presentations are associated with marked weakness and may compromise respiration.

HypoPP presents with episodes of focal or generalized skeletal muscle paralyses that can last hours to days, associated with concomitant hypokalemia with potassium level less than 2.5 mEq/L. Many develop myopathy, and the myopathy can be progressive. Muscle weakness primarily affects the proximal muscles of the lower extremities. There is an increased risk for pre- and postanesthetic weakness.

HyperPP presents with attacks of limb weakness and an increase in serum potassium during an attack, although normal potassium levels can be seen in some patients. In about 50% of patients, symptoms start in the first decade of life. Common triggers include potassium-rich diet, rest after exercise, fasting, exposure to cold, and emotional stress. Muscle stiffness is a common symptom in between attacks. Attacks in HyperPP are typically more frequent and shorter in duration than attacks in HypoPP. Myopathy with permanent weakness can be seen, and some patients can develop chronic progressive myopathy.

Anderson-Tawil syndrome presents with episodic flaccid muscle weakness, cardiac abnormalities, and distinctive skeletal features with low-set ears, wide-spaced eyes, small mandible, toe syndactyly, and fifth-digit clinodactyly. Weakness typically occurs following rest after exertion or prolonged rest. Attacks of weakness can be associated with high, normal, or low potassium levels. Cardiac complications with prolonged QT interval and ventricular arrhythmia are common and potentially fatal, although syncope and cardiac arrest are rare. Cardiac symptoms include palpitations and syncope.

Laboratory Findings

Serum CK levels can be normal or mildly elevated. Genetic testing demonstrating mutations in causative genes is essential in establishing diagnosis and determining medical treatment. All periodic paralyses are inherited in an autosomal dominant manner. CACNA1S and SCN4A are the most commonly associated genes in HypoPP, and SCN4A is also associated with HyperPP. KCNJ2 is responsible for the majority of Anderson-Tawil syndrome. When genetic testing is unrevealing, diagnosis can be made based on clinical presentations. Evidence of changes in muscle fiber excitability are characteristic findings on EMG. In patients with HyperPP, positive sharp wave and myotonia can be seen. A reduction in CMAP amplitude is typically seen after the long exercise test when a focal attack of paralysis is induced by exercise of a single muscle.

▶ Differential Diagnosis

Differential diagnoses include secondary episodic paralysis (eg, thyrotoxicosis) or blood potassium deficiency or excess, and for initial presentation, one should consider Guillain-Barré syndrome, stroke, postictal paralysis, or spinal cord injury.

▶ Complications

Swallowing difficulty and respiratory deficiency are complications during severe attacks. Cardiac complications can be seen especially in Anderson-Tawil syndrome, with ventricular arrhythmia being most common and potentially fatal.

▶ Treatment

Current medical therapies for the periodic paralyses include patient education and lifestyle changes to minimize triggers, followed by potassium therapy (either supplement or avoidance based on the type of periodic paralysis). Consultation with a dietician is beneficial. When the potassium level during an attack is unknown, behavioral strategies can be used for acute attacks (eg, mild exercise at attack onset can be helpful to abort attacks or reduce the severity of attacks).

Pharmacologic interventions consist of therapies to abort acute attacks and chronic preventive therapy. Carbonic anhydrase inhibitors have been used as empiric treatment for both HypoPP and HyperPP, with about 50% of patients responding to treatment and the response deferred by genotypes. Acetazolamide is most commonly used. HypoPP with the CACNA1S mutation responds better to acetazolamide treatment than HypoPP with the SCN4A mutation. Patients could have worsening symptoms with acetazolamide treatment, and some patients subsequently respond well to treatment with dichlorphenamide. Dichlorphenamide is approved by the US Food and Drug Administration for both HypoPP and HyperPP. In addition, potassium-sparing diuretics are a potential option for treatment of HypoPP. Thiazide diuretics have been used for HyperPP treatment, with hydrochlorothiazide being the drug of choice. Potassium-sparing diuretics should be avoided in HyperPP. Patients with Anderson-Tawil syndrome require a coordinated approach from both a neurologist and cardiologist. Treatment depends on the potassium levels during acute attacks and should be individualized.

In addition, cardiac considerations are a critical part of medical management. Antiarrhythmic agent should be considered for significant ventricular arrhythmias in the setting of compromised left ventricular function. Flecainide, a type 1c antiarrhythmic, may reduce cardiac arrhythmia in Anderson-Tawil syndrome. Beta-blockers, calcium channel blockers, and amiodarone were also reported to have potential benefits for suppressing ventricular arrhythmias. However, some antiarrhythmic drugs (eg, lidocaine, mexiletine) may paradoxically exacerbate neuromuscular symptoms and should be used with caution in patients with Anderson-Tawil syndrome. Patients also should be cautioned to avoid medications known to cause prolonged QT intervals.

BIBLIOGRAPHY

Al-Ghamdi F, Darras BT, Ghosh PS. Spectrum of nondystrophic skeletal muscle channelopathies in children. *Pediatr Neurol.* 2017;70:26-33.

Jitpimolmard N, Matthews E, Fialho D. Treatment updates for neuromuscular channelopathies. *Curr Treat Options Neurol.* 2020;22(10):34.

Matthews E, Fialho D, Tan SV, et al. The non-dystrophic myotonias: molecular pathogenesis, diagnosis and treatment. *Brain.* 2010;133(1):9-22.

Statland JM, Fontaine B, Hanna MG, et al. Review of the diagnosis and treatment of periodic paralysis. *Muscle Nerve.* 2018;57(4):522-530.

Stunnenberg BC, LoRusso S, Arnold WD, et al. Guidelines on clinical presentation and management of nondystrophic myotonias. *Muscle Nerve.* 2020;62(4):430-444.

Hereditary Peripheral Neuropathies

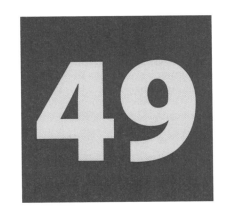

49

Cuixia Tian, MD

Hereditary peripheral neuropathies are a large group of genetic diseases with an overall prevalence of 1 in 2500; they include Charcot-Marie-Tooth (CMT) disease, hereditary sensory neuropathy, hereditary motor neuropathy, and hereditary neuropathy with liability to pressure palsies (HNPP). Here we focus on CMT disease and HNPP.

CHARCOT-MARIE-TOOTH DISEASE

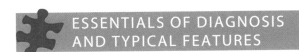

ESSENTIALS OF DIAGNOSIS AND TYPICAL FEATURES

▶ A heterogeneous group of hereditary sensory and motor neuropathies

▶ The most common genetic neuromuscular disorder in children

▶ Clinically presents with distal muscle weakness and atrophy and foot deformity that is often associated with sensory loss

▶ Medical management is primarily supportive in nature

CMT disease refers to a group of genetic disorders characterized by a chronic motor and sensory polyneuropathy, also known as hereditary motor and sensory neuropathy (HMSN). It is the most prevalent genetic neuromuscular disease in children and traditionally divided into 3 groups: demyelinating, axonal, and dominant intermediate types.

Mutations in more than 80 genes have been identified to date, with the peripheral myelin 22 (*PMP22*) gene duplication in CMT1A being most common, which accounts for about 50% of all CMT diseases. Inheritances of this heterogeneous group of genes range from autosomal dominant and

autosomal recessive to X-linked dominant or recessive types. A gene-based classification of hereditary neuropathies was proposed in 2018 by Magy and colleagues to provide more complete and informative classification, including descriptions of mode of inheritance, neuropathy type, and causative genes.

▶ Clinical Findings

Symptoms and Signs

Patients typically present with symmetric, slowly progressive distal motor neuropathy of the arms and legs that results in weakness and atrophy of the distal muscles, especially weak ankle dorsiflexion, diminished deep tendon reflexes, and feet deformities (eg, pes cavus). The majority of affected individuals have symptoms beginning in the first to second decade of life. There is often associated mild-to-moderate distal sensory loss and, in some patients, associated pain.

The demyelinating neuropathy type is typically slowly progressive with symptoms of both distal weakness and sensory loss. Foot deformities with pes cavus are common, and patients may have bilateral foot drop. About 5% of patients become wheelchair dependent, with a normal life span expected. The axonal neuropathy type presents primarily with progressive distal weakness and muscle atrophy, with typically less severe symptoms and less sensory loss compared to the demyelinating neuropathy type. It is worth noting that in the less common third group, which is the dominant intermediate type, the neuropathy varies, with some affected members of the same family being axonal and others being demyelinating.

Laboratory Findings

Serum creatinine kinase levels may be normal or mildly elevated. Electromyography (EMG) and nerve conduction studies (NCSs) are abnormal with demyelinating and/or axonal neuropathic features. Demyelinating is defined as a nerve conduction velocity (NCV) less than 35 m/s, axonal is defined as an NCV greater than 45 m/s, and dominant intermediate is defined as an NCV of 35 to 45 m/s. Genetic testing demonstrating mutations in causative genes is essential for diagnosis. Although nerve biopsy is not routinely carried out in CMT neuropathies, it may show characteristic features, which can guide genetic testing and aid in establishing the diagnosis when genetic testing is unrevealing.

Differential Diagnosis

Differential diagnoses include broad categories such as systemic disorders with neuropathy, other hereditary neuropathies, distal myopathies, motor neuron diseases, and metabolic neuropathies.

Complications

Foot deformity, hip dysplasia, neuromuscular scoliosis, musculoskeletal pain, and neuropathic pain are common complications; vocal cord paralysis can be seen in some patients with potential risk for airway obstruction.

Treatment

Supportive treatment is managed through several medical disciplines and provided typically through a multidisciplinary pediatric neuromuscular care center. The management is typically orchestrated by a pediatric neurologist, in collaboration with other specialties, such as orthopedics, genetics, rehabilitation medicine, physical therapy, and occupational therapy.

Ankle/foot orthoses are helpful to correct foot drop with walking. Some patients may need assistant devices for walking. Orthopedic surgery may be required to correct severe pes cavus foot deformity. Exercise is encouraged as tolerated to remain as physically active as possible. Daily heel cord stretching and hand gripping exercises are recommended to prevent ankle Achilles tendon contractures and improve hand strength.

For patients with risk for vocal cord paralysis, close monitoring for symptoms and consultation with an otolaryngology specialist are required. Hoarseness and/or stridor are typical symptoms of vocal cord paralysis, and development of these symptoms warrants prompt evaluation by an otolaryngologist to assess for degree of airway obstruction.

Neuropathic pain may be treated with gabapentin, carbamazepine, or tricyclic antidepressants (eg, amitriptyline). Musculoskeletal pain can be treated with acetaminophen or nonsteroidal anti-inflammatory drugs. Particular caution is recommended to avoid medications that are potentially neurotoxic.

HEREDITARY NEUROPATHY WITH LIABILITY TO PRESSURE PALSIES

 ESSENTIALS OF DIAGNOSIS AND TYPICAL FEATURES

▶ Clinically present with recurrent acute sensory and motor neuropathy in individual nerves due to nerve entrapment

▶ Mutation in *PMP22* gene is identified in the majority of cases

▶ NCS shows focal conduction abnormalities at entrapment sides

▶ Treatment is supportive in nature

HNPP is an autosomal dominant genetic disease affecting peripheral nerves, with nerve injury secondary to entrapment that leads to episodes of muscle weakness, numbness, tingling, and pain in the limbs affected. It is caused primarily by mutations in the *PMP22* gene. Symptoms typically start in adolescence or young adulthood. Besides the clinical features, genetic testing is essential in the diagnosis. EMG, NCS, and nerve biopsy can aid in diagnosis if genetic testing is unrevealing. Management is provided by a multidisciplinary neuromuscular team. To date, only symptomatic supportive treatment is available.

Clinical Findings

Symptoms and Signs

Symptoms start in the second or third decade of life, mostly during adolescence or young adulthood. Symptoms are numbness, tingling, muscle weakness, and pain in limbs, most commonly affecting the legs, feet, elbows, wrists, or hands. Myelin damage occurs with pressure, stretch, or repetitive movements that lead to muscle weakness. Severity is variable. Symptoms are episodic, and initial presentation usually is an acute onset of a focal sensory and motor neuropathy in a single nerve. An episode can last from minutes to months. In most cases, symptoms resolve completely, but sometimes, there are partial recoveries, although typically, the remaining symptoms are mild. Deep tendon reflexes are usually depressed or absent distal to the entrapment site.

Laboratory Findings

NCS shows features with focal conduction abnormalities of prolongation of distal nerve conduction latencies (eg, common peroneal nerve at fibular head). NCV may be delayed at the site of compression with conduction block. Genetic testing demonstrating mutations in causative genes is essential in establishing the diagnosis.

Imaging and Other Findings

Magnetic resonance imaging may show asymmetric nerve swelling or an enlarged nerve at the entrapment site. Characteristic sausage-like swellings of the myelin sheath can be seen on nerve biopsy.

▶ Differential Diagnosis

Differential diagnoses include acquired neuropathies (eg, neuropathy with diabetes mellitus), chronic inflammatory demyelinating polyneuropathy, compression neuropathies, and CMT and other hereditary neuropathies.

▶ Complications

Incomplete recovery leads to permanent muscle weakness in some patients, causing disability and frustration. Chronic neuropathic pain is commonly seen.

▶ Treatment

Supportive treatment is managed through several medical disciplines and provided typically through a multidisciplinary neuromuscular care center. The management is typically orchestrated by a neurologist, in collaboration with other specialties, including genetics, rehabilitation medicine, physical therapy, and occupational therapy.

Transient bracing (eg, wrist splint or ankle/foot orthosis) may be needed to assist with proper motor function and help to improve pain. Sometimes, patients may need permanent use of an ankle/foot orthosis due to foot drop. Medications for pain are beneficial and range from topical analgesics to systemic neuropathic pain medications (eg, gabapentin, carbamazepine). The benefits of surgery are controversial because spontaneous recovery is common and there is a lack of controlled studies on surgical interventions.

Preventive measures are recommended, such as wearing protective pads for elbows or knees and avoiding high-risk activities including sitting with legs crossed for a prolonged time, prolonged leaning on elbows, wearing a heavy backpack on the shoulders, and repetitive wrist movements. It is recommended to avoid medications that are potentially neurotoxic. Particular care needs to be taken during surgery to avoid positions that could cause nerve injury.

BIBLIOGRAPHY

Attarian S, Fatehi F, Rajabally YA, et al. Hereditary neuropathy with liability to pressure palsies. *J Neurol*. 2020;267;2198-206.

Chrestian N, Adam MP, Mirzaa GM, et al. Hereditary neuropathy with liability to pressure palsies. *GeneReviews* [Internet]. 1998-2020. Accessed July 25, 2022. https://pubmed.ncbi.nlm.nih.gov/20301566/

Jani-Acsadi A, Ounpuu S, Pierz K, et al. Pediatric Charcot-Marie-Tooth disease. *Pediatr Clin North Am*. 2015;62(3):767-786.

Magy L, Mathis S, Le Masson G, et al. Updating the classification of inherited neuropathies: results of an international survey. *Neurology*. 2018;90:e870-876.

van Paassen BW, van der Kooi AJ, van Spaendonck-Zwarts KY, et al. PMP22 related neuropathies: Charcot-Marie-Tooth disease type 1A and hereditary neuropathy type 1 and hereditary neuropathy with liability to pressure palsies. *Orphanet J Rare Dis*. 2014;9:38.

Index

Note: Page numbers followed by b indicate boxed material; those followed by f indicate figures; those followed by t indicate tables.